What Managed Care is Doing to Outpatient Mental Health

A Look Behind the Veil of Secrecy

By Ivan J. Miller, Ph. D.

Published by Boulder Psychotherapists' Press, Inc.
© Copyright 1994
Boulder Psychotherapists' Press, Inc.
350 Broadway, Suite 210
Boulder, Colorado 80303
Printed in the United States of America

Acknowledgments

This book could not have been written without the encouragement, constructive criticism, and editorial advice of my colleagues and friends: Dr. Carol Atkinson, Dr. Evelyn Bassoff, Dr. Lyn Gullette, Dr. Martha L. Hipp, Julie Phillips, Dr. Wayne Phillips, Dr. John Rifkin, Dr. Susan Rosewell-Jackson, Dr. Jed Shapiro, and Don Williams. A note of special appreciation goes to my wife, Millie, who not only offered encouragement, constructive criticism, and editorial advice but also general assistance, support, and comfort. The political cartoon was artistically presented by Millie Miller. Dorothy Rankin of Apropos Graphics provided editorial advice and the graphics, design, and layout. The American Psychological Association, in particular Neela Argawalla, was extremely helpful in finding data about managed care. I must also thank my librarian, Marilyn Rogers-Rothman, who is a sort of private detective specializing in library information. She takes the pain out of trying to locate obscure journals.

Table of Contents

1. The Healthcare Crisis and Managed Outpatient Health Care	1
2. Understanding the Managed Care Solution	4
The managed care solution	4
Where's the fat in outpatient mental health?	5
The evolution of managed care	7
The economic structure of managed care	10
Is there any difference between managed care psychotherapy and other psychotherapy?	15
What is traditional patient-focused psychotherapy?	17
How does managed care alter psychotherapy? - strategies for invisible rationing	19
3. Managed Care Issues	27
How much of managed care's savings is an accountant's illusion?	27
Shouldn't psychotherapists be more businesslike in psychotherapy?	29
Isn't short term treatment a good idea?	29
Isn't it a good idea to have a professional utilization review person determine that the patient is receiving the best treatment?	30
Psychotherapy is a target because the system is opportunistic	32
Hostility toward patients	34
Important decisions are made without consulting consumers	34
Recommendations to consumers	35
How can consumers with managed care make the best of their treatment?	35
Therapy outside of managed care can be affordable!	37
A Sunshine Law for managed care and insurance companies	38
Is there a better alternative than managed care for cost containment?	39
Is managed care good for any mental health services?	41
4. Conclusion	43
5. Endnotes	46
Order Form	

1 The healthcare crisis and managed outpatient mental health

Healthcare costs have reached the point where our nation can no longer afford to pay the bill, and millions of people are turning to managed care to alleviate the financial strain. This new industry promises to provide all medically necessary treatment at an affordable price. Managed care's solution to the financial crisis is to use innovative business techniques to contain costs and eliminate waste. It replaces inefficient with efficient treatment. When treatment choices are equal, it chooses the cheaper one, and it removes incentives for excessive testing and treatment. Sounds wonderful, doesn't it?

This new industry promises to provide all medically necessary treatment at an affordable price.

Not to psychotherapists, who are increasingly distressed about the effects of managed care on outpatient treatment. They are seeing that necessary treatment for patients is cut short, and standards for high quality treatment are undermined. Managed care directs therapists to overlook emotional problems that are difficult to treat and lets severely depressed patients linger on long waiting lists. It threatens psychotherapists with loss of future contracts unless they end treatment prematurely. Confronting these harmful practices, psychotherapists across the nation are protesting the abuses and publicly pointing out the problems with managed care.

In spite of the controversy, the managed-care industry continues to grow at a phenomenal rate. Eighty percent of all mental health coverage in California[1] is delivered under managed care, and the trend is spreading across the country. The national trade journals predict that in a few years almost all psychotherapy will be delivered either under managed care or contracts dictated by managed care to large self-managing groups.[2] Although the first generation of managed care programs did not save money in outpatient treatment, now, the second and third generations have become lucrative businesses.

Managed care is promising not only to provide all the mental health care needs for the country, but is also predicting that the number of therapists needed in the future will be cut in half.[3] Many of the remaining half will be in bureaucratic utilization review positions and no longer delivering services. No one is claiming that as a nation our mental health will have improved, just that the new delivery system won't cost much money. How will they accomplish this miracle?

The picture has been confusing for nearly everyone. I, like most people, had hoped that managed care would cut the fat out of healthcare and make it a more effective system available to more people. As managed care began eating into my psychology practice, however, I was thrown off-balance. The utilization reviewers made no effort to find waste but instead cut effective treatment and demonstrated a shocking disregard for both patients and psychotherapy.

Neither trade journals nor the popular press clearly explained why outpatient managed mental health treatment functions so poorly. In order to understand the reasons for the problems, I decided that I needed to undertake my own investigation. This book is the report of my findings and is intended to inform both concerned citizens and psychotherapy practitioners.

Although the report is unfavorable to managed care, it is not intended as a criticism of everyone who works in the system. There are many psychotherapists and employees of managed care organizations who struggle daily to provide competent and constructive treatment within a system that is dysfunctional.

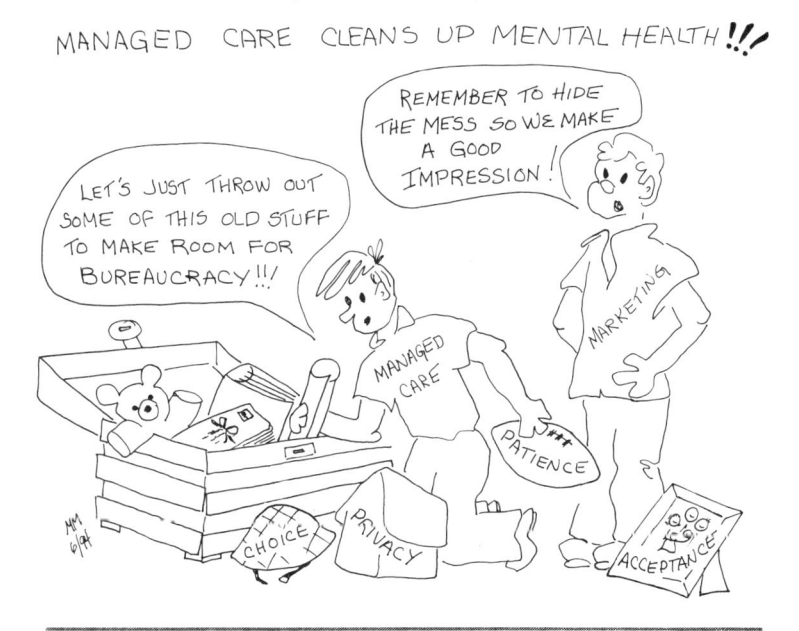

2 Understanding the Managed Care Solution

The managed care solution

The free market system is based on a simple principle – the consumer purchases products or services by evaluating the products or services and weighing their value against the cost. The old healthcare system, most often, did not follow the free market principle. Insurance companies, rather than consumers, paid for healthcare. As a result, nothing stopped the consumer and provider from escalating costs in the pursuit of more valuable services.

> *The ... management company evaluates both the cost and the value – the consumer is removed from the decision-making loop.*

Managed care offered a solution. One party, the insurance company or management company, evaluates both the cost and the value – the consumer is removed from the decision making loop. The management or insurance company decides the value of types of treatment, the value of the provider, and how much can be paid for treatment. In this system the consumer is involved only in picking the management or insurance company by weighing the cost and value of the *total management service*.

The managed care solution does not follow the free market principle either. In the free market, the consumer, not the management company, weighs the value against the cost. Unfortunately, the management company frequently looks at value differently than does the consumer. For the management company, all money withheld from treatment contributes to profit and all money spent on a consumer's treatment is an expense. The term used by management companies for the possibility that healthcare will be provided is "risk." To a management company "risk" does not apply to the risk that the consumer will be sick, but the risk that the management company will spend money.

Where's the fat in outpatient mental health?

The promise of managed care is that so much money can be saved by removing the fat and waste from healthcare, that there will be enough left to provide treatment for everyone at an affordable price. In outpatient mental healthcare, managed care published some flashy examples of ways to cut expenses:
- Stop the California syndrome – Stop paying for people who want to talk and grow.
- Stop the New Yorker syndrome – Replace expensive treatments like psychoanalysis.
- Stop the rich doctor syndrome – Bargain for lower fees from wealthy providers.
- Stop the Woody Allen syndrome – Stop excessively long and unproductive treatment.

Although each of these conditions exists, outpatient mental health already had cost controls[4] that prevented the cost escalation that happened in other types of healthcare.

Most insurance policies had a high copayment for outpatient mental health services, often as much as 50%. Because the consumer paid much of the cost, the free market principle of comparing the value of the service to cost of the service was operating.

The movement toward briefer therapy had been taking place for 30 years anyway. But brief therapy doesn't solve every mental health problem.

... outpatient mental health already had cost controls that prevented the cost escalation that happened in other types of healthcare.

Most insurance policies already had limits on the number of sessions per year, often under 30 sessions, which prevented excessively long treatment.

Many kinds of professionals competed for psychotherapy patients: psychiatrists, psychologists, social workers, professional counselors, and family counselors. This competition kept fees down so that the psychotherapy profession was rarely a road to riches.

Because of cost controls and policy limitations, there has not been much fat in outpatient mental health. Furthermore, outpatient mental healthcare did not contribute to the escalation of healthcare costs but remained at a constant three to four percent of healthcare expenses for 20 years in spite of serving increasing numbers of patients.[5]

The evolution of managed care

The policies and procedures of managed care companies vary greatly. Some companies seem to maintain high quality treatment focused on the patient's needs, while others seem to undermine quality. At the beginning of my study, I was tempted to push for regulation requiring high quality treatment standards. However, once I understood the evolutionary trend of the industry, I realized that there is a pattern that can't be solved by regulation. The managed care industry has not been able to simultaneously control costs and maintain the quality of services. High standards for quality treatment belonged to the first generation of managed care which, unfortunately, could not control costs. The second and third generations have developed aggressive cost-containing strategies, but these dramatically curtail the quality and amount of treatment provided.

First Generation Managed Care.

Originally, managed care made a serious effort to provide requested and needed treatment. It offered only small reductions in the copayment and bargained for a small fee reduction from providers. The main cost-control strategies were to encourage briefer therapies, limit the choice of providers, and establish gatekeeping obstacles which discouraged patients from seeking treatment. Although first generation managed

Although first generation managed care generally maintained quality, it greatly increased paperwork and didn't save enough money to justify its own bureaucracy.

care generally maintained quality, it greatly increased paperwork and didn't save enough money to justify its own bureaucracy. Additionally, because the copayment was only slightly reduced for using therapists within the managed system, many consumers preferred the option of choosing their own therapists outside the system and making a slightly higher copayment.

Second Generation Managed Care.

To justify itself, managed care must reduce the cost of healthcare and this pressure is pushing the industry into a more aggressive and controlling second generation. In order to control treatment, consumers are locked into this system with a very low copayment for seeing therapists within the system and no insurance benefits for seeing therapists outside the system. Once consumers are locked in, the system prevents treatment by *invisible rationing* – a combination of policies and procedures that make treatment inaccessible and/or undesirable. The rationing is invisible because treatment is not overtly denied, but is effectively undermined. The invisible rationing is combined with drastic cuts in therapists' fees, which results in a drift to lower quality providers. This generation cuts quality, reduces the amount of treatment provided, and greatly increases bureaucracy, but, in contrast to the first generation, succeeds in limiting healthcare expenses.

Third Generation Managed Care.

The success of the second generation proves that outpatient mental health services can be curtailed or prevented. A problem with the second generation has been that the financial incentives of the management companies are in conflict with those of the provider - the payer (the managed care or insurance company) makes a profit when treatment is limited, and the provider makes a profit when treatment is provided. This conflict encourages time-consuming disagreements between payer and provider over the amount of treatment. Third generation managed care resolves the conflict by splitting with the providers the money saved through treatment limitation. The professional trade journals predict that this will typically be accomplished with "capitated" contracts[6] with groups, not solo practitioners. Capitated means that a set fee is paid to a care provider group for each person treated. For example, a company might pay $190.00 per episode. If the patient is seen once, the provider group earns $190/hr., but if the patient is seen ten times, the provider group earns only $19/hr. In this new system, the provider group assumes responsibility for the invisible rationing as well as for the group management. Within the group, the forces of peer pressure and group support give each member additional motivation to curtail the patient's treatment. In this arrangement, the provider's financial incentive to provide treatment is replaced by a powerful financial incentive to limit treatment. This generation is just now developing, but it promises to be highly effective at reducing costs.

> *In this arrangement, the provider's financial incentive to provide treatment is replaced by a powerful financial incentive to limit treatment.*

The economic structure of managed care

The key to understanding managed care is knowing about its underlying economic structure. Simply speaking, there is not enough money to pay for all that managed care promises, and therefore sacrifices are made. The economics can be understood most easily by looking at an example of changing from a traditional copayment cost-control program to a managed care cost-control program.

Example of the Enticement to Transfer from Traditional to Second Generation Managed Care

The managed care solution can be offered in a way that makes it look awfully good.

- **The employer's cost for insurance premiums is lowered; in our example it is lowered 20%.**[7]
- **The consumer's copayment is lowered; in our example it is decreased from $40.00 to $10.00.**
- **Provider's fees are lowered giving the appearance of less expensive services; in our example the provider's fee is decreased from $80.00 to $65.00 per session.**

How much treatment does managed care actually provide?

Managed care looks as if it offers a wonderful service – making outpatient mental healthcare available to many more people because of lower fees. Everyone seems to win except the provider, who concedes to a fee discount. Here's the rest of the story.

- Management services are very expensive and consume a large portion of the healthcare dollar. In this example, 12.5% of the mental healthcare dollar is consumed by the managed care company[8]

- Managed care promises to reduce the overall cost of the insurance premiums in order to sell their services to employers. In this example, the managed care company promises a 20% reduction.

As a result of these two managed care expenses, only 67.5% of the original insurance fund remains to provide services. But there is one more financial problem for managed care.

To make the managed care finances balance, managed care must eliminate 51% of the psychotherapy.

- Each hour of psychotherapy costs the management company more than it cost the insurance companies prior to managed care. In the old system, insurance paid half of an $80.00 fee or $40.00. Because the copayment is only $10.00 in the new system, the management company pays $55.00 of the $65.00 fee. Each hour of psychotherapy costs the managed care company $15.00 more. The result is that less mental health treatment can be provided.

In fact, as the chart below demonstrates, once all of these financial factors are considered, only 49% of the mental health service available before managed care can be purchased after managed care. To make the promises of lowered cost and lowered copayment come true, something must be sacrificed. What is sacrificed is treatment. To make the managed care finances balance, managed care must eliminate 51% of the psychotherapy.

How Much Treatment Does Managed Care Provide?

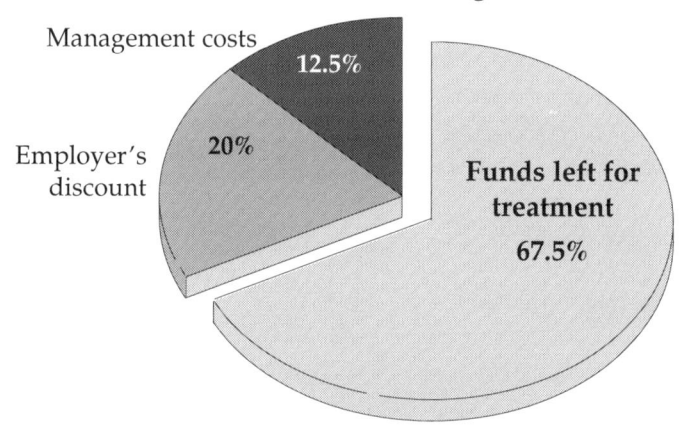

- Management costs: 12.5%
- Employer's discount: 20%
- Funds left for treatment: 67.5%

After the 20% discount is given to the employer and the 12.5% administrative expenses are subtracted from the mental healthcare dollar, only 67.5% of the money is left for treatment. Each hour of psychotherapy costs the managed care company more than before managed care. The result is that after managed care, 51% of mental health treatment is eliminated.

Unfortunately, in this example treatment is reduced to 49% of pre-managed care service levels. This is just the minimum necessary to gain a contract. Because another company may offer greater savings, a competitive company needs to be prepared to prevent even more treatment units.

The 51 cent solution for the 20 cent problem

Now there is enough information to understand the problem. Because there have always been cost controls on outpatient mental health, there is little fat. In addition, I have not been able to find anyone who recommends that our nation needs to provide fewer mental health services. However, for the sake of argument, in this example we will presume there is 20% excess or unnecessary treatment. To solve the problem of 20% fat, the managed care solution is to eliminate 51% of the treatment. Because managed care has promised to provide all necessary mental health treatment, it must maintain the appearance of offering mental health services while actually reducing the amount of treatment. To resolve this dilemma, the industry has developed policies and procedures that covertly prevent or invisibly ration treatment.

> ... *the industry has developed policies and procedures that covertly prevent or **invisibly ration** treatment.*

The core problem with managed care is that the economic structure makes it unworkable. No matter how conscientious, well-intentioned, or thoughtful a managed care employee may be, a 51 cent solution for a 20 cent problem is destructive.

Does managed care reduce the cost of treatment?

In outpatient mental health, managed care maintains an illusion of greatly decreased costs. The actual case is reduced services.

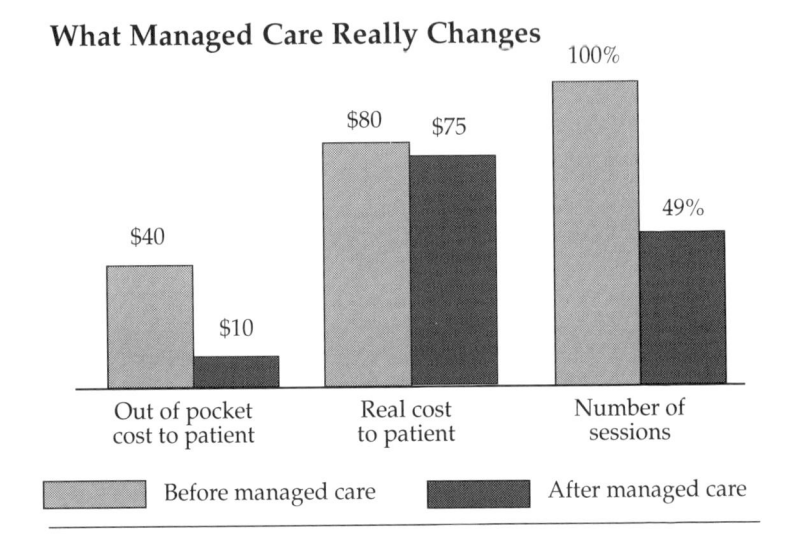

What Managed Care Really Changes

	Out of pocket cost to patient	Real cost to patient	Number of sessions
Before managed care	$40	$80	100%
After managed care	$10	$75	49%

- The first set of columns displays the lowered out-of-pocket copayment. For this example, before managed care the patient paid 50% or $40.00. After managed care, the patient pays only $10.00. At first it seems as though the consumer's cost was cut drastically.

- However, the consumer's true cost (second set of columns) combines the insurance premium money given "in trust" to the insurance company and the out-of-pocket expense. The "trust" refers to the promise from insurance to return the money to pay for healthcare. Under managed care, more of the "trust funds" are required for an hour of psychotherapy. Once money from the "trust" is included, the cost of each hour of psychotherapy is actually $75. This is only a 6% decrease in the cost to the consumer.

- The third set of columns demonstrates the drastic reduction in the amount of service provided. There is 51% less mental health service to achieve a savings of 6% in the cost of an hour of psychotherapy.

The illusion of a greatly reduced out-of-pocket expense makes it appear as if managed care has made psychotherapy more accessible. The reality is that the cost of treatment has been reduced a mere 6%. But most importantly, the quantity of mental health services was so drastically reduced that access for everyone is lowered. The low copayment is not a method of increasing access.

> ... *the quantity of mental health services was so drastically reduced that access for everyone is lowered.*

The copayment is low so that the consumer feels there is no affordable alternative to the managed care system.

Is there any difference between managed care psychotherapy and other psychotherapy?

In 1970 Ralph Nader's study group wrote an exposé which included a story on practices of the baby food industry.[9] Originally, baby food jars contained the meat, fruit or vegetable described on the label. As the cost of these real ingredients increased, some of the nutritious ingredients were replaced by less expensive starches and sugars. Salt and monosodium glutamate were added to make the food more appealing to mothers, who tested the taste for their babies. Then it was discovered that if some of the baby's saliva was transferred by the spoon to the contents of the baby food jar, the saliva digested the starch and turned it to water. The baby food company solved this problem by using a starch that could not be digested by saliva, even though some experts pointed out that a baby's digestive system was not capable of fully digesting the new starch. The result was a product that was called food and looked and tasted like food. But when the secret processes of removing nutrients and adding chemicals became known, few mothers would allow their babies to eat the chemical brew.

A similar story can be told about managed care and outpatient mental health. The processes and procedures of managed care are to a great extent secret. Managed care companies won't reveal the specific guidelines regarding selection of their providers, the specific guidelines for deciding the continuation of treatment, or the specific details of their influence on treatment. These are trade secrets! However, the therapists experienced with managed care witness on an ongoing basis the alteration of psychotherapy by the managed care industry. The next two sections outline first, the nature of traditional patient-focused psychotherapy and second, how the managed care industry adds undesirable conditions, while removing many essential ingredients in the invisible rationing process.

What is Traditional Patient-Focused Psychotherapy?

Psychotherapy is a time-honored, powerful, and proven method for healing the heart and soul. It is important in healing the psychological wounds of life and in treating mental illness. It is vital in the prevention of many of the social tragedies of our time, including: domestic violence, child abuse, school failure, suicide, substance abuse, and depression. Psychotherapy is based on both the science of psychology and on the art of understanding, teaching, nurturing, and confronting.

A special kind of relationship between patient and therapist is central to the effectiveness of psychotherapy. For everyone, feelings of shame hinder self-awareness and openness. To be successful, the therapist must support the patient and avoid any shaming and judging. The patient needs to trust that the therapist will be able to provide this support even when discussing behavior about which the patient and/or therapist may disapprove.

The trust a patient places in a psychotherapist requires openness and honesty about their relationship. Any deception or secretiveness about the nature of psychotherapy or secret agreements with third parties can undermine this trust.

Medically Necessary Treatment

The managed care company retains the right to determine "medically necessary treatment." In spite of how powerful and scientific this phrase sounds, it has no definition and allows the company to do almost anything.

Confidentiality and privacy are both basic tenets for the development of a therapeutic relationship. Confidentiality means the information divulged in therapy cannot be released without permission. However, if permission to release information is required by managed care companies, then privacy is lost. Each erosion of privacy undermines psychotherapy's potential to help patients honestly explore themselves.

Each person's therapy moves according to a different clock. An important principle in psychotherapy is that interventions must be timed according to the patient's readiness to use the information. As it turns out, the fastest type of effective psychotherapy is the one that moves at the patient's speed.

Human beings have the amazing ability to control or change the course of their lives. Furthermore, we are biologically programmed to control and change our fate most effectively when we discuss our feelings with a helping person. This is why talking to another person makes so much more difference in how we feel than just talking to ourselves. Psychotherapy uses the skills and knowledge of psychology and gains power by using the healing relationship, built over time, between patient and therapist.

Research verifies that with trained, empathic, and experienced therapists, people can make great improvements in their personal, emotional, occupational, and interpersonal lives.[10] In fact, millions of people have benefited from psychotherapy.

The psychotherapeutic relationship is powerful, but it is also very fragile. If the relationship or conditions of acceptance, privacy, confidentiality, and patience are changed, therapy can become just a conversation, a discussion, a class, or a lecture. If we tamper with psychotherapy we must take care not to eliminate or dilute its essential ingredients.

How does managed care alter psychotherapy? – strategies for invisible rationing

Each of the strategies used for *invisible rationing* cuts expenses by eliminating treatment sessions but also changes the nature of patient-focused psychotherapy. I think that being a purist about psychotherapy is impractical. At times, some alterations of psychotherapy are necessary and acceptable. However, after I listed all of the ways managed care has partially removed essential ingredients of therapy and added noxious conditions, its therapy seems as altered as the baby food of 1970.

Gatekeeping. A gatekeeper is an employee of managed care who must authorize treatment prior to the first session. Sometimes the gatekeeper is the family physician and other times a telephone referral person. A few companies use a full initial evaluation by a psychotherapist in their organization to decide if treatment is recommended. Managed care claims to need gatekeeping to prevent the unnecessary use of specialists. And, as their name implies, gatekeepers function as a one-directional barrier to keep patients out of psychotherapy. The reasoning behind gatekeeping sounds solid, but in practice it doesn't work. Family doctors often don't feel qualified to make decisions about psychotherapy. A phone conversation between the consumer and gatekeeper is too superficial to determine the need for treatment. But gatekeeping does keep some people out of treatment; which reduces expenses for the managed care company! Many people feel shame about asking for help and want as few people to know about their personal lives as possible. For some of these people, just the idea that their requests for help may be challenged will keep them from asking. Additional cost savings come from blocking the non-assertive or confused patients who are easily discouraged. But for everyone, gatekeeping begins to set the unwelcoming tone of managed care.

Developing consumer "unfriendliness." When people go to a doctor or psychotherapist they want a person who is "user or consumer friendly" - a professional who is welcoming, listens with understanding to their symptoms, has time for them, is willing to provide treatment, and offers a promising treatment plan. Gatekeepers, extra personnel the patient must contact, forms to be completed, cold attitudes, overly busy offices, and rushed providers are unpleasant and often drive patients away. Consumer unfriendliness is the most extreme in some HMOs which maintain a small, understaffed, and overworked in-house mental health service. These overworked staff get some relief when their unfriendliness drives away new intakes and discourages old patients from returning.

Using unpopular providers. The trade journals and leaders of managed care[11] all agree that managed care is selecting providers who see their patients the fewest number of times. A therapist may see patients for very few sessions because he or she is highly skilled and can treat patients faster than other therapists. But it is also a strong possibility that therapy is brief when the patient is

BOULDER PSYCHOTHERAPISTS' PRESS, INC.
350 Broadway, Suite 210
Boulder, Colorado 80303
303-444-1036 FAX 303-494-3837

Erratum

After the final proofreading and without our permission, the computer threw away the line at the top of page 21. This page should begin with the line "unsatisfied and leaves treatment pre-."

Ivan J. Miller, Ph. D.

maturely. Because the patients do not return to these providers, the managed care treatment costs are reduced.

Restricting providers. Managed care companies maintain restricted lists of participating providers. In my interviews with consumers of psychotherapy, I have found that most people feel more comfortable about seeing a therapist who is recommended by someone they know. Because they may not find the recommended therapist on the managed care list, they may forego therapy altogether. This is another way that managed care cuts costs!

Coerced Medication

Many emotional problems can be treated with either medication or psychotherapy. Medication, of course, takes effect more quickly but may not last as long and has side effects. Many times managed care companies refuse to provide treatment unless the patient also takes medication, even when there are indications that psychotherapy is the treatment of choice. This is an example of how the values of the company can be very different than the values of the patient.

Ironically, medication is not always cheaper. A year's worth of Prozac can be over $1360.00[12] without considering the cost of the visit to the physician. Medication may be promoted more frequently because the managed care company is not responsible for medication costs which accounting places under another budget.

Lowering the quality of providers. The working conditions of managed care are driving away quality providers. The managed care combination of fee reductions and increased paperwork cause income reductions for psychotherapists that can easily be as large as 40%.[13] Additionally, most professionals find it insulting to have treatment directed by a management company employee who is less qualified, less concerned about the patient, less experienced, and has not had contact with the patient. Many times psychotherapists face an ethical problem when they believe the managed care company is making treatment decisions that are not in the best interest of the patient. Highly qualified psychotherapists who can find other ways to make a living are frequently refusing to work under these conditions. Many previously successful psychotherapists are leaving their profession. On the other hand, some psychotherapists who have not succeeded in the past in the consumer-controlled marketplace are finding success with managed care. As was noted above, being unpopular with consumers has advantages under managed care.

Preventing the treatment of personality problems. Many of the psychological and emotional problems that cause distress are a result of long-term personality patterns. Psychotherapy helps a person change these patterns, but a 20- or 30-year pattern does not change in a few weeks. Biologically speaking, the neurons in the brain take many months to develop healthy new pathways for handling emotions. Many companies refuse to treat people with personality disorders; others direct the provider to treat only symptoms that will change in a few weeks and to ignore the underlying issues. Because personality patterns require more than brief treatment, management companies save by discouraging the diagnosis and treatment of these disorders.

Preventing a trusting relationship. We are able to heal ourselves and change our personal direction more effectively when we talk about ourselves with a trusted person. Expressing our thoughts and feelings to a managed care psychotherapist who shows the most concern for limiting the number of sessions is just not the same as sharing our feelings with an understanding and trusted confidant. The development of this trusting, accepting, and healing relationship is one of the essential ingredients in psychotherapy. Once the relationship has developed, the therapist becomes someone a patient can trust. This relationship is necessary for making many of the major changes patients are seeking in psychotherapy

Because personality patterns require more than brief treatment, money can be saved by policies that discourage the diagnosis and treatment of these disorders.

Managed care discourages emotional and long-lasting relationships between patients and therapists because they are deemed to promote unhealthy dependency [14] But research findings time and again show that the trusting relationship between patient and therapist is essential to successful treatment. Undermining the therapeutic relationship is another way that managed care undermines psychotherapy and reduces costs.

Undermining privacy. Talking about one's innermost thoughts and feelings requires some degree of privacy. This privacy has historically been protected by guarantees of confidentiality – which means that the information revealed in therapy could not be shared without the patient's permission. Now, with managed care, payment for therapy depends upon the patient releasing confidential details of his or her innermost thoughts, worries, fears, and behavior to a group of care managers. This group maintains records, some of which are in computer data banks, and its role is to pass judgment about whether therapy should continue. In order to justify therapy, the therapist must give this group information that emphasizes the patient's most severe dysfunction. Technically speaking, confidentiality is still maintained because the patient's signature is required. In fact, however, *privacy is seriously compromised.* Another essential ingredient of psychotherapy is altered. Again, as therapy becomes less desirable, fewer sessions will be billed to the insurance company.

Disrupting the timing. One of my early lessons in psychotherapy was that timing is essential. By learning to understand the patient's own speed and knowing when to provide an intervention, therapy was shorter and remarkably more effective. On the other hand, the greatest techniques and most brilliant interventions had little power when presented at a time when the patient was not emotionally receptive. Managed care develops businesslike schedules for treatment and encourages therapists to speed the presentation of techniques. Such policies create clear records of the treatment provided and abbreviate therapy, which proceeds in a businesslike manner. Managed care therapy ends when techniques have been taught to the patient and the targeted number of sessions are completed, not when the patient's problems are solved. This diminishes another essential ingredient of psychotherapy – working at the patient's optimal speed.

Judging and shaming the patient. Mental health advocates have spent years teaching that it is healthy to admit to having an emotional problem, ask for help, and solve the problem. Still, it is difficult for most patients to overcome feelings of shame or embarrassment when seeing a therapist. They are filled with inner doubts: "Do I deserve help?"; "Am I making too much of my own problems and needs?"; "Am I hopeless?"; "Should I just accept my failure?"; "Will I be rejected if I ask for help?"; or "Will I be ridiculed if I admit a weakness?" An essential ingredient in psychotherapy is accepting a patient's feelings in a non-judgmental, non-blaming, and non-shaming manner.

> *This diminishes another essential ingredient of psychotherapy – working at the patient's optimal speed.*

Managed care utilizes a periodic review of treatment, usually every four to six sessions, to determine if the treatment will continue to be authorized. These reviews set a judgmental and shaming tone. Each time, the reviewer decides if the patient is deserving of continued treatment. Because managed care advertises that it will provide all necessary treatment, it usually does not accept responsibility for refusing treatment. Instead it rationalizes that the patient is responsible; either the patient was not responding fast enough, was wanting too much, was not motivated enough, or had a personality problem that insurance is not responsible for treating. In each of these cases the managed care company criticizes the patient who asks for help.

By introducing a judgmental evaluation every four to six sessions, managed care has passed a cloud of shame over psychotherapy that further weakens another essential ingredient of psychotherapy.

Does Research Show When Managed Care Works?

Not now, and it won't in the near future. Unfortunately, good outcome research is very difficult, expensive, and takes years. On the other hand, easy-to-prepare research frequently exaggerates the benefits of therapy and shows that just about anything works. Many managed care companies are collecting the kind of easy data that inflates the benefits of their treatment. While this may help their marketing staff, it doesn't seriously answer the question about their treatment's effectiveness.

3 Managed Care Issues

How much of managed care's savings is an accountant's illusion?

The insurance industry calls managed care and similar services that are responsible for only a portion of healthcare delivery, "carve outs." In mental health, the management company measures the cost savings solely in the behavioral health budget that is "carved out" and separated from other healthcare expenses. However, many of the so-called savings of managed mental health care actually shift expenses to another part of the healthcare system. [15]

- Many studies show that appropriate use of mental health services reduces the use of related medical care to such an extent that the mental health services pay for themselves. Other analyses question whether the reduction completely pays for the mental health services but acknowledge that without mental health treatment many medical treatment expenses are increased.[16]

- Frequently, patients go to their primary care physicians to talk about an emotional problem or request psychiatric medication.[17] While it looks like managed care saves money by keeping these patients out of therapy, the cost of treatment is just shifted to the family doctor.

- Mental health management companies are often responsible only for containing the costs of seeing providers and not for the expense of medication. By using more medication to shorten treatment, the managed care company can claim credit for the briefer treatment. But some other part of the healthcare budget must carry the burden of the considerable expense for medication, which may be long term.

> *The illusions of managed care result in more than invisible rationing, they also result in invisible cost shifting.*

Managed care prevents consumers from receiving appropriate quality psychotherapy. This has many costs. Some of these are human costs felt by the consumers and their families. These can't easily be measured in dollars. Some of the costs show up as increased sick days and on-the-job injury.[18] These costs are carried by the employer. But much of the so-called savings of managed care is simply cost shifting to other parts of the healthcare budget. The illusions of managed care result in more than invisible rationing; they also result in invisible cost shifting.

Shouldn't psychotherapists be more businesslike in psychotherapy?

Psychotherapists are told that they have not met the business community's desire for clearly defined treatment outcomes, brief time limits on treatment, and standardized procedures. This is the way business people approach problems. But if business people knew how to solve mental health problems, patients would go talk with a business person, not a psychotherapist.

Psychotherapists know the most effective approach to mental health problems is respecting the patient's personal treatment goals even when they are abstract, moving at each patient's optimal speed, and placing the patient's individuality above the standardized treatment package.

Many managed care companies respond to the business community by emphasizing the clear, time limited, and standardized treatment packages. In this way they are selling what the business market thinks it wants. However, the true desire of business people is the most effective and valuable treatment for the money. A more reasonable approach would be to educate business people about why effective psychotherapy often does not proceed like a good business plan.

Isn't short term treatment a good idea?

Yes – but it's not new. Managed care advertises savings by using therapists who do not want to treat everyone for years. Sounds good, but most therapists already do short term treatment when it is appropriate.

The movement toward shorter therapy has been taking place for 30 to 40 years. For the past 25 years brief therapy consisting of just a few sessions has been taught in professional schools and at workshops. Seventy percent of patients are seen for six or fewer sessions. Only 10% of patients are seen for more than 24 sessions a year.[19] Brief therapy has had its impact, and therapists who think everyone should be treated for years are not dominating the profession.

Trying to force all patients into brief therapy is not a good idea.

When the approach is patient-focused, then long term therapy is appropriate for many. The research indicates – as common sense would also suggest – that brief therapy is effective for the less severe problem, and long term therapy is indicated for the more severe problems.[20] Trying to force all patients into brief therapy is not a good idea.

Isn't it a good idea to have a professional reviewer determine that the patient is receiving the best treatment?

Managed care often advertises the advantage of a professional reviewer who watches over the patient's treatment. It claims that the reviewer assures the highest quality treatment. While this sounds reassuring, the reality is different. The apparent benefits of review are based on four false assumptions.

First, this advertising assumes that patients can be categorized by a precise and accurate diagnosis. Mental health diagnoses are usually not that clear cut. Sometimes patients have multiple diagnoses; sometimes professionals disagree about the diagnosis. Most often, individual differences and circumstances are more important than the diagnosis. It actually shouldn't be that surprising that real patients don't fit easily into diagnostic boxes. Intuitively, most people know that an individual's unique circumstances are very important in mental health.

Second, the advertising assumes that research has determined the specific treatment of choice for each diagnostic category. This is not true in many areas of healthcare[21] and especially not true in mental health. While there are some guidelines for treatment, research has answered very few of the questions about which treatment is best.[22] The judgment and experience of the psychotherapist is still the best guide.

Third, the advertising assumes that the utilization review person will be a helpful instructor for the provider. This argument portrays the utilization review person as the expert and the psychotherapist as a student. In reality, the expertise is reversed. Most utilization review staff have fewer credentials and less experience than the professionals whom they review.

Fourth, the advertising assumes there is an advantage to a brief second-hand review of treatment. But this is actually a disadvantage. Whereas the psychotherapist may spend hours with a patient, reviewers have only a few minutes for each patient. Whereas the psychotherapist sees the patient first hand, the reviewer gets only selected second-hand information. It is hard to believe that a reviewer with these disadvantages would know best.

While the illusion of expert professional review is a persuasive marketing tool, the advertised advantages are not the purpose or function of utilization review. The real function of a reviewer is to introduce cost consciousness into decision making. When economic incentives have created extensive fat and waste, the utilization review person can save money without harming the quality of treatment. This is not the case with outpatient mental health.

Psychotherapy is a target because the managed care system is opportunistic

Psychotherapists often ask me why the managed care system seems to be attacking our profession. After all, it is well documented that outpatient psychotherapy is not one of the factors that has led to rapidly escalating healthcare costs.[23] We have cost containment mechanisms in place. Many studies document that the money spent on psychotherapy is more than reimbursed by the long-term benefits[24] – fewer work days lost to illness, fewer visits to the medical doctor, less stress related illness, and less money spent on divorces. It doesn't seem fair that managed care would be so hard on our profession.

If they can't prove the short-term savings, they may not be players after healthcare reform.

Unfortunately, our contributions don't protect us. The human benefits resulting from less stress, less family strife, fewer jobs lost, fewer divorces, fewer sick days, and higher productivity only slightly impress managed care companies. They are more concerned about proving that they can save money in the short-term. If they can't prove the short-term savings, they may not be players after healthcare reform is set in place.

The primary task of managed care is to find ways to avoid spending money. From the perspective of the bottom line, the dollar saved by not treating a depressed, isolated person is just as green as the dollar saved by eliminating fat and waste. Managed care cuts where the opportunity arises, and psychotherapy offers a great opportunity for three reasons:

- **Psychotherapy is an abstract service** that is poorly understood by most consumers. If a concrete service like medications were cut, this loss would be visible and consumers would complain. The changes managed care makes in psychotherapy are so abstract that they are invisible to most consumers.

- **There is little chance of legal reprisal.** Lawsuits require proof that the actions of managed care caused specific damage to the patient. This kind of causation has always been difficult to prove regarding the effects of psychotherapy. Lawsuits also require major injuries with large enough damages to pay the attorney's fee. The most likely result of too little psychotherapy is individual or family stress and suffering, not major, tangible, measurable injury.

- **Psychotherapy patients won't complain in public.** Most patients want their psychotherapy to be private and may hesitate to admit publicly to having felt the need for treatment. Any patient who considers complaining is caught between looking like a "whiner" who wants to be indulged with more treatment or a "really disturbed person" who desperately needs more treatment. It's no wonder few complaints are voiced.

Hostility toward patients

A colleague told me the story of a day he visited an HMO mental health unit. One of the staff boasted about how he had gotten rid of a patient with a severe personality problem in just one session. The rest of the team seemed duly impressed. Because of an excessive workload, the staff developed hostility toward the patients who needed their help the most.

Important decisions are made without consumers

During my study of managed care I had a revelation after reading a 30 page manual written to help therapists thrive while working under managed care. As I put the manual down, I realized that it never mentioned including the patient in decisions about therapy. The entire manual covered closed-door negotiations between the payer (insurance or managed care company) and the provider about how to direct treatment. The implication was that all important treatment decisions could be made before the consumer entered the office. When managed care and treatment providers make secret decisions about treatment, the consumer is disempowered.

> ...all important treatment decisions could be made before the consumer entered the office.

How can consumers with managed care make the best of their treatment?

Many consumers feel they are locked into managed care because it is part of their insurance contract and their copayment is so small they must try to use it. Fortunately, consumers can take steps to protect themselves. In spite of the trend toward secret contracts between payers and providers, psychotherapists have codes of ethics that require them to be honest with patients. Consumers can ask directly what kind of arrangement their therapist has with managed care. Consumers should not trust the therapist who won't give specifics. If the therapist says the managed care company has only the consumer's interests in mind, the therapist is either easily fooled or not straightforward. The best therapists will be open and honest about the interference managed care may present to treatment and will commit themselves to keep clients informed about what is happening with managed care programs.

Recommendations to consumers

Try to understand what your benefits really are. If your company promises so many benefits at such a low cost that it seems too good to be true, it probably is not true. There is no free lunch! It is okay to ask your therapist what the benefits really are. Ask if the therapist tries to target an average number of sessions. You may directly inquire about any policies that may encourage limiting your treatment.

Find out what financial arrangements exist between the therapist and the managed care company. It is important to know if the therapist is on a capitated contract. (Captitated contracts were explained earlier – in these, the healthcare provider makes a set amount regardless of how much treatment is provided.) If the therapist won't tell you about the arrangements, be wary. It is unethical for most psychotherapists to have secret arrangements with third parties about your personal medical care.

Ask your managed care therapist what treatment he or she or other professionals might recommend if you were paying your own fees. Managed care severely limits treatment options, and a good managed care therapist will inform you about the potential choices. Watch out for the therapist who tells you the managed care company offers only the best treatment.

If you choose to go ahead with a managed care therapist, don't give up hope. While the system as a whole offers a lesser good to the greatest number, there are still many patients who benefit, many skilled and caring therapists who work for managed care, and many successful treatment episodes. Managed care works best for those who want just a few sessions. On the other hand, if you think your therapist wants to avoid deep-seated problems, it may be true. If you think your therapist is eager to get rid of you or is a little unfriendly, don't take it as a personal rejection; moving patients out of treatment quickly may be just a way to make money.

And if the therapy just isn't helpful, consider looking for therapy outside of managed care.

Most importantly, if you have any questions about your treatment, get a second opinion. Ask someone whom you trust and who also knows psychotherapists to refer you to a psychotherapist for an independent second opinion. Occasionally insurance companies can be persuaded to follow the outside opinion. But even if they won't honor an independent opinion, at least you will know the score. In addition, you will have the opportunity to discuss your treatment with someone who does not have a conflict of interest.

Therapy outside of managed care can be affordable!

In our society many of us have come to assume that insurance will pay for mental health care and psychotherapy. But now, many consumers are finding that they must pay for therapy out of their own pockets. Psychotherapy services are within the reach of many consumers. Quite a few therapists are lowering their fees or offering a sliding scale. If the fee is a problem, consumers can call several therapists and ask about fees in order to locate an affordable therapist. Many times the investment of a moderate amount of money in therapy can be personally worthwhile.

A sunshine law for managed care and insurance companies

Many of the problems with managed care result from companies operating behind a veil of secrecy. Specific policies and procedures of managed care companies are classified as trade secrets. Managed care budgets are not open to public review. The decisions and explanations of managed care are usually communicated over the telephone with few written records. In most states managed care is considered neither treatment nor insurance and is unregulated by laws governing these businesses. Because the internal operations of managed care are secret, they might as well be invisible.

Legislation is being introduced in Colorado requiring that all managed care company policies and procedures that affect a consumer's personal healthcare must be open to public review. The legislation would require the disclosure of financial reports that provide an accounting of the money entrusted to the managed care company.

The arguments supporting this legislation are threefold. First, as a participant in personal healthcare decisions, managed care should follow the medical tradition of full disclosure. This includes the disclosure of policies that affect the choice of treatment and provider. Second, in order for the free market to function properly, the consumer must be able to compare cost to the value of the service. The value of the psychotherapy benefit is known only when information is available about policies, procedures, treatment choices, and the selection of providers. Third, insurance is a trust. Money is given in trust through premiums with the understanding it will be returned when the consumer is in need of healthcare. This trust should be open to the consumer's review.

In the future, companion legislation may be proposed for a health insurance tax designated to fund a consumer organization similar to *Consumer's Reports*. This organization would evaluate and rate health insurance and managed care companies on consumer issues. The Sunshine Legislation would guarantee that enough information is available for meaningful evaluation. While this involves a new tax, the tax is likely to reduce the cost of healthcare and result in a savings for the consumer.

These two pieces of legislation are alternatives to regulation. Insurance and managed care companies would retain freedom to operate in the most effective way. The consumer organization could thoroughly research and evaluate the insurance and possibly the healthcare industry. By reporting the results to the consumer, the consumer will again be empowered in the marketplace.

Is there a better alternative than managed care for cost containment?

Yes – returning to straightforward cost control methods is better. Managed care relies on illusions to hide invisible rationing and invisible cost shifting. It just isn't right to fool the consumer. I believe that all controls should be visible to the consumer and that the consumer is in a better position to evaluate costs and benefits than a managed care company.

The Coalition of Mental Health Professionals and Consumers, Inc., has proposed a basic plan that uses copayment, session limits, and a fixed treatment payment to control costs. [25]

- Set a fixed reimbursement rate that the insurance companies pay for psychotherapy. The copayment is added to this fixed rate. In our example we will use $40.00/hour.

- Allow patients to negotiate with the provider for a copayment on a sliding scale. If the provider has a good reputation or strong credentials, the provider could ask for a greater copayment. If the patient has a low income, the patient could ask for a lower copayment. For example, a psychotherapist with excellent qualifications may ask for a $60.00 copayment in addition to the $40.00 insurance reimbursement. Or, a socially conscious provider may see a low income patient for a copayment of $10.00 in addition to the $40.00 insurance reimbursement.

The New Language of Managed Care

Managed care has changed the language of mental health care so that sometimes it is hard to understand what is being said. Sometimes things may be called the opposite of what they are.

Examples:
Quality assurance programs may actually be programs that primarily focus on reducing costs.

Focused therapy may mean focusing on the superficial problem while failing to diagnose and treat the important underlying condition, one that would require more extensive treatment.

- Place a cap on the annual reimbursement in order to protect the insurance company from excessive financial risk. If treatment must be limited[26], a cap of $960.00 or 24 hours of psychotherapy yields the same 20% cost savings used in the example of a second generation managed care company presented earlier. [27]

Managed care may argue that their program has an advantage over visible rationing because it can use its judgment to provide more than 24 sessions to those truly in need. But in practice, the financial reality of the situation makes this very rare. Because of the drastic limitation on the amount of treatment, very few of those with second and third generation managed care receive treatment beyond 24 sessions. This advantage for these few people doesn't justify the negative consequences of managed care for the great majority of users.

> *Compared to managed care, straightforward limits offer the greatest good for the greatest number of patients.*

This proposal provides 62.5% more treatment than the managed care proposal for the same cost to the purchaser of insurance.[28] Compared to managed care, straightforward limits offer the greatest good for the greatest number of patients.

Is managed care good for any mental health services?

Yes. There are two areas that require management. First, inpatient mental health care has a history of tremendous waste, abuse, and excessive expenses. The economics of inpatient managed care are different because there is enough waste to finance quality managed care. Managed care has been very effective at curtailing the escalating costs of inpatient care.

Second, chronically mentally ill patients need extensive services that require some management to contain costs. Copayments and session limits cannot be used because these patients are so severely disabled that treatment cannot be stopped or refused. However, these patients can easily be exploited and are too vulnerable to have their treatment managed by a profit-making corporation. Nonprofit community mental health centers are in the best position to balance the needs of these patients against cost containment.

There are quality of care problems with managed inpatient treatment and services to the chronically mentally ill. Some of these problems occur because managed care creates incentives for under-treatment. At other times, quality problems, particularly with community mental health centers, are the result of inadequate funding. However, there is not room here for a full discussion of managed care in these areas.

4 Conclusion

Managed care promises too much to too many people. It promises to reduce the cost of insurance, reduce the out-of-pocket copayment from the patient, and provide all needed mental health services. The marketing professionals who advertise managed care make it sound wonderful. However, once their operations and finances are brought out into the sunlight, the picture is different. There just isn't enough fat and waste in the outpatient mental health system to pay for all of those promises. As a result, managed care severely limits services and cuts much of the substance and heart out of psychotherapy.

> *The bottom line is that faulty economics undermine the quality of outpatient managed mental healthcare.*

At times managed care companies may endorse thoughtful and well-intentioned plans to maintain quality. These efforts and ideas cannot overcome the economic problems created by a 51 cent solution for a 20 cent problem. The bottom line is that faulty economics undermine the quality of outpatient managed mental healthcare.

There will always be some managed care, if only for inpatient services. The system will function better if all rationing of healthcare is visible to the consumer. To guarantee that rationing is visible and that consumers are empowered to control managed care, we must have Sunshine Legislation.

I believe that, whenever possible, consumers must be in charge of the mental health delivery system. As a psychotherapist and psychologist, I find the current system controlled by insurance and managed care companies distressing and am working with others for change.

Endnotes

1. "Therapy under siege," *New Age Journal*, May/June 1994, pp. 90-101.
2. Kathleen McCarthy, "Psychologists Explore Larger Group Practices," *American Psychological Association Monitor*, May 1994, p. 34; and "Issues in Managed Care," *Psychotherapy Finances*, Jupiter FL., 1993.
3. Vicki Meade, "Psychologists Forecast Future of the Profession," *American Psychological Association Monitor*, May 1994, p. 14.
4. In 1988, 95% of insurance plans had controls on outpatient visits. E. Eckholm, *Solving America's Health-Care Crisis: A Guide to Understanding the Greatest Threat to Your Family's Economic Security*, New York: Random House, 1993, p. 224.
5. D. C. Ackley, "Employee Health Insurance Benefits. A Comparison of Managed Care with Traditional Mental Health Care: Costs and Results," *The Independent Practitioner*, Vol. 13(1), Washington, DC: American Psychological Association, 1993, pp. 49-53..
6. "Issues in Managed Care," *Psychotherapy Finances*, Jupiter, FL., 1993.
7. *How to Resolve the Health Care Crisis: Affordable Protection for All Americans*, Yonkers, NY: Consumer's Union of United States, 1992, p. 112. The managed mental healthcare industry reports that they can save 20-50% on expenditures in the first year. The lower end of this range was chosen because the upper end probably refers to inpatient care where greater savings are possible.
8. The portion of the healthcare dollar consumed by managed care is one of the facts hidden behind the veil of secrecy. In my extensive search for data on managed mental health care, I couldn't find a single clear report of the portion of healthcare expenses that pay management costs. The General Accounting Office ran into similar frustration, concluding that the industry doesn't provide enough inside data to determine how or if they produce healthcare savings ("Managed Health Care: Effect on Employers' Costs Difficult to Measure." GAO/HRD-94-3, 1993).
The best estimate of the administrative costs of managed outpatient mental health care was available through a consultant with the American Psychological Association, Ron Finch. He had investigated the mental health managed care industry both as a purchaser of managed care for a large corporation and for testimony to Congress on managed mental healthcare and healthcare reform. He estimated that an outpatient mental health management system with the features used in our example (exensive utilization review and developing a provider network) would consume 10-15% of the mental healthcare dollar. I chose the midpoint of this range, 12.5%, for the sake of the example. (Personal communication, 7/11/94, Ron Finch, Coopers and Lybrand, 1155 Peach Tree Street, Suite 1100, Atlanta, GA.)
9. J. S. Turner, *The Chemical Feast*, New York: Grossman Publishers, 1970. pp. 86-87.
10. M. L. Smith, G. V. Glass, & T. I. Miller, *The Benefits of Psychotherapy*, Baltimore: The John Hopkins University Press, 1980.
11. "Issues in Managed Care," *Psychotherapy Finances*, Jupiter, FL. 1993.
12. The therapeutic dosage of Prozac is 1-4 tablets per day. Because it is fairly common for a patient to take two tablets daily, this daily dose was used for the estimate. The Boulder Table Mesa King Sooper's grocery store and pharmacy quoted a price of $112.40 for 60 tablets. This is over $1360.00 per year.
13. This estimate uses the $15.00 per hour fee reduction in the example. Because overhead on a private practice is approximately $20.00 per hour, only $60.00 of the hourly fee of $80.00 is income. The $15.00 fee reduction lowers the income to $45.00. In addition, managed care administration time can easily consume 15 minutes per patient hour. The new income is $45.00 for 1.25 hours or $36.00 per hour. This is 40% below the prior figure of $60.00 per hour.

14. "Working with a Managed Care Company." *Network Connection: A Newsletter for HAI/AHP Behavioral Health Providers*, Nov./Dec. 1993.
15. "Pro & Con: What Does the Future Hold for Managed Behavioral Health Programs?" *Open Minds*, Gettysburg, PA., Vol. 3(11). 1991.
16. D. C. Ackley, "Employee Health Insurance Benefits. A Comparison of Managed Care with Traditional Mental Health Care: Costs and Results," *The Independent Practitioner*, Vol. 13(1). Washington, DC: American Psychological Association, 1993.
17. J. Kirzay, E. Brawn, & Monica E. Oss, *Outpatient Behavioral Health Care in the United States A Statistical Manual of Physician Office Visits for Treatment of Mental Illness and Chemical Dependency*. Gettysburg, PA: Behavioral Health Industry News, Inc., 1991.
18. "Industry Statistics: Reduced Employer Costs Result from Chemical Dependency Treatment in Most Cases," Gettysburg, PA: *Open Minds*, Gettysburg, Vol. 3 (6), 1990.
19. C. A. Taube, H. H. Goldman, B. J. Burns, & L. G. Kessler, "High users of outpatient mental health services, I: Definition and characteristics." *American Journal of Psychiatry*, Vol. 145, pp. 19-24.
20. M. P. Koss & J. Shiang, "Research on Brief Psychotherapy," *In Handbook of Psychotherapy and Behavior Change, Fourth Edition*, A. E. Bergin & S. L. Garfield (Eds.) New York: John Wiley & Sons, Inc., 1994. In a thorough review of the literature the authors find that brief therapy is not the treatment of choice for patients with more severe problems, substance abuse problems or personality problems.
21. M. D. Reagan, *Curing the Crisis: Options for America's Health Care,* Boulder, CO: Westview Press. Boulder, CO. p. 125.
22. S. L. Garfield & A. E. Bergen, *Handbook of Psychotherapy and Behavior Change, Third Edition*, New York: John Wiley & Sons, 1986.
23. D. C. Ackley, "Employee Health Insurance Benefits. A Comparison of Managed Care with Traditional Mental Health Care: Costs and Results," *The Independent Practitioner*, Vol. 13(1), Washington, DC: American Psychological Association, 1993, pp. 49-53.
24. Ibid.
25. "Outpatient Psychotherapy Plan Based Upon 'Managed Cooperation.'" Coalition of Mental Health Professionals and Consumers, P. O. Box 438, Commack, NY. 11725. 3/14/94. This proposal is essentially the same as the Australian single payer system.
26. I am not recommending curtailing outpatient visits to 24 per year. This number was selected only because it allows comparison between the Coalition's plan and the managed care example. Some rationing of mental healthcare is a reality, and few patients have full coverage. Full coverage for mental healthcare should include a minimum of 52 psychotherapy sessions a year.
27. This estimate is based on data from C. A. Taube, H. H. Goldman, B. J. Burns, & L. G. Kessler, "High users of outpatient mental health services, I: Definition and characteristics." *American Journal of Psychiatry*, Vol. 145, pp. 19-24. They reported on a National Medical Care Utilization and Expenditure Survey which determined the proportion of the users of outpatient mental health services who made over 24 visits per year. Extrapolating from their data, it can be estimated that the 24 session per year limit will result in a 20% reduction of services.
28. This estimate is based on the costs listed in the managed care example listed earlier. The managed care company pays $55.00 per session, and the cost of the company's overhead was estimated at $10.00. This is a total cost of $65.00 per session. When the cost is lowered to $40.00 in the example here, 62.5% more sessions can be provided.

The Boulder Psychotherapists' Press, Inc. is an organization that promotes traditional, confidential, and patient-focused psychotherapy. Informing the public about the status of outpatient psychotherapy and managed care is a central part of our mission. You may help by purchasing copies of this booklet and distributing them. Because the sale of this booklet is a necessary part of our fund raising, we request that you honor our copyright and purchase the booklets from us so that we can afford to continue our work.

PRICE LIST

Number	Price	Postage and Handling
1 copy	$4.70 each	$2.00
2-5 copies	4.30 each	4.00
6-10 copies	3.90 each	6.00
11 + copies	3.50 each	8.00

Colorado residents add 3% sales tax.

Please send me ___ copies of
What Managed Care Is Doing to Outpatient Mental Health: A Look Behind the Veil of Secrecy.

Number of Books: _____   Price Each: _____   Total Price: _____
Tax (3% if purchased in Colorado) _____
Postage & Handling _____
Total Enclosed _____

Send to:
_____
_____
_____

Credit Card Information:

☐ Visa   ☐ MasterCard

_____
Name
_____
Card #
_____
Exp. Date
_____
Signature

Make check payable and mail to:
Boulder Psychotherapists' Press, Inc.
350 Broadway, Suite 210
Boulder, CO 80303

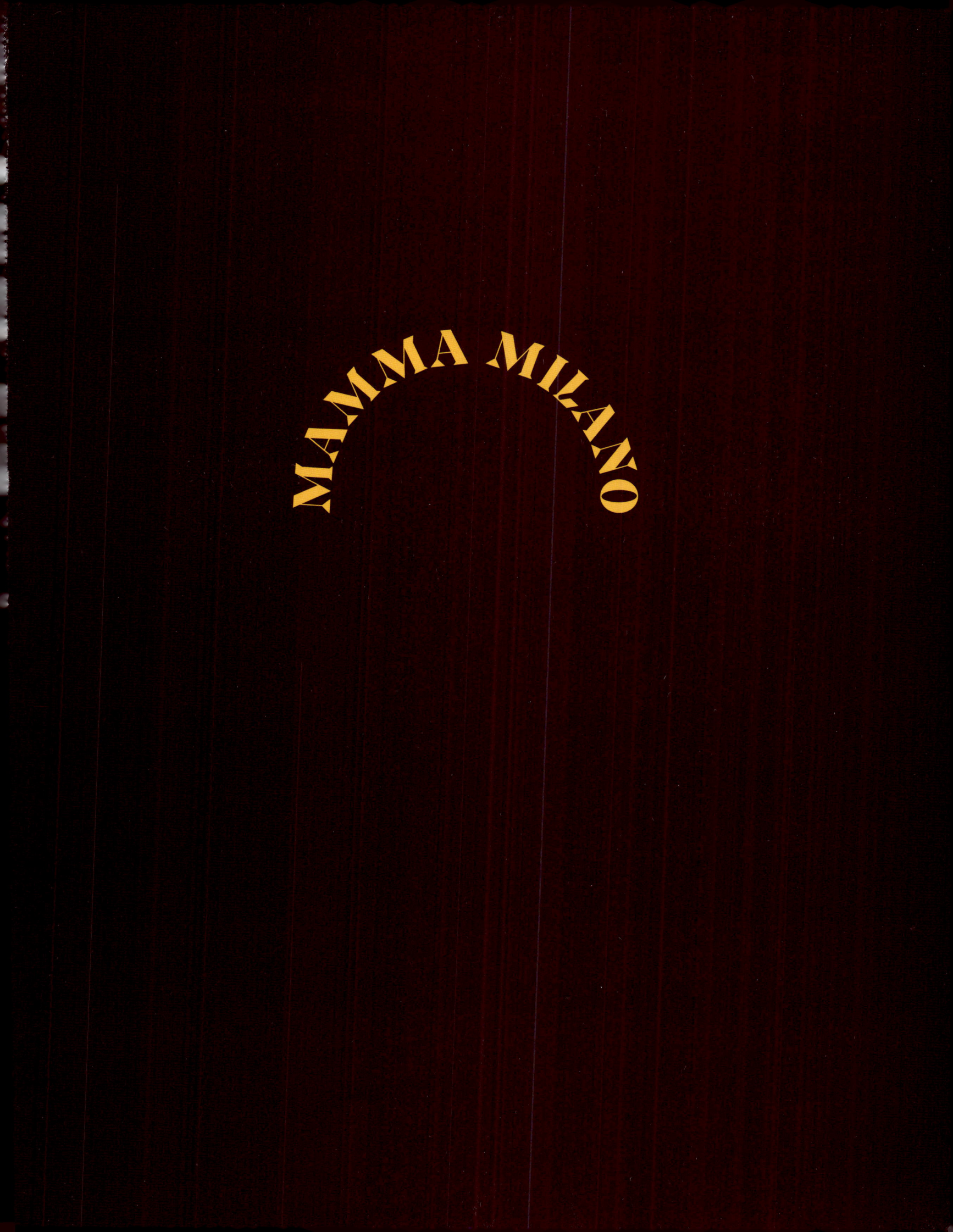

MAMMA MILANO

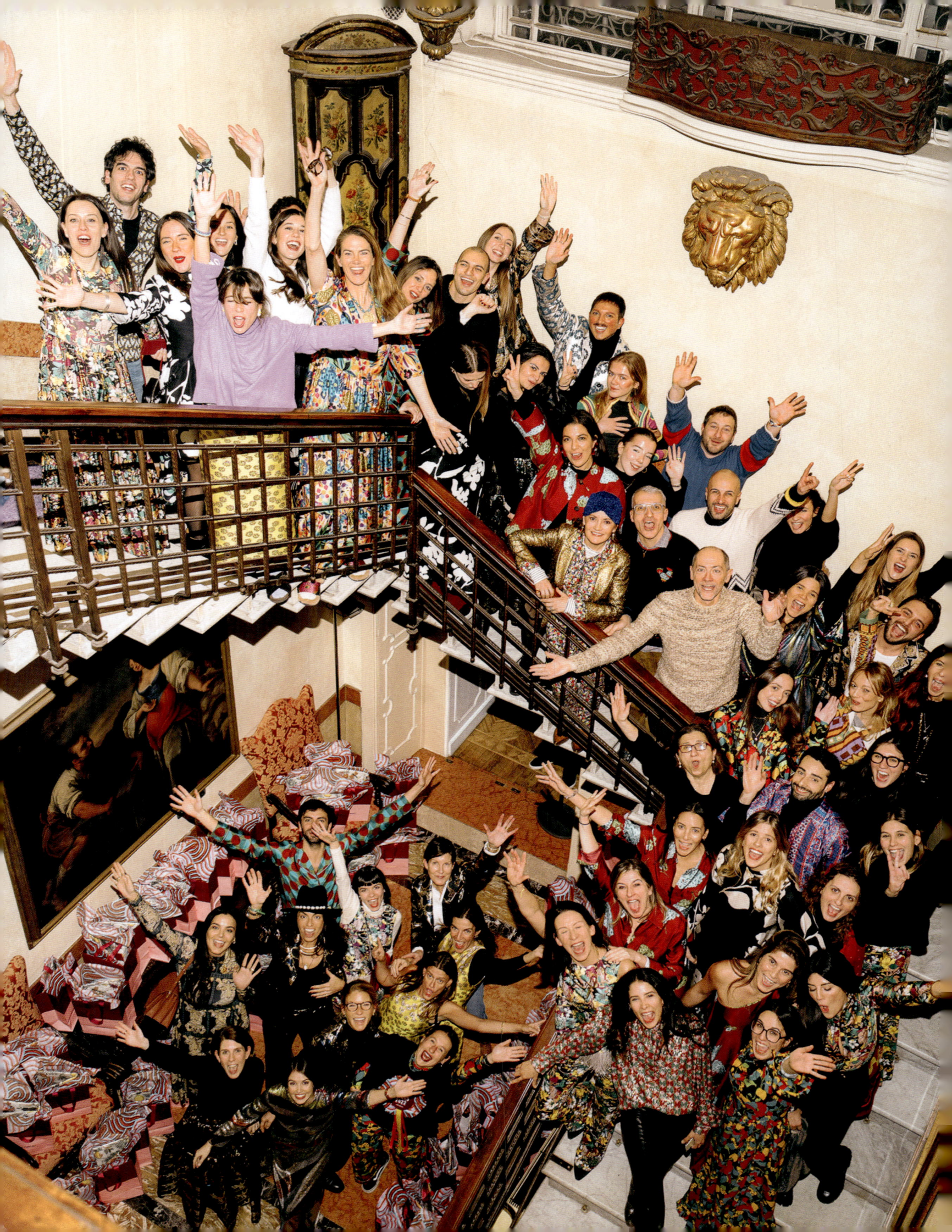

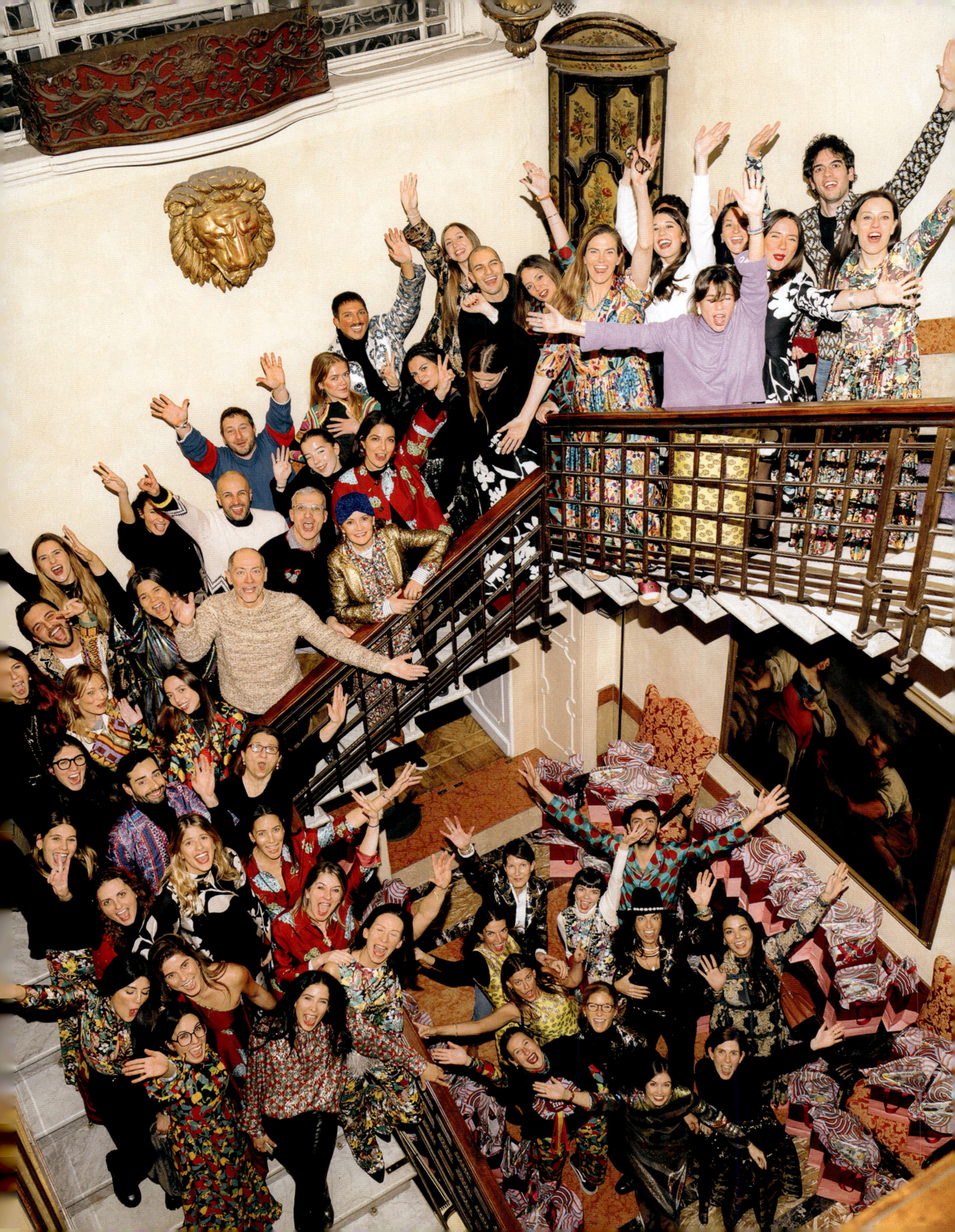

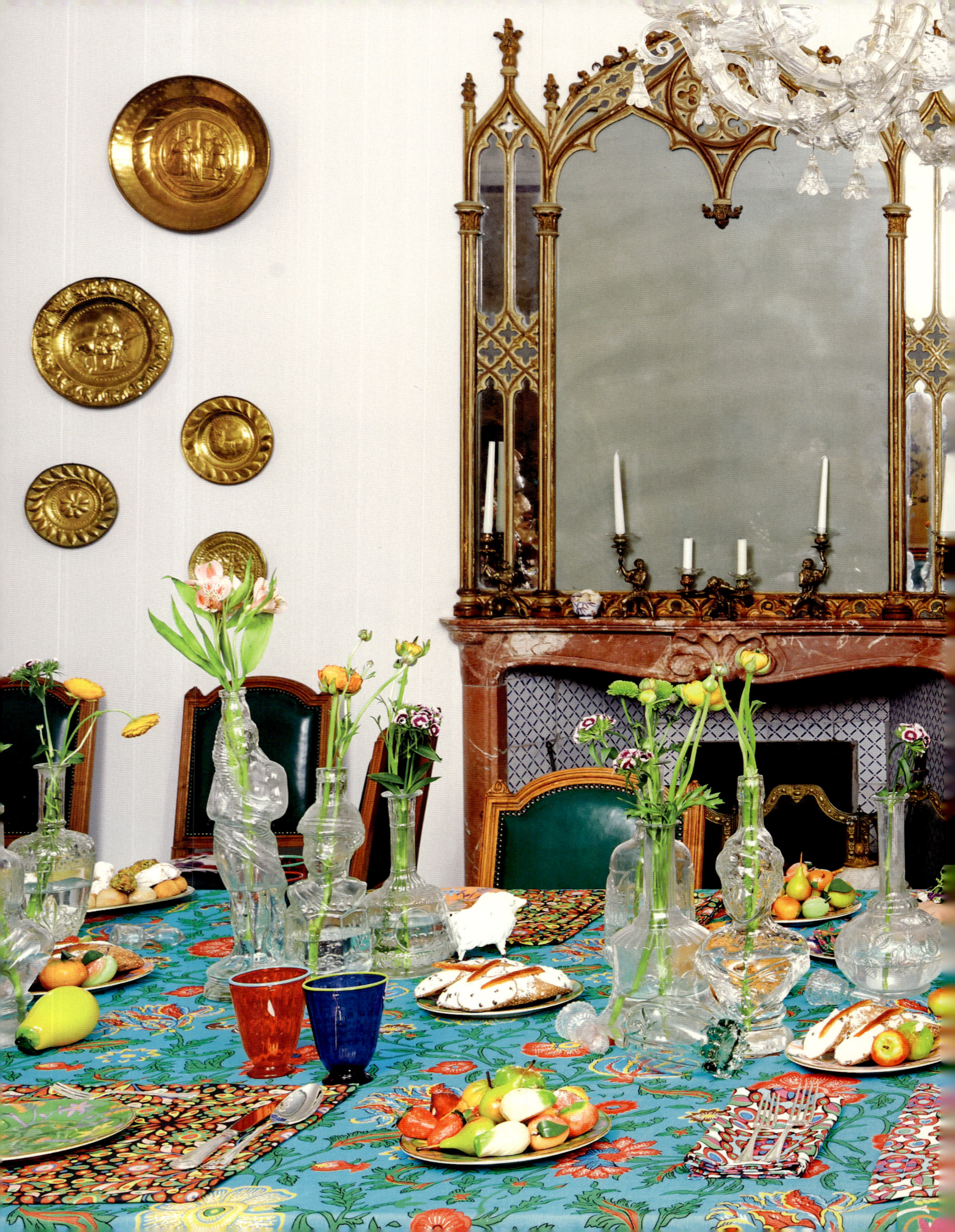

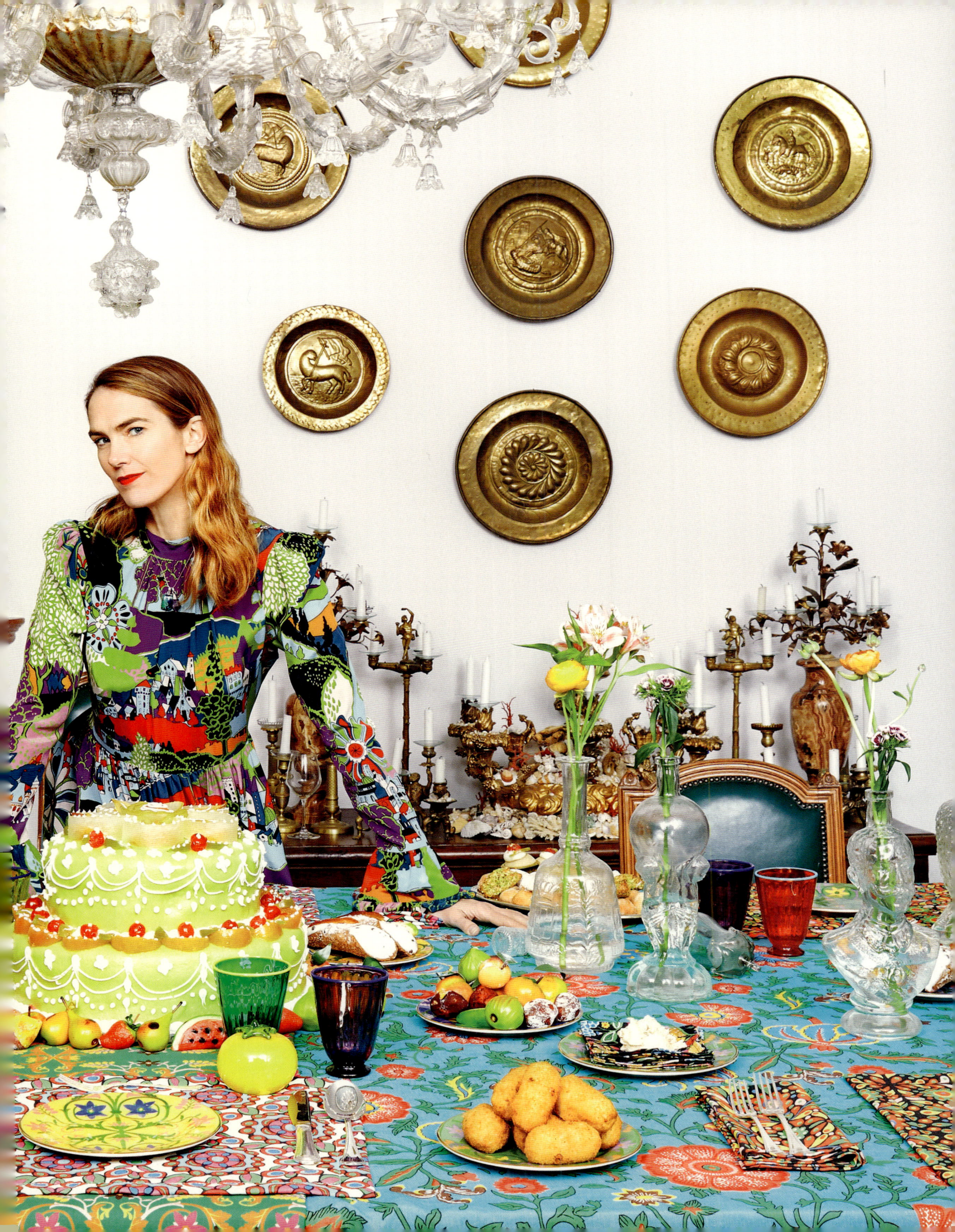

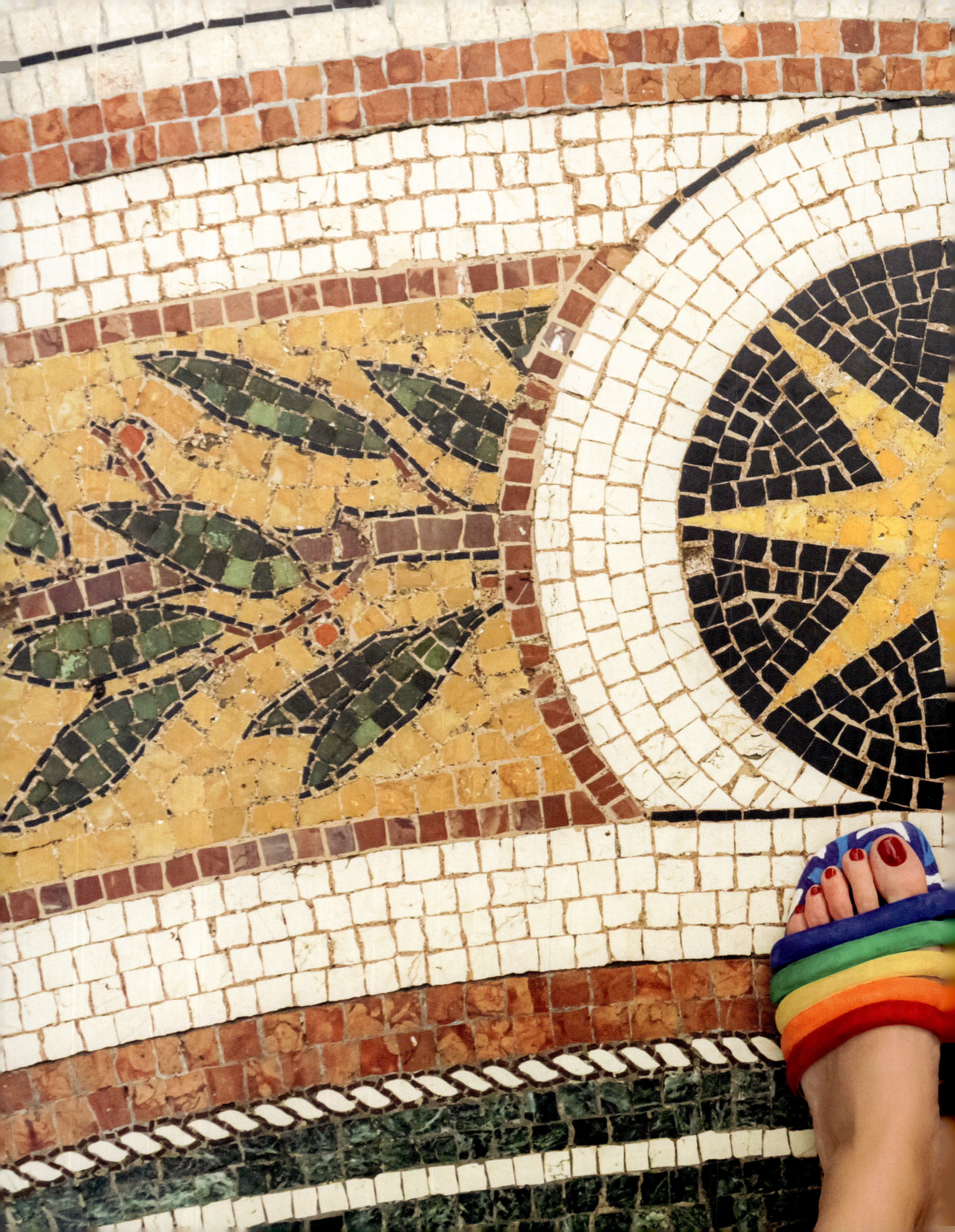

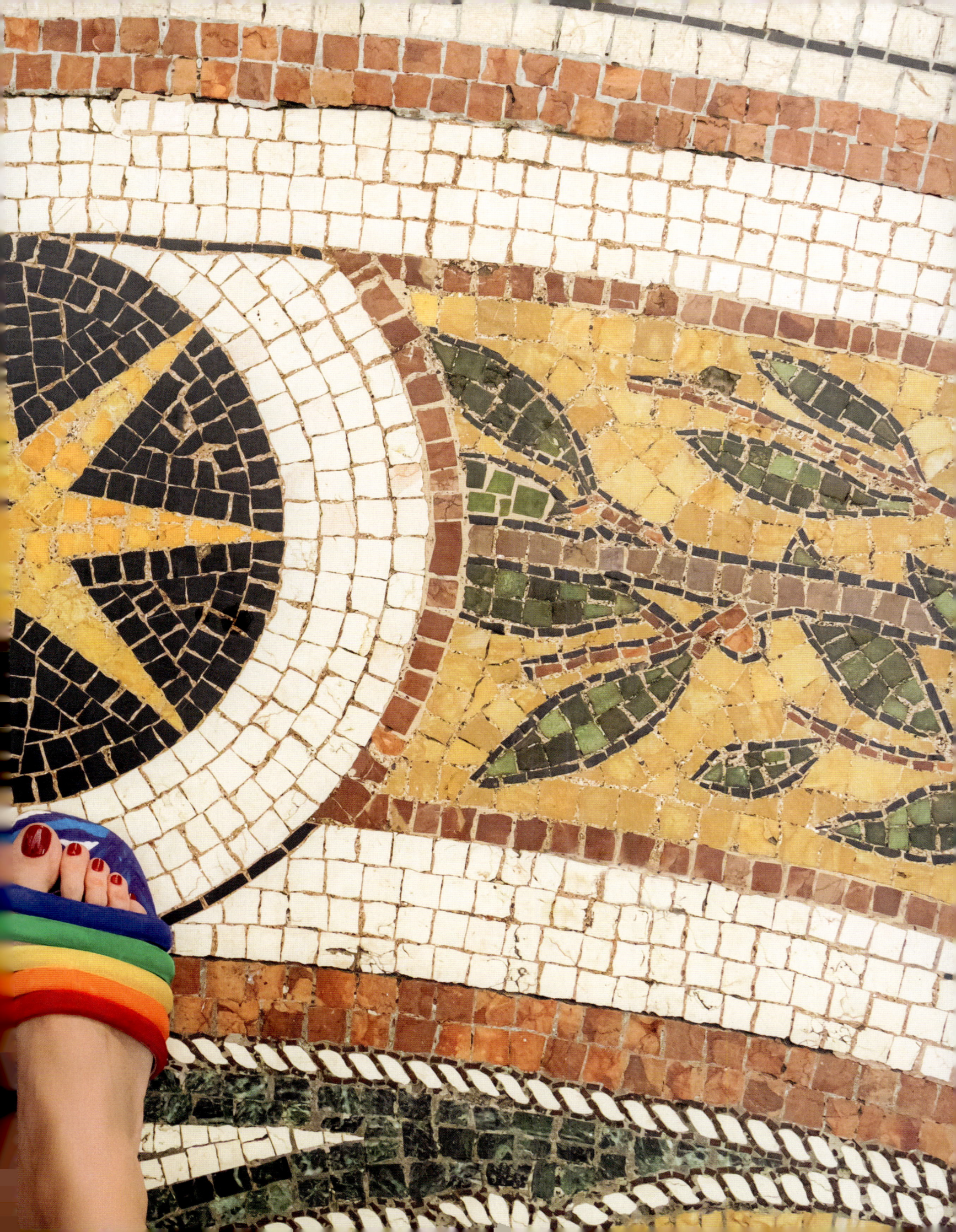

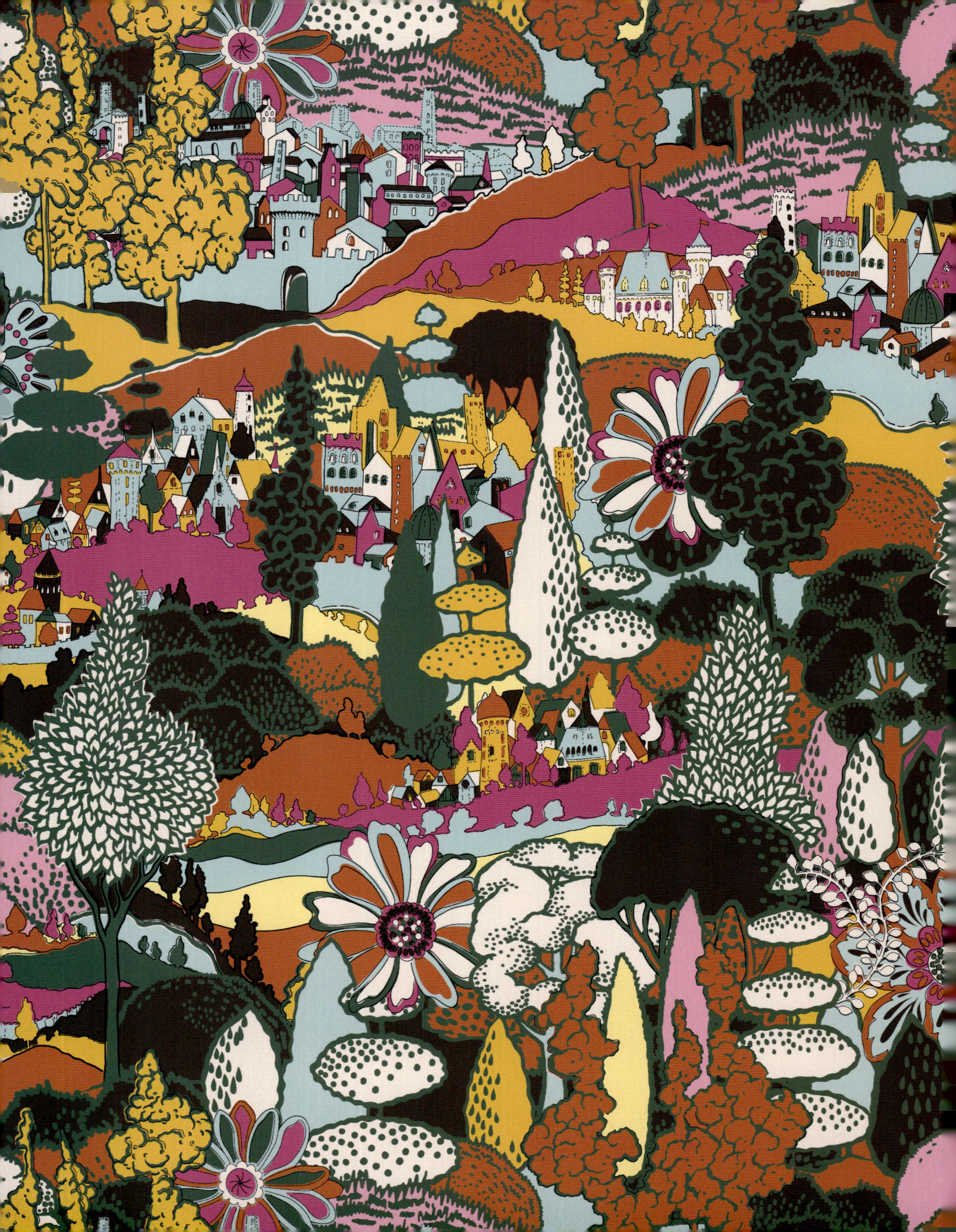

MAMMA MILANO

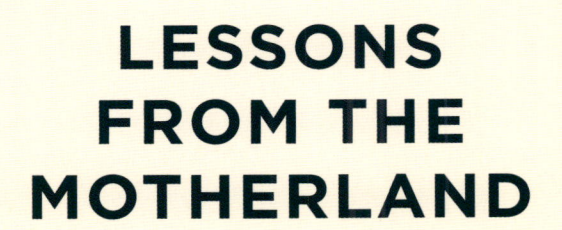

LESSONS FROM THE MOTHERLAND

How Italy taught me to bask in her beauty, slow down, glow up, create consciously, flirt shamelessly, live joyfully, laugh my palazzo pants off, and birth a company out of her marvelous, maximalist, chaotic, Big Mamma energy.

J.J. Martin

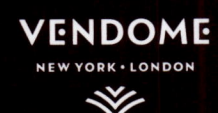

VENDOME
NEW YORK · LONDON

*Dedicated to the Divine Mother everywhere,
in all her magical forms*

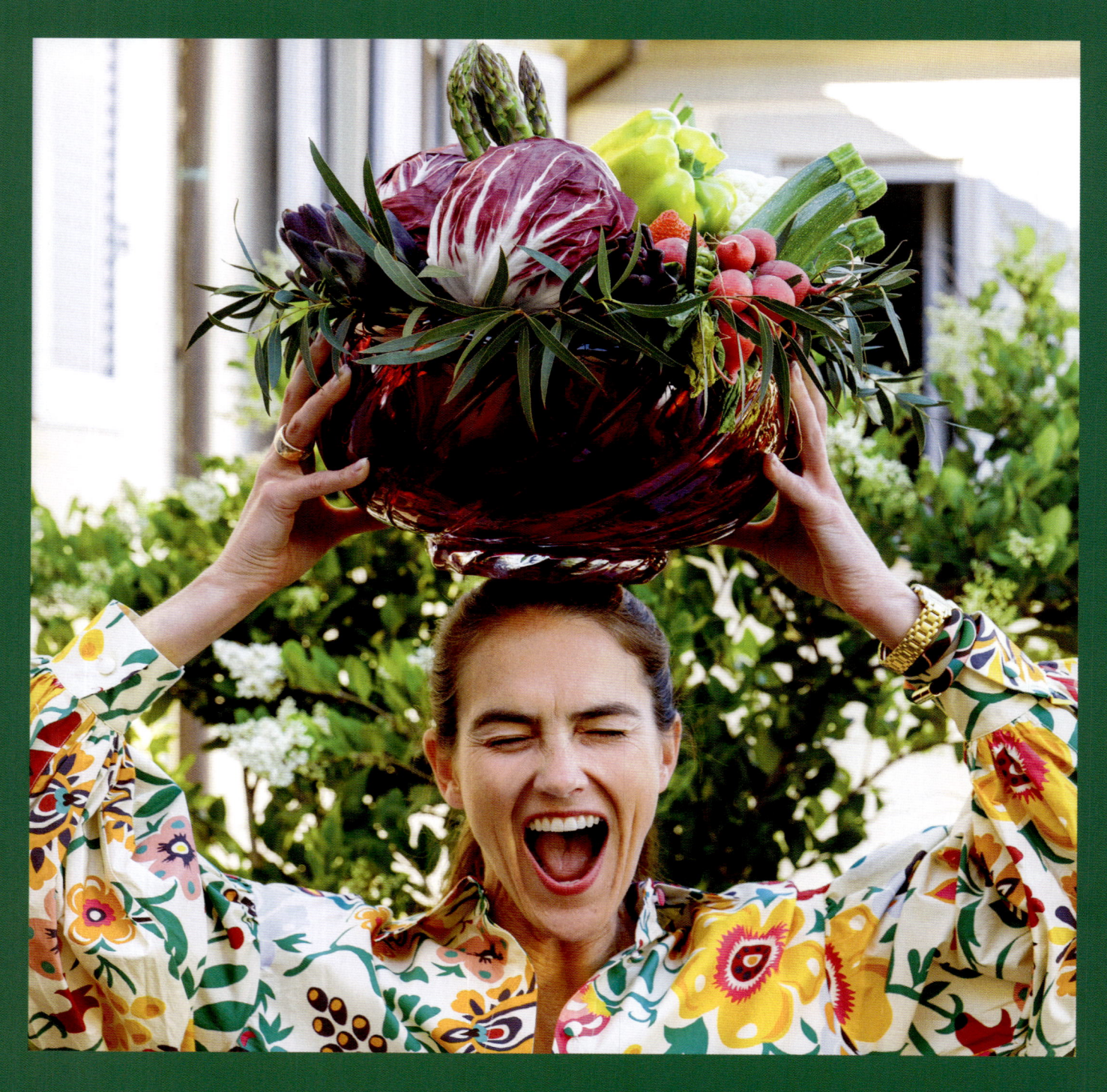

I
INTRODUCTION
A FEW THINGS YOU NEED TO KNOW FIRST, RAGAZZI!

II
ITALIAN LESSONS

How Mamma Milano schooled me in the art of living patiently, passionately, open-heartedly, and with all my senses soaking in her flamboyant beauty

III
ABBONDANZA!

Creating a life inspired by Milan's magnificent and prolific people, places, and things

IV
BORN TO BE WILD

The not-so-immaculate birth and marvelous, magnetic, to-the-maximalist life of La DoubleJ

V
RAISE YOUR VIBRATION

Using Divine Mother energy to flip your creative switch

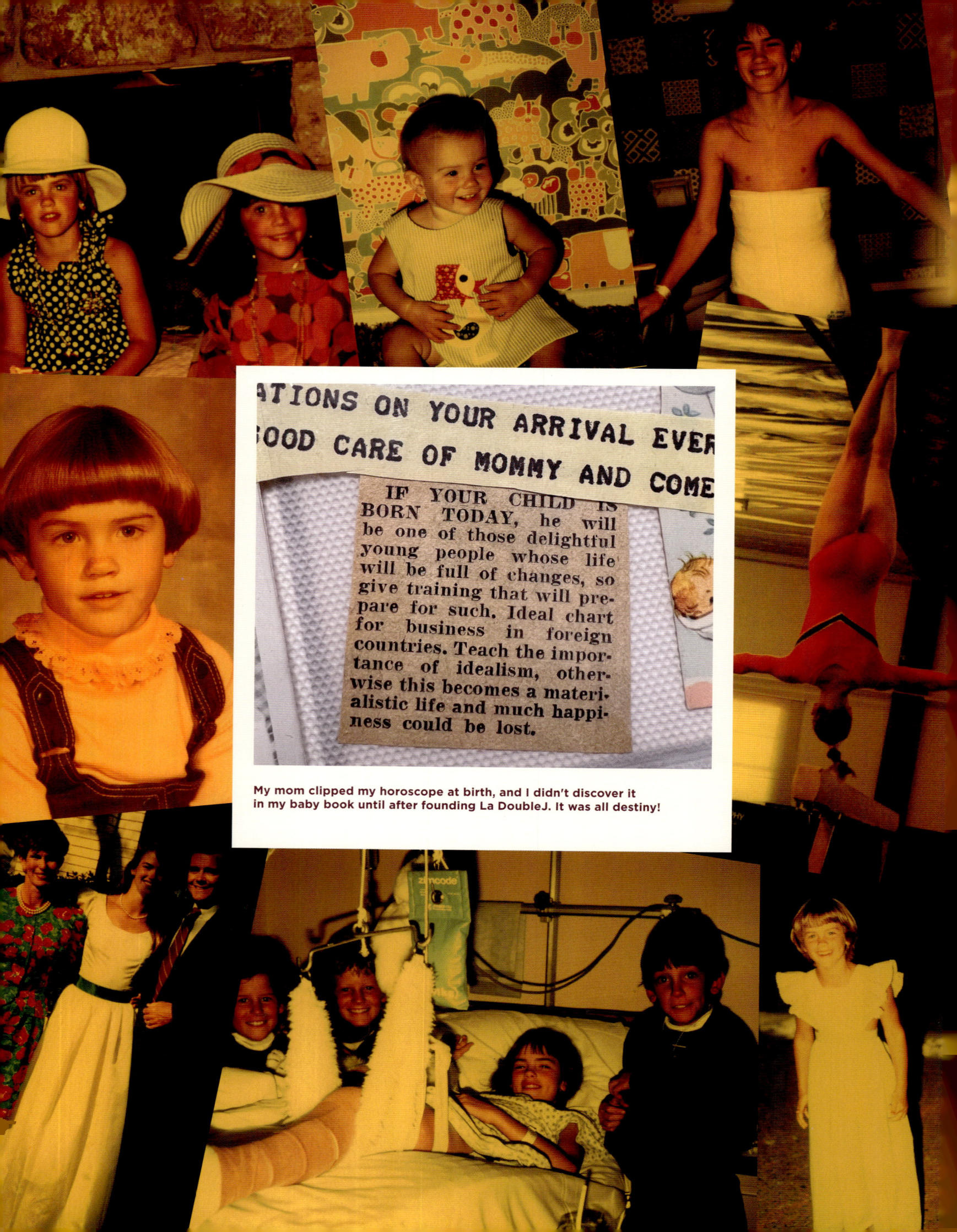

IF YOUR CHILD IS BORN TODAY, he will be one of those delightful young people whose life will be full of changes, so give training that will prepare for such. Ideal chart for business in foreign countries. Teach the importance of idealism, otherwise this becomes a materialistic life and much happiness could be lost.

My mom clipped my horoscope at birth, and I didn't discover it in my baby book until after founding La DoubleJ. It was all destiny!

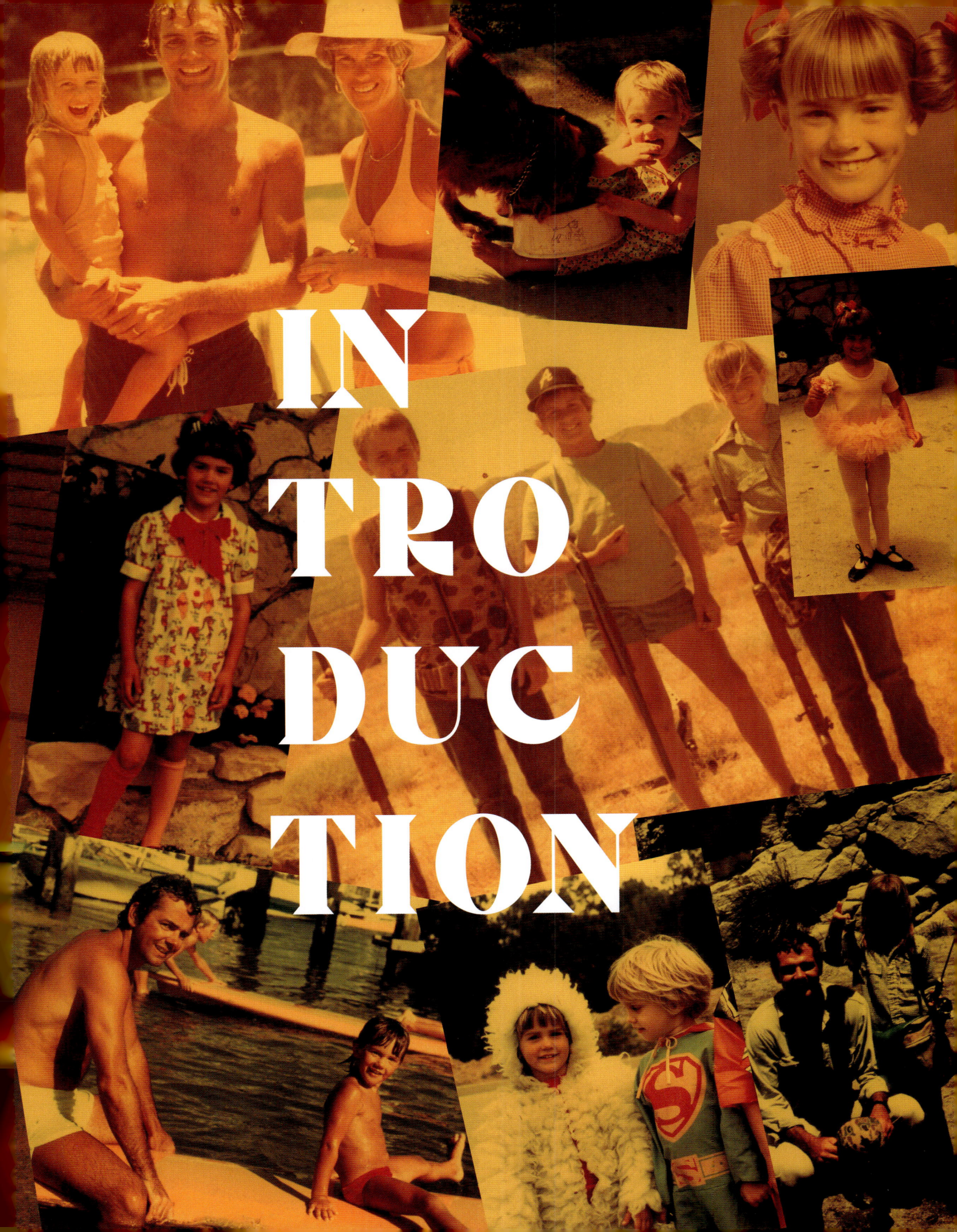

INTRODUCTION

THIS IS A DIFFERENT STORY ABOUT ITALY

You've undoubtedly seen the sensational palazzi and gilded churches, the glittering gowns and piles of pasta with oozing *burrata* produced in this sun-splashed corner of the world (and don't worry—you'll find those here, too). But this is really a tale about the spirit of a nation that became my first Spiritual Teacher. You could say it's about births and rebirths: the transformation of an uptight, compulsive, complaining American (me) into a buoyant, joy-seeking, cheerleader for my adopted homeland. A chiaroscuro of chaos and confusion into sparkling inspiration. A seed of an idea into a flourishing company, La DoubleJ, that wears feathers in her hair and does high kicks for fun.

It's also a love story—my reluctant seduction by, and surrender to, this beautiful boot of a country and its people. Italy gradually and gently took me in with her Big Mamma energy: fed me, spoiled me, taught me, tickled me, and cracked my armored heart wide open. Like any good teacher, Italy's boot also kicked me in the ass more times than I care to count, because I was going about things all wrong, like approaching a wolf—Italy's national spirit animal—with a harness and leash, rather than a glistening piece of tenderloin and a blood-pumping call of the wild.

Along the way, I'll share the trials and takeaways from this bumpy relationship—reinventing a home, a career (twice!) and a marriage; building a network of friends and family and creating a company from nothing; easing my iron grip and giving myself over to Italy's comical levels of illogic, fogginess, and disorder; opening my heart, rewiring my head, and activating my senses until out swirled an irrepressible creative force. Plus, there'll be lessons I've absorbed over twenty years of living among the tenderhearted, carefree, beauty- and quality-obsessed Italians—about the vibration-raising daily practice of joy and generosity, patience and playfulness, creativity and serendipity. And, above all, about trusting that some unseen universal force always puts you *exactly* in the place that you need to be.

The name of this cosmic force, this divine teacher? I call her Mamma Milano.

MY LIFE IN ITALY DID NOT START SMOOTHLY OR GRACEFULLY.

When I landed in Milan in August 2001—having dropped my entire life in New York to follow my Italian boyfriend, Andrea, to his motherland—I stepped out into a pizza oven. The heat was causing the street signs to wobble and shimmer. My heels sank into the pavement with every step I took; yes, the Milanese sidewalks were literally melting. Not a single restaurant was open. The fruit vendors had shuttered their *tapparelle* and hightailed it to the beach. Every Italian, from the freshly pressed little old ladies at the bus stops to the tuxedo-suited waiters at the cafés, was doing what they do best: vacationing.

When the Milanese locals finally returned from their nationally sanctioned month of snoozing and sunbathing, they waltzed back into town rested, refreshed, and carefree. I, meanwhile, was having my own kind of meltdown. Besides Andrea, I didn't know a soul. I didn't speak the language, couldn't get a job, and was unable even to feed myself (I didn't cook, and delivery service was non-existent at the time). There was no AC in our house, or anywhere for that matter, as the Italians feared it would make them sick within seconds of it being turned on. WiFi? Not really.

You could find an ATM, but it was never working, so I'd wind up standing in line at the bank for hours. There was no coffee to-go. No salad bars. I couldn't jog without tripping on a wayward cobblestone or getting stared down for exercising in public. When I finally found a gym, it was basically a tiny, down-at-the-heels disco with '80s music and equally dated fitness trends.

So, I did what we Americans do best: I got busy. I pushed my misery down into my belly and slogged through six hours of Italian lessons a day, until I could sputter out cogent-enough phrases to keep me from getting drunk and face-planting into my plate of *penne* during four-hour, all-in-Italian dinners with Andrea's friends and family.

I felt like I'd tumbled down a steep flight of stairs from my old life in New York. I'd just left high-stakes, high-shakes, high-heeled Manhattan where I was marketing director at boutique ad agencies in San Francisco and New York, then two years inside Calvin, toiling for a conglomerate that was the pinnacle of cool, but which felt like a cavernously empty hall of justice for fashion. Everyone and everything was done up in minimalist black and white, down to the Post-its, while I would show up in a car crash of bright vintage prints victoriously plundered from the Chelsea Flea Market. (It wasn't just that I loved color—the flea market had the best prices in town.) But I was burned out and sucked dry, living in my bite-sized New York apartment and getting up at 6:00 a.m. to jog an hour on the icy streets next to a frozen river just to empty my emotional garbage bag. I was caught in a storm of pure doing, in a city that prizes those who do the most.

I met my Italian guy, a management consultant in black leather pants (I kid you not), at a party downtown. Andrea and I began a long-distance relationship—helped by my

"OH MY GOD, YOU'RE LIVING MY DREAM!"

Calvin Klein. (It was A.C.B.—After Carolyn Bessette—but Calvin Klein still showed up from time to time for the five or so people he would design to see. Which was not me.) It was the kind of job I'd been clamoring my way towards my whole life, having grown up wearing the hand-me-down denim (and the alarmingly similar bowl cuts) of my two older brothers in an athletic, outdoorsy family from LA's Pacific Palisades—with parents for whom vacation was never about visiting European art museums, but driving across the border to Mexicali to hunt and camp in an ammo-filled Chevy Suburban. My childhood trained me to keep up: to be just as strong, just as fast, just as loud, and just as unflappable as anyone. We were a family of exceptional doers in a country that excels in doing.

I graduated from UC Berkeley and spent four years karate-chopping through the creative wonder-hubs of start-up frequent work trips to Europe. After ten months of this, I decided to quit my job, offload my apartment, and follow him to Milan—a city that, in the years since its dominance in the 1980s, was now sneered at by fashion editors for its not-hotness. I had nothing lined up. But my body was eerily relaxed, and in that peaceful silence, my gut said yes. So I jumped.

"Oh my god, you're living my dream!" shrieked every American woman I knew.

BUT WHAT KIND OF DREAM WAS THIS?

Andrea was acting more American than I was, working maniacally at his consulting firm, pleased enough with a giant wedge of *parmigiano* in the fridge for our 10:00 p.m.

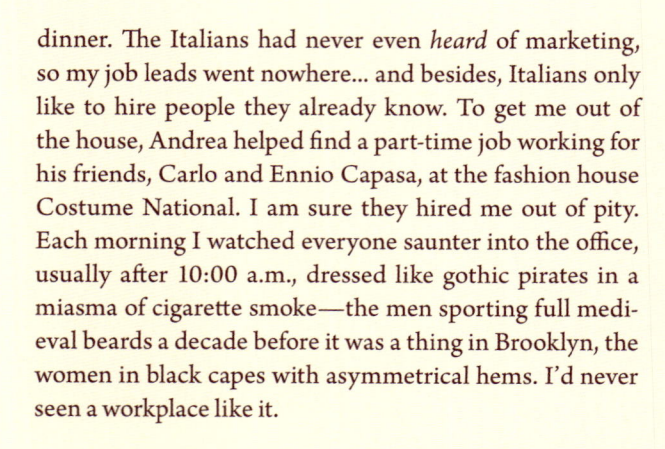

dinner. The Italians had never even *heard* of marketing, so my job leads went nowhere... and besides, Italians only like to hire people they already know. To get me out of the house, Andrea helped find a part-time job working for his friends, Carlo and Ennio Capasa, at the fashion house Costume National. I am sure they hired me out of pity. Each morning I watched everyone saunter into the office, usually after 10:00 a.m., dressed like gothic pirates in a miasma of cigarette smoke—the men sporting full medieval beards a decade before it was a thing in Brooklyn, the women in black capes with asymmetrical hems. I'd never seen a workplace like it.

One day, I got a foot in another door—more like jammed it in, American-style. I was invited to designer Stephen Fairchild's fashion presentation at Milan's Hotel Diana. At the bar I met Godfrey Deeny, the salty Irish editor of *Fashion Wire Daily*. He was the former bureau chief of *WWD* Paris and was now helming the world's first online fashion news service. But the Italians could not have cared less—most barely even had the internet. He hired me with zero journalism experience and threw me into the Neil Barrett show, after which I spent six hours anxiously wringing out my first five-hundred-word review. I passed the test.

It then became my daily job to write about everything under the Milanese sun: Moschino's show, Gucci's new store opening, Prada's financial results, and who got fired from Bally. I was delivering seven pieces of five-hundred-word news every day during Milan's four annual fashion weeks, and yet I existed at the bottom of the slimy barrel, standing in the twenty-fifth row behind someone's grandmother at the Dolce & Gabbana show. Over two years, I cranked out four hundred reviews and articles, shamelessly asking Posh Spice about what she ate for breakfast or interviewing Alberta Ferretti backstage about her show inspiration, typing it all out on my Sony Vaio from the backseat of a taxi before running into a hotel to hook up to their dial-up modem. My office was a table at Pasticceria Cucchi on Corso Genova. The genteel owner behind the cash register eyed me and my computer with deep suspicion and considerable pity.

PR agents never rolled out the red carpet for me in those early years in Milan. And no one, as far as I could tell, read a word I wrote. I felt invisible, lame, thoroughly irritated. But, as fashion fate would have it, there was one person who was watching and reading. And that was *International Herald Tribune* fashion editor Suzy Menkes, who liked my scoops and asked me to write for her.

It was a miraculous golden lifeline.

Suddenly, I was yanked up from the bottom to one of the industry's most esteemed positions. The Italians worshipped Suzy and adored the *Tribune*. My byline there led to Kristina O'Neill and Amanda Ross from *Harper's Bazaar* USA discovering me one day during fashion week in the corner of the Four Seasons Hotel, hooked up to an outlet and furiously filing copy. The next month, they hired me to join their team, led by Glenda Bailey, as *Bazaar's* editor in Italy.

During my first years clawing at the well-shod feet of the Italian fashion scene, I still found myself scoffing at the old-fashioned ways of my adopted country. I wanted to boss the Italians around, improve them, modernize them, speed them up, and tone their soft, ab-less stomachs. I was determined to wake them up, make them more efficient. Make them *better*. When I would bump up against the oddball hours of small shops that were never open at the moment I wanted to go, I stomped my feet and snorted.

Back then, I was always at the bank. Italians were forever patiently spending an hour in line to do very simple things, like deposit a check, that Americans did in fifteen seconds at their outdoor ATMs that always worked. No one seemed to have a problem with this epic waste of time, except me. One day, just as I got up to the friendly faced yet totally time-challenged bank teller who I'd been mentally mind-bombing, I was ready to shoot off some American-style self-righteousness about his poor line management. The sweet man saw me and my scarlet face about to burst... and handed me a crumpled brown paper bag of ripe *fagiolini*. Green beans. "They're fresh from my garden this morning!" he declared proudly.

The twinkle in his eye shot through my skin and penetrated the shellacked shell armoring my heart. Those homegrown green beans planted a powerful seed, the first of many that Italy would bury in me. In that very moment, I did something Americans hardly ever do: *I surrendered*.

ITALY, YOU WIN!

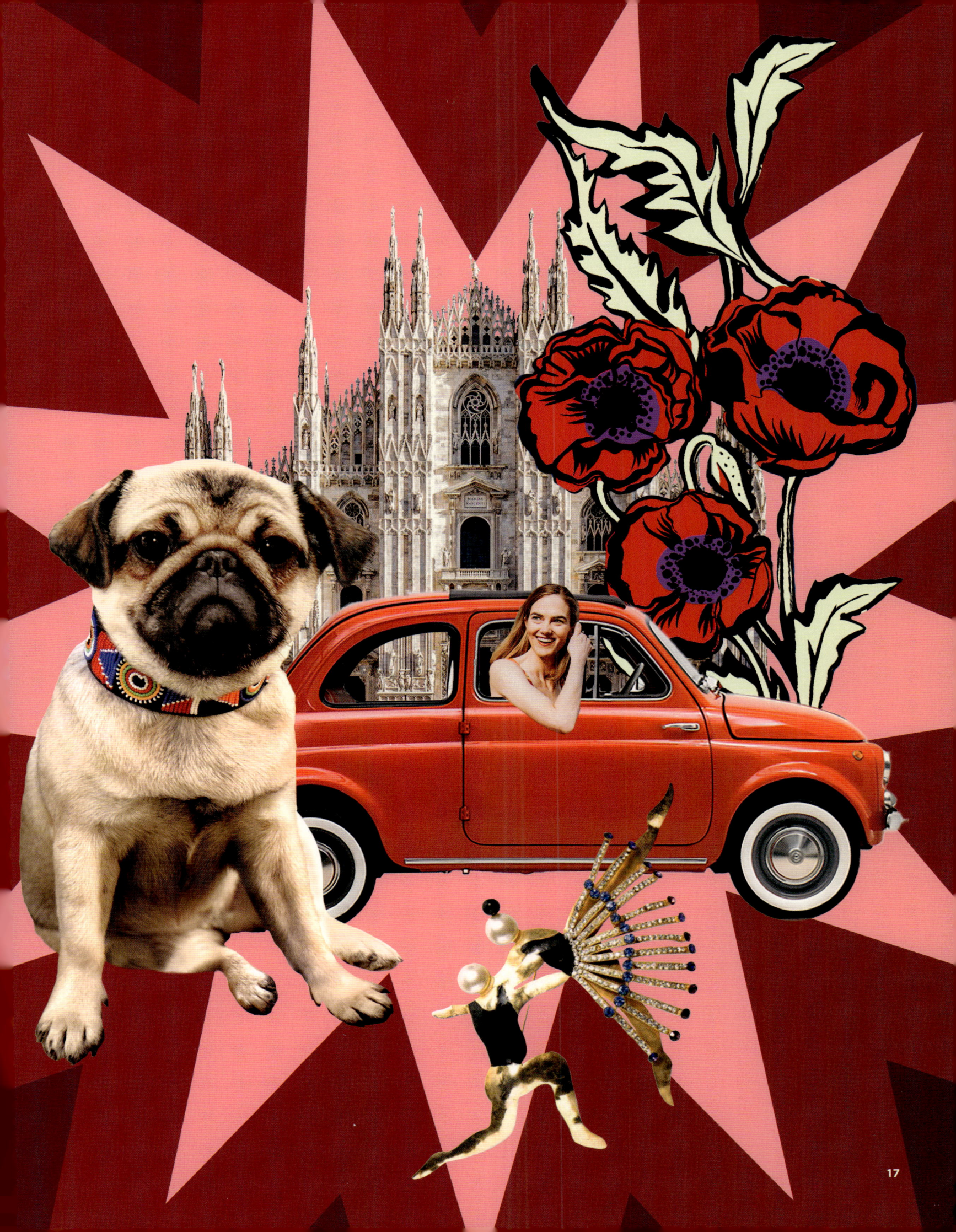

MY SURRENDER wasn't just a thought.

It was a deeper knowing, a flash of insight that I felt inside my millions of tiny molecules. This country—its customs, its backwards everything, its long lines, its slow rhythms, and its constantly-on-a-lunch-break store owners—was all just exactly as it should be. I couldn't change it. In that moment of understanding that everything was very right that I had thought was so wrong, I caved to the power of this great country.

I finally began to see her for the queen she actually is and the wise mother who was giving me exactly what I needed.

The student was ready. Mamma Milano—muse and messenger from the motherland—had arrived.

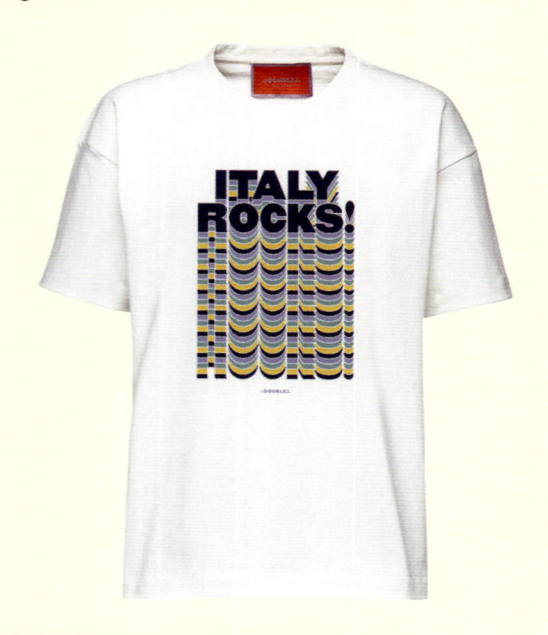

MAMMA MILANO SOFTENED ME AND SOFTENED MY HEART.

Her lessons came gently, without the drill-sergeanting or rah-rah majorette-ing we Americans expect, or even crave, from a spiritual makeover. I began to see things I'd never noticed. I fell in love deep and hard with Italy's beauty and serendipity, her magnificent traditions of artisanal creativity, her cool, dark churches with candlelit Tintorettos, and her sun-drenched pebbly beaches where the roly-poly *nonne* and tanned children spend all day picnicking under candy-striped umbrellas. She trained me to slow down and admire the *fruttivendolo*'s glistening produce, to flirt back with policemen in their cornflower-blue uniforms and auto-mechanics wielding their wrenches like Michelangelo with his chisel, and to be dazzled by the kaleidoscopic mosaic floors and soaring ceilings of the city's entryways.

Mamma Milano showed me how to stop fighting with the general order of things, and instead tap into the ambient joy, ease, and creative spirit that she doles out in gorgeous golden waves.

It was this nurturing environment that provided the safe, warm womb for my own creativity to take root and grow—birthing a vibrant journalism career, and then a bouncing, beautiful baby called La DoubleJ.

La DoubleJ was conceived not from any left-brained logic or business plan, but out of pure joy. She started in 2015 as an online magazine selling vintage fashion and jewelry, and she beguiled from the start. She has blossomed into an amazing team of seventy full-timers and twenty freelancers, creating maximalist fashion and homeware collections inspired by Italy's vibrant colors and artisanal traditions. Everything we do is 100 percent made in Italy. We've achieved this by creating a wide collaborative universe, shining a light on the work of decades-old fabric producers and heritage artisans, from the Mantero silk archives founded in Lake Como in 1829 to Salviati, our glassware manufacturer that has been blowing glass in Murano since 1859.

My creative muses for this project have been the Italians themselves: from the architects, interior designers, stylists, and photographers I was lucky enough to meet, to Milan's *sciure* (stylish "housewives"), and everyone who took me by the arm and showed me how it's done. I have been a grateful guest, a lucky visitor, and a faithful student in Italy's majestic homes, artistic ateliers, sacred spaces, and light-filled landscapes, drinking in its slow rhythms and time-honored customs—not to mention its epic food secrets.

La DoubleJ became the canvas for all of this learning. She was, and still is, my energy baby. She is so sensitive that whenever I misbehave and act too American—too bossy, too controlling, or too judgmental of people or situations—she swirls back and slaps me in the face: someone will quit, a project will fall apart, a gray cloud will turn into a supersize, gravity-sucking black hole. The truth is, I lose control when I try to control. I swear that my company is a sentient being, not a business enterprise. She has feelings. She loves creativity. She loves laughter.

INTRODUCTION

She loves collaboration. She loves the unexpected. She performs only when the conditions are right. In that way, she's just like Italy and Mamma Milano. Later in my spiritual practice (honed by a small army of healers, teachers, shamans, and psychics), I learned that not only do people, spaces, words, and actions carry energies, but countries do, too.

Italy is a very feminine-energy country, while America's can-do spirit is resoundingly masculine. Italians are beautifully and naturally attuned to the state of just *being*; their homeland is very maternal. You might even say that Italy *is* the Divine Mother—she is receptive and accepting, soft and lovely. What Italy first taught me was then mirrored back and confirmed by my energy practice: you have to respect the Mother. You have to go with the flow and accept the dark chaos that may come with her, as I did in trying to establish a life, and a business, in Italy. But feminine energy is also the deepest dark, the most fertile ground for sowing the fecund jungle of your life, your soul, your dreams.

When I stopped blaming and fighting with Italy, Italy stopped fighting with me. When I did less, I got more.

Now, of course, Italy has take-out food, high-speed internet, ATMs, decent yoga studios, and a city full of young creative people in Milan. You might think I just got lucky in terms of timing. But I know I got everything I ever wanted merely by stopping my insistence on having it.

How does that work? You let go. You stop trying to control. You listen. You wait. You let Mamma Milano—or your own Divine Mother with her unique, wild wisdom—slowly take you by the hand and lead you. *Dai, andiamo!*

With love,
J.J.

A BILLION REASONS TO LOVE THIS BRILLIANT COUNTRY:

VINTAGE FIAT CINQUECENTOS
TINY ARTISANS WITH MASSIVE TALENT
THE MEN
THE APERITIVO SNACKS
THE CREATIVE CRAFTMANSHIP
THE APEROL SPRITZES
EVERYONE THRIVES ON CHAOS
THE HAND GESTURES
MONEY COUNTS LESS THAN RELATIONSHIPS
THE MOTTO: PIANO, PIANO
GRANDPAS WHO STILL FLIRT
LE NONNE WHO ALWAYS SAY EAT, EAT, EAT!
MORE IS ALWAYS MERRIER
CHILDREN ARE THE BOSS
RELAXING IS A NATIONAL BIRTHRIGHT
NO ONE WEARS SWEATPANTS OUT OF THE HOUSE
THE MOZZARELLA
THE WAITERS ACTUALLY CARE IF YOU ENJOY YOUR MEAL
ROOFLESS CAPRI TAXIS
EMERGENCIES BRING OUT THE CREATIVE BEST IN EVERYONE
EVEN STRAIGHT MEN KNOW ABOUT GOOD FASHION
IT'S ALWAYS IL COLPO D'ARIA'S FAULT
TOMATOES THAT TASTE LIKE SUGAR
MEN WHO RIDE BICYCLES IN BRIONI SUITS
LE SCIURE
THE SEA COLOR IN PANTELLERIA
THE SALONE DEL MOBILE TURNS MILAN INTO AN EPIC PARTY
HOTEL IL PELLICANO
BAROQUE SICILIAN CHURCHES
EVERYONE MAKES OLIVE OIL OR KNOWS SOMEONE WHO DOES
NO ONE IS PISSED OFF FOREVER
THE MONTH OF AUGUST IT ALL TURNS OFF

ITALY, TI AMIAMO TANTO & SEMPRE!

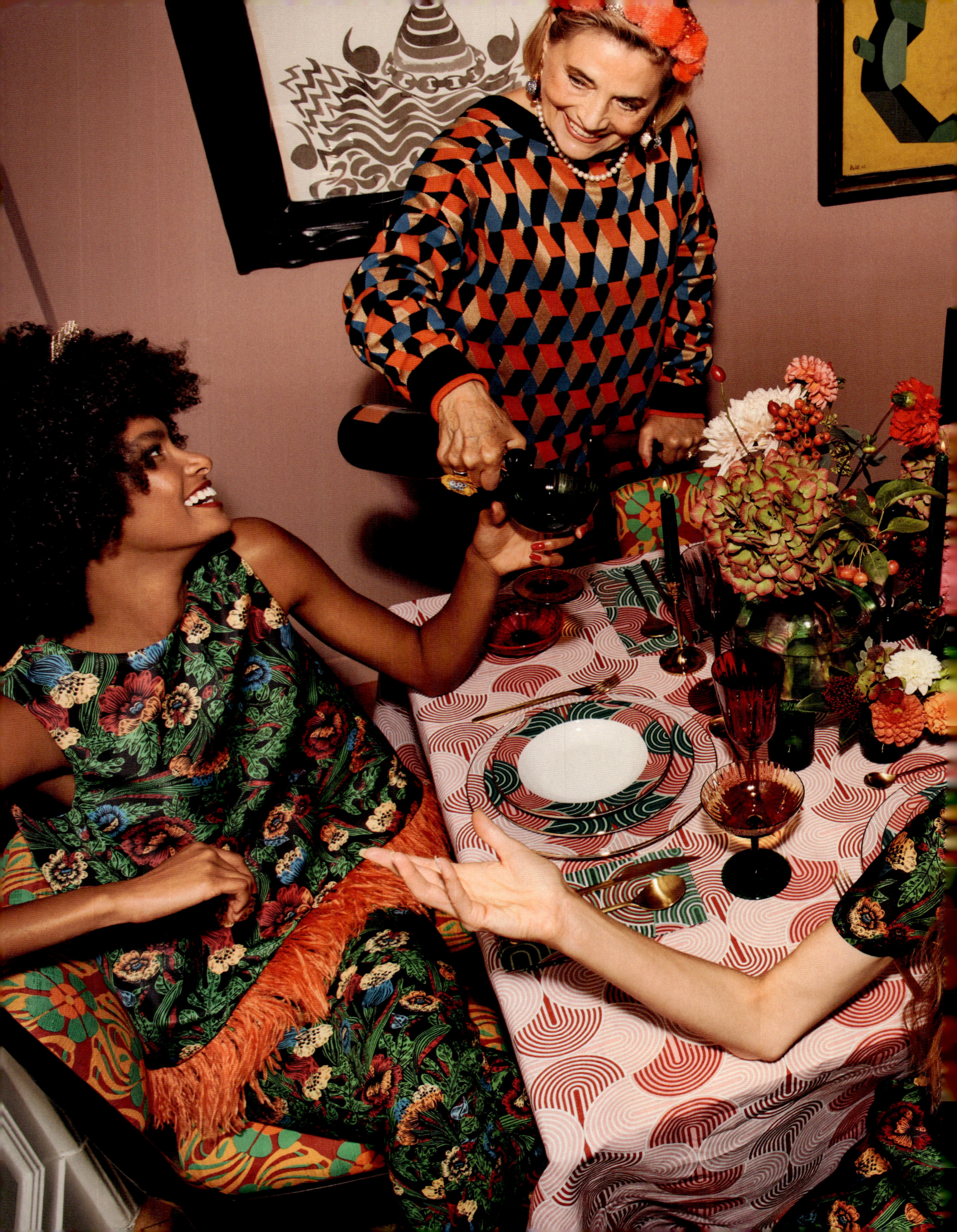

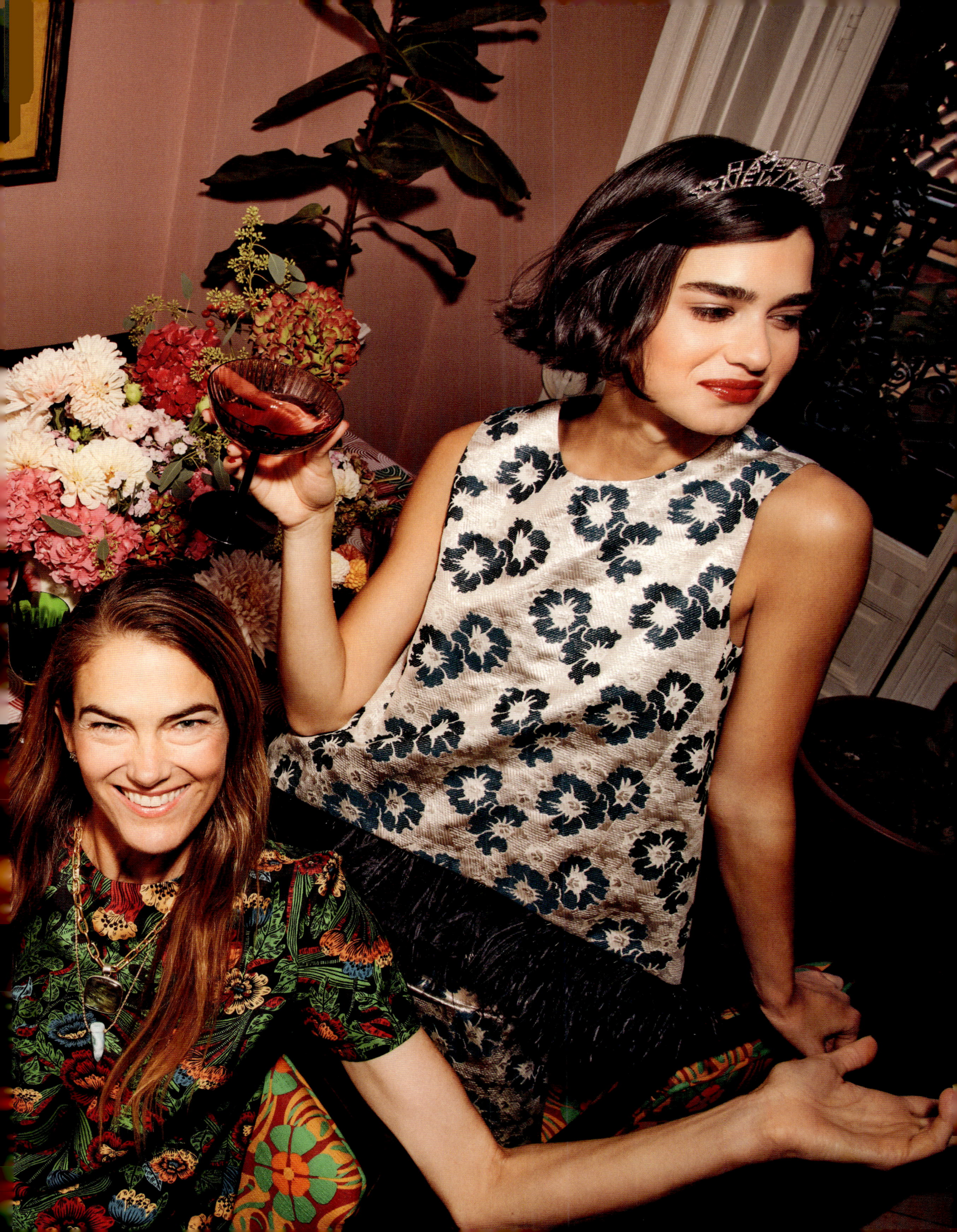

ITAL
LES

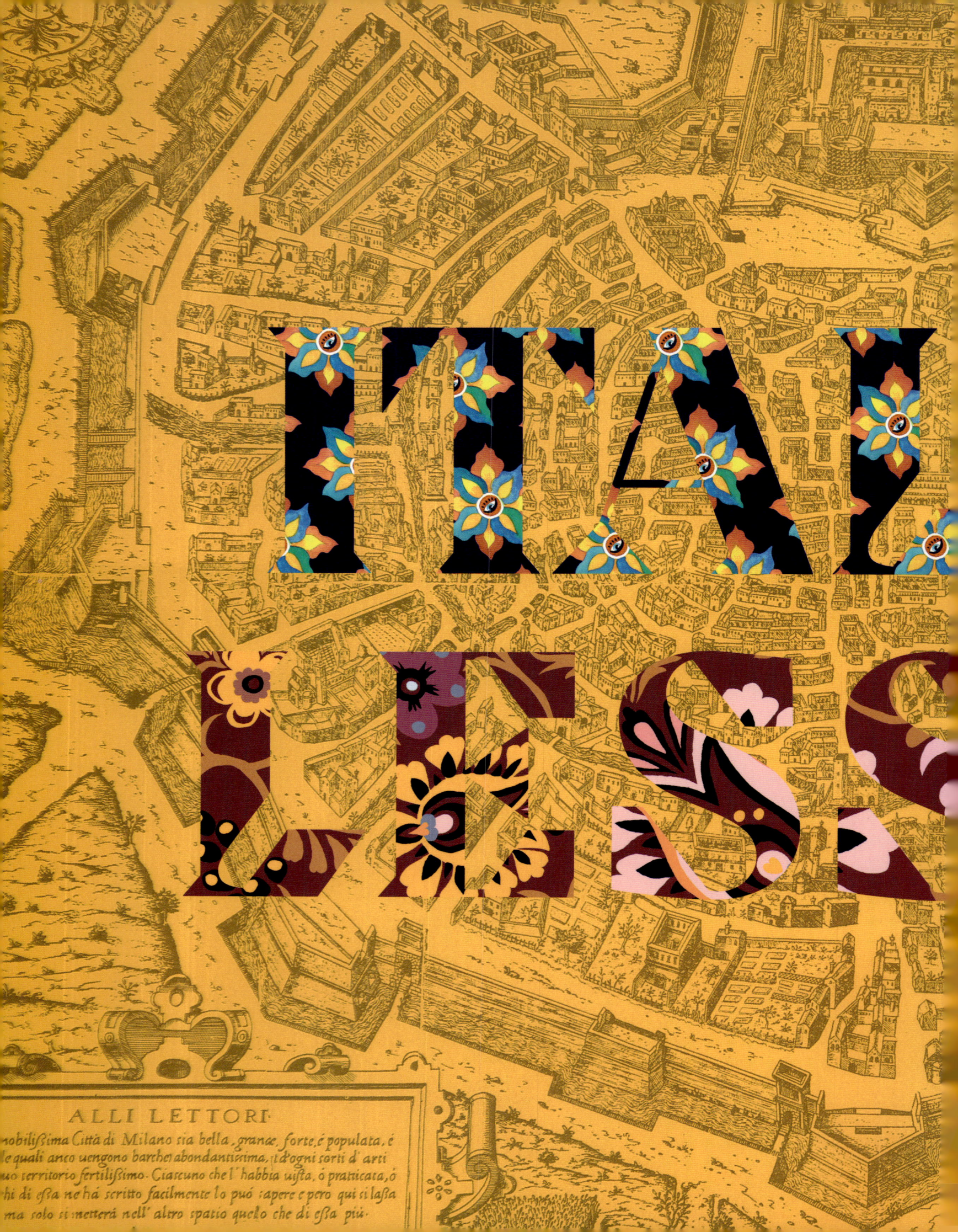

ALLI LETTORI.
nobilissima Città di Milano sia bella, grande, forte, è populata, è
le quali anco uengono barche abondantissima, d'ogni sorti d'arti
uo territorio fertilissimo. Ciascuno che l'habbia uista, ò praticata, ò
hi di essa ne hà scritto facilmente lo può sapere e pero qui si lassa
ma solo si metterà nell'altro spatio quelo che di essa più

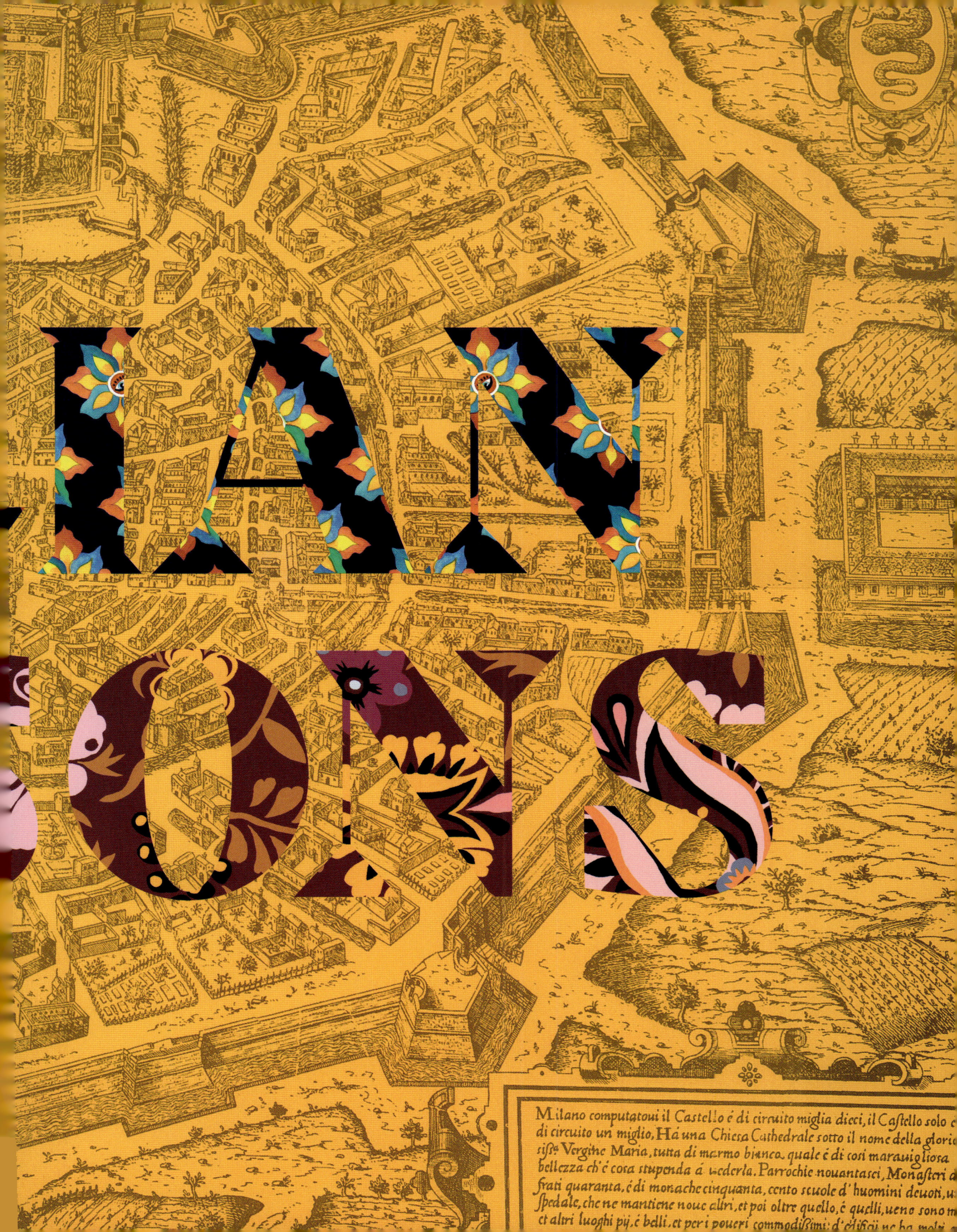

Milano computatoui il Castello é di circuito miglia dieci, il Castello solo
di circuito un miglio. Ha una Chiesa Cathedrale sotto il nome della glorio
sissª Vergine Maria, tutta di marmo bianco, quale é di cosi marauigliosa
bellezza ch'é cosa stupenda á vederla. Parrochie nouantaséi, Monasteri d
frati quaranta, é di monache cinquanta, cento scuole d'huomini deuoti, u
spedale, che ne mantiene noue altri, et poi oltre quello, é quelli, ueno sono m
et altri luoghi pij, é belli, et per i poueri commodissimi: d'edificij ne ha molti

LESSON 1

LIKE FAMIGLIA

In Italy, family and personal relationships rule absolutely everything

I landed in Italy twenty years ago knowing exactly one person: Andrea. (For those who skipped the Introduction: Andrea was my boyfriend, eventually my husband, and then—spoiler—business partner and ex-husband.) His family lived three hours away by train. I had no friends, no job, and no one to show me the ropes, from how to find an electrician to how to order pizza. Wading into this new culture meant steeping myself in the mother tongue—not just the language, though I barely spoke a word of it—but the mother mindset.

Almost more important to finding my way was learning a whole new mode of relating to the world around me and the people who would pull me into a gleamingly supportive web of connection—and, eventually up into Mamma Milano's warm, padded, and stylish lap.

From making doctors' appointments to making friends, I soon learned that everything magical that coalesces around you in Italy is powered by relationships—who you know, who you're related to, whose cousin went to nursery school with the friend who is going to be your hook-up for a house rental in Capri. If there's one thing that bonds all Italians together, it's their devotion to family. And on the highest throne sits the Italian mother. This family orientation extends far beyond DNA, with good friends gaining status as quasi-family members, and everyone from bankers to handymen being treated like longtime friends.

This was a strange concept for someone who had just arrived from the most transactional country on the planet. "Can't I just pay for better service?!" I would think as my waiter ran by for the seventh time without even looking in my direction. "Can't I just get the information I need in an email?" No, you can't. Italy is not a culture of tipping or doing business with strangers.

Things happen not because you pay more or ask for it nicely (or get pushy and demand it). They happen because you chat, you listen, you share, you appreciate what someone has made or done, and everyone bounces home happier and better than when they arrived.

This is the art of relationships, a mutual give-and-take, rooted in a nurturing feminine energetic. And no one does it better or more intuitively than the Italians.

> **EVERYONE BOUNCES HOME HAPPIER AND BETTER THAN WHEN THEY ARRIVED.**

ITALIAN LESSONS

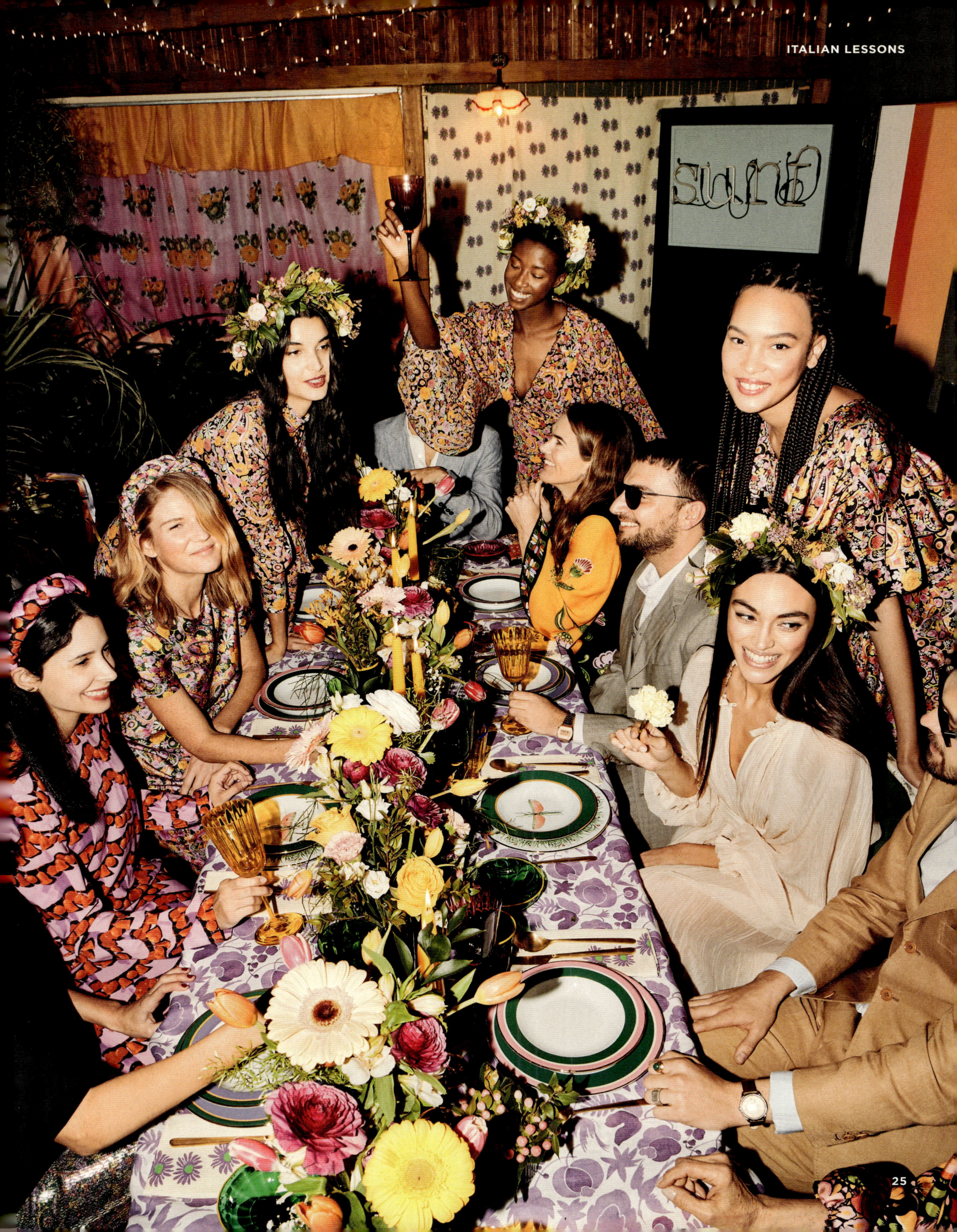

MAMMA MILANO

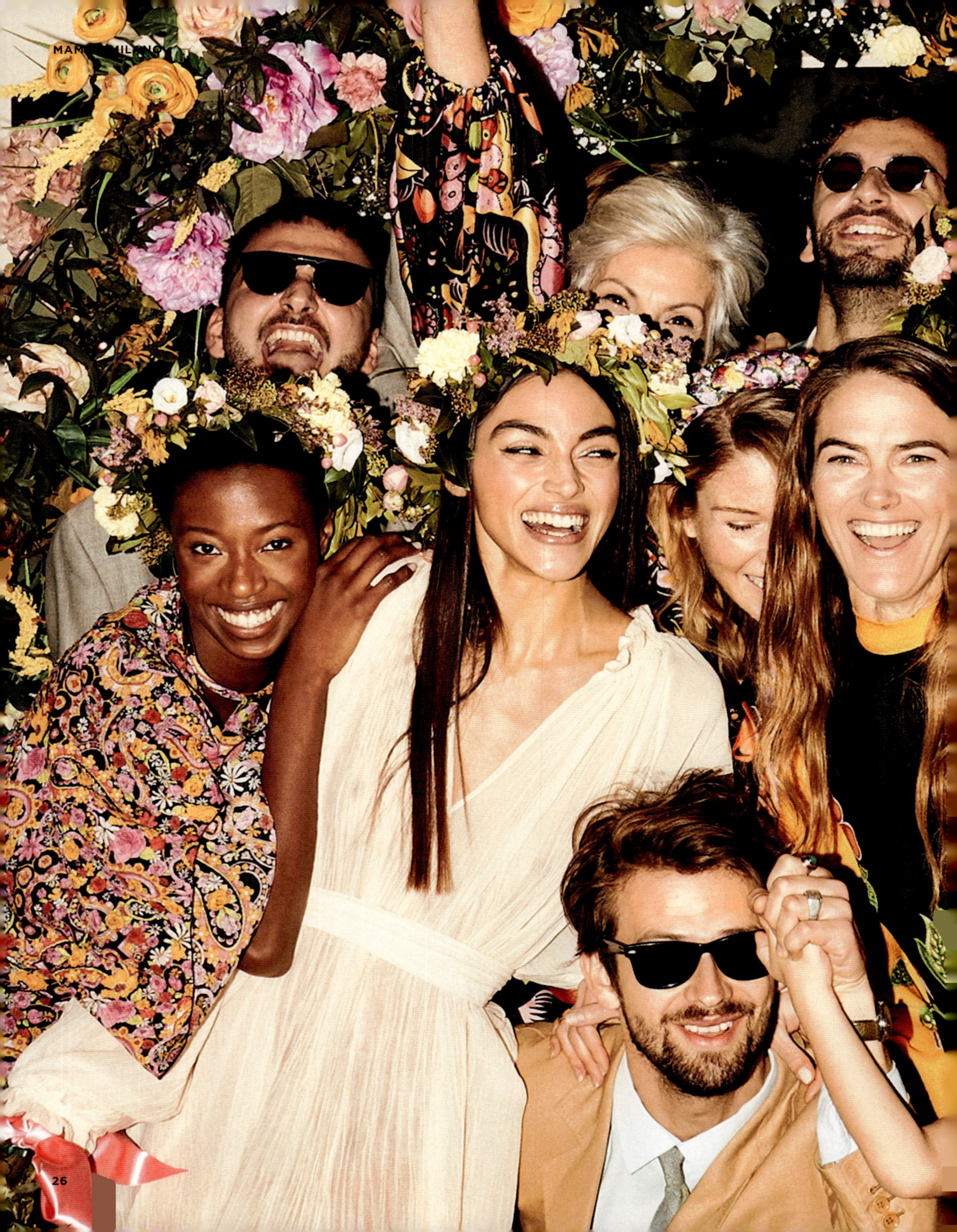

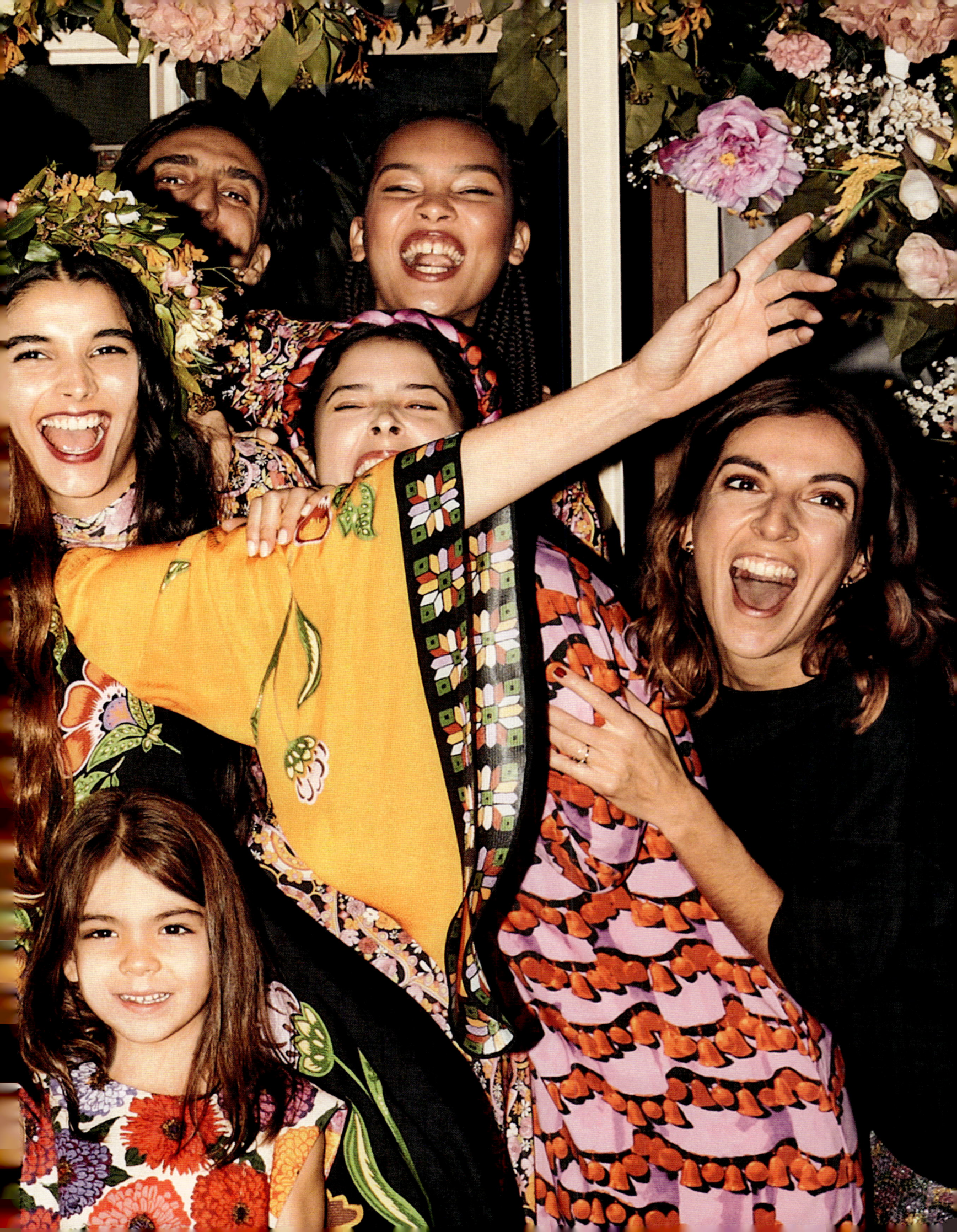

MAMMA MILANO

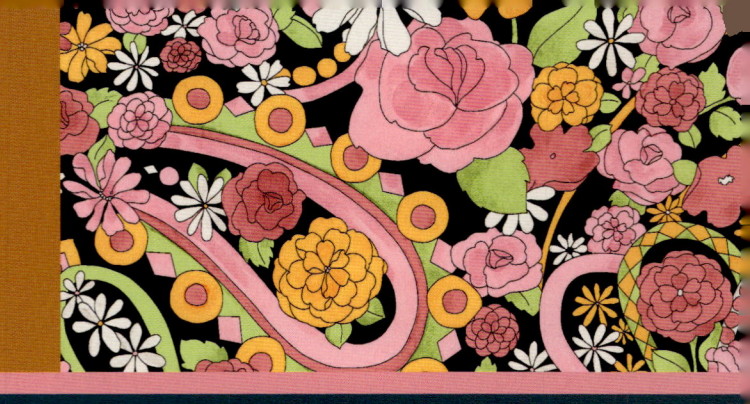

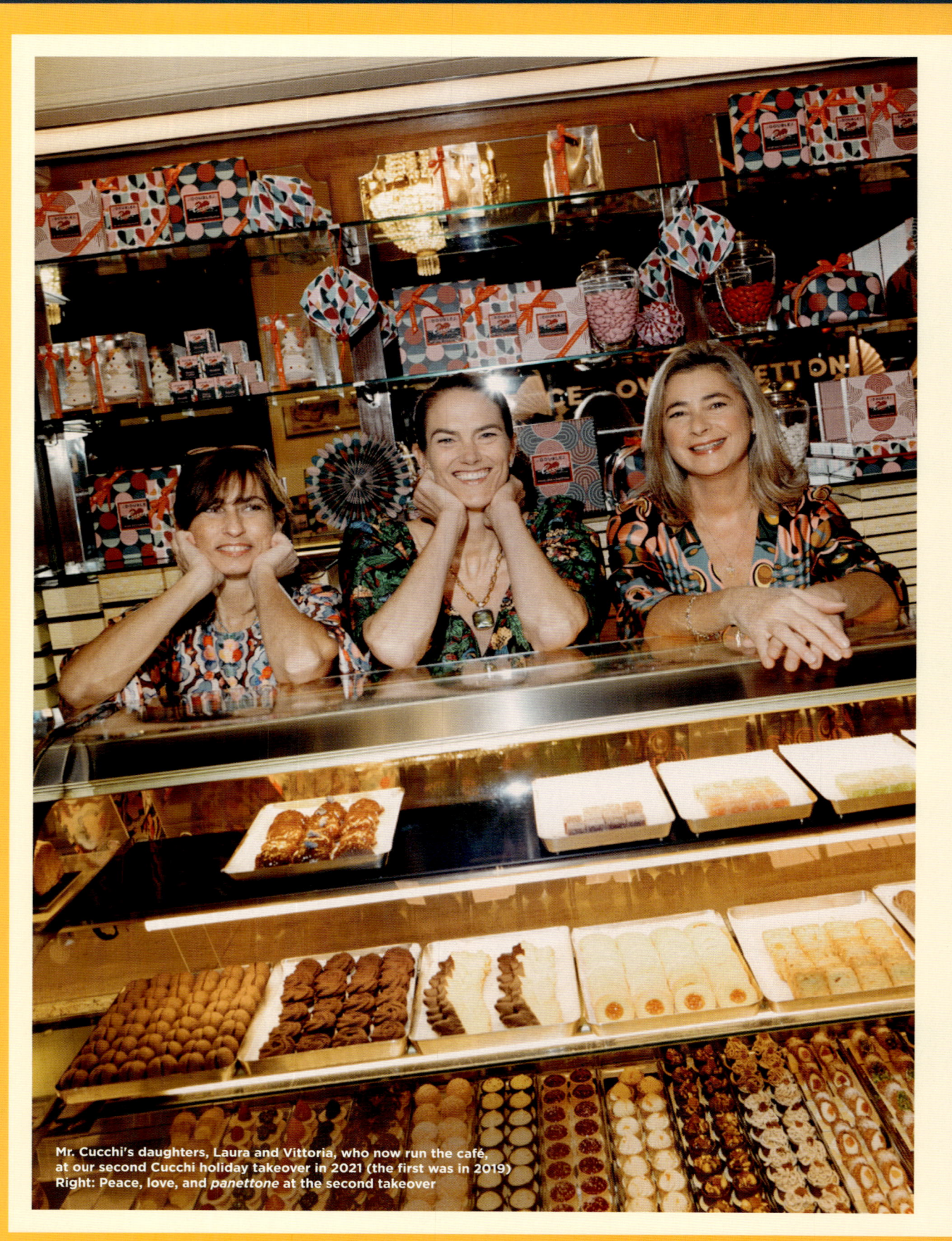

Mr. Cucchi's daughters, Laura and Vittoria, who now run the café, at our second Cucchi holiday takeover in 2021 (the first was in 2019)
Right: Peace, love, and *panettone* at the second takeover

ITALIAN LESSONS

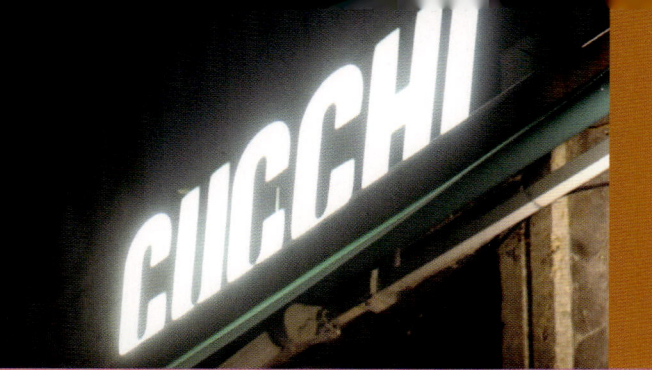

JOINING THE CUCCHI FAMILY

LESSON 2

I first observed the power of relationships at Pasticceria Cucchi, a traditional café with damask buttercup-yellow tablecloths and dusty chandeliers, located a few blocks from my first apartment in Milan.

During my early years in the city working as a journalist, I would show up daily and do what New Yorkers do: work. I sat down, opened up my Sony Vaio, and kept my nose down for five-hour writing sprees, oblivious to everyone and everything around me. When I did look up, I would notice the staff staring at me—not so much in judgment, but with deep pity and a genuine concern that seemed to ask, "Doesn't she have anywhere else to go—and where are her friends?" I would return their curiosity with my own death stare that said, "Why don't you have WiFi and why does my waiter never refill my coffee cup?!!"

This was not a relationship. It was a transaction. I treated their beloved café like my all-day office with janitors. No Italian wants that. So, the impeccably starched staff and stately Mr. Cucchi—stationed behind his cash register in suit, tie, and pocket square just as his family forebears had done since 1936—kept their distance every time I came to the till to pay.

One day a few years later, a bald philosopher with crooked teeth named Franco began showing up at the café several times a week. He, too, had a computer! I felt an immediate kinship. As we edged closer together over time, Franco showed me the ropes. Order just one cappuccino—but never after 12:00 noon. If you come at *aperitivo* time, have just one drink, even if you stay three hours. And always keep up a stream of lively banter. When I wasn't on a tight deadline, I would follow Franco into the day's bubbly, lively conversation. Franco knew the first name of each waiter and would laugh, play, and joke around with them. They were not staff, they were friends. Soon, I noticed that the faces at Cucchi brightened as I came in and greeted everyone by name, later telling them how marvelous today's *sfoglia di mela* was. (It truly *was* a life-changing pastry. I had just never thought to tell them how much I loved it.)

My veneer continued to crack over the next few years, until one evening it crumbled completely. I had stopped into the café around 7:00 p.m. to use the restroom. As I was walking out, patriarch Cesare Cucchi was there, alone in the middle of the brightly lit bar, wearing a tweed coat, purple-and-burgundy striped tie, and brown lace-up shoes. I had never seen him out from behind the register before. He stopped me, and for a moment I wondered if I had forgotten to pay my bill earlier that day.

"My dear," he announced, taking my hand, "today I am eighty years old." Pride beamed from behind his frameless, Italian-made glasses. "You don't look a day over sixty," I replied. "That's what *everyone* tells me," he said, kicking up a heel like he wanted to waltz. He then poured me a glass of fizzy Ca'del Bosco and we stood there alone, drinking together, admiring the giant brioche

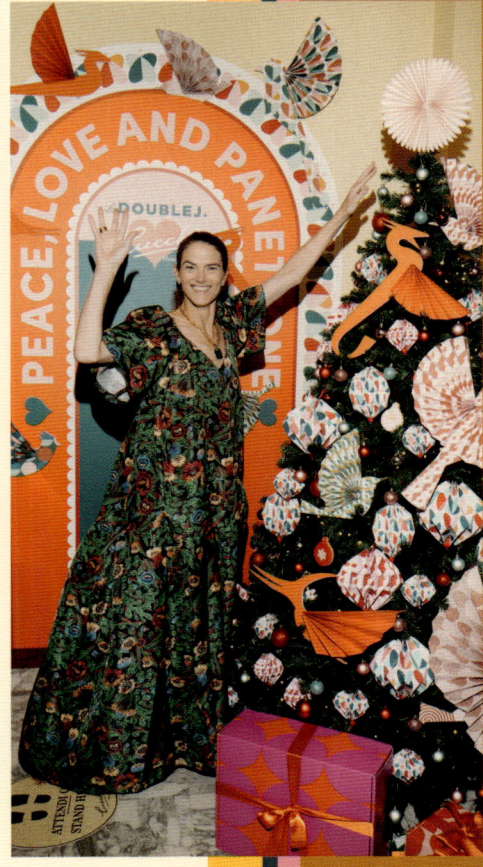

29

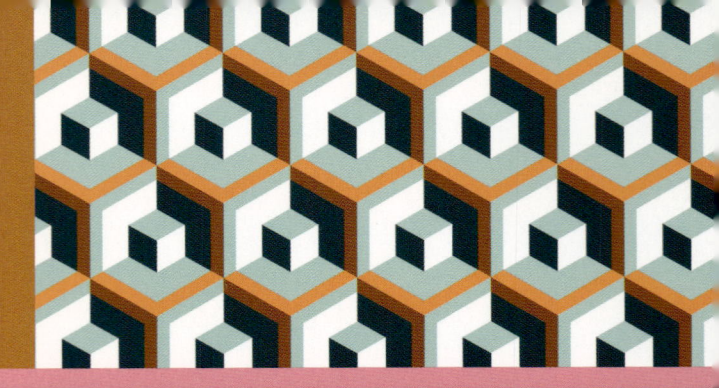

his pastry chef had made him with a big 80 in drippy lettering. When I left, my body was pulsating. An eighty-year-old Italian had just invited me to his birthday party! I was now part of the Cucchi family. It had only taken a decade.

As the years passed, Cucchi became a home—a mothership of sorts, that fed me emotionally, energetically, and physically. The service was still spotty, the new WiFi never worked... and it never mattered. The staff treated my pug, Pepper, like a celebrity (and never got upset when she ran into their kitchen). They looked out for my vintage Cinquecento when the meter maid came by.

One day, Mr. Cucchi's daughters Laura and Vittoria asked me to festoon the entire café with La DoubleJ prints for the holiday season. We designed a full takeover, and for two months our printed fabrics and patterns lined every table, shelf, and chocolate box. Mr. Cucchi had sadly passed away a few years earlier, but we toasted Cesare on our opening night and repeated the whole operation the next year.

Pepper, the Cinquecento, and I are now more than well-known regulars; we are part of the Royal Family at one of Milan's oldest cafés.

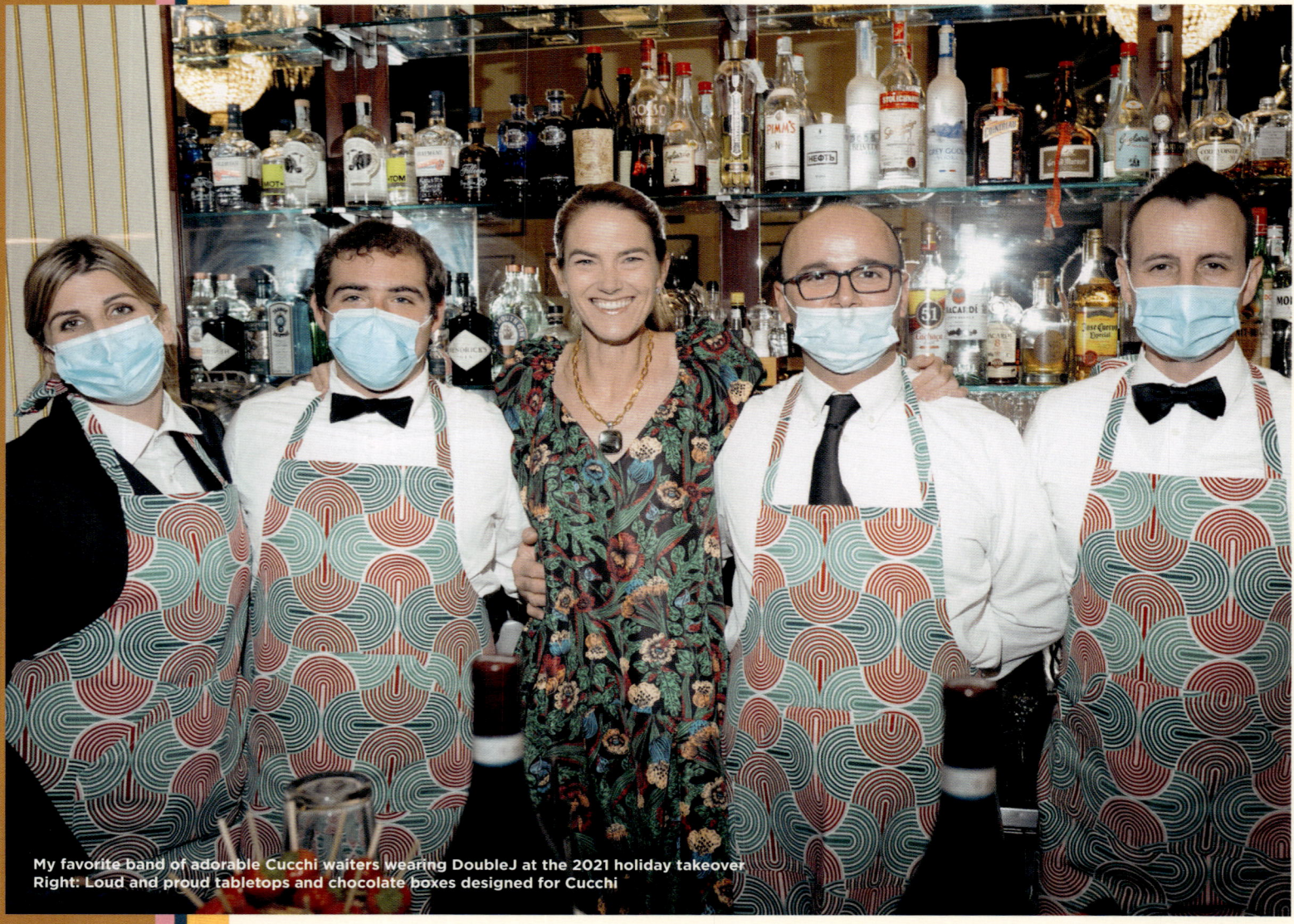

My favorite band of adorable Cucchi waiters wearing DoubleJ at the 2021 holiday takeover
Right: Loud and proud tabletops and chocolate boxes designed for Cucchi

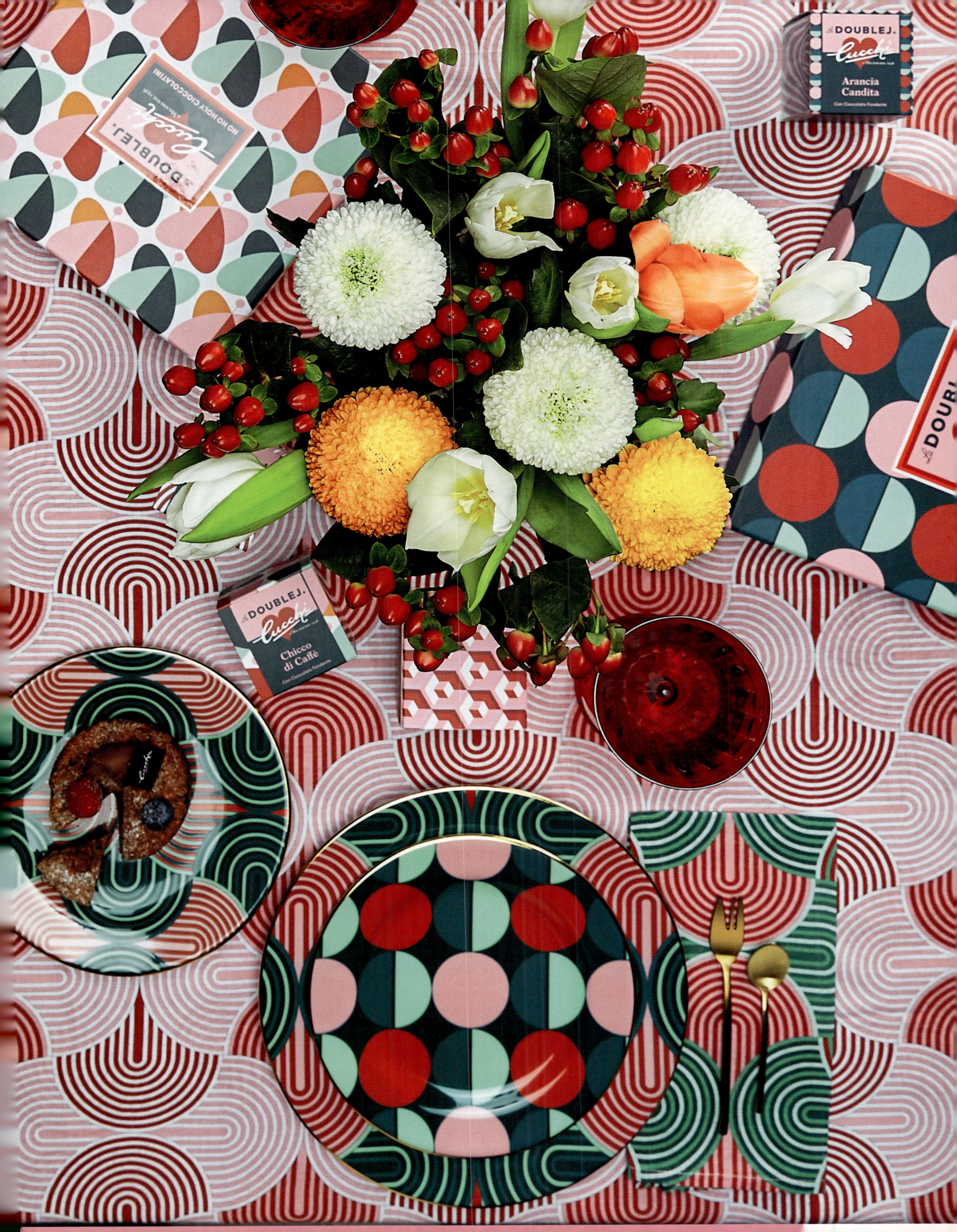
DOUBLEJ.
Arancia
Candita
DOUBLEJ.
Chicco
di Caffè
DOUBLEJ.

MAMMA MILANO

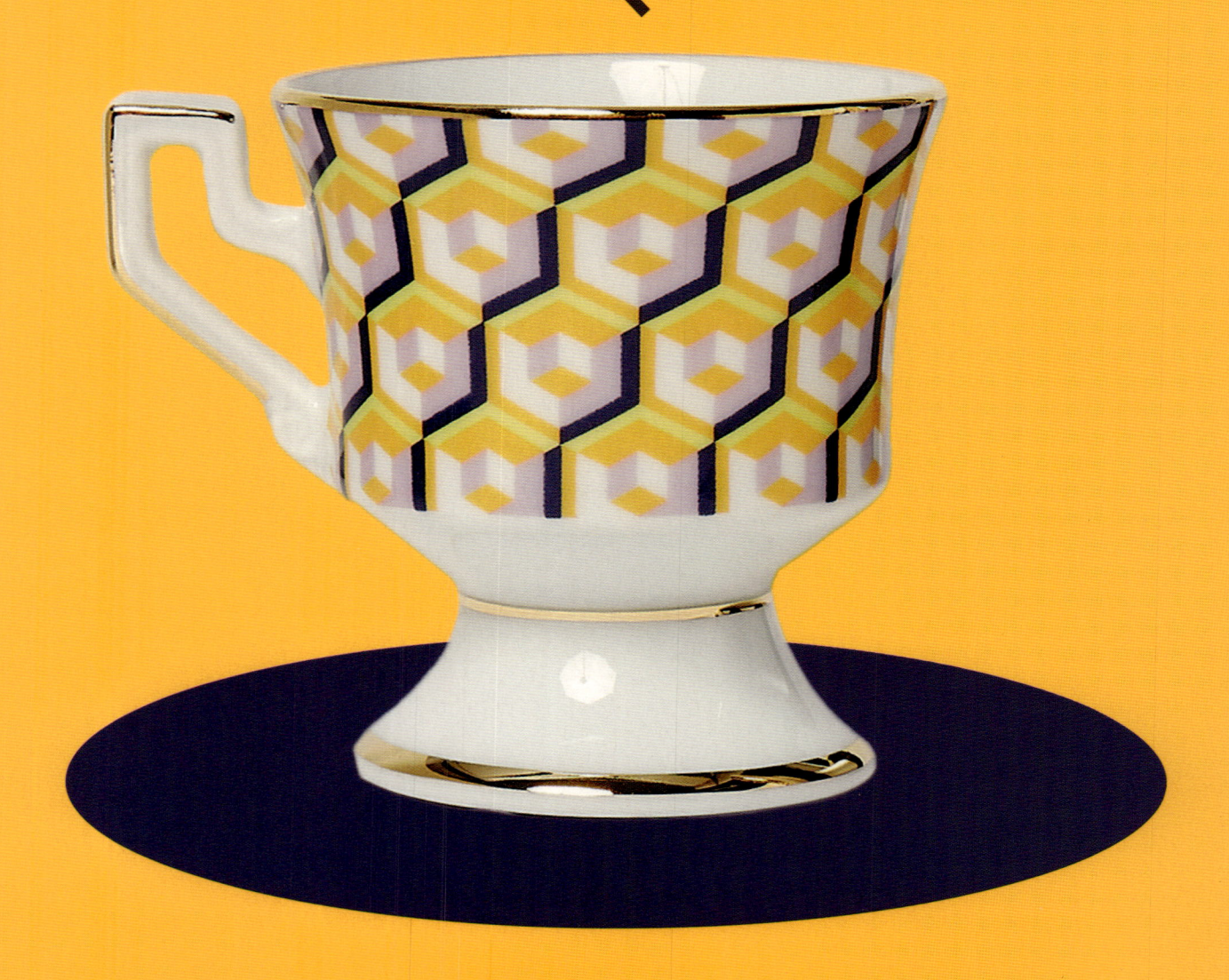

LESSON
3

The right way to order coffee in Italy

32

The Italians drink coffee like a dog laps water—all day long. But Big Coffee doesn't exist. They drink tiny thimblefuls of a rich brown espresso brew (known simply as *un caffè*), sometimes dotted with a macchiato foam. These are most often taken standing up at the bar where, if you're alone, you are expected to converse with the barman or strangers around you. You sit at a table—and pay more for it—only if you want to have an hour of conversation with someone. A cappuccino is a breakfast drink only, and only one can be drunk per day. Do not order a cappuccino after dinner; you will scare the waiter and shame yourself. Milk is full fat and full cow, though recently soy milk has come onto the scene. If you want American-style coffee, you'll have to order a *caffè lungo*, an espresso drowned in water. But don't try to drink it like an American in a to-go cup. Though they started offering them during Covid, no self-respecting Italian would ever be caught walking down the street with their coffee cup.

MAMMA MILANO

BUILDING RELATIONSHIPS, ITALIAN-STYLE

In Italy, where connections are key, I consciously cultivated each one—from butchers and mechanics to high-flying designers and Milan's stylish social gatekeepers

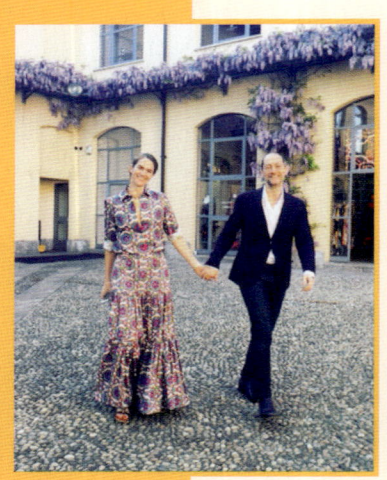

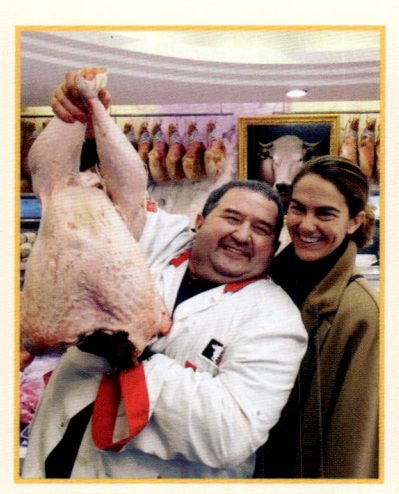

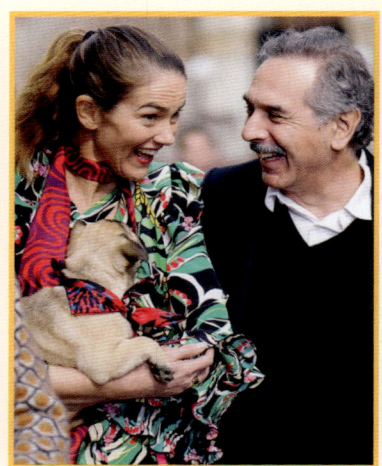

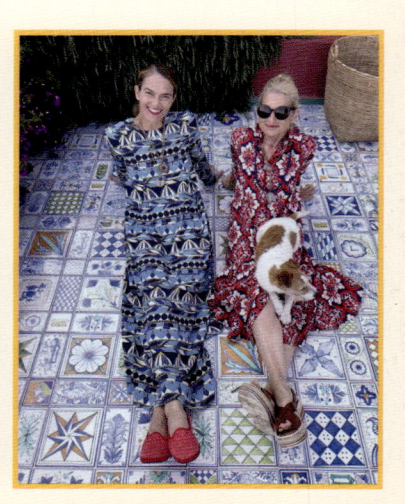

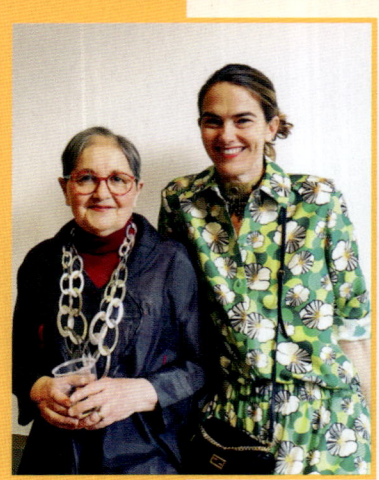

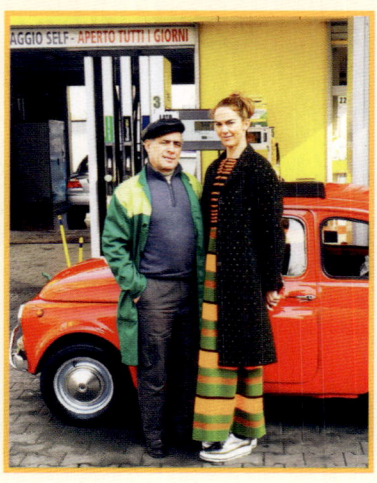

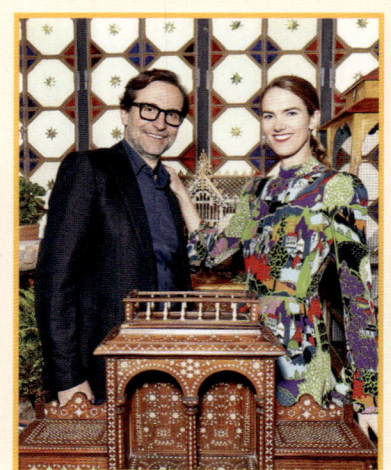

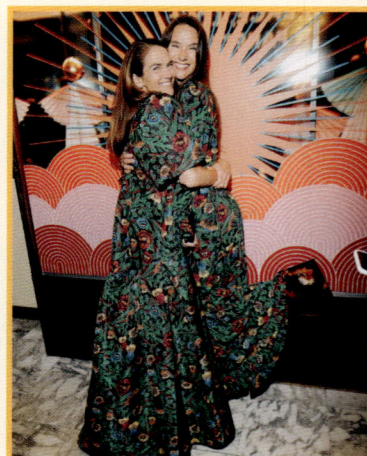

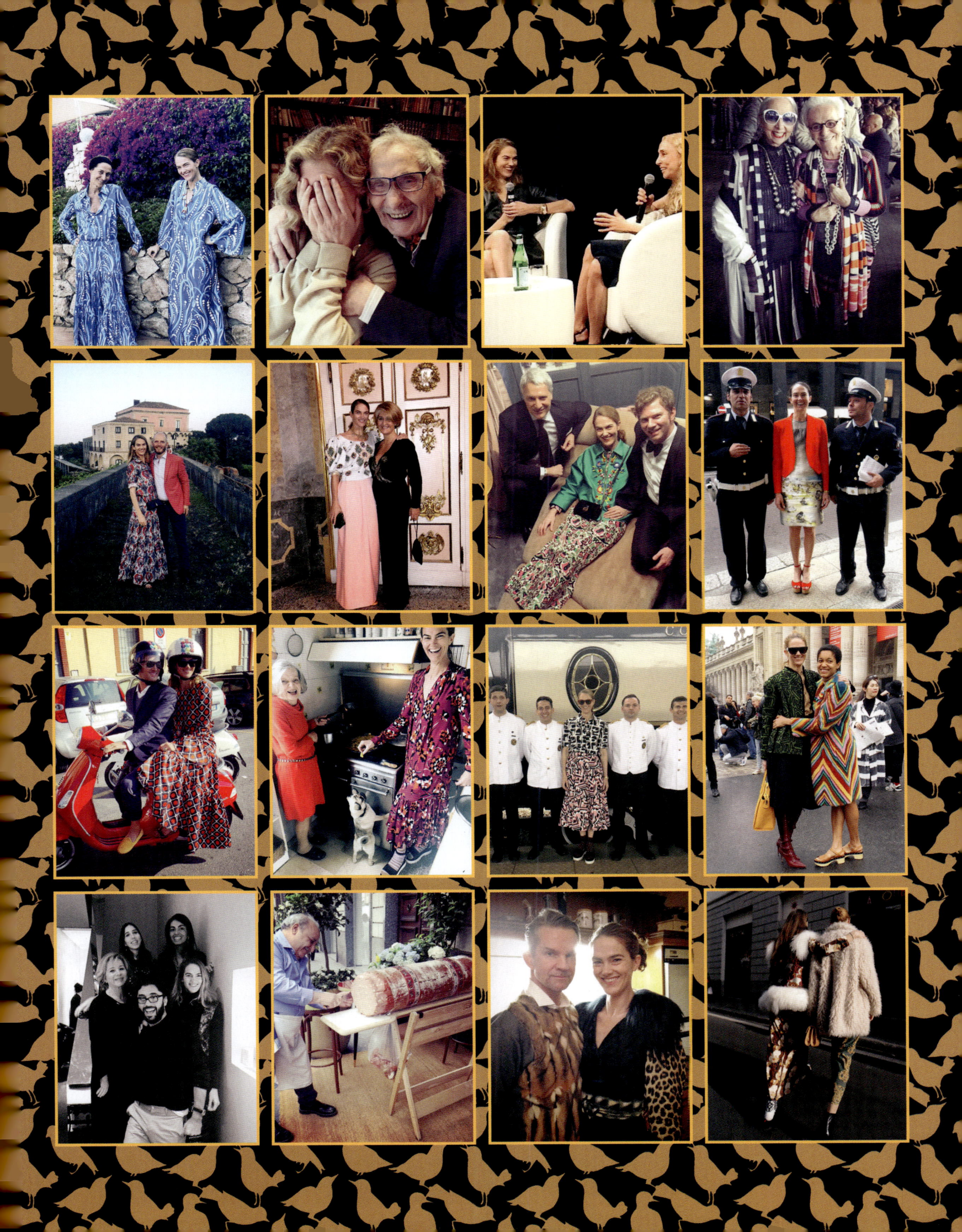

MAMMA MILANO

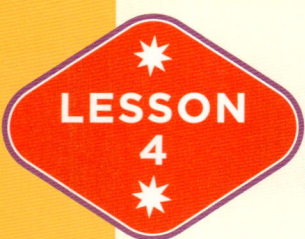

LESSON 4

SHOW YOU REALLY, REALLY CARE

Italians can be dismissive of tourists who blaze through the country's beauty and wonder in a trail of consumption. However, they love it when you value quality and care about what they do. When I first moved to Milan, there was a fabulous *fruttivendolo* (greengrocer) called Faravelli near my home with prized jeweled fruit, who kept giving me sub-par specimens. The fourth time this happened, a surge of anger boomeranged me back to their door. "I am not a tourist!" I protested in my brand-new Italian. "I live around the corner, and you keep giving me the bad stuff! I want the beautiful things you have!"

From that moment on, the fruit people were my friends. If you compliment an Italian and let them know you recognize superior quality, you will always get the best from them—even if you are a visitor. When a director friend of mine, shooting a movie in Rome, told a restaurant owner he was in town for two weeks and wanted to eat there every night, he was immediately embraced like a longtime regular.

LESSON 5

WHATEVER IT IS, DO IT IN PERSON

Italians prefer not to do anything over the phone or email. They ask to meet over coffee, a two-hour lunch—or, even better, in the comfort of their own home, where both parties can sink into the *pesto* sauce and coax the work part out with ease and grace. For years, this drove me nuts. I couldn't believe that the PR woman of that A-list fashion house couldn't give me the answers I wanted RIGHT NOW by phone. I was on a deadline! No, she had to be seated before a starched linen tablecloth for any helpful information to flow.

Once I gave in to this practice, its wisdom became clear. The Italians are not big on action items. The final objective may be an exchange of information or a deal, but it unfolds through having an enjoyable time and making a real connection. And all of that chatting, laughing, and eating cooks up something that we rarely have time to savor in America—a relationship.

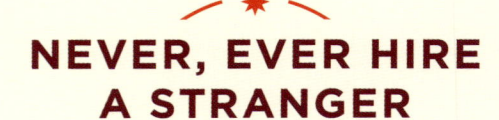

NEVER, EVER HIRE A STRANGER

When the bathtub in our first apartment sprung a leak, I pulled out the dusty yellow pages (this was pre-smartphone) and flipped to the "I" section looking for *idraulico*. After eight tries, I finally found a plumber who understood my bathroom was rapidly filling up like an aquarium and did not put me off to the following week. My great find arrived two hours later, resolved the problem in twenty minutes, then slapped me with a 200-euro bill that I happily paid. When Andrea came home that night, he excoriated me for calling a stranger who had clearly ripped me off. "The yellow pages?!" he exclaimed. "Throw that thing away!"

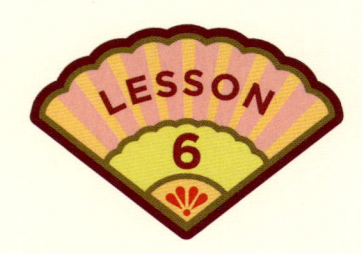

LESSON 6

Italians, I quickly learned, never call strangers. Strangers will probably cheat you. You need a referral, whether it's your carpenter, your hairdresser, your fishmonger, your lawyer, and, above all, your auto-mechanic. Then this person is inextricably bound to give you good service, a great product, and a fair price, otherwise he risks losing favor with the person who referred you, who has undoubtedly done business with him for the last twenty years. That's how it works.

Now my door lady Mariela is my friend and I only ask her who she recommends for any household job. No one ever rips me off and I always get top service. She also makes me the most amazing homemade *lasagna*.

Bonus tip: in Italy, you should always ask for discounts. It's not a sign of stinginess, it's an expression that the seller respects you enough to give you a good price and doesn't think you're dumb enough to accept a bad one. A discount shows that you have moved into "friend" territory. At DoubleJ, we receive special treatment from suppliers and collaborators who are friends, and we in turn always extend discounts to them and our other non-business friends. A friend in Italy always expects a special honorific.

ITALIAN LESSONS

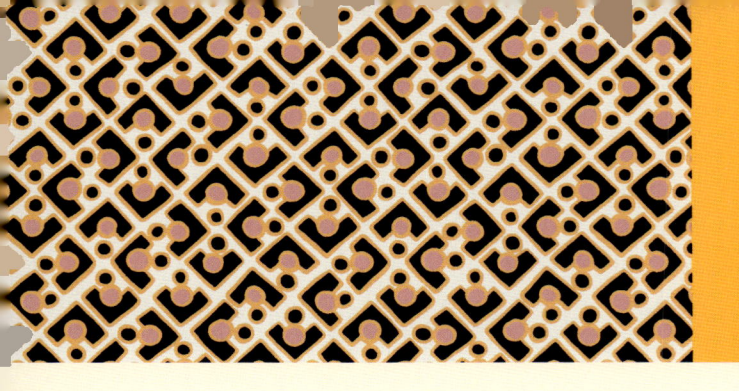

FLIRT WITH THE PLUMBER

LESSON 7

Flirting is now officially illegal in the United States, but it's alive and well in Italy. This is a good thing. I used to roll my eyes at the spellbound looks, piled-on compliments, and spicy chatter that Italian men and women toss at each other. Everyone—from plumbers to doctors, restaurant owners to eighty-year-old doormen—does it. I have had elderly men gaze at me, stop their afternoon stroll in mid-stride, and point their canes and arms to the heavens to proclaim, "MA BELLEZZA!!!" as if thanking God for the vision of beauty before them.

So now I'm a full convert. Flirting in Italy is about noticing and openly appreciating the best qualities of another person—anyone!—in a playful way. It is not about cheating on your partner, and it comes with no strings attached.

"Ninety-nine percent of flirting in America is meant to land you in the bedroom; ninety-nine percent of Italian flirting is not," explained an Italian friend who is a champion flirt, not to mention a happily married father.

Flirting is also an excellent catalyst in business exchanges. This type of banter rarely has anything to do with sex or objectification. Generally, it means being fun and friendly in your dialogue, treating the other person with lightness, appreciation, and affection, and inviting them into your field of positivity, solution, and gratitude. It is not fake niceness; it is genuine and comes from the heart. (Maybe it shouldn't even be called flirting!) It makes everyone's lives better and more fun—and is one of the fine, proven oils that lubricates most Italian relationships.

◦◇• PHRASEBOOK •◇◦

FIGLIO DI: SON OF...

Usage: Who are you related to that you got this job?!

When I dropped my bright and shiny journalism career for the slippery black hole of entrepreneurial life, my Italian friends looked at me like I was nuts. Why would I give up all of those hard-won relationships to move into an untested, friendless space? Besides, I was not a Figlia di Qualcuno Importante: the daughter of someone important (who could help me in this new business). The idea of being a figlio/a di in Italy is still a strong one. Many Italians feel that they have less social and professional mobility if they are born outside of certain circles, important families or classes, and that there is less opportunity for outsiders. As an American, I never had that inhibition. I was brought up in a country that says we can do anything we set our mind to, so I went into my new business enterprise with both trust and naivete.

I do believe a lot of my success has to do with the fact that I was not pre-programmed with fear and inhibition about where I do or don't belong. I love to lather some of this can-do "American-ness" on young Italians when they feel they don't have the power to motorize their own ascent—of course you do, go for it!

HIT THE JACK

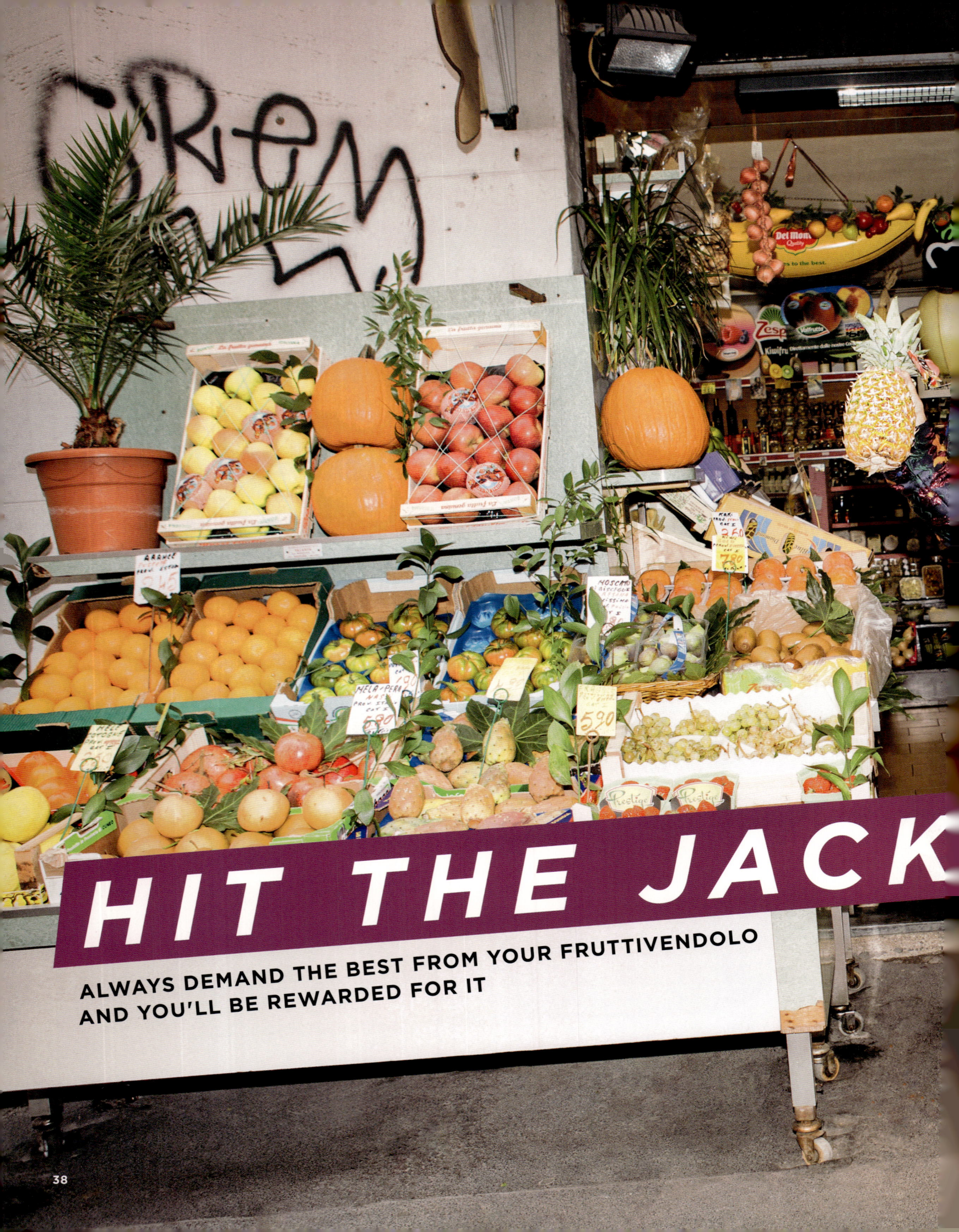

ALWAYS DEMAND THE BEST FROM YOUR FRUTTIVENDOLO
AND YOU'LL BE REWARDED FOR IT

OT!

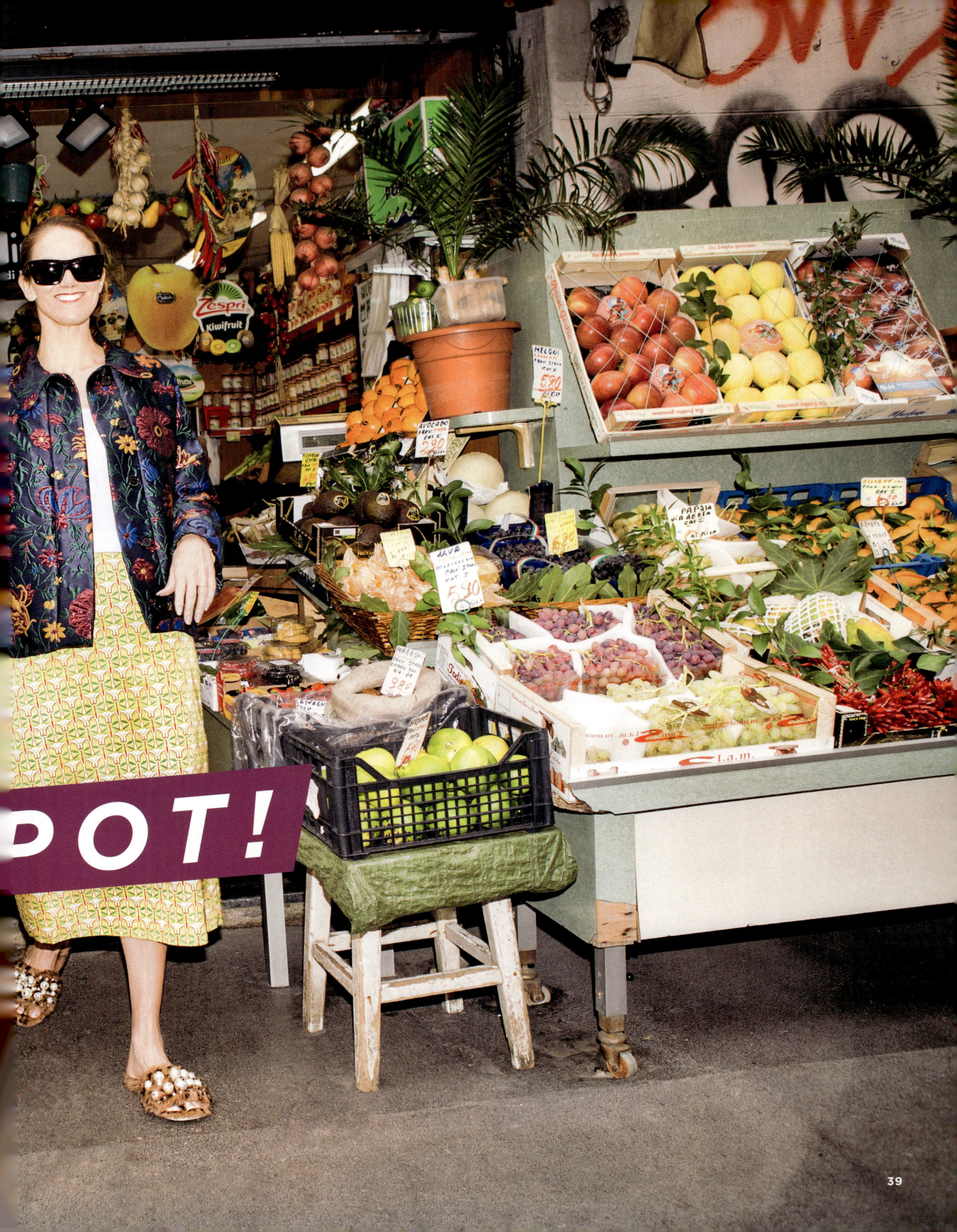

39

MAMMA MILANO

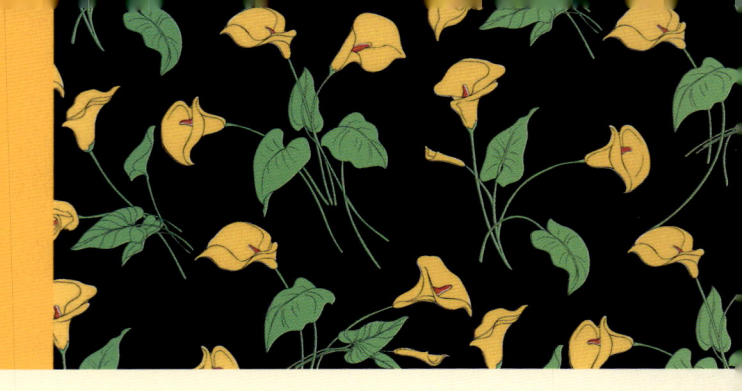

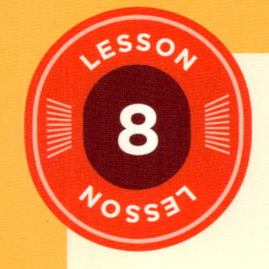

LESSON 8

DROP KINDNESS BOMBS

As I have mentioned, during my early days in Milan, I spent an inordinate amount of time at the bank. I'd be parked in a non-moving line, as the on-duty tellers smiled and chatted sympathetically with their clients, oblivious to the thirty-three people waiting behind them. No one else but me seemed to be ruffled by the inefficiency. Good customer service in Italy means taking care of the person in front of you, and never worrying about the impatient ones behind them. Once I realized this, I marveled at the old-world elegance of this errand: the teller could have been writing in his ledger with an ink quill, it took so long.

One time, finally arriving at the window, I murmured to the young banker that in America I could've just slipped my check into an ATM rather than wait to deal with him. He looked up with an open face, his wide-knotted orange tie brilliant against a sky-blue jacquard shirt, and smiled: "But then we wouldn't get to know you." Then he asked if I was American or English, and launched into a story about his recent trip to London. Just then, a little old lady in a round tweed coat and square-heeled lace-ups approached the teller next to mine and handed over a rumpled brown bag full of fresh oranges. "To juice," she announced, before waddling off.

MAKE A FRIEND IN ITALY AND YOU'VE MADE A FRIEND FOR LIFE

Care about people and they will care for you. Real friendships with people you choose to create your life around take more time to develop in Italy than they do in America. But once you've moved past cocktail banter, been to their house or them to yours, you will be astounded by an Italian friend's devotion. I have maintained many of my closest Italian friends since the beginning.

Italian friends came to my rescue when I had business troubles, and sent medicine to my home when I was sick. They will make a call any time of day or night to connect me with their network of allies and helpers, and, above all, make introductions to other friends of theirs.

They are also outstandingly generous—inviting your out-of-town friends or family who they don't even know to their home for a meal, or inviting you to their home on vacation. I've been everywhere from Capri, Palermo, and Puglia to Portofino, Como, and Tuscany with people I did not know well. I have even been handed the keys to empty vacation homes. When an Italian says you should come visit them at their house by the seaside, they're not just being nice (and insincere) like a New Yorker. They mean it.

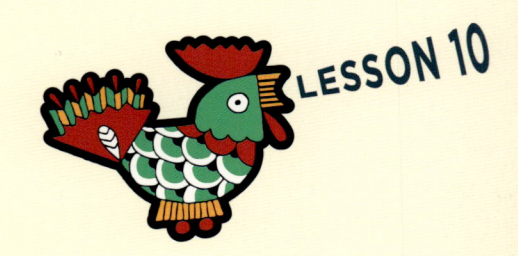

LESSON 10

ABOVE ALL, TREAT LIFE LIKE SHE'S YOUR BEST FRIEND

"I've always thought of life as my best friend. And just like my best friend, sometimes life disappointments me. But I still love her." So said my friend Claudio, a perennially sunny Italian PR for Tod's, who I was sitting with at a fashion-week dinner in Villa Necchi several years back. He continued: "And so I ask myself: what is life trying to tell me? What can I learn? *La vita* is upset with something and is trying to communicate with me. So I listen to her. And I ask, what have I not given you? What do you need from me?"

This outlook is so Italian, so kind and so wise. It can be instinctive to lash out when a friend, or life, disappoints us. For so long, I was screaming at Italy for not giving me ease, functionality, or speed—not to mention take-out food, air conditioning, yoga classes, or a working ATM machine. When I finally caved in to her unpredictability, I realized she was functioning on a totally different operating platform. I was being flooded with abundance, but I just didn't see it. What happens when you turn it around and ask how you can be of service to a friend, and to the flow of life?

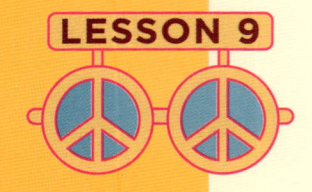

LESSON 9

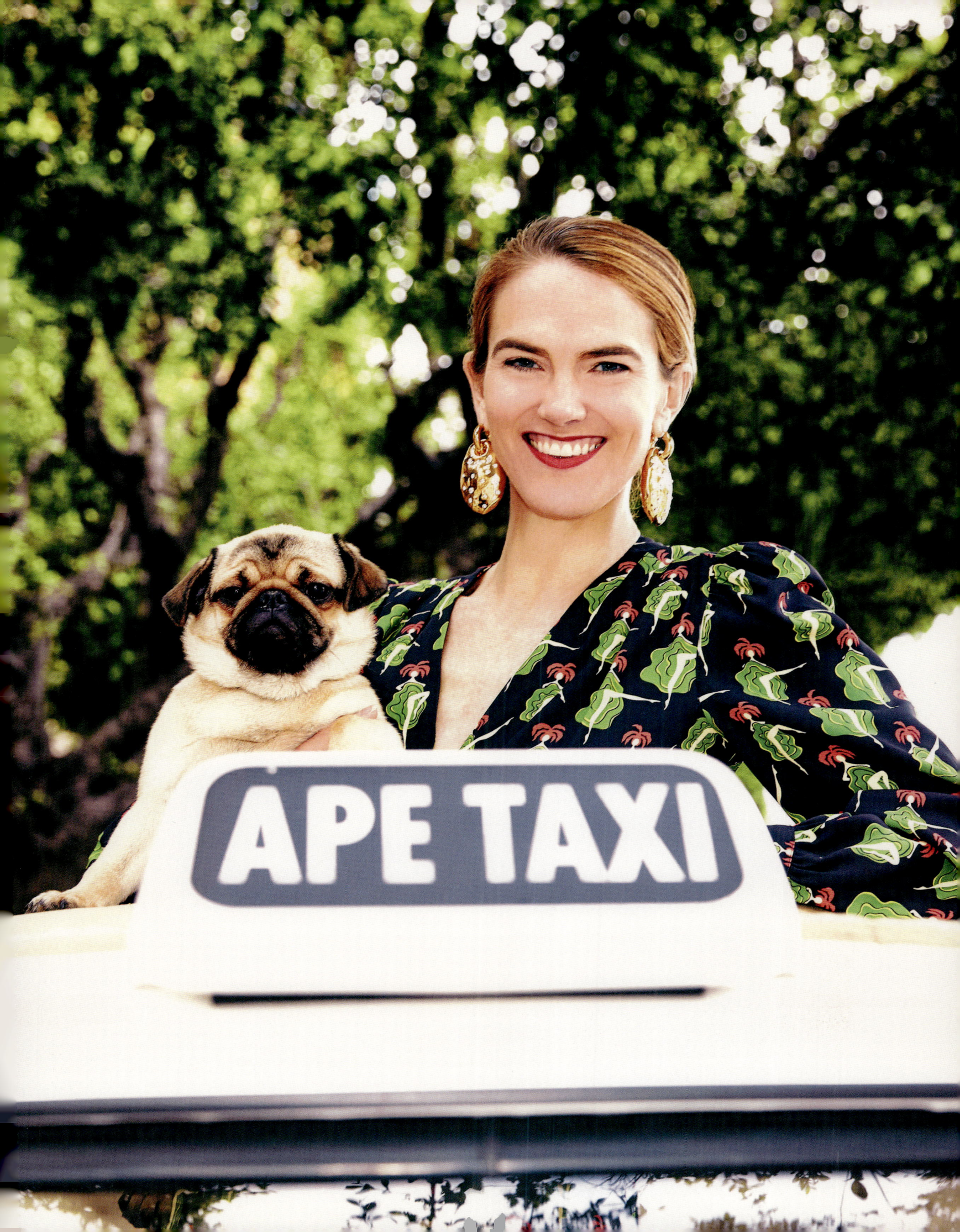

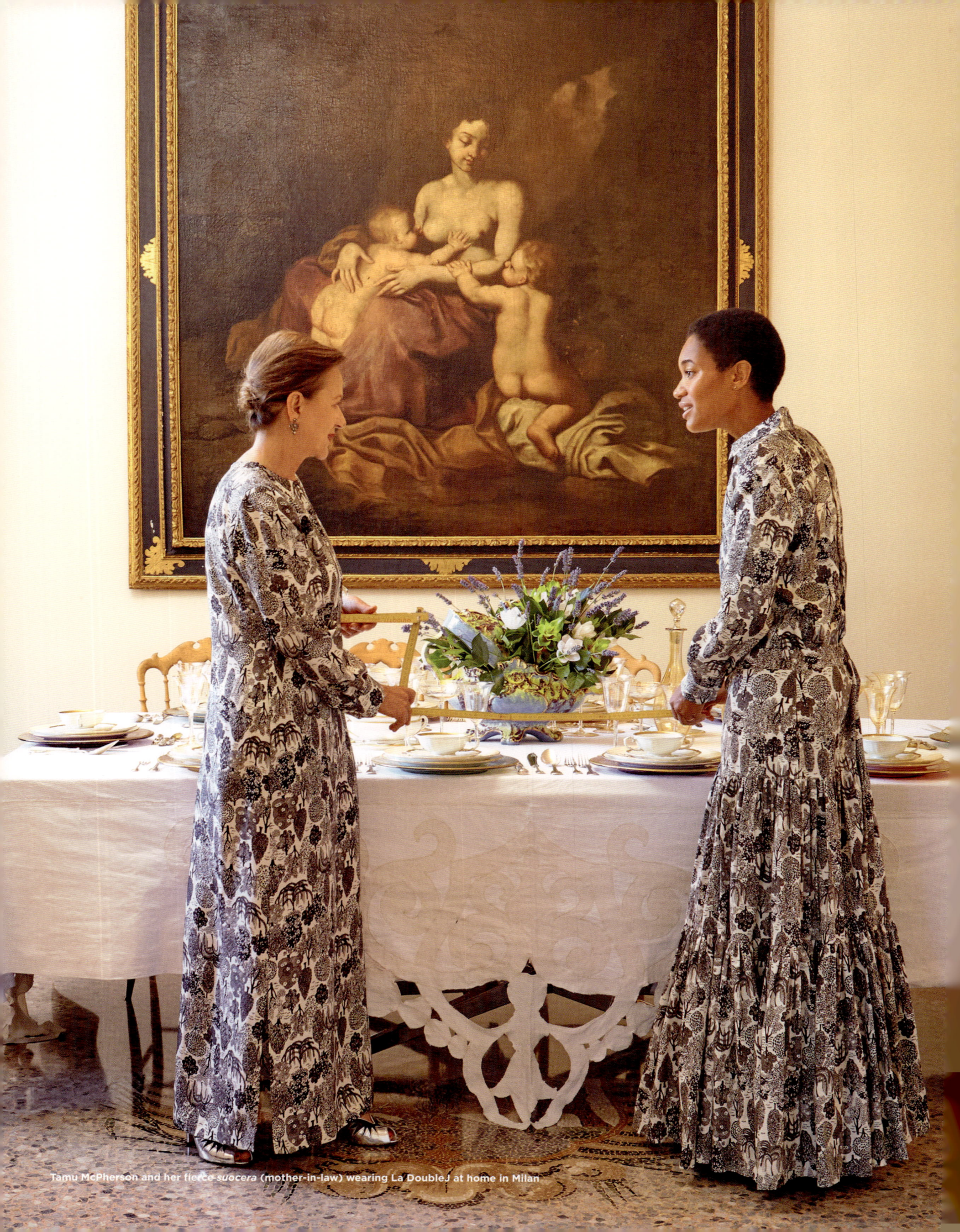

Tamu McPherson and her *fierce suocera* (mother-in-law) wearing La DoubleJ at home in Milan

ITALIAN LESSONS

THE MAGNIFICENT, MAGNETIC, GROUNDING FORCE OF THE ITALIAN MOTHER

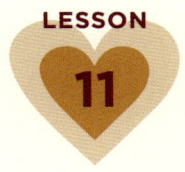

LESSON 11

If relationships are what grease the entire magical Italian operation, and if Italians learn this art of connection and glue inside their own family unit, then the big boss of that love empire is the Italian mother herself.

The mother's role in Italy is paramount. Mothers are the stars around which all Italians circle: a goddess, a captain, a boss, a bosom, and an all-powerful magnetic pull back to the home. This role is honored across all social classes in Italy. It is, no doubt, the force that underlies the Italians' orientation towards clannish loyalty and their endemic sense of tenderness, love, play, and mercy—all key attributes of divine feminine energy, which Italy is swimming in.

I used to laugh when landing at an airport and every passenger's cell phone sprung to life: *"Ciao Mamma!"* everyone would exclaim in unison, assuring their mother of their safe arrival while also confirming their presence at next Sunday's three-hour lunch. I wondered why these mothers weren't kicking their kids out of the house at age eighteen like mine did, why they were happily harboring forty-year-olds (like my future brother-in-law) in their childhood bedrooms—and complaining that people weren't eating enough or they never saw their children enough (only once a week in the flesh!).

Now I revel in the Italian mother's central role. I see how powerful her force actually is. This feminine energetic anchors the family down around a table, a hearth, or a home. She often has a simple message: more food, more family time. But she also typically provides safety, nurture, and nourishment. She is revered for this, even if Italians can be outwardly dismissive of their mothers when they are being offered their fifth helping of homemade *tagliatelle*. But the connection is undeniable. And so is the love.

As a result, I've observed that the Italians carry less obvious emotional baggage than Americans do. You rarely see or hear an Italian blaming their parents for their fucked-up life or wounded psyche. There is little absent parent syndrome, because their parents can't wait to have them over to eat.

More importantly, the mothers in Italy instill a basic tenet of Divine Mother energy: acceptance. From the moment children arrive, they are screaming, laughing, running wild under dinner tables and across hotel lobbies, and turning the house upside down. Early on, I found my face turning purple as I watched Italian parents doing nothing as their children wreaked vocal and visual havoc in public settings.

But marinating in these juices for several years tenderized my eyes. I saw that the Italians are the most tolerant human beings I've ever encountered, at ease with themselves and accepting of others. I came to see this as a trait that could be traced back out to the gentle arms in which they were raised.

LESSON 12

CHE CASINO!

You'll need a huge, tender heart to laugh at life and thrive amidst the chaos

Have you ever driven on an Italian autostrada? Apart from the Autogrill—the freeway fast-food chain that sells finely aged *parmigiano*, glistening legs of salt-cured *prosciutto*, and bottles of red wine—there is absolutely nothing functional about it. It's a miracle if you can even get on the right one; the signs give you towns accompanied by two arrows pointing in completely opposite directions. Bologna to the right. Or to the left. The choice is yours. Once you're on the roaring road where speeding cars come up behind you like schoolyard bullies, just try to get off it again. The exit sign flashes a totem pole of fourteen different towns whose names are impossible to read at 120 km per hour.

It is no better when an Italian gives you verbal directions on how to get to their home. "Go towards the water and after a few hundred meters, turn right at the big tree," is as precise a route as you can hope to receive. Everything in Italy is approximate, indefinite, subjective. Consequently, Italians allow for error—within themselves and others. They won't blast you on the facts, act as sticklers for rules, nor insist that their way is the right way.

Efficiency—more action, bigger and better results in less time—may be paramount in America, but it is not so prized in Italy. The journey—no matter where it goes and how long it takes you—is much more important than the arrival. Italians, therefore, are both zealously impassioned and rigorously laid-back. They are creatively heroic yet organizationally doomed.

When I arrived in 2001, I was bound by an alternative universe known as LET'S GET IT DONE. Mamma Milano's ancient buildings, ornate interiors, and soaring churches may have tried to bewitch me, but I spent my first years in Milan ruminating on why the bank lines were endless, train schedules ignored, and stores closed. Why couldn't I find good avocados, a great mani-pedi, cilantro, or a single coffee in a large to-go cup? Where the fuck to buy a hairdryer? A warrior at heart, I was first in line to combat all of Italy's inefficiencies, galloping ahead and swinging a two-ton sword. This made me even angrier, not to mention anxious, scared, and emotionally lost, while I circled around myself as if on an endless autostrada, never reaching my destination.

It soon became blindingly clear that Italy and its people possessed everything that I did not: incredible patience, boundless forgiveness, and supreme flexibility. Once I stopped criticizing the Italians, I started marveling at them.

◦◊◦ PHRASEBOOK ◦◊◦

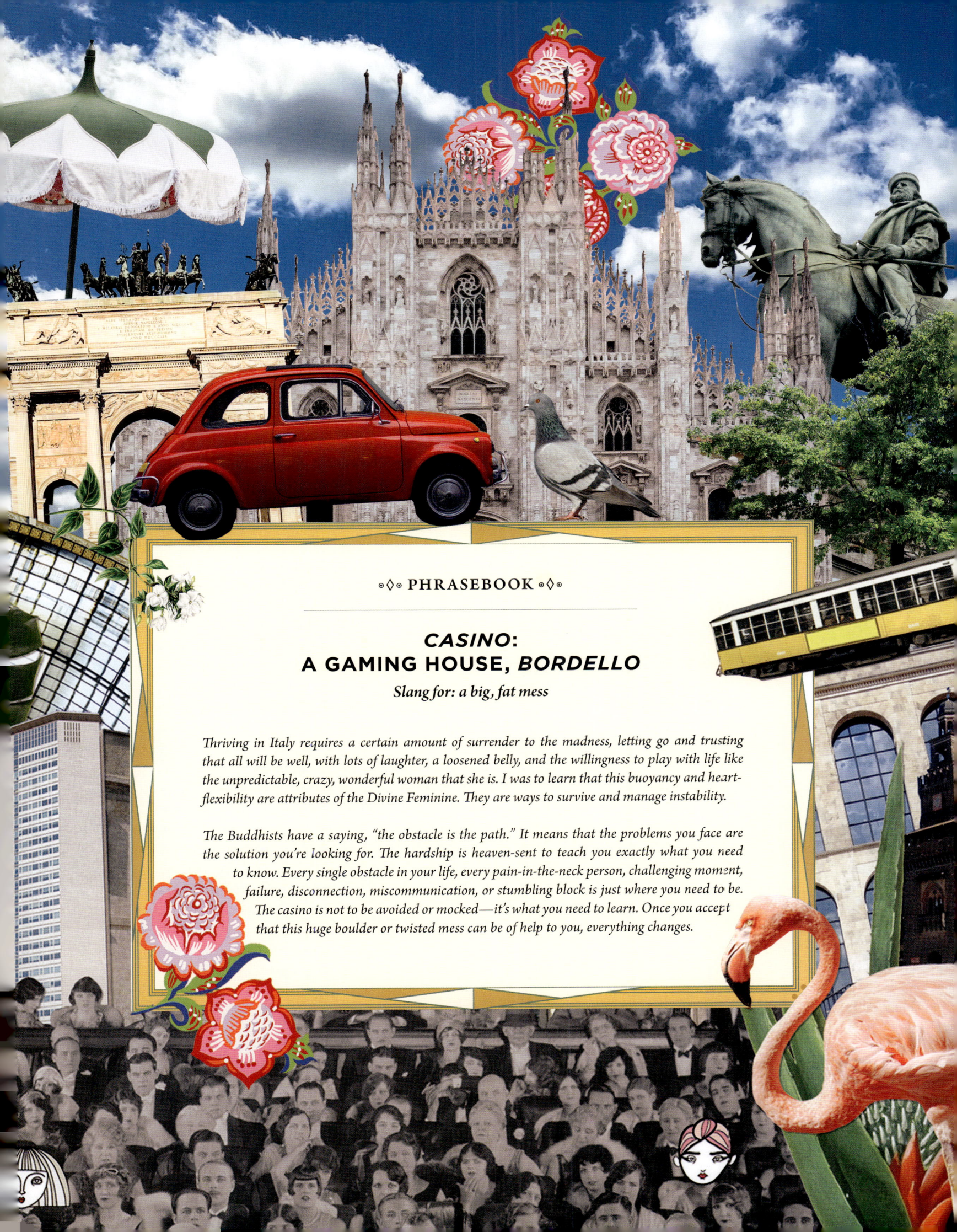

CASINO: A GAMING HOUSE, *BORDELLO*

Slang for: a big, fat mess

Thriving in Italy requires a certain amount of surrender to the madness, letting go and trusting that all will be well, with lots of laughter, a loosened belly, and the willingness to play with life like the unpredictable, crazy, wonderful woman that she is. I was to learn that this buoyancy and heart-flexibility are attributes of the Divine Feminine. They are ways to survive and manage instability.

The Buddhists have a saying, "the obstacle is the path." It means that the problems you face are the solution you're looking for. The hardship is heaven-sent to teach you exactly what you need to know. Every single obstacle in your life, every pain-in-the-neck person, challenging moment, failure, disconnection, miscommunication, or stumbling block is just where you need to be. The casino is not to be avoided or mocked—it's what you need to learn. Once you accept that this huge boulder or twisted mess can be of help to you, everything changes.

LESSON 13
KEEPING MY COOL ON TRENITALIA

One day many summers ago, I boarded a train in sweltering mid-July heat to go to Portofino on the Ligurian coast, only to discover that, for the fifth weekend in a row, the air conditioning was broken onboard.

I exploded with a sense of civic duty. "This is NOT a third-world country!" I shouted at the top of my lungs, hoping to start a mini-revolution, or at least snap my Italian seatmates out of their sweaty complacency. "We paid 200 euro in first class for this miserable trip! I will not be treated like cattle! This is unacceptable. Let's go find the captain and demand our money back!" The Italians looked at me, the unhinged American, with a mixture of bemusement and pity. There was no judgment at all.

Of course, my hollering got me nowhere. Not on that day when I could not galvanize a revolt onboard Trenitalia, nor any day thereafter. My complaining only served to alienate me from my host country, from its sweet-tempered citizens, and most of all from myself. It had wrapped me in a hot, scratchy, wool blanket of negativity, where I twitched and itched for years.

I watched my fellow passengers accept the unfortunate situation with grace. They embraced it as they would a wailing child: "There's nothing to be done," whispered the spirit of Mamma Milano in my ear. So, I focused on the one single mantra that truly mattered at that moment: "Thank God for Portofino." Beauty and tranquility are never far off.

"There's nothing to be done," whispered the spirit of Mamma Milano in my ear

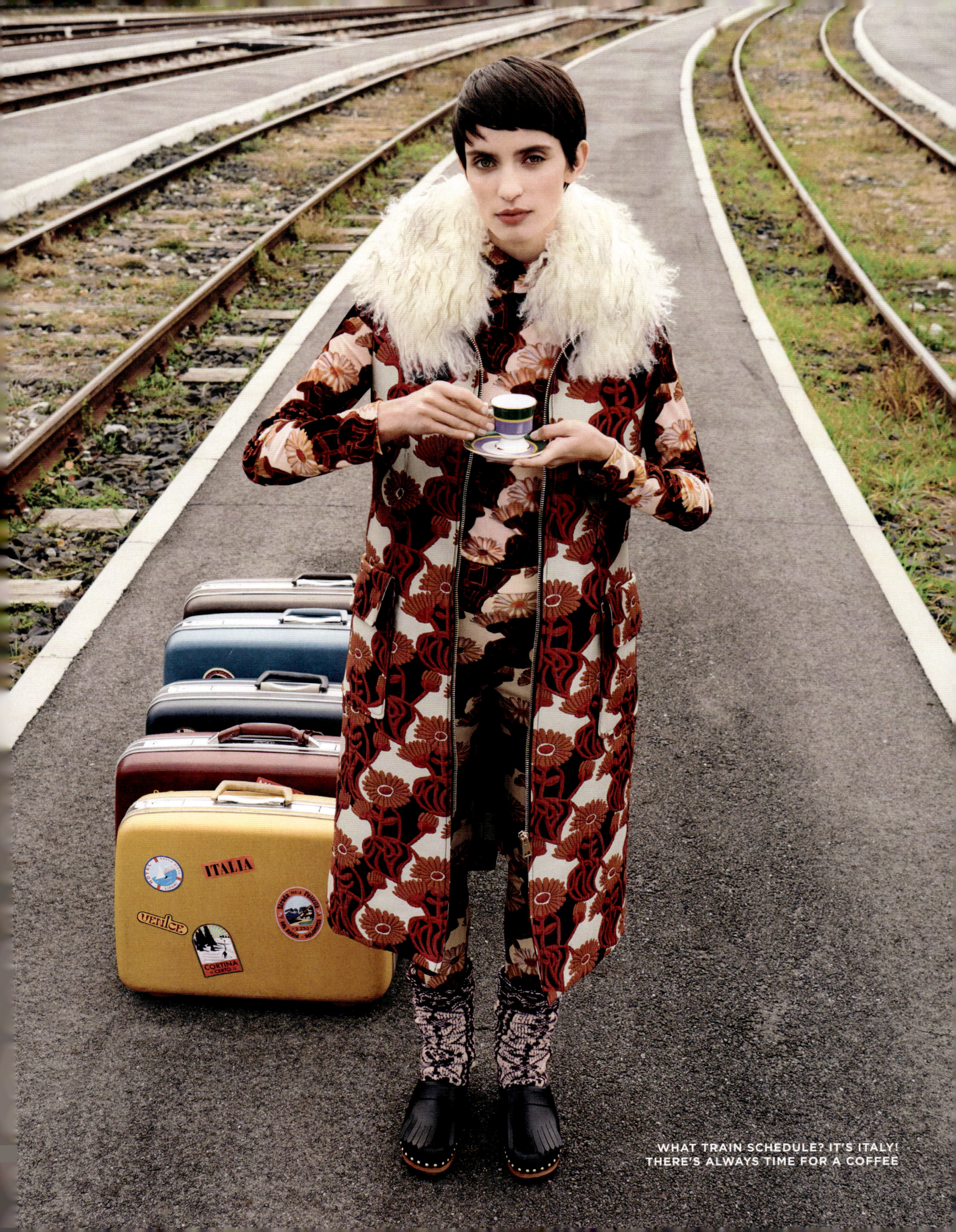

WHAT TRAIN SCHEDULE? IT'S ITALY! THERE'S ALWAYS TIME FOR A COFFEE

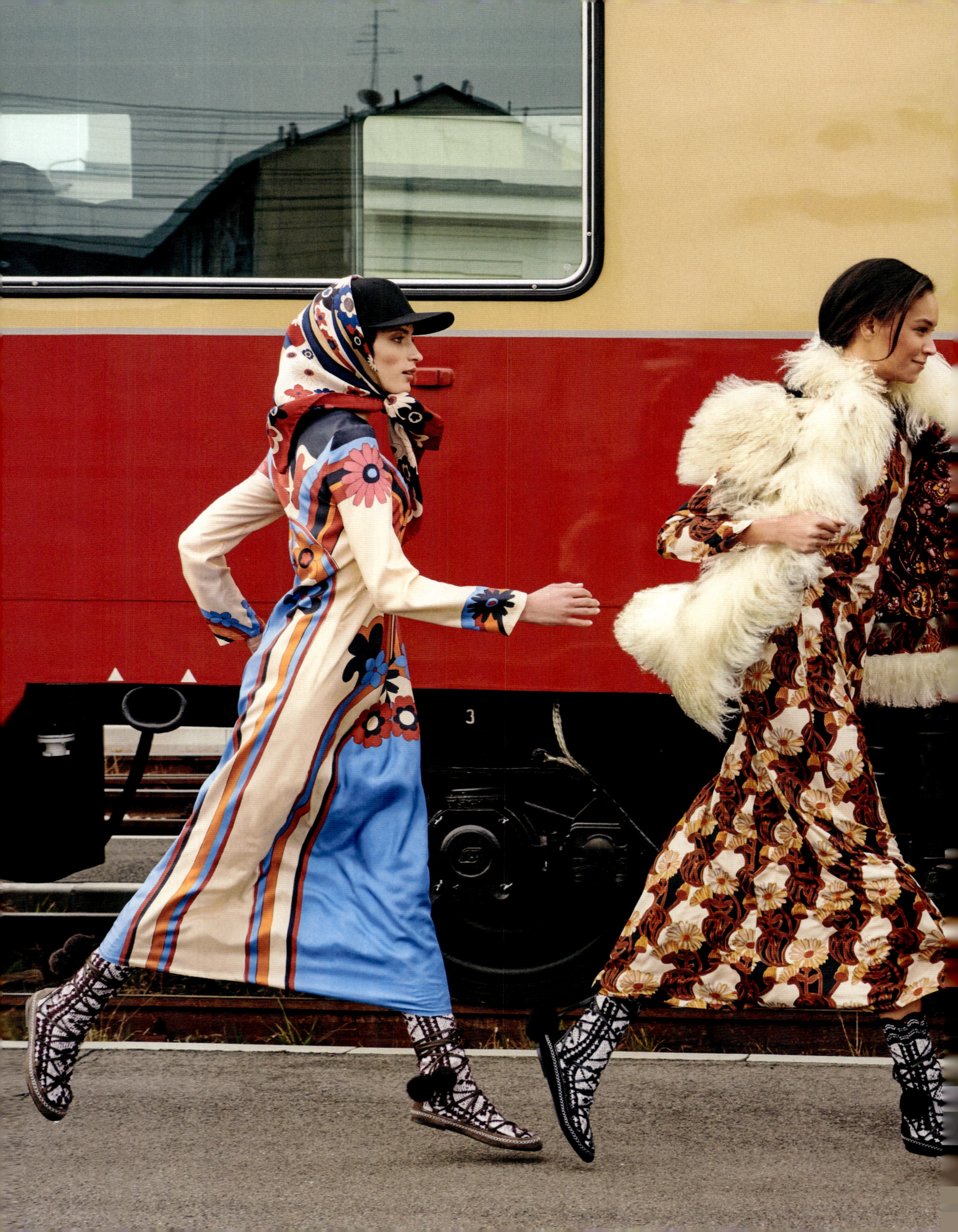

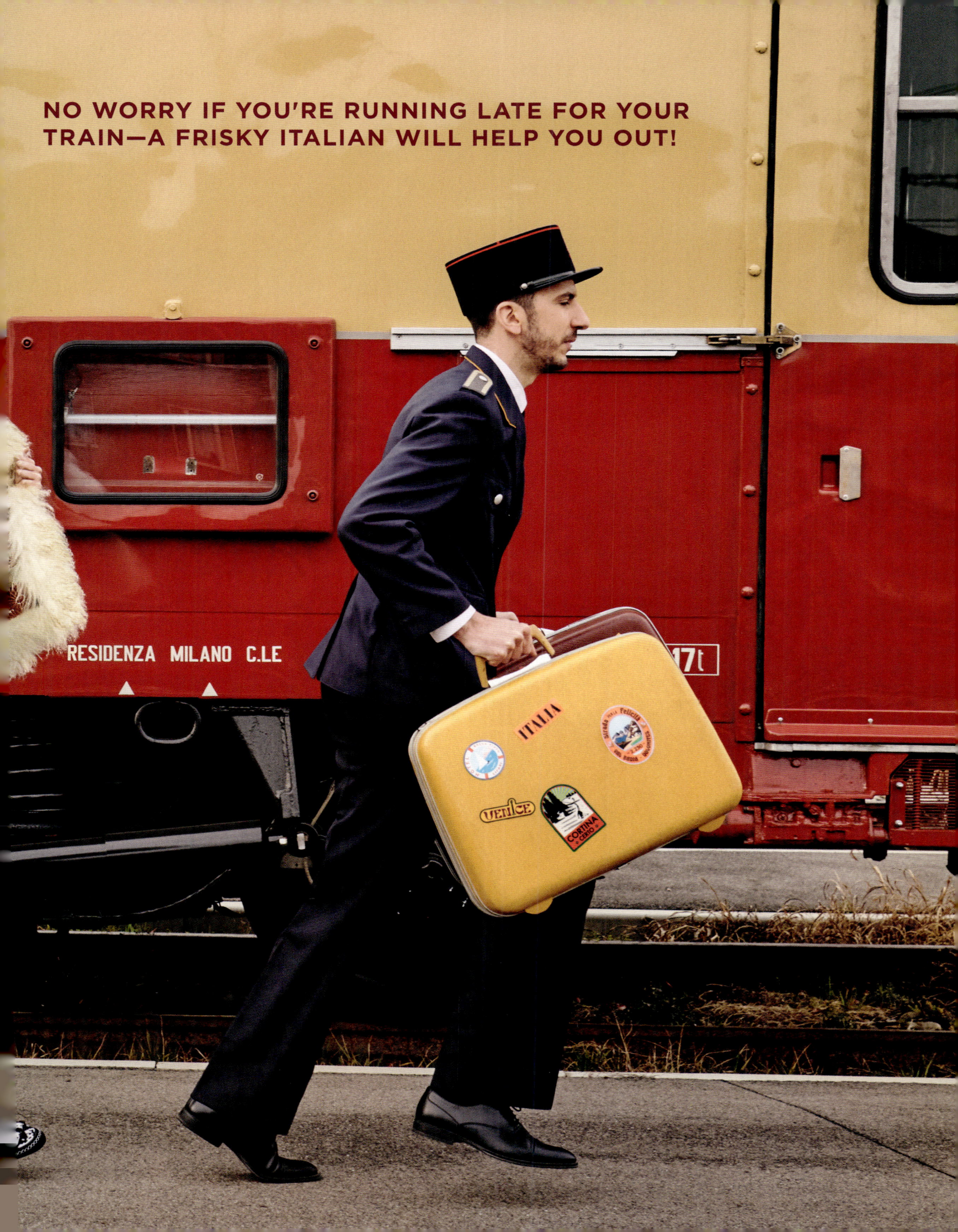

NO WORRY IF YOU'RE RUNNING LATE FOR YOUR TRAIN—A FRISKY ITALIAN WILL HELP YOU OUT!

YOU ARE NOW ENTERING THE HEARTLAND

As a newcomer in Milan, I needed to learn how to relax. I also needed to learn flexibility, patience, and presence, and the ability to laugh off frustration and shake off anger. These are Italian superpowers that come from inflating the heart and using it as a life raft to bounce along life's chaotic waters. Here are the lessons that helped me…

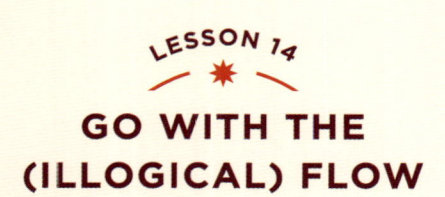

LESSON 14

GO WITH THE (ILLOGICAL) FLOW

Transportation of every kind truly is a metaphor for Italy's disorder and illogic. In Milan's city center, cars swim like fish across the roads. During fashion week, our *Bazaar* fashion team had a driver from Naples who we nicknamed "Foxy." He wore a winter overcoat with a huge fox collar. If we were late to an Armani or Ferragamo show, he would ignore the rules and confidently drive down the streets backwards.

In Milan, you will often find cars double-parked, with their hazard lights flashing, as if to say, *Hey, I'll be back in five minutes—I'm just getting a gelato with my kid.*

The Italians ski in the same way that they drive or park. There are no organized lines in front of the lifts; everyone just packs into the funnel like happy cattle. That's what happens in disorder: a lot of socializing and kindness. Smiles not shouts. If I walk inadvertently in a bike lane, I hear someone's charming, twinkly bike bell behind me rather than an avalanche of cursing, as in America.

There are many routes to get to where you want to go, but some are slower than others. Eventually, you will get there. This looseness permeates all aspects of Italian life, not just their freeways and their sense of direction. An inner softening makes the journey much easier.

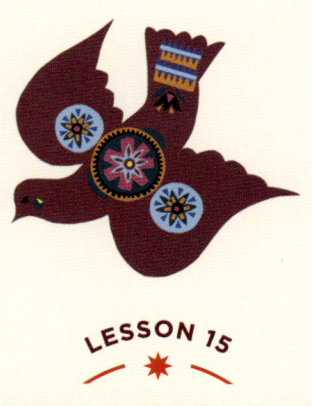

LESSON 15

SPONTANEITY IS THE SPECIAL SAUCE OF LIFE

Italians hate planning. If you invite them to a dinner three weeks ahead, they'll look puzzled and say, "I have no idea what I'm doing or where I'll be in three weeks."

What they don't say is that they have no idea how they will *feel* in three weeks. They love an unexpected invitation a couple of days prior to any event. They know how they're feeling and if they're up for it. This doesn't stress them out; it excites them. *Look what life has magically delivered!* Even exotic vacations are planned within days or hours of departure. (I was still getting RSVPs to my wedding a week before—which was fine, since the Italian wedding planner understood that no one could possibly know how they would be feeling before that.)

I've now sided with the Italians. Too much planning can stifle the magic of a moment; you miss the mysterious sauce of life that wants to swirl around you and carry you off to unexpected happiness—if you are open to it.

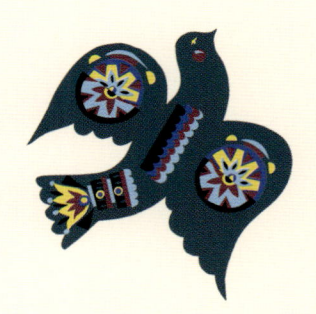

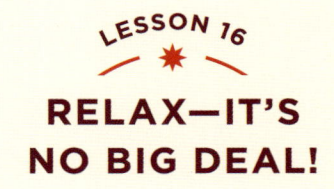

LESSON 16

RELAX—IT'S NO BIG DEAL!

When I first arrived and was mangling the language at every turn, I was never met with the judgment I got in France during my university study year abroad. Instead, I was offered enthusiasm for even trying to speak the language: "*Piano, piano,*" they would tell me whenever I slapped my own wrist for not being better. Slowly, slowly. Take it easy. There's no rush.

Italian tenderness is so beautiful it breaks my heart. (This patience is also the underlying principle for any deep, mysterious spiritual practice to flow forth. The Italians just happen to do it naturally.) Just like a blindly loving mother, Italians are tolerant of children running wild at dinner parties, restaurants, and hotel lobbies, causing a *casino* wherever they go. They are truly loved, indulged, and given free rein to play.

Italians are also very indulgent of animals. Your dog can go anywhere with you, except for a museum or a large supermarket. My dog Pepper is welcome at the dentist and the accountant, virtually every restaurant, and even at the Prada boutique, where she is fed a bone and given her own bowl of water. Animals make Italians happy, and whatever makes this nation happy becomes a prize to covet and coddle.

For such a Catholic country—more than three quarters of citizens identify that way—the majority of Italians don't moralize or get on their high horse about right and wrong. They never verbally massacre each other over politics, abortion, or vaccines. America had some pretty charged political moments after 9/11 and through the Trump presidency, and I never once heard an Italian berate me about it. They looked genuinely perplexed and then wanted to have a friendly debate.

This mood of tolerance is everywhere. After all, half of Italy's couples pop out kids without being married, grandmas sit back on Sundays taking in the view of the topless women on the beach, and children and pregnant women are regularly offered wine with dinner.

I once admitted to an Italian doctor that I smoked. "How much per day?" he asked. "Three a day," I replied, embarrassed and ready for a big fat moralistic slap on the face. "Packs?" he asked, not lifting his eyes from his paper. "Uh, no. Individual cigarettes." "Oh, come on," he said, putting the cap back on his pen and waving his arm in the air. "That's no big deal. Don't worry about it."

Italians are big on personal freedom. What you do (within reasonable limits) is your choice. They don't have a sense of retribution and punishment or try to put you in your place. Italians are easy on others, and most of all, they are easy on themselves. This allows the heart to stay open so that everyone can sit down to properly enjoy a plate of pasta together.

MAMMA MILANO

◦◊◦ PHRASEBOOK ◦◊◦

PIANO, PIANO: SLOWLY, GENTLY, CAREFULLY, GRADUALLY, LEISURELY

*In other words: chill the *F* out*

Italians are not critical of slow-moving enterprises or efforts. This means they are often late for appointments or dinner—it's all good. Also, it's no big deal if you're an occasional slacker, if you don't exercise, or if you stop working because it interferes with your well-being. They are preternaturally at peace with themselves and others.

◦◦◊◦◦

NON SI PUÒ: IT IS NOT DONE

Accompained with wagging index finger and a tongue cluck from a pouty mouth

Although extraordinarily liberal most of the time, Italians are ridiculously rigid when it comes to form and style. There are some no-nos that I tripped over. When swimming: never sit around in a wet swimsuit, or you'll get stomach pain. And don't swim after lunch. When eating: never sprinkle parmesan on a seafood pasta or put different foods on the same plate. And never, ever walk around barefoot (never, ever).
Of course, I still do most of these.

LESSON 17
EMOTE ENDLESSLY

The Italian talent for argument is a built-in trait, a national source of pride. If the conversation doesn't get heated over dinner, it's the fallen soufflé of all evenings: a total downer. Mad hysteria and red-faced screaming are effortlessly followed by a calm double-kiss and a civilized sit-down lunch, where talk turns to the vintage of the wine, the ricŸess of the broth, the vision of this weekend's sapphire water bath in Capri. Everything is fine.

The first time I witnessed this, I was working at Costume National. The CEO, Carlo Capasa, started shouting at the sky, unleashing a torrent of feelings about a business deal all over the conference room table. I was shaking in my shoes. I thought we were going to get fired. I was also a bit offended. But as soon as his eruption ended, he shook off the lava rocks, smiled, and said, "Let's go get lunch, guys!" in a genuinely friendly tone. We all walked out of the office and sat down to a two-course meal without a trace of negativity soiling the starched white tablecloths.

The fire of the Italian heart is strong and free, bubbling up in equal measures from excitement, sadness, joy, or rage, and everything is allowed. They wear their big noisy emotions on their beautiful silk sleeves. Grown, heterosexual men hug closely and kiss each other warmly on the cheeks. They cry during soccer matches. Romantic love is screamed from the roofs and written in graffiti. Couples of all ages unself-consiously make out in public. Grandmothers nod in approval when they see love in action, and open their soft arms when anyone is upset or in pain.

I've seen people scream on the street, in restaurants, and in offices. It's totally normal. What's not normal is holding a grudge about it.

Italians are fantastic at this heart elasticity. I began to wonder why I couldn't express the same degree of feeling—or come down from it quickly. I was judging myself for even *having* the emotion. If you do it like an Italian, you just let the feeling spew forth like a geyser, without any judgment or self-awareness. This was a huge lesson in letting emotions burst and glide, rather than clamp or cling. Imagine if the whole world recuperated and reconciled this fast, too?

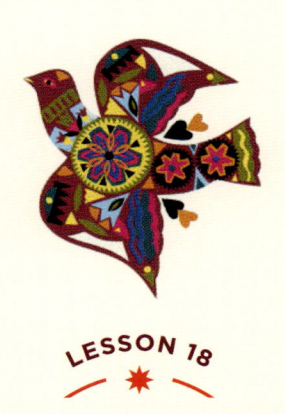

LESSON 18
...AND LAUGH ABOUT IT

Laughter is the sound of the heart. The Italians, you won't be surprised to learn, laugh frequently. When the metro breaks down, when they get utterly lost, when their kid knocks over the waiter's tray, they don't turn to stone or lash out. They let laugher pour out of their bellies, turning life's tragedies into comedies.

LESSON 19
PLAY YOUR PANTS OFF

For many years, I spent the weekends in my husband's hometown of Pesaro. Here, the Italians spend their summer in the knee-deep, bathtub-warm sea, chat under the sun, and watch their nutmeg-skinned babies splashing around. Teenagers, meanwhile, spend three months as a pile of writhing limbs under striped umbrellas.

"Why don't Italian teenagers have summer jobs?!" I asked my friend Massimo Giorgetti, founder of the MSGM fashion label. He laughed. "While you Americans were out running after your first internship at age sixteen, we just played all day." I pondered this. Massimo did not wind up a slacker. He is one of the hardest-working people I know.

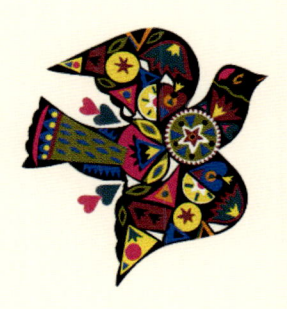

The benefits of play are foreign to Americans, who firmly believe in "no pain no gain." The Italians place much more importance on enjoying life than on parlaying it into a fortune or a corner-office career. Play is a relaxant, a lubricant, and puts you in a receptive state that says to the universe, "I want to flow with life and enjoy it."

Once you splash in those juicy waters long enough, it will flood out and begin to soften your interactions, your work, and virtually every aspect of your life.

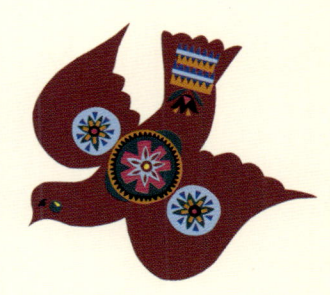

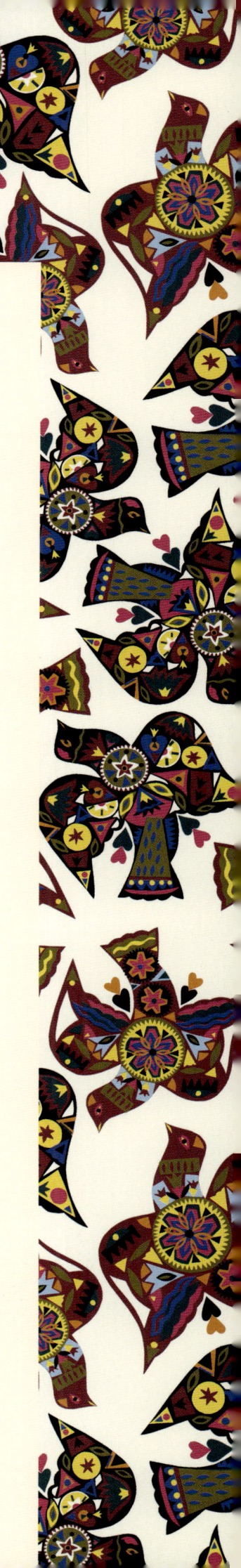

INTERMEZZO

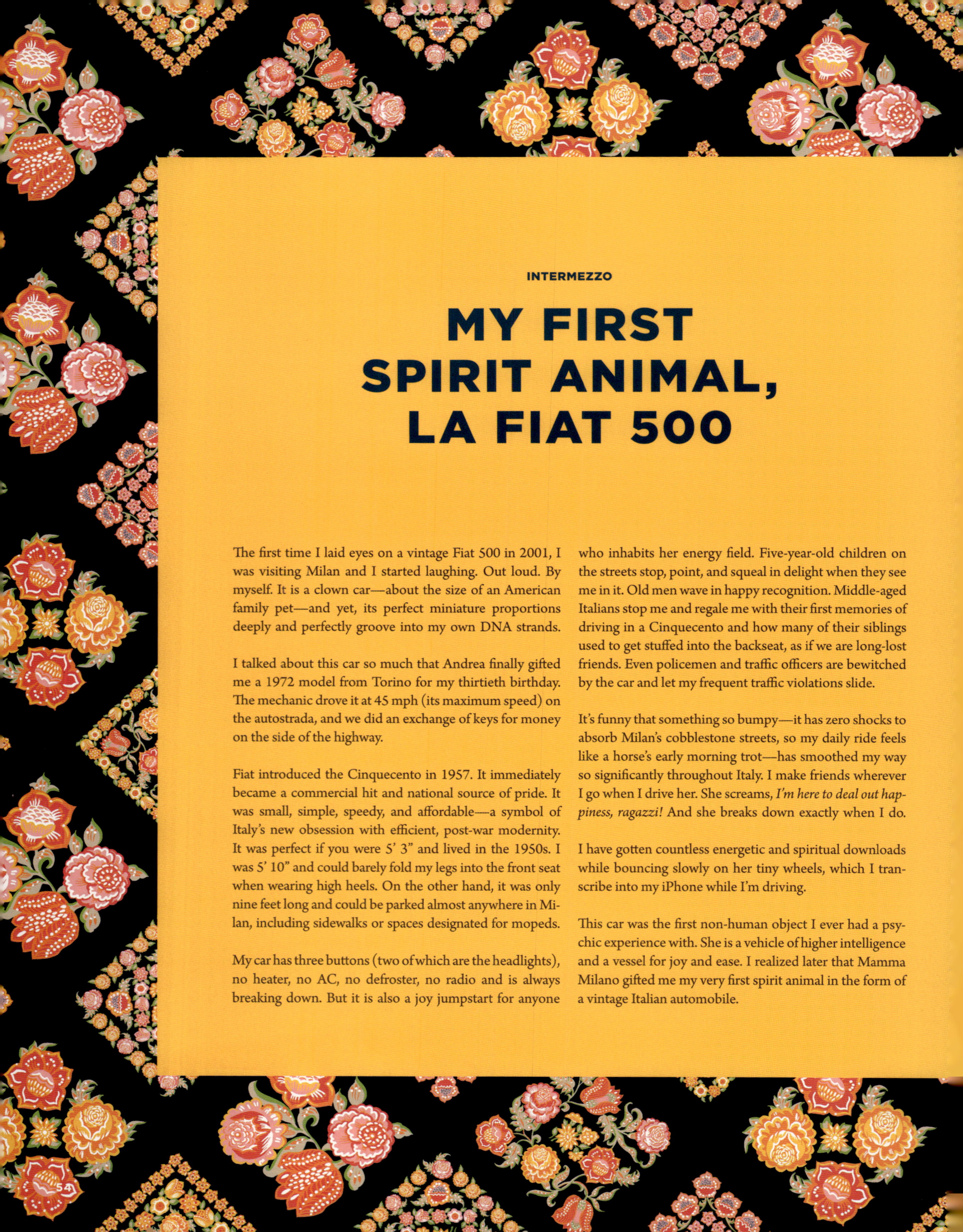

MY FIRST SPIRIT ANIMAL, LA FIAT 500

The first time I laid eyes on a vintage Fiat 500 in 2001, I was visiting Milan and I started laughing. Out loud. By myself. It is a clown car—about the size of an American family pet—and yet, its perfect miniature proportions deeply and perfectly groove into my own DNA strands.

I talked about this car so much that Andrea finally gifted me a 1972 model from Torino for my thirtieth birthday. The mechanic drove it at 45 mph (its maximum speed) on the autostrada, and we did an exchange of keys for money on the side of the highway.

Fiat introduced the Cinquecento in 1957. It immediately became a commercial hit and national source of pride. It was small, simple, speedy, and affordable—a symbol of Italy's new obsession with efficient, post-war modernity. It was perfect if you were 5' 3" and lived in the 1950s. I was 5' 10" and could barely fold my legs into the front seat when wearing high heels. On the other hand, it was only nine feet long and could be parked almost anywhere in Milan, including sidewalks or spaces designated for mopeds.

My car has three buttons (two of which are the headlights), no heater, no AC, no defroster, no radio and is always breaking down. But it is also a joy jumpstart for anyone who inhabits her energy field. Five-year-old children on the streets stop, point, and squeal in delight when they see me in it. Old men wave in happy recognition. Middle-aged Italians stop me and regale me with their first memories of driving in a Cinquecento and how many of their siblings used to get stuffed into the backseat, as if we are long-lost friends. Even policemen and traffic officers are bewitched by the car and let my frequent traffic violations slide.

It's funny that something so bumpy—it has zero shocks to absorb Milan's cobblestone streets, so my daily ride feels like a horse's early morning trot—has smoothed my way so significantly throughout Italy. I make friends wherever I go when I drive her. She screams, *I'm here to deal out happiness, ragazzi!* And she breaks down exactly when I do.

I have gotten countless energetic and spiritual downloads while bouncing slowly on her tiny wheels, which I transcribe into my iPhone while I'm driving.

This car was the first non-human object I ever had a psychic experience with. She is a vehicle of higher intelligence and a vessel for joy and ease. I realized later that Mamma Milano gifted me my very first spirit animal in the form of a vintage Italian automobile.

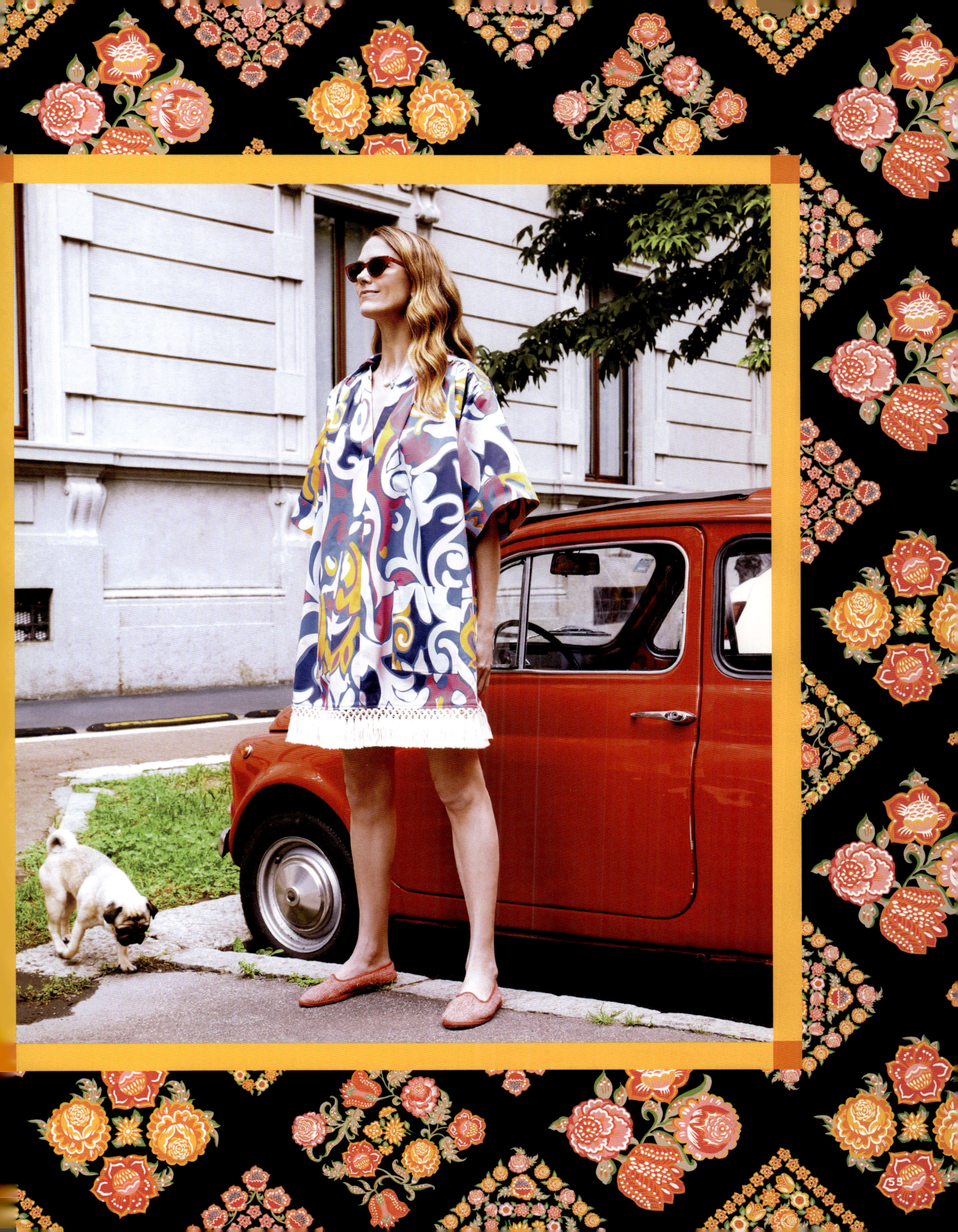

LESSON 20

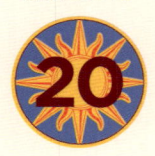

THE DOLCE ART OF DOING ABSOLUTELY *NIENTE*

Slow down and open your pleasure pores

Dolce far niente—the sweetness of doing nothing—should be Italy's national motto. When an Italian goes on vacation, whether it's a weekend trip or a four-week sponsored August break, they almost never go with a list of goals or a schedule. They arrive with the desire to melt into their sunbeds, entirely surrendering to their surroundings.

I've noticed that Americans are not nearly as good at vacations as the Italians. This is because they very seldom do what an Italian does... which is absolutely nothing. Rest is hard for us go-getters. We feel guilty, weak, lazy, or lost when we allow ourselves to chill.

But in Italy, I grasped that stillness is not the same as nothingness—it is rich with potential. Pausing from the busyness allows your being to process, recharge, and prepare for its magnificent future creations. To rest is to exist in the present, and it prepares a refreshed, fertile space in which more magic can unfold.

Americans now practice stillness on a meditation pillow, something the Italians do naturally without any guru, app, or yoga mat. They are unaware that in doing so, they are receiving the divine feminine—embracing the slowness, the stillness, and the wonderful powerful human energetic state of simply being.

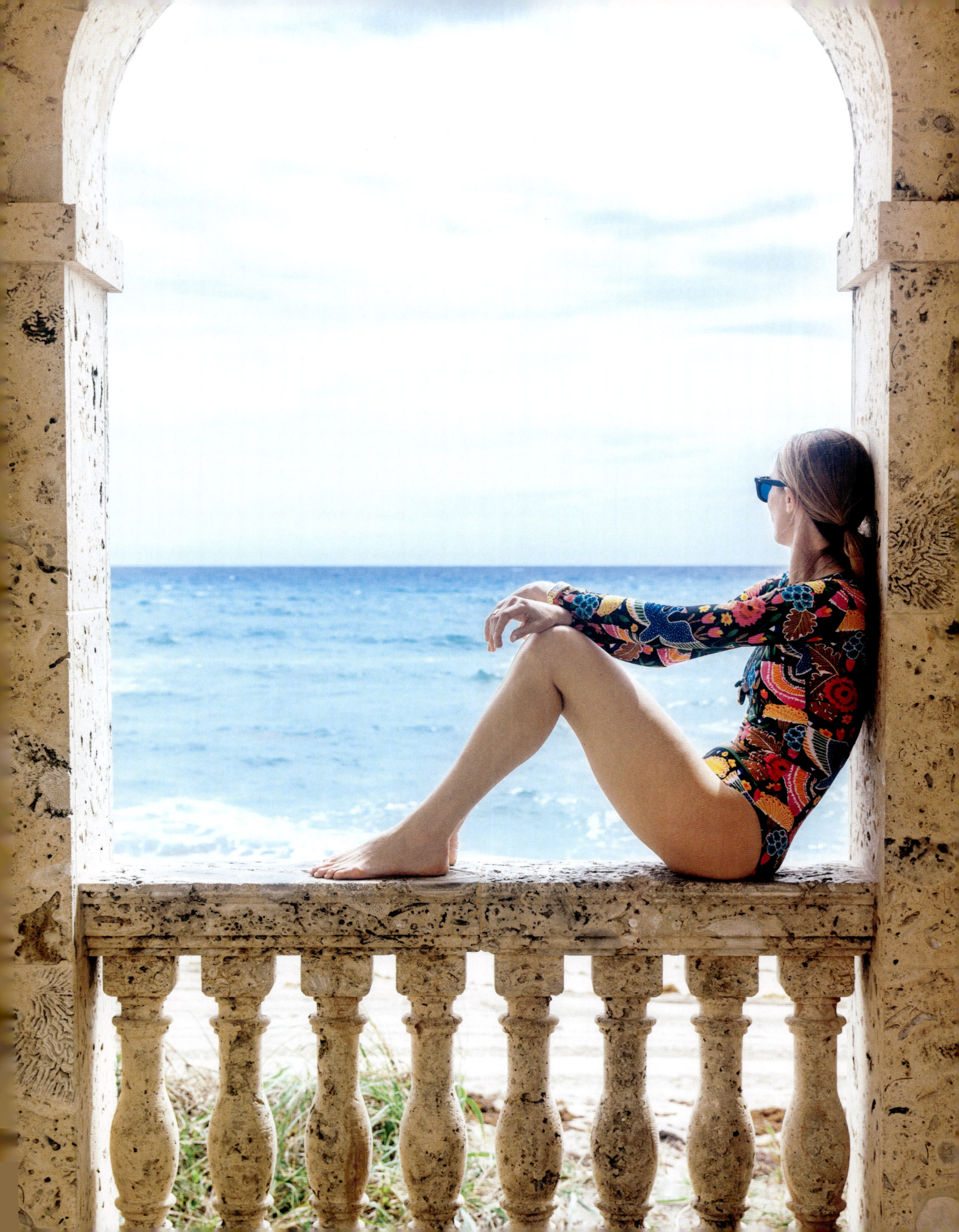

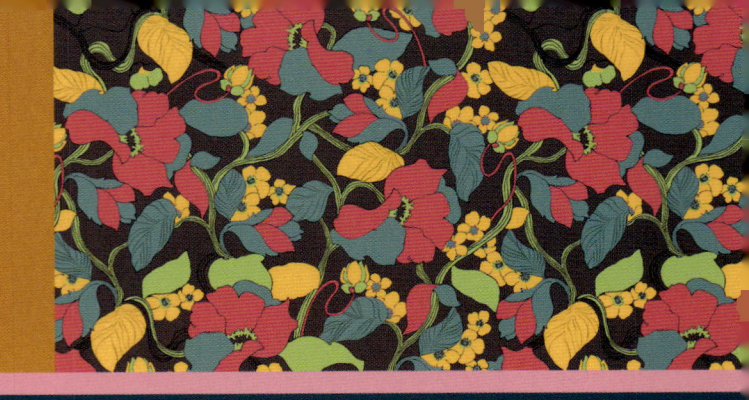

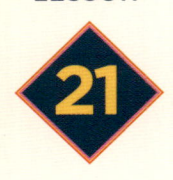

LESSON 21
SINKING INTO THE PLEASURES OF PESARO

My first teacher in the art of not doing much was Pesaro, a small town on the Adriatic coast where my husband's family lived. Like all good teachers, she showed me exactly what I needed to learn.

The first lesson was on looks. While almost everything in Italy is knee-crumplingly gorgeous, Pesaro is an ugly duckling. The sea is flat, low, and murky instead of clear emerald; the coastline was built up quickly and cheaply in the 1960s with a lot of badly designed hotels. Snobby Italians from more sophisticated areas look down their noses at the *popolo della provincia*—the masses of regular people (babies in diapers, women with huge bellies in giant bikinis, families unwrapping their homemade *panini*) who colonize a maze of sunbeds. The brightly striped beach umbrellas are charming, but Pesaro is definitely not posh Portofino or glittering Forte dei Marmi.

Pesaro is, nonetheless, packed in peak season. Everyone cycles—from the old ladies in their square cotton house-dresses to lanky five-year-olds in their bathing suits and plastic shoes. They are not on bicycles to exercise; they go about three miles per hour max, and no one wears a helmet.

I used to mock them; then I got myself a bicycle and began my own leisurely bike wanderings. I discovered scores of elegant, pastel-painted seaside villas built in the 1910s, tucked away on leafy streets or next to a bad disco-blaring bar, including Villa Ruggeri, a Liberty-era jewel covered in delicious lacy meringue plasterwork.

It was as if the town was purposefully hiding its magnetic treasures. The food was like that, too. There were very few attractive restaurants, but the meals were sensational. Families would come up from the shore with sandy legs and sit at plastic seaside tables to be served massive *risotto di mare* platters for 9 euro, or heaping plates of homemade tomato-sauced meat *tortellini*, or huge bowls of steaming mussels. Emerald-green mint ices sat next to watermelon slices the size of handbags. These little pop-up restaurants were more like shacks. At the back they would pitch a homemade tent where tubs of food were laid out.

The pace in Pesaro is honey-drip. No one is in a hurry, even during the work week: the cruising is leisurely, the roads are 100 percent flat. The biggest weekly drama in Pesaro is when a toddler loses their parent at the beach. A message is broadcast over a loudspeaker: "We've found a little boy in a red swimsuit in Bagni Wanda! Come over and get him!"

Deeper lessons in Pesaro occurred back in the household. For over fifteen years, my in-laws waited on my husband and me like indentured servants. His father would huff and puff his way up the stairs with our bags, while his mother would lock herself in the kitchen at 7:00 a.m. to handmake the *tagliatelle*, the *piadine*, and the rest of the day's provisions. We were not allowed to help. We were not supposed to clean up. We couldn't even make the beds. I grew up with lists of chores left in my bathroom every Saturday morning that had to be completely done before leaving the house: I sometimes felt like a ward in my parents' home, but I definitely had a role. I was doing rather than receiving.

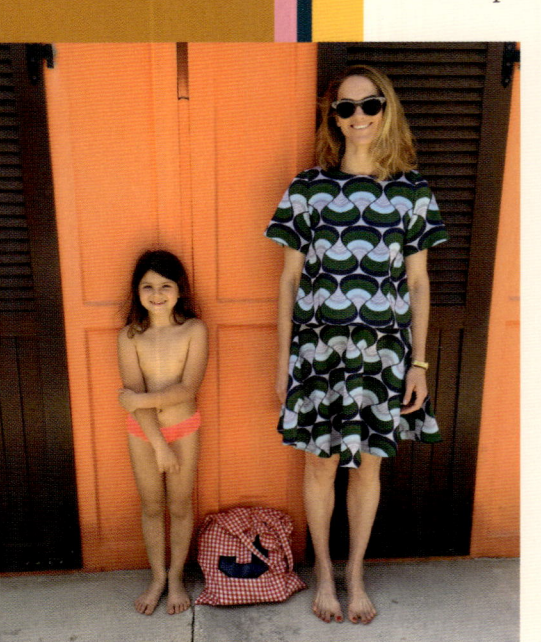

ITALIAN LESSONS

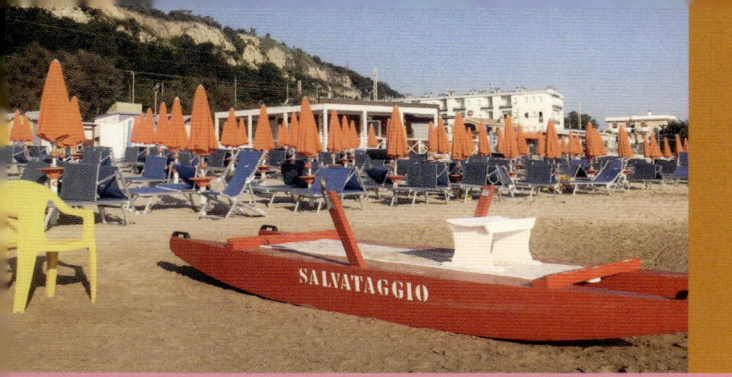

I really had no idea how to connect with pure Italian givers. What to do when your only role is to watch other people do very simple things, such as a whole morning spent rolling out the pasta or an hour walking to the market?

Then, one day, I decided to just submit completely to the pampering. On arrival, I assumed a horizontal position on my in-laws' fifty-year-old leather couch, burying myself in a magazine until lunch was on the table and I could begin my single required duty as a daughter-in-law: joyfully eating. This, at last, gave my mother-in-law the acknowledgement and receipt of her gifts that she wanted.

Around the time I finally began to relax in and surrender to Pesaro, the town's first chic seaside hotel, the Excelsior, suddenly opened, changing my entire experience there. I also discovered the town's only (and fabulous) vintage furniture store, Zucca, befriending the owners and spending every weekend visiting them as I did most of my vintage contacts. And I got to know the owners of Ratti, a hundred-year-old boutique and one of Italy's best multi brands. (Yes, in the middle of nowhere in Italy, you will find a four-story emporium of chic that has one of the best selections of luxury designers in the world!)

Several years later, Silvana Ratti and her daughter Mathilde came to Milan to buy La DoubleJ for their shop, and a few years after that, DoubleJ had its own pop-up under the frescoed ceilings of their *piano-nobile* top floor.

I went from knowing no one in Pesaro to being featured in, and friends with, the best shop in the Le Marche region. I went from disliking Pesaro to craving the sweet, soft normalcy and gentle arms it held me in.

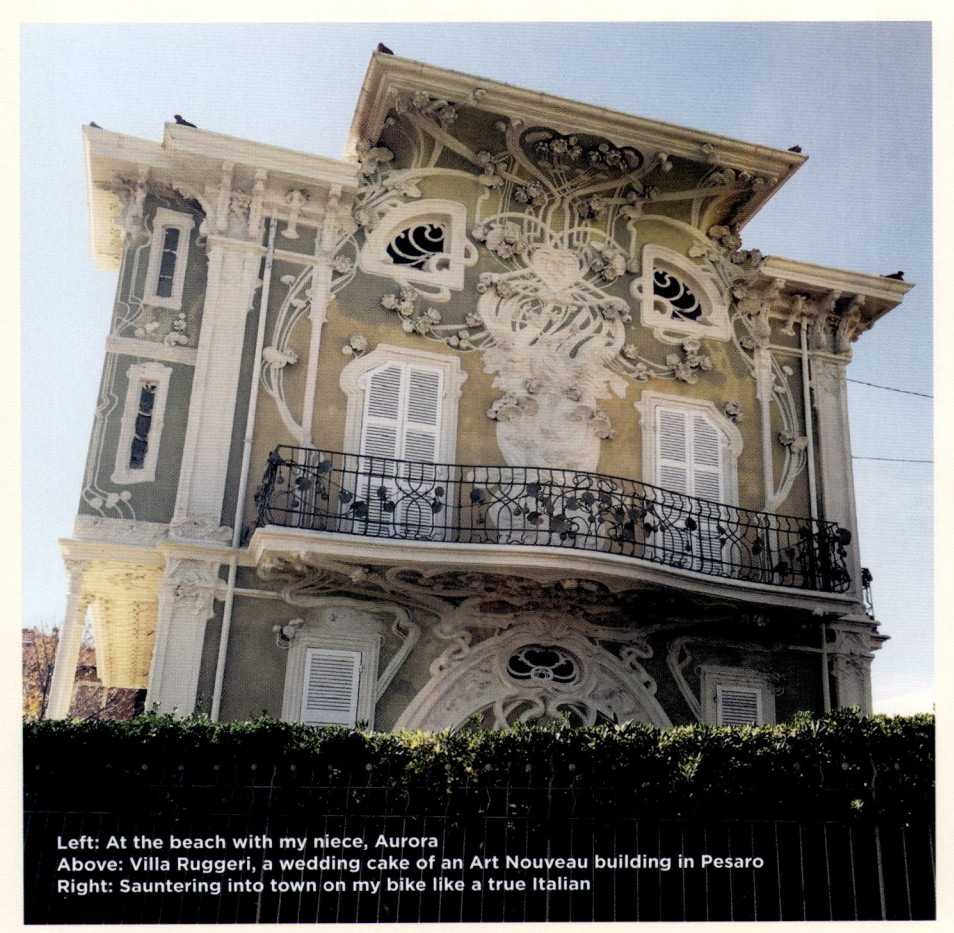

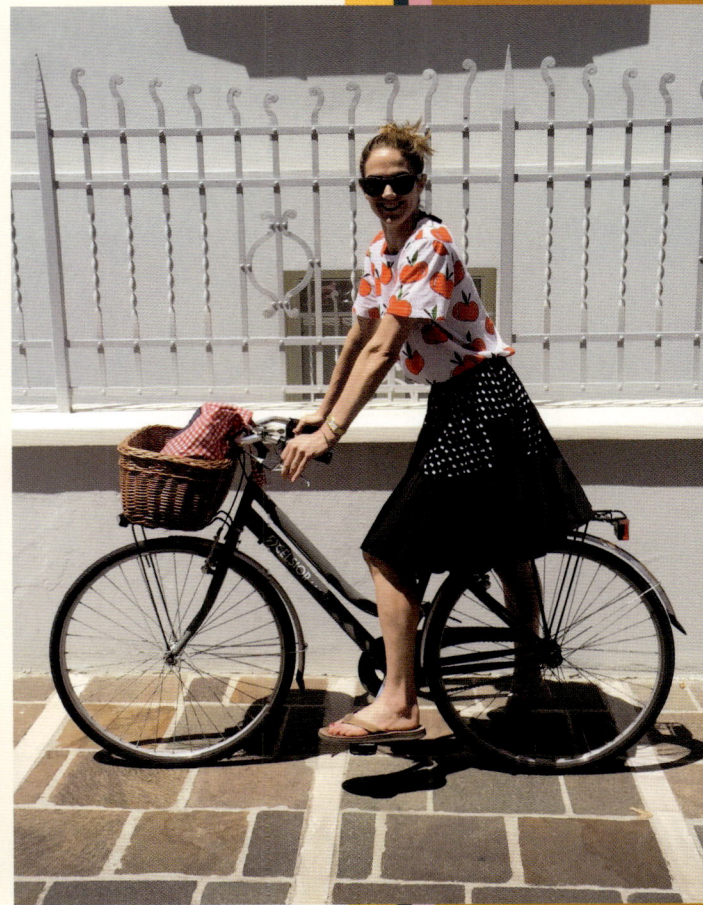

Left: At the beach with my niece, Aurora
Above: Villa Ruggeri, a wedding cake of an Art Nouveau building in Pesaro
Right: Sauntering into town on my bike like a true Italian

MAMMA MILANO

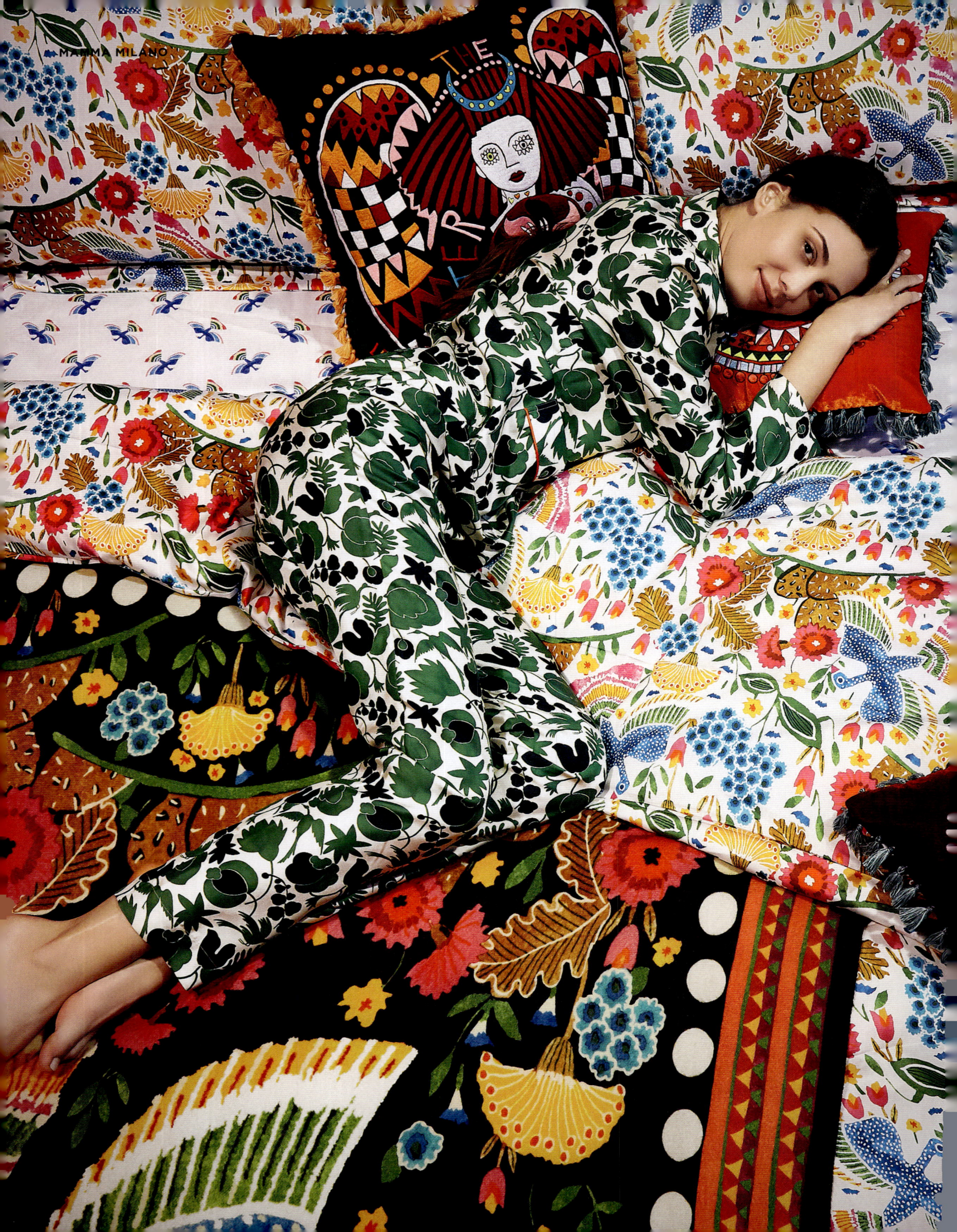

SLOWING IT WAY DOWN

Learn the Italian art of doing a whole lot of absolutely nothing

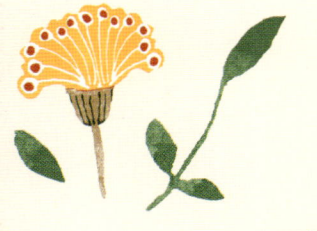

LESSON 22
SEE WHERE STILLNESS LEADS

Italy taught me the flip side of my nostril-flaring Californian impatience: how to slow down and enjoy—even *melt into*—the moment, the splendor of experience.

If a waiter is slow, you have time to look around the restaurant and notice its beautiful woodwork and vintage glass chandeliers. When you discover a certain shop is closed again and you can't chop through your to-do list, you may find you're standing next to a church you've never seen before, that's hiding astonishing Renaissance masterpieces flickering in honeyed candlelight.

Or you can just take a nap—like my dog does. Pepper is thoroughly Italian. Food and play are fundamental to her. When either of these are unavailable, she just collapses on the ground with a giant sigh and falls deeply asleep. As an American, I hadn't napped since I was six years old. Then somewhere along the line, I learned to relish a long, delicious afternoon snooze and began to hear my body speaking to me in the silence. I just had to slow down enough to listen to it.

Part of learning to slow down was being able to sit for three hours at a lunch table on a Sunday, when I was invited to a family meal. At first, I found this torturous: I would get ants in my pants while everyone heaped third helpings on their plate and opened yet another bottle of wine. But after several years of training, I acquiesced. Plus, there was nothing else for me to do on a Sunday, with everything closed. Of course, once I learned how to melt into my house and not leave it for an entire day, businesses in Milan began to stay open on Sundays, along with the gym. But Mamma Milano's golden lesson was carved into my cells anyway.

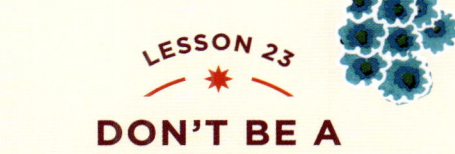

LESSON 23
DON'T BE A MOLTO-MULTITASKER

As a freelance journalist, I found myself doing my job in odd places. When someone called early for an interview and I was in my car, I would pull over, yank out my computer, and begin typing from the front seat, my legs dangling over the passenger side. I once did a phone interview for a style story in the gym bathroom, seated on a toilet, the only place without pumping club music.

Italians found my behavior very odd, because they never do more than one thing at once. You're never going to see an Italian walking down the street with a coffee cup—walking and drinking don't happen simultaneously. I'll never fully give up my American, eight-armed multitasking ways, but you may now find me walking down the street doing nothing except losing myself in my surroundings.

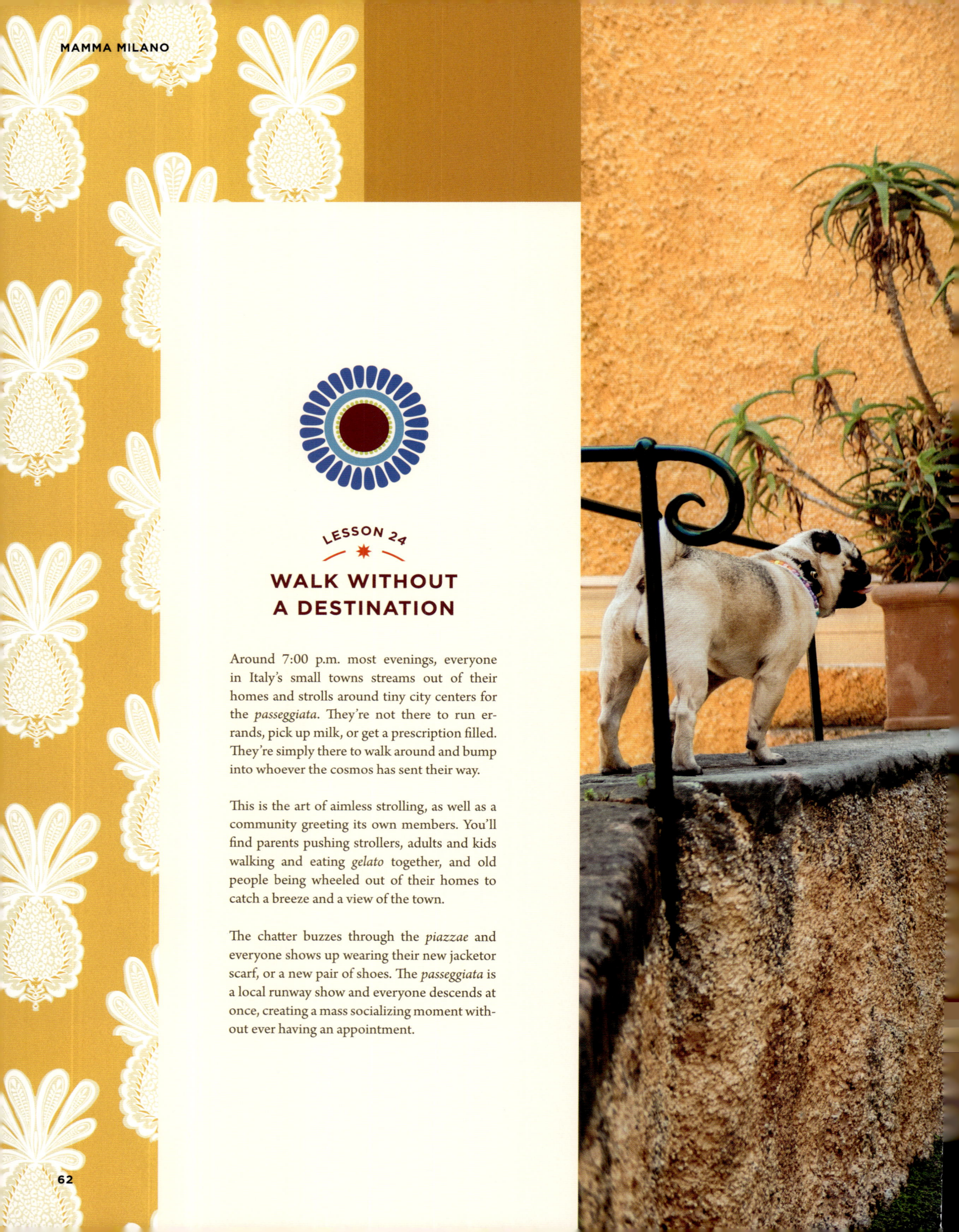

MAMMA MILANO

LESSON 24

WALK WITHOUT A DESTINATION

Around 7:00 p.m. most evenings, everyone in Italy's small towns streams out of their homes and strolls around tiny city centers for the *passeggiata*. They're not there to run errands, pick up milk, or get a prescription filled. They're simply there to walk around and bump into whoever the cosmos has sent their way.

This is the art of aimless strolling, as well as a community greeting its own members. You'll find parents pushing strollers, adults and kids walking and eating *gelato* together, and old people being wheeled out of their homes to catch a breeze and a view of the town.

The chatter buzzes through the *piazzae* and everyone shows up wearing their new jacketor scarf, or a new pair of shoes. The *passeggiata* is a local runway show and everyone descends at once, creating a mass socializing moment without ever having an appointment.

ITALIAN LESSONS

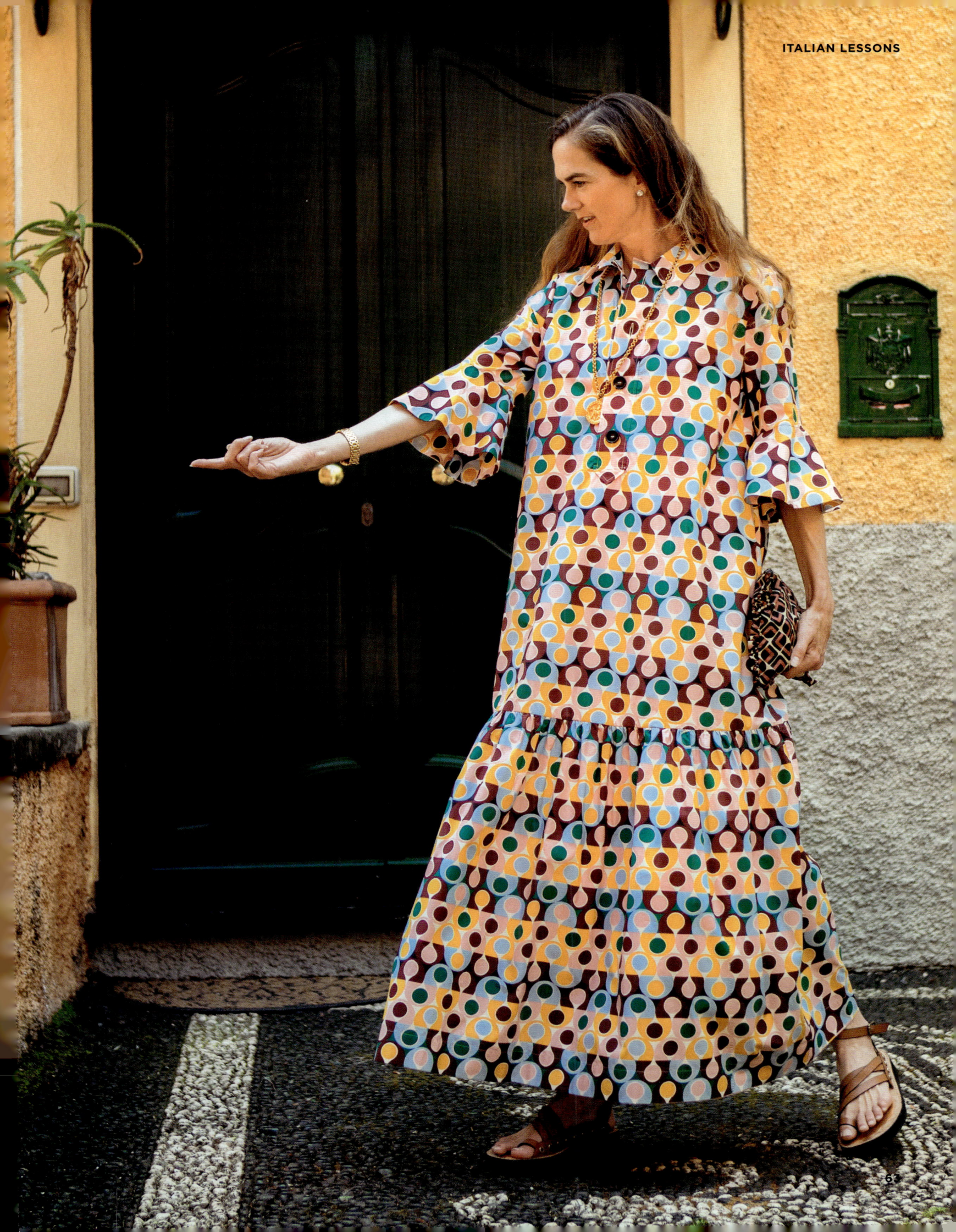

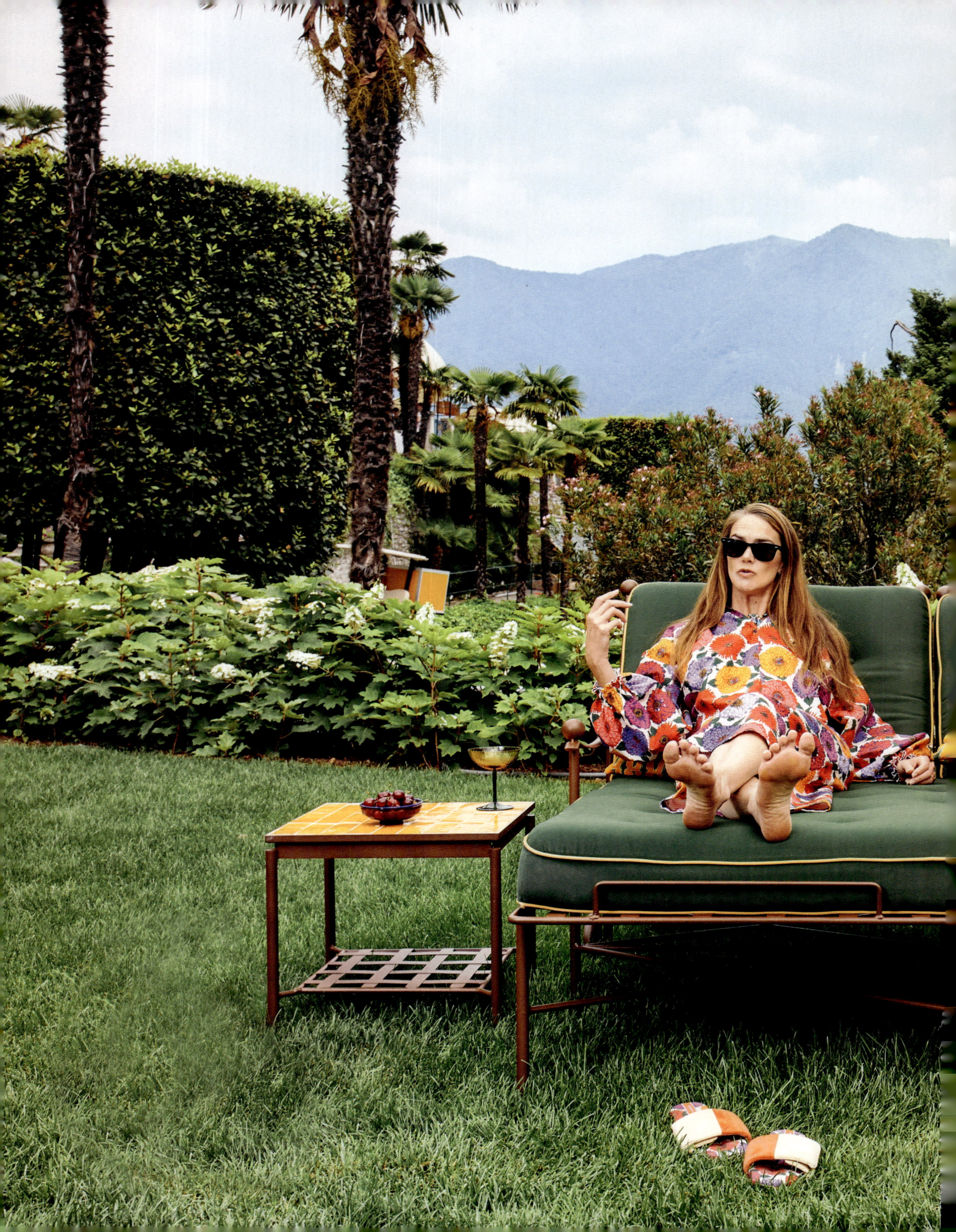

ANDIAMO!

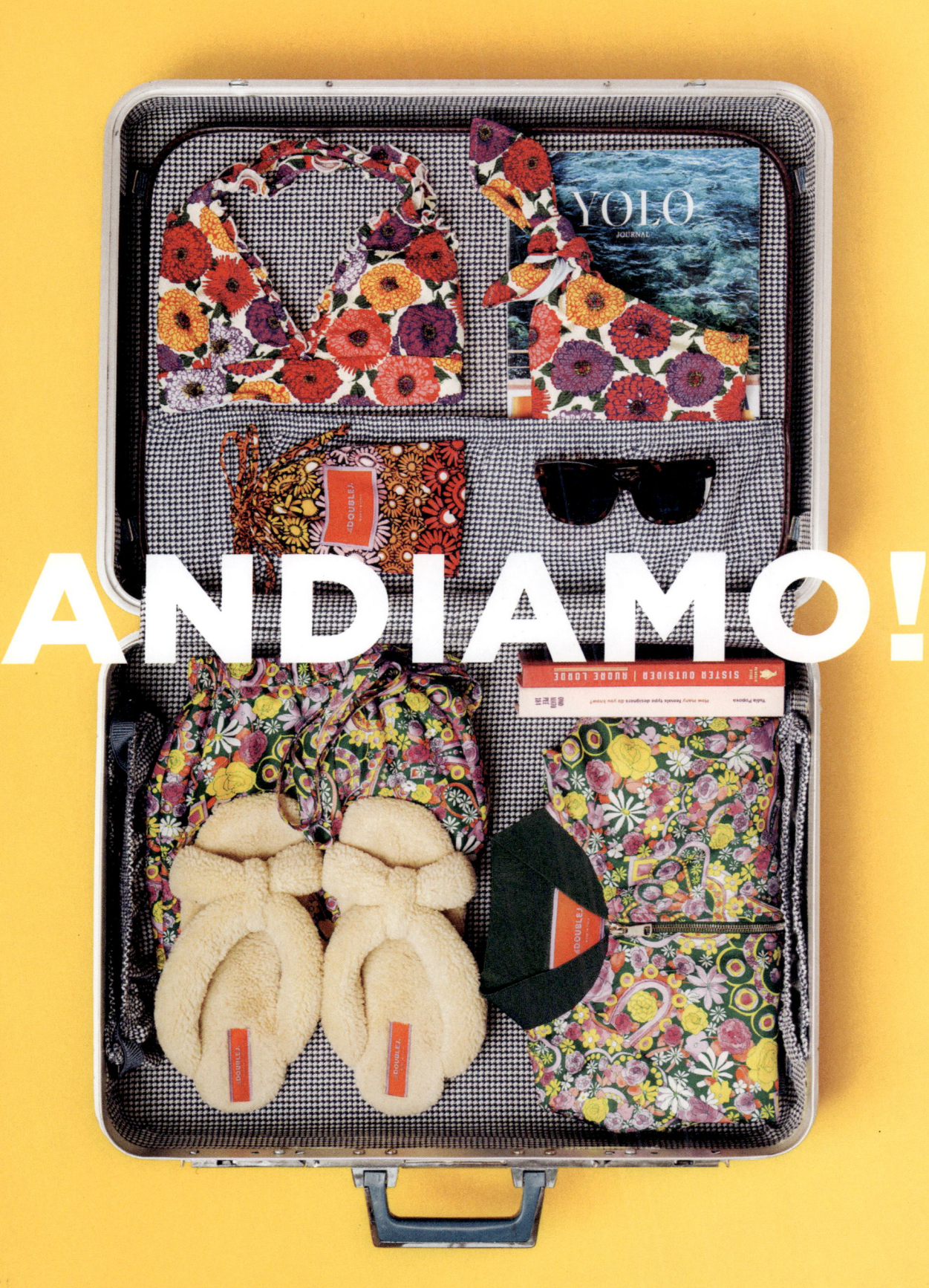

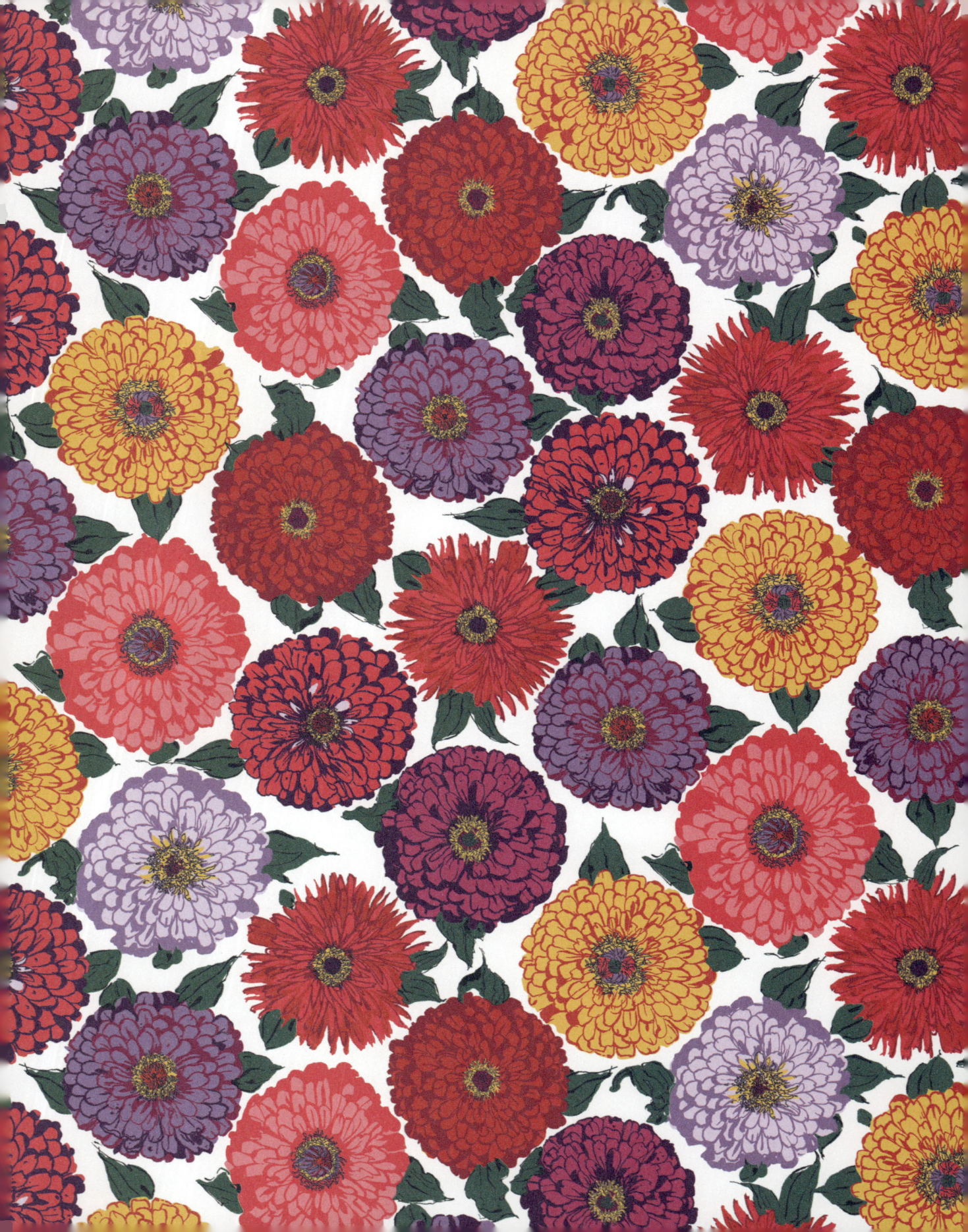

VACATION NATION: WHAT I LEARNED FROM BEING A HOUSE GUEST

Over two decades in Italy, I've visited almost every corner of this great country. The best way to travel here, I've learned, is as a guest. Since most Italians have a second home—even a small shed with a bed—you almost always end up having the opportunity to be hosted by a friend. All of these places taught me their local customs, charms, rhythms, and pace. I watched, I tasted, I listened, and I learned. These are a few sacred spots in Italy where I've had my heart cracked open.

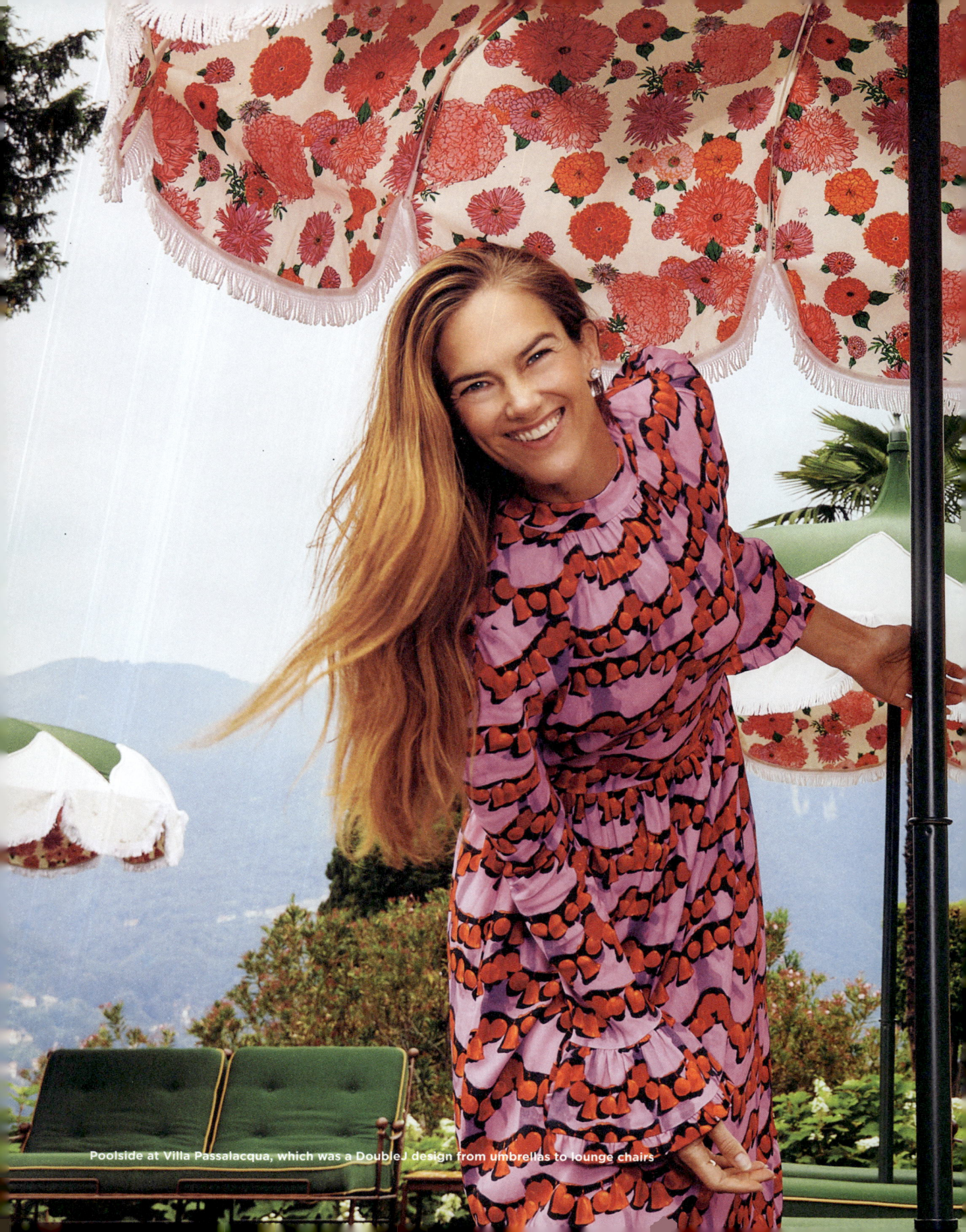

Poolside at Villa Passalacqua, which was a Double J design from umbrellas to lounge chairs

LAKE COMO

I can get to Lake Como from my doorstep in Milan in forty-four minutes flat. That is less time than I've spent in a taxi going from uptown Manhattan to Brooklyn. The proximity is incredible, and yet many Milanese people do not frequent this jewel. Why not? This was the response I got from my Milanese friends: "It's sleepy! It's sad! It's depressing! And there's nothing to do!" Wait, what?! Lake Como is one of the most gorgeous corners of Italy—covered in sloping terraces and vibrant gardens that pour down into the lake—but the Italians are so spoiled for beauty that they can afford to find a less expensive slice of their country's bounty.

The real reason that the Milanese don't love the lake is that there aren't many places to actually gather and be Italian: no beaches where they can all pile on top of each other, or shallow waters where they can plant themselves, or a defined town center around which they can all do their *passeggiata*. The lake is a mysterious, deep, powerfully dark body of water. And it's really best enjoyed from a lakefront villa. So, naturally, I became a guest.

One weekend, I was in Como at a hotel I didn't like. I suddenly became very Italian and contacted my friend Emily FitzRoy in London, who knows all things travel-related in Italy, to see if she could help me out. She instantly snapped into Italian mode (her grandmother is Neapolitan) and called her friend Valentina De Santis, who just happened to own a gorgeous hotel down the lake called the Grand Hotel Tremezzo. A few hours later, I found myself on a captained Riva landing on her orange-striped shores and being greeted by her hotel manager, Silvio.

Valentina told me she was a fan of LaDoubleJ, so I sent her a dress. A few months later, she asked me if DoubleJ would decorate the pool and lounge area of a new twenty-four-room villa she was opening the following year. When it opened in June 2022, Villa Passalacqua quickly became one of Como's most magical corners, and we were able to shower a small slice of it with our signature prints and joyful designs.

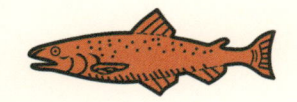

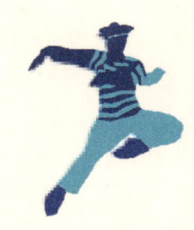

PORTOFINO

Only two hours from Milan on the Ligurian coast, Portofino surprises people because, for all of its globally glamorous reputation, it's actually the size of a peanut. It bangs a lot of beauty into its tiny frame, but this also means it's packed with tourists.

I got married in Portofino. I learned, by watching the locals, how to navigate this special little jewel: skip the stores and go for a hike up on Il Monte above the port; walk to San Fruttuoso, a magnificent abbey unreachable by car; avoid the crowded beaches and rent a little boat (not a flashy super yacht!) to go to a little cove with a supply of *panini* from the tiny bakery in town; never go in July or August; always stay on a Sunday night in spring or fall when the *piazza* empties out.

Although it appears to be a playground for the superrich, Portofino is actually filled with lovely, modest homes that dot the Monte, inhabited by people who just want to enjoy their little corner of paradise. Seeing friends in town doesn't require much—you'll just bump into them at 7:00 p.m. in the *piazza* and then you can make a plan for a boat the next morning.

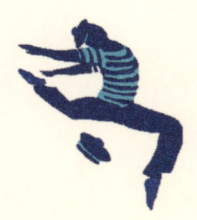

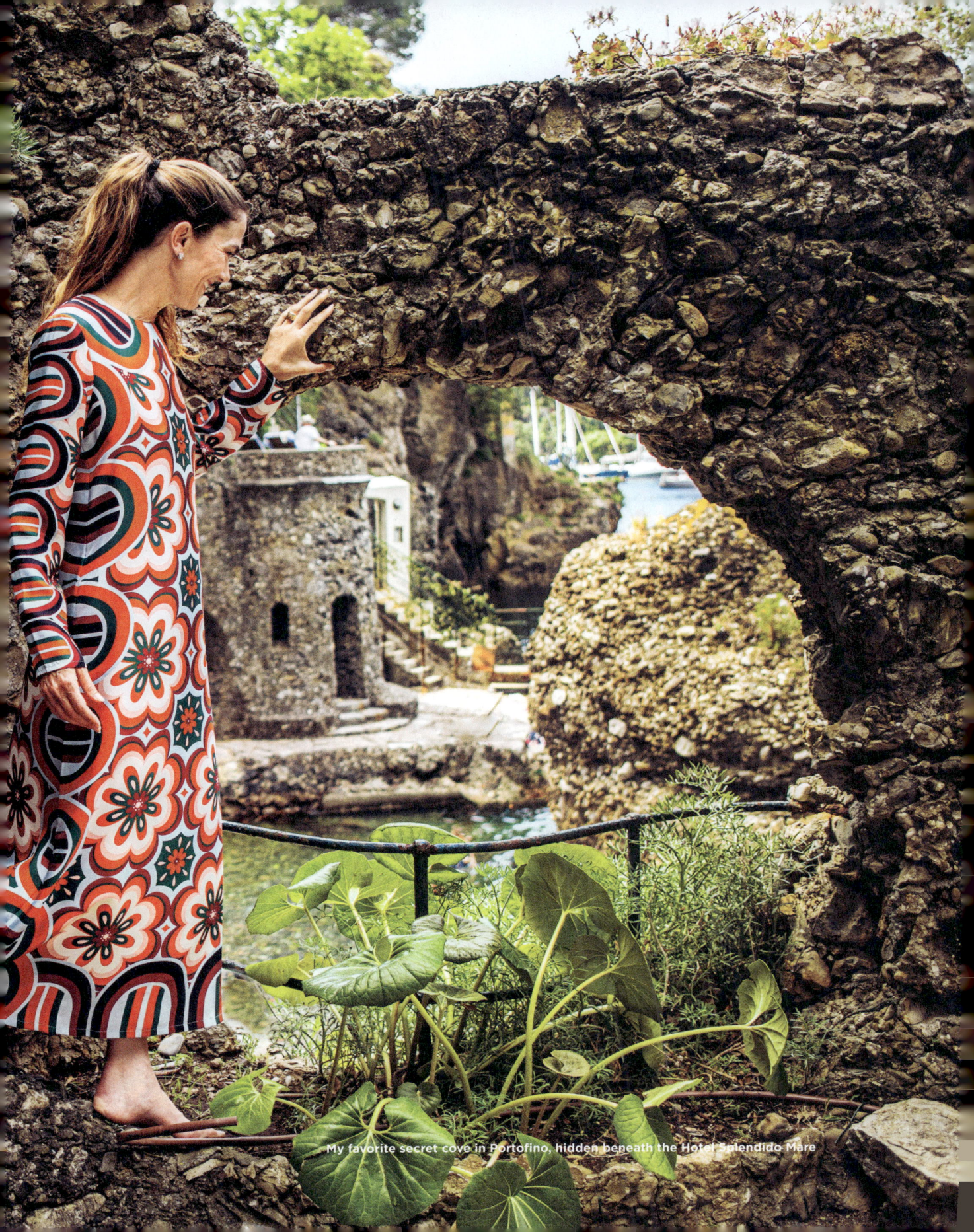

My favorite secret cove in Portofino, hidden beneath the Hotel Splendido Mare

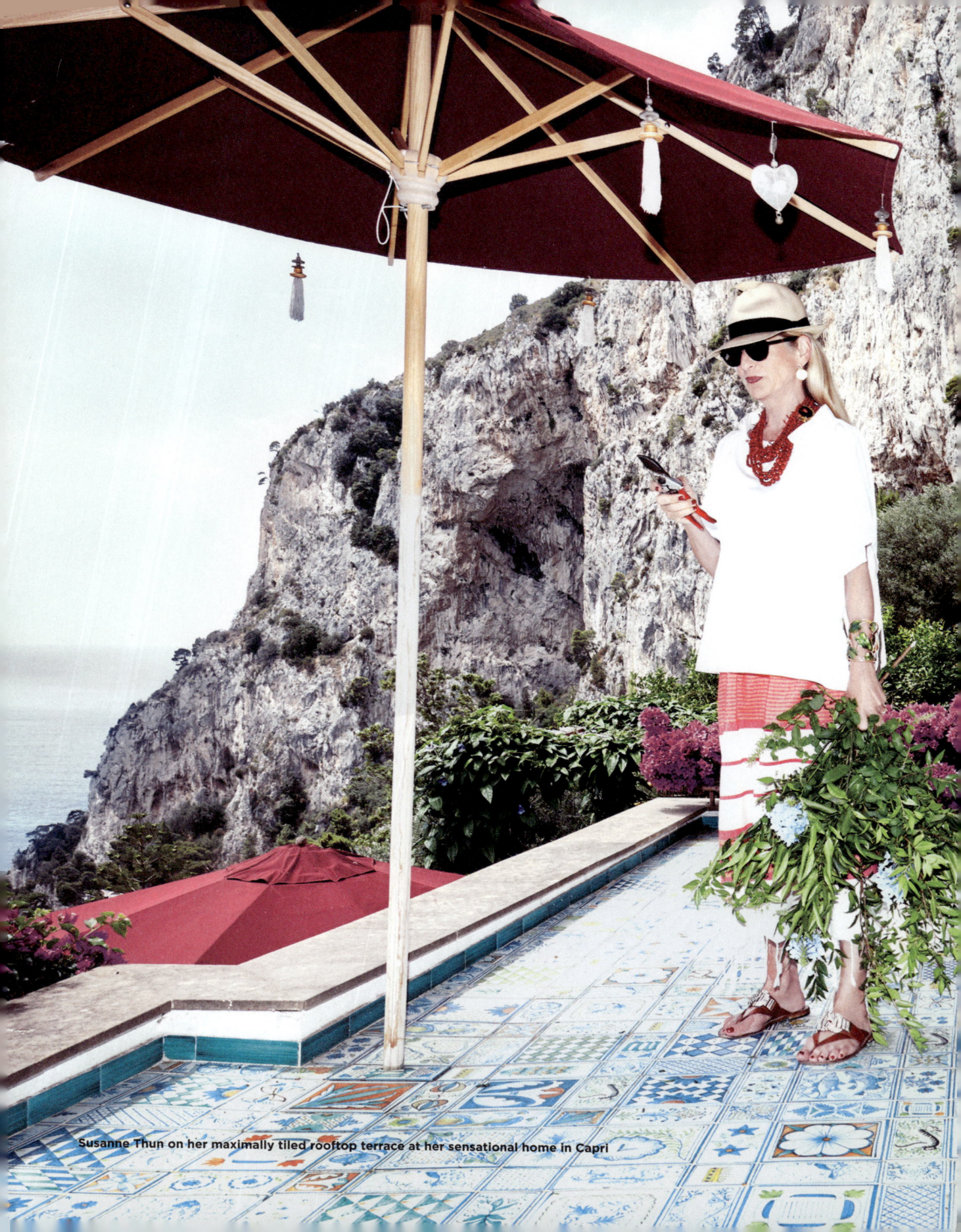

Susanne Thun on her maximally tiled rooftop terrace at her sensational home in Capri

CAPRI

Carpeted in magenta bougainvillea, with tangles of rosemary and lemons and surrounded by transparent turquoise and emerald waters, Capri is a stunner of an island in the Bay of Naples. Crowds of visitors swim, boat, eat, and shop here. I've been invited each summer by my friends Susanne Thun, a former stylist and decorator, and her architect husband, Matteo. Their home, which Matteo designed, is built into a vertical slab of rock that overlooks Marina Piccola and the two most romantic arched rocks in the world: *i Faraglioni*.

The house is an Edenic paradise surrounded by a grove of olive trees and exploding bushes of white roses. It was here that I studied Susanne as she decorated, organized, entertained, hosted, dressed, cooked, shopped, and personified the very way to live like an Italian.

And it was also here that I finally connected to the incredible, bright-green heart of Capri sliced into Monte Solaro, which most visitors never see. Matteo and I would make it up to the top just as the sun rose over a small church. I learned to crave sinking into the ivy-floored ground and the silence at the top of the *monte*, light years away from the bustle below.

Capri has now become bloated and bruised by tourists. You would do well to skip June through August. Now when I go, it's in the magic months of May and September, when the crowds slip out and you're left with the pure magic of this hypnotic island's energy.

Inside a glorious, gilded villa in Palermo

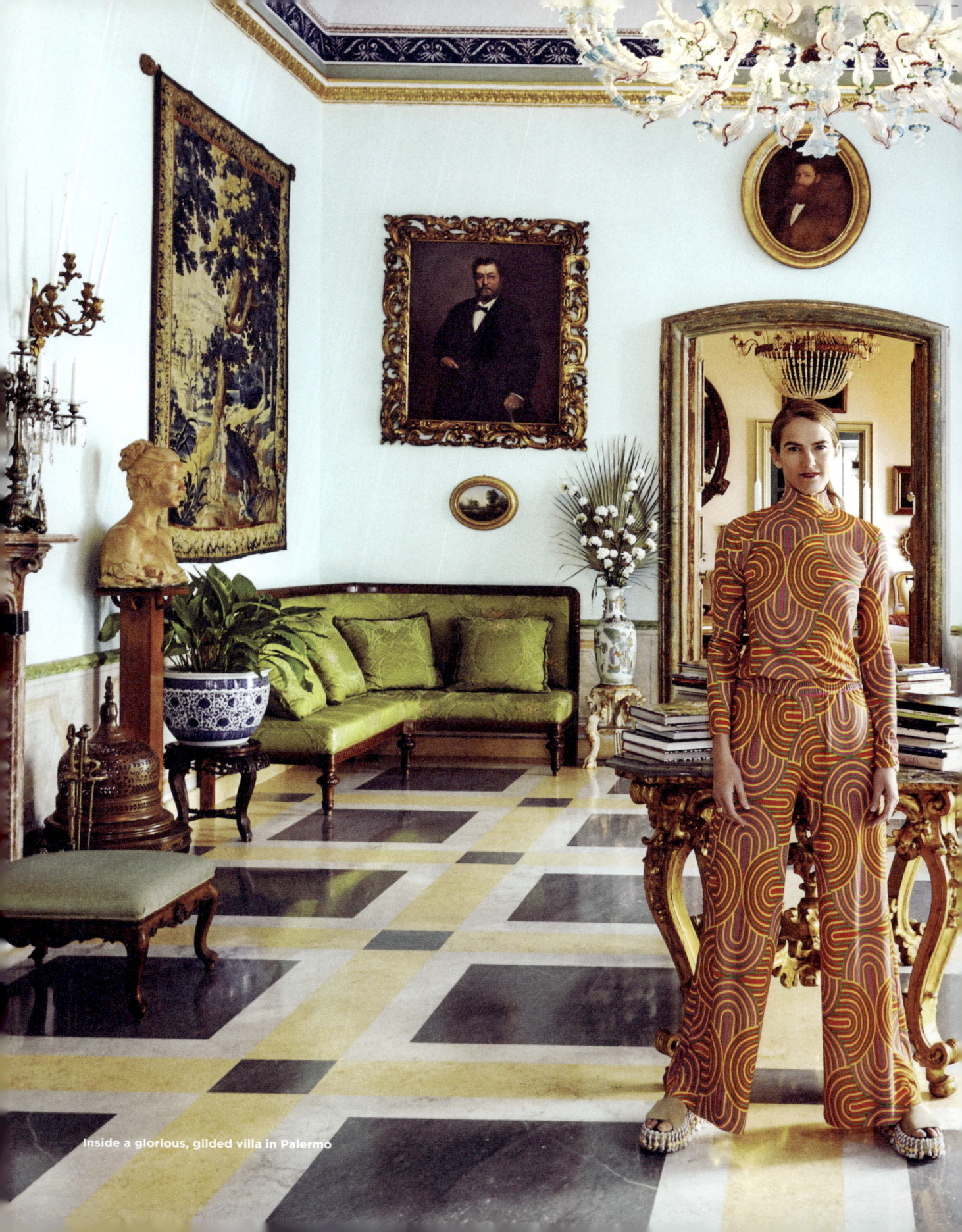

SICILY

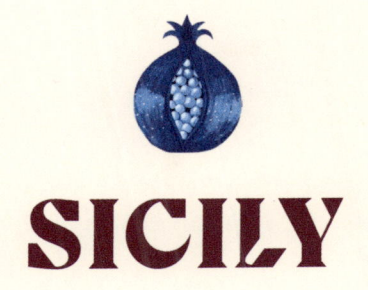

If Italy is a soft ball of *mozzarella*, then Sicily is an oozy pile of *burrata*—even softer, even warmer, even richer. Richer in calories (you will gain ten pounds for each week you stay), richer in ornamentation (the Baroque churches are simply sensational), and above all, richer in feeling. Sicily is literally hot with its southern temperatures, but also in its fiery, open hearts that give love freely. Sicilians are the friendliest, nicest, most uncomplicated people you will ever meet. They are also wildly generous. Doors fling open wherever you go; you're always invited. You can be a friend of a friend of a friend, and a Sicilian will make it their absolute duty to entertain you, take care of you, and make you feel welcome and pampered in their hometown.

PALERMO

Palermo is an intoxicating shake-up of east and west, beauty and grit, formal and informal. It is a highly traditional city, where classic rules around form, style, and manners are still very much honored, and yet a rumbling of wildness and exotic extravagance vibrates under everything.

I was introduced to this special place by Mario Dell'Oglio, a supremely well-dressed local who went to business school with Andrea and whose family has lived in Palermo for generations. We didn't know him well, but he put us up in his extra apartment, brought us to three-hour lunches overlooking the sea at his friend's Planeta winery, and ushered us on a tour of the famed Palazzo Gangi—the mammoth gilded site of Visconti's *Il Gattopardo* (*The Leopard*). It was closed to the public, but friends of his were restoring it. (Of course they were.)

Several years later, when I started La DoubleJ, Mario was the first retailer in town to pick up our label, and he launched us as only a Sicilian would. He rented an enormous palazzo, invited every chic woman in town for lunch, organized our Legendary Lady photo shoots, and threw a party in his store. Being hosted by a Sicilian became the most decadent experience of my life.

SCICLI

Over Christmas 2015, I visited my friends Alberto and Laura Biagetti in Scicli, a town in south-eastern Sicily with a population of 20,000. Scicli is not a rich city, but it has a noble, elegant past and is dotted with many beautiful *palazzi* bearing elegant, wave-like facades and intricate iron balconies. In the small town's twisting streets, ancient ruins date to the Bronze Age, and there are more than a hundred churches. The entire city is built from a sandy, rose-colored stone that illuminates like a pristine, pink-yellow backlit stage when the sun hits it every morning. From afar, the city appears like a mass of small cubes in a tight, tidy formation, as if the inside of the mountain had been scooped out like rough eggplant flesh, diced up, and then reassembled inside its matching skin.

I had come to Scicli exhausted—mentally, physically, emotionally, spiritually—having launched my company a year earlier, and it had been a wild circus ride. So I turned my back on her completely and didn't answer a single work email for seven days, a personal lifetime record. I was becoming an Italian!

Scicli reminded me of the sacredness in the small. The good energy of this magical, humble place spun around me. It wound around the narrow, steep stone pathways where tiny doors led to small, poor homes built under the rock. It blew under the groups of old men who congregated every morning and late afternoon on street corners, many of them missing teeth, but all of them dressed with care and flair. They wore collared sweaters buttoned up to the neck, sturdy wool jackets, and driving hats. In poor areas in the south of Italy, I could sense despondence and defeat in the men who stood outside, waiting for something to happen and yet knowing it never would. But in Scicli, there was a buoyancy and internal brightness to many of the locals. Their eyes twinkled with a sense of purpose—there was hope and faith that everything would be just fine.

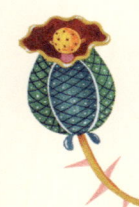

It was inside the empty, magnificent churches of this humble, small town that I slowly began to rebuild my heart and connect to the raw Mother power available to me, and all of us.

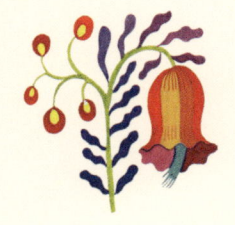

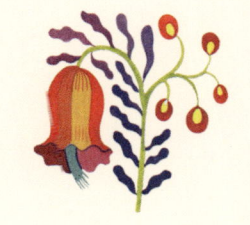

MT. ETNA

Rocca delle Tre Contrade is a spectacular villa at the base of Mount Etna owned by two friends, Jon and Marco, who spent years refurbishing the property. The surrounding towns and seaside of this villa are nothing to write home about. But once you've been whisked into the grounds, you don't care. The gardens are a wild Eden with views of the volcano, which was spitting fiery sparks one time I came. The twelve bedrooms used to be for a noble family—now Jon and Marco rent it out as an ultra-luxe B&B, or for cooking-class retreats, or as a gathering place for friends.

Everything swirls around their cook, Dora, the blood pumper of the entire operation. She handmakes everything in their professional kitchen, sending out a fleet of freshly made quiches, eggplant pastas, and the best fava bean and fresh pea soup you've ever had in your life. You come here on vacation and you rest, read, sleep, eat, and repeat. Then when you get home, you can't button your pants up anymore.

PANTELLERIA

I first learned about Pantelleria from Giorgio Armani, who built a home here in the 1990s before anyone had heard of it. He intrigued me with tales of this wild, raw, unpredictable place with no hotels, no beaches, no taxis, no chic places for cocktails, no sand, no shade, and none of the creature comforts of regular Italian vacationing. This volcanic island, south of Sicily and just north of Tunisia, is scorching hot in the summer, harshly windy all year round, and a pain in the neck to get to. It is a vertiginous pile of obsidian (a crystal rock known for its powerful energetic qualities). The island pulsates with undeniable power, which Armani cautioned me about, offering me the keys to his house for a stay some years ago. Later, I became a guest of Scasicia Gambaccini and her husband, Wayne Maser, at their sensational, sprawling compound and learned how the locals truly live life there. Then the island offered its gifts freely—I rolled around in the high-mineral mud at the island's central lake, pulling in waves of potent energy into my cells; I connected to the stones, crystals, and water at seaside yoga with the sunrise.

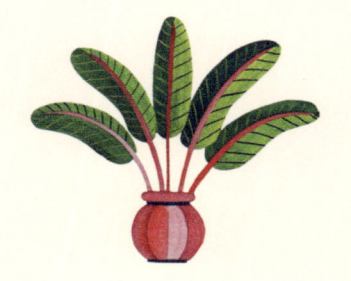

PUGLIA

Puglia is arid and, in many places, eerily empty. You might arrive and wonder, "Where am I and why am I here?" It's not lush Liguria or romantic Tuscany. You've got a little work to do in order to penetrate its magic and beauty. In fact, you really need to be guided here to get anchored down into its beautiful roots. I was a guest in the Otranto family home of Carlo and Ennio Capasa—my friends from Costume National—probably fifty times. This was a place where I learned to cook many things (see the next chapter!), and where I ate warm sheep's ricotta for the first time, freshly made by a farmer down the road. Many years later, I had solo adventures in this corner of Puglia, discovering caves built into the sea and practicing energy and meditation work inside their craggy cavities.

◦◊◦ PHRASEBOOK ◦◊◦

GODITI IL MOMENTO: ENJOY THE MOMENT

Usage: When you're trapped in a line somewhere beautiful or lost in a maze of tiny, narrow streets that Google maps has never heard of.

Clockwise from top left: Carlo & Ennio Capasa's masseria in Puglia, Athena McAlpine's masseria in Puglia, the Otranto Coast, Valentine de Santis at Passalacqua in Lake Como, Ennio Capasa in Puglia, a Palermo palazzo, and with Sciascia Gambaccini in Pantelleria.

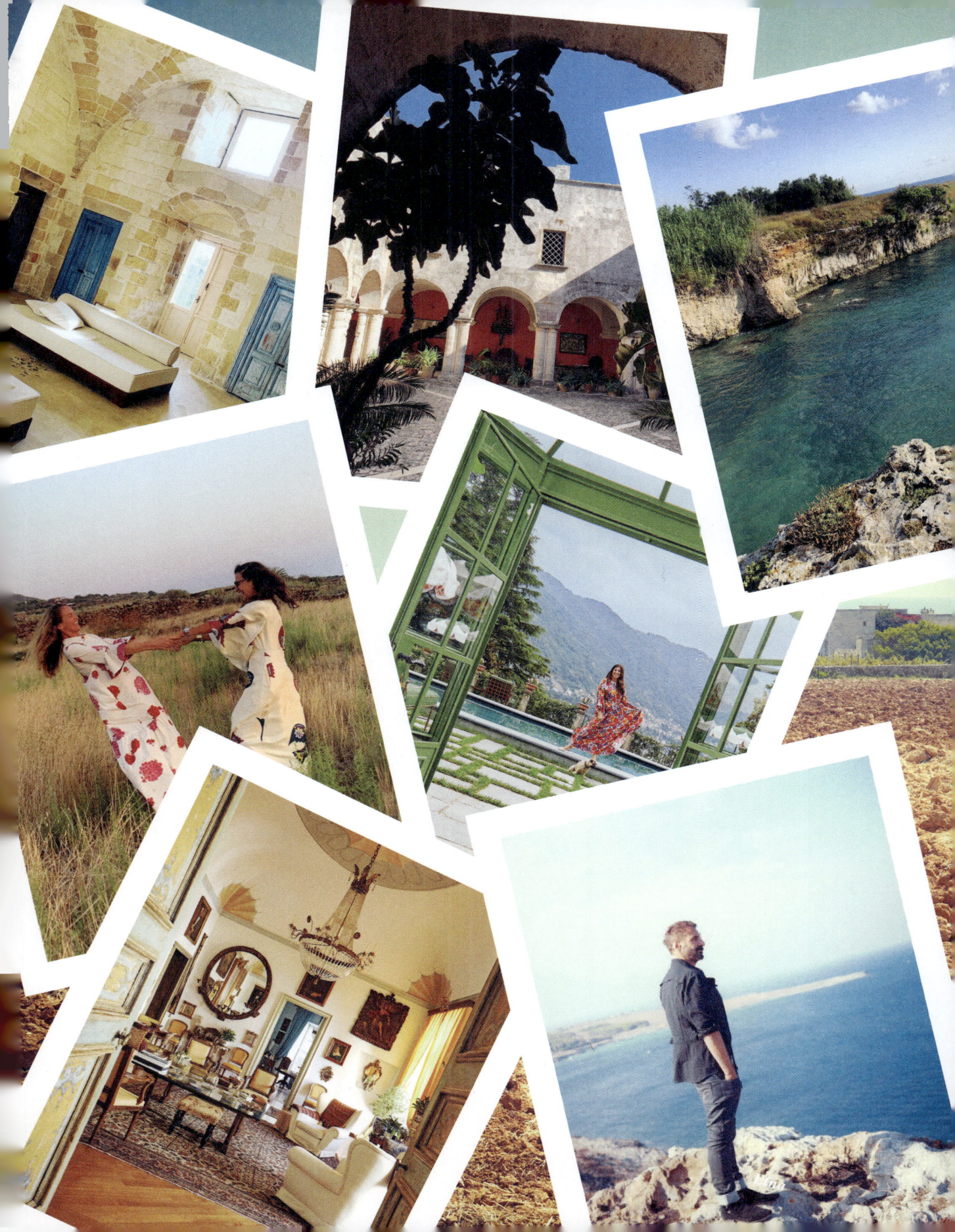

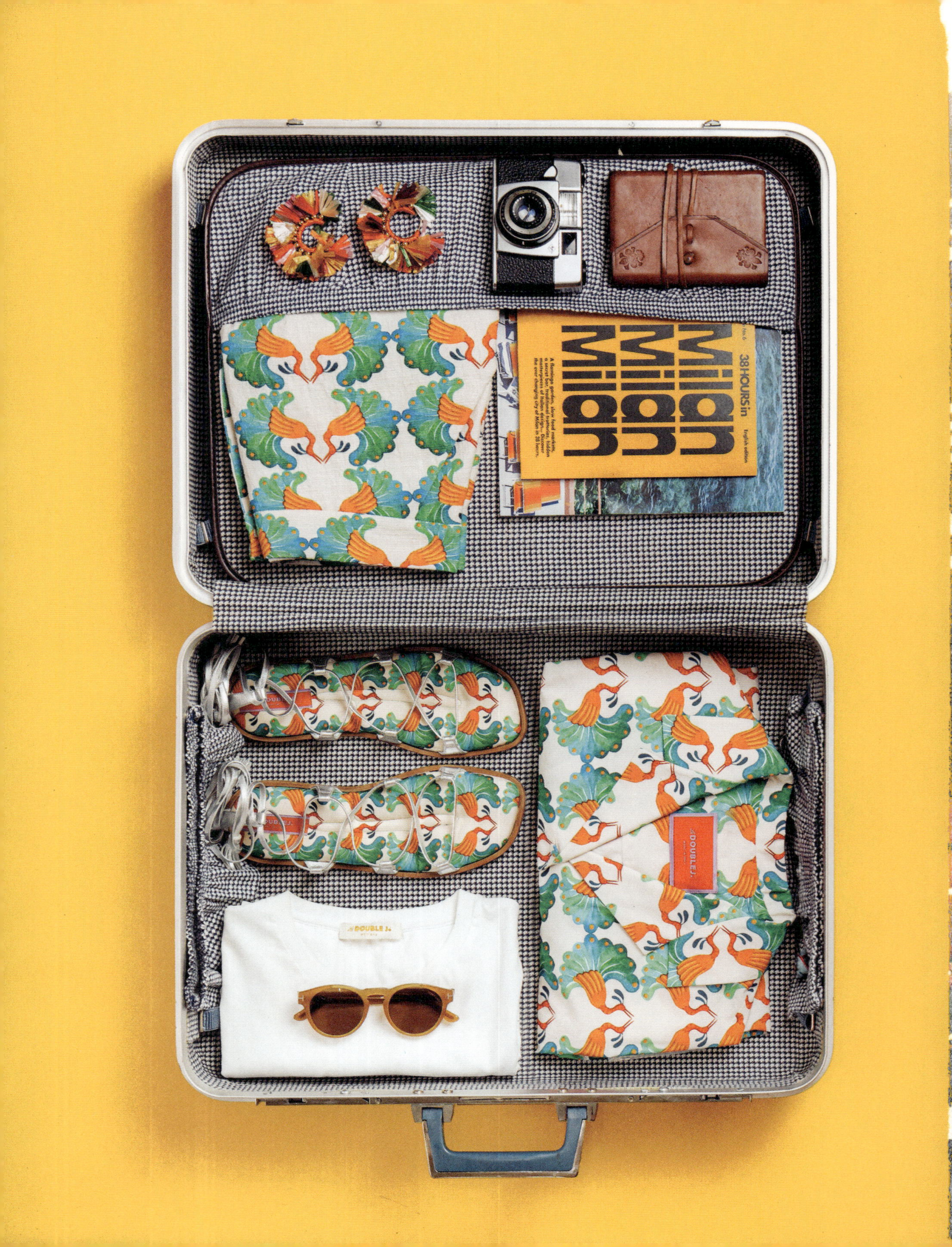
38 HOURS in
Milan
Milan
Milan

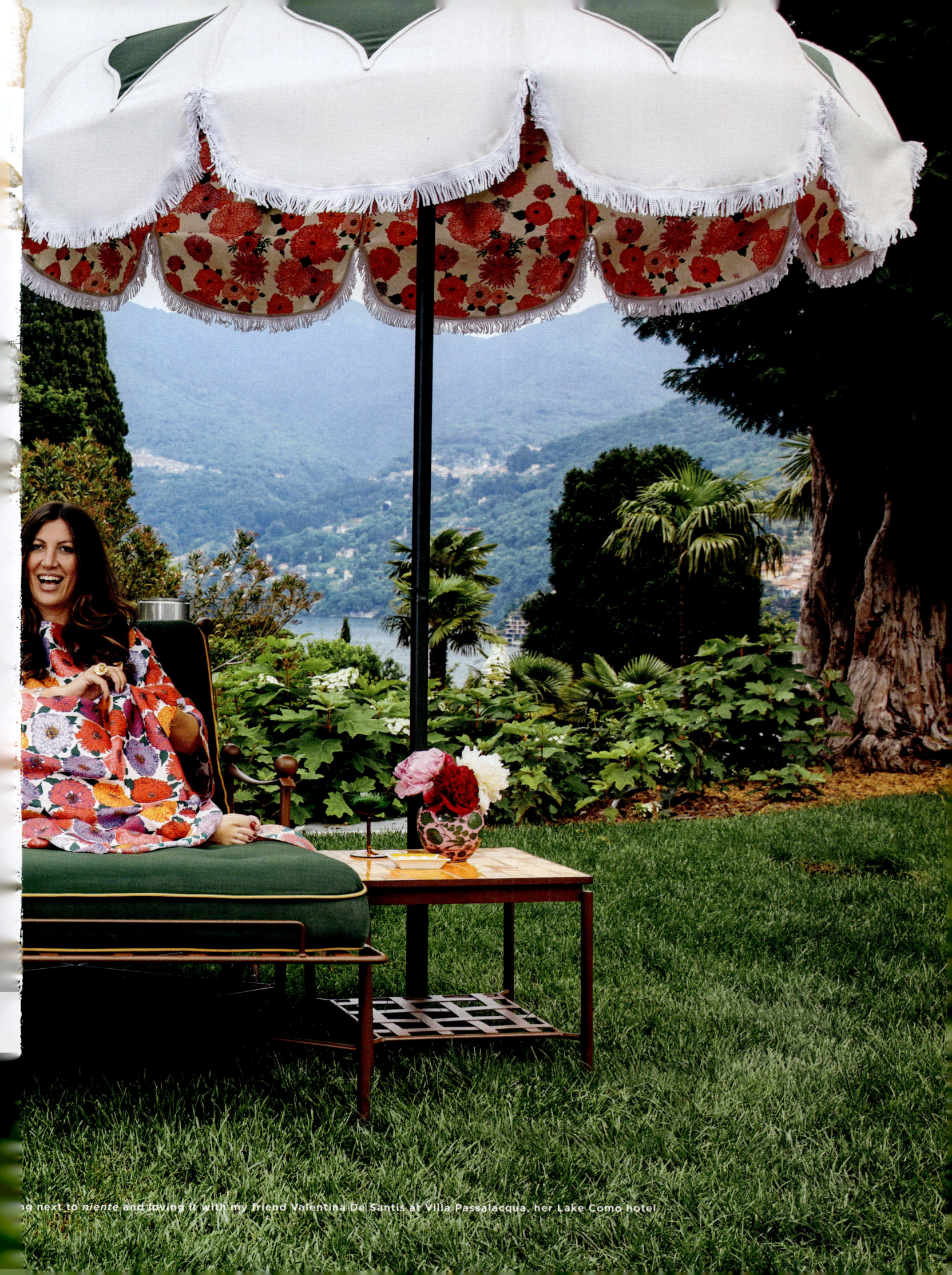

...ng next to niente and loving it with my friend Valentina De Santis at Villa Passalacqua, her Lake Como hotel

LESSON 25

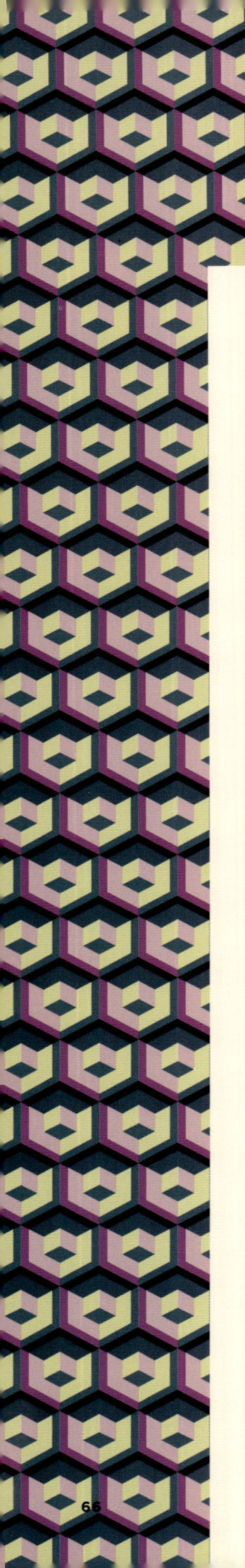

MANGIA!

Eating and feeding in Italy is really all about love

Cooking in Italy is resolutely an art, not a science. You will get laughed out of town if you tell anyone that you've made your meal from a recipe. I know this is true because it has happened to me—many times. "What? You mean this was the first time you've ever made it?" exclaimed one guest at my home after I admitted that the pork loin stuffed with escarole, raisins, olives, and pine nuts that we had just eaten had come from a cookbook I'd picked up in Pesaro. I am positive she was giving me the Italian no-no-no finger wag under the table.

When I first moved to Milan, I couldn't cook at all. There was no take-out food or prepared meals at the grocery store. I ate out at a restaurant every single night except Sundays, when I splurged on a pizza (the only food Italians deemed appropriate for delivery). Growing up in LA in the '80s and '90s, my brothers and I were busy with our sports schedules and were sent to school with giant Gelson's market bags stuffed with two sandwiches, chips, cookies, fruit, and a thermos filled with hot Stouffer's *fettuccine Alfredo* that I woolfed down at 5:00 p.m. every day in the car before my three-hour daily gymnastics practice. Food was fuel, it was eaten fast, and later in my college years, it was fraught with judgment (bad = fatty, good = sugar free).

But I was a high achiever, so when I got to Italy, I ordered the *Dean & Deluca Cookbook* and devoured it every night in bed like a romance novel. I spent hours studying these twenty-five-ingredient concoctions, not understanding that this was merely America's idea of what Italian cooking should be. In Italy, cooking comes from the heart, from the belly; never from the head. It is an intimate, slowly savored, seated-at-a-table experience of giving and receiving.

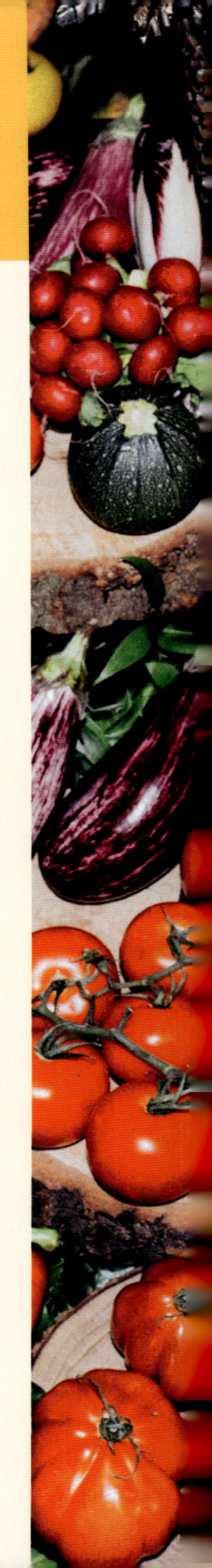

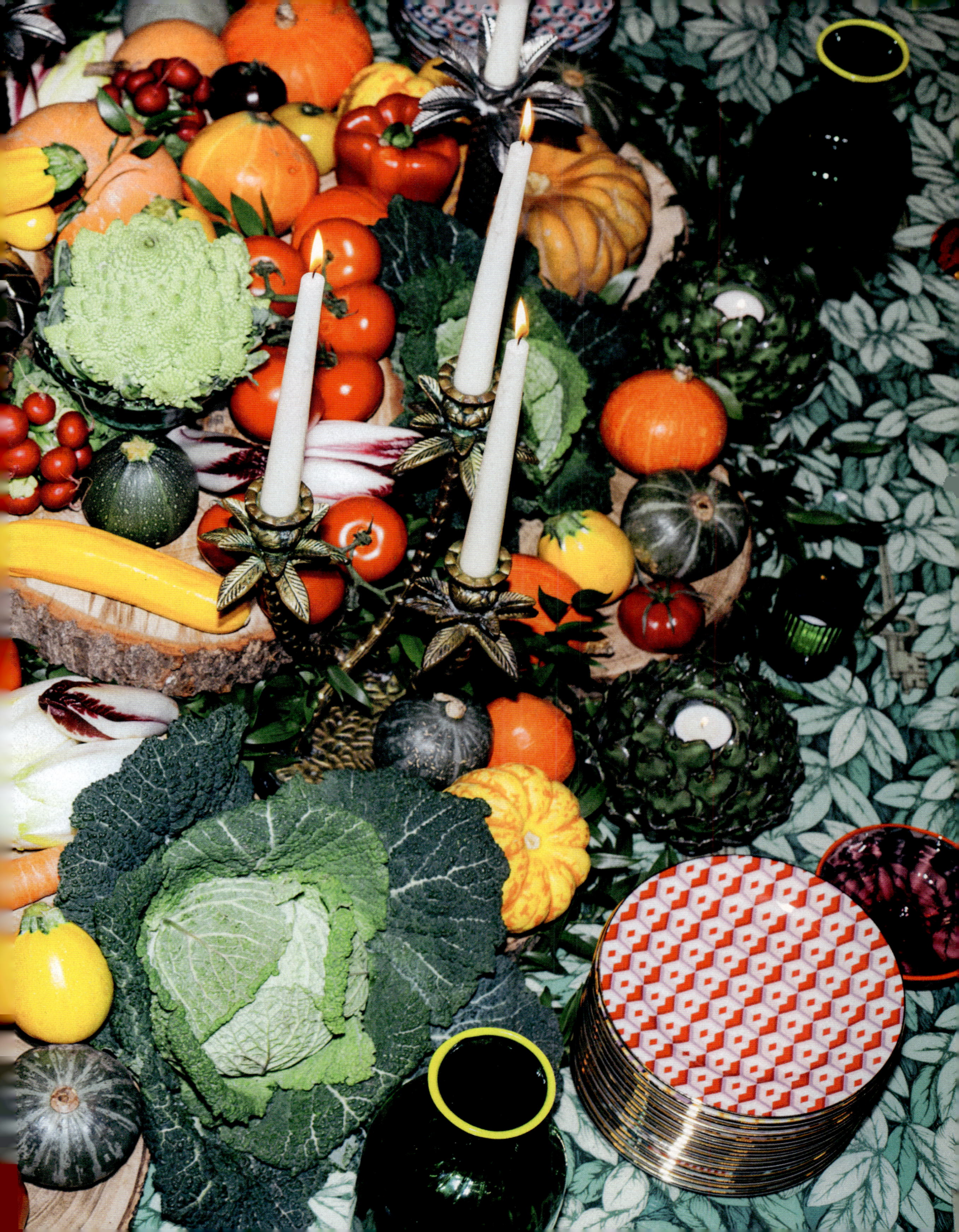

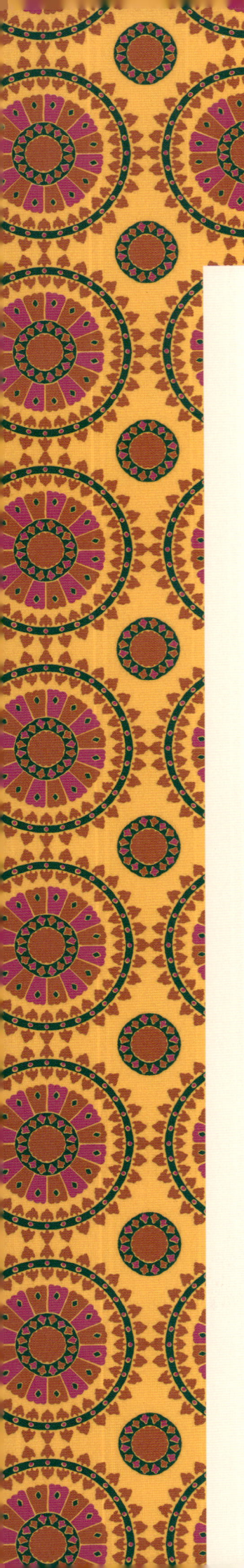

Every self-respecting Italian knows how to cook, *obviously*. Their mother taught them how to whip up dinner blindfolded by the age of ten. Then their grandmother brought out the black-belt family recipes of homemade pastas without even a bowl or a measuring spoon in sight. Cooking is a legacy, and a gift from one family member to the next.

Food in Italy is strictly localized. Whatever grandmothers are making in Puglia, grandmothers in Liguria have never heard of, never tasted, and definitely wouldn't like. There is immense pride in the local fifty-mile radius of culinary traditions. Is your *piadina* made with olive oil or *strutto*? Did you add oregano to the sauce? You did? Why?! Everyone is convinced of the superiority of their local *sughi*, the shape of their handmade pasta, and the aroma of their mother's *brodo*. Do not attempt to convince them otherwise.

ninety-three consists of cookies dunked in milk, or sweet croissants called brioche or, in the south, *cornetti* in big bowls of milky coffee.)

The way Italians make food is the same way they make friends or approach their free time: they go with the flow, they follow their hearts. They are guided by the seasons of Mother Nature, moving with their stomachs, not their heads. Sometimes it's messy, or late, or imperfect, but feeling your way through the process is the gift of it.

Italians don't like big supermarkets. They want to have a relationship with the person who sells them their meat, their cheese, their vegetables, and their fish; none of these people are found under a single roof. They don't want to be pinned down to a plan, a timetable, or the number of guests who will arrive for a meal. That's why they always

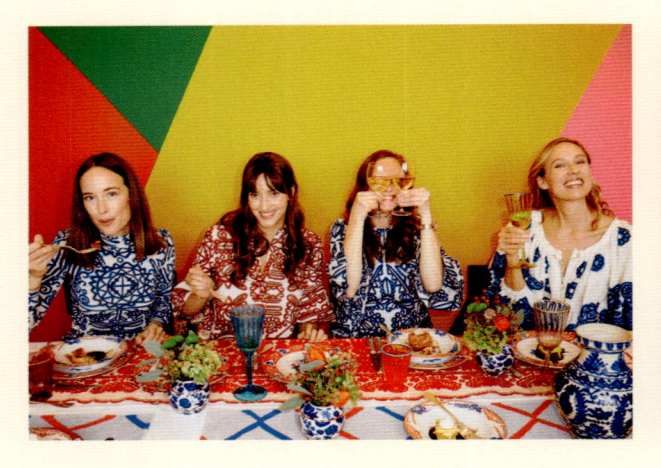

When we talk about food in Italy, we are taking about something more than just sustenance or nutrition. It is nourishment. It is nurturing! It is another expression of the Divine Mother, who glues Italians together in her sticky web of perfectly al dente pasta and forces them to sit together, stay, relax, and receive.

Food is also a portal to opening all the sensory receptors in your own body, letting your taste buds come alive with the flavors and fragrances of Italy. The magnificent, sweet ruby-red tomatoes and the warm nuttiness of an artichoke is an earthly delight. And there's no better place to allow this to unfold than in Italy. (The exception is breakfast! The first meal of the day for all Italians aged three to

prepare extra and why plus-ones were always showing up to my home unannounced, whether I was having a big buffet for forty or a sit-down dinner for ten. That unpredictability used to frustrate me no end. But, eventually, I realized that food is actually a special member of the family, as beloved and essential as *La Nonna*.

It is here in Italy that I have learned the true taste of food: that tomatoes can be as sweet as pears, that fresh egg yolks are actually orange in color, that olive oil can be more seductive than a lover.

And the way you learn to cook in Italy is by watching the Italians in action.

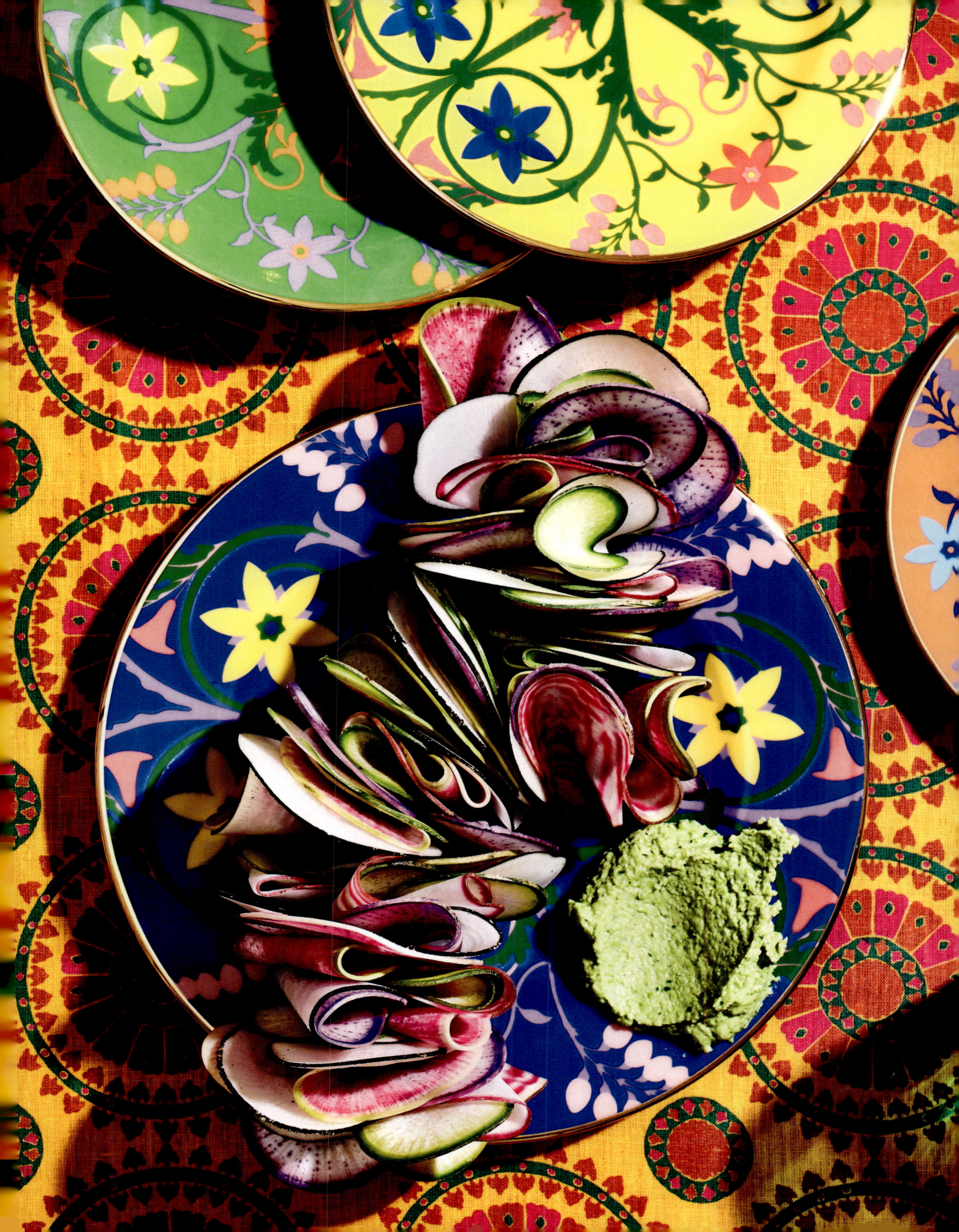

MAMMA MILANO

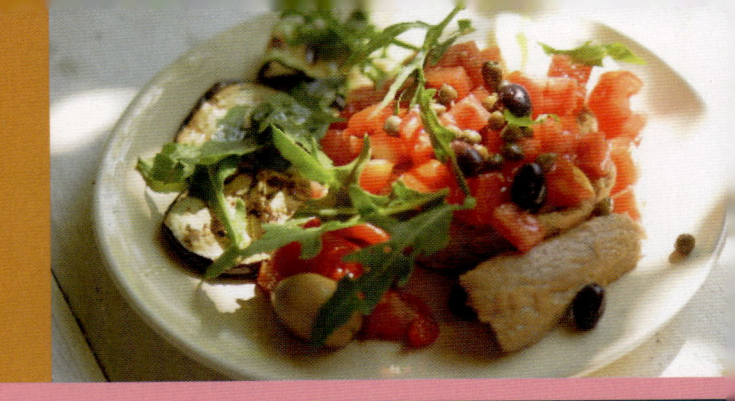

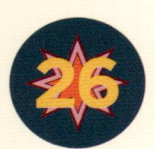

LESSON 26
IN THE KITCHEN WITH THE *ZIE*

Built from huge slabs of local stone, *masserie* are centuries-old block-like structures unique to Puglia, with tiny windows and unembellished, often crumbling, exteriors. Sometimes they have the grand air of a medieval fortress, other times they appear to be nothing more than a bombed-out war shelter. But they are spectacular in their simplistic beauty. Inside, the scene is often majestic, with seventeenth-century soaring vaulted ceilings, airy rooms, and the natural temperature regulation system unique to buildings with walls that are five feet thick.

My favorite *masseria* has a rare, prized position right on the emerald sea in Otranto. It belongs to Carlo and Ennio Capasa, who founded the Italian fashion label Costume National (where I worked for my first nine months in Milan). Though the south of Italy is packed with men oozing machismo through their bronzed pores, deep down everyone knows it's the women who run the show.

All the power in this soaring citadel is ceded to four silver-haired grandmothers, built like blocks of limestone and sheathed exclusively in black.

The matriarch of the group is Maria Luisa, an eighty-year-old woman with a magnificent Roman nose and a virtually lineless face, quenched for nearly a century with gallons of raw extra virgin olive oil. She is Carlo and Ennio's mother, and commands the *masseria* as if it were her own stone castle. In reality, she is a widow who lives in the Baroque city of Lecce, where she ran a high-fashion boutique called Smart for fifty years. On my first trip here almost twenty years ago, we ate fresh fava beans and enormous pea pods pulled out from the wild vegetable patch that runs alongside the house. Maria Luisa had driven forty-five minutes from Lecce just to shuck those beans and make her sons' soup. After brief instructions—the *ricotta* was NOT to be put in the refrigerator under any circumstances—she returned home.

The food in Puglia is my favorite in all of Italy. It is a vegetarian's paradise: crunchy *friselle di orzo* that are dunked in water, lathered in pungent olive oil and sea salt, then drizzled with candy sweet tomatoes and spicy arugula; the two-hours-old warm sheep's *ricotta* that you spoon directly into your mouth for breakfast; the authentic, tooth-cracking *taralli* crackers (an essential ingredient to any successful *aperitivo* spread). And Carlo and Ennio's three *zie* (aunts), scattered across Italy's heel, are the best cooks in the region.

Anytime the brothers came down for the weekend, alone or with twenty other relatives (only a quarter of the full Capasa clan), plates of freshly prepared food magically started appearing throughout the day. A rich pizza *rustica* on a huge tray made by Zia Annunziata with flour that's been ground the week before by a neighbor in Otranto. Twenty pounds of tissue-thin *lasagna*, a 150-year-old

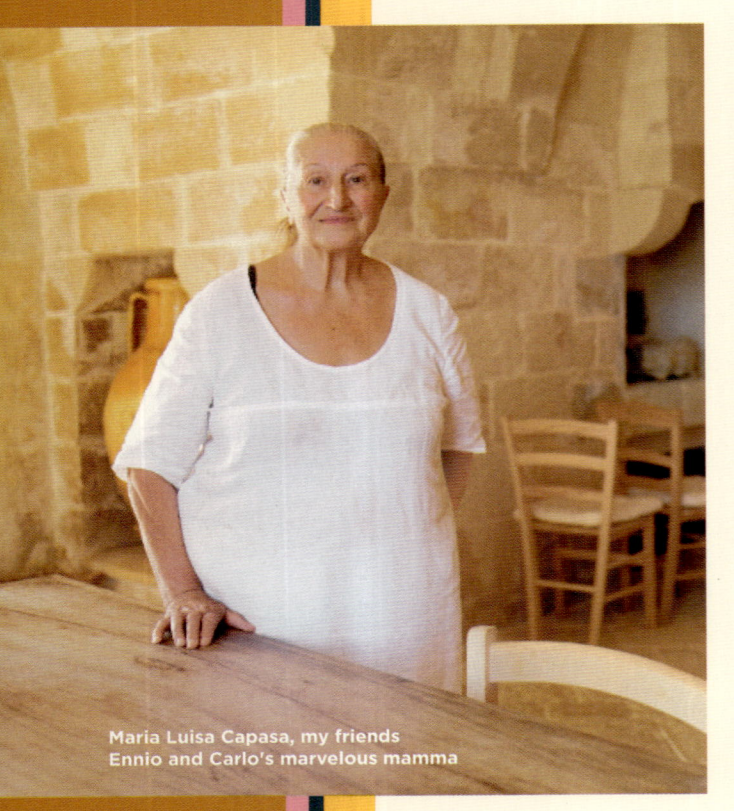

Maria Luisa Capasa, my friends Ennio and Carlo's marvelous mamma

70

ITALIAN LESSONS

recipe with three cheeses, meatballs, *mortadella*, and pasta that Zia Franca rolls out herself. A big pot of olive and caper-flavored *peperonata*. I would stand in the kitchen and watch Maria Louisa dig her hands into mountains of raw ground veal to make her pan-fried meatballs, or squeeze fat chunks of lamb to make her *agnello agli agrumi*. These are hugely time-consuming culinary constructions that the *zie* managed to whip up with half an eye open before breakfast, never consulting any sort of written recipe.

The very first thing I ever learned to cook in Italy was a traditional *peperonata* (sweet bell peppers cooked in olive oil), taught to me by the seventy-something Zia Annunziata while we sat on the beach—her smoking a cigarette in a bikini, me trying desperately to decode her vague instructions... *Just start with some oil in the pan, as much as you need. Some capers, some* taggiasche *olives, a sprinkling of breadcrumbs.* How much, exactly? *Just eyeball it*, she insisted. I never did get precise quantities, but went home, pulled out my pans, approximated the whole thing, and in spite of my doubts, it worked out beautifully. In that moment of following my gut, reaching into my own body's instinctive recipe system, I was initiated in the art of Italian cooking.

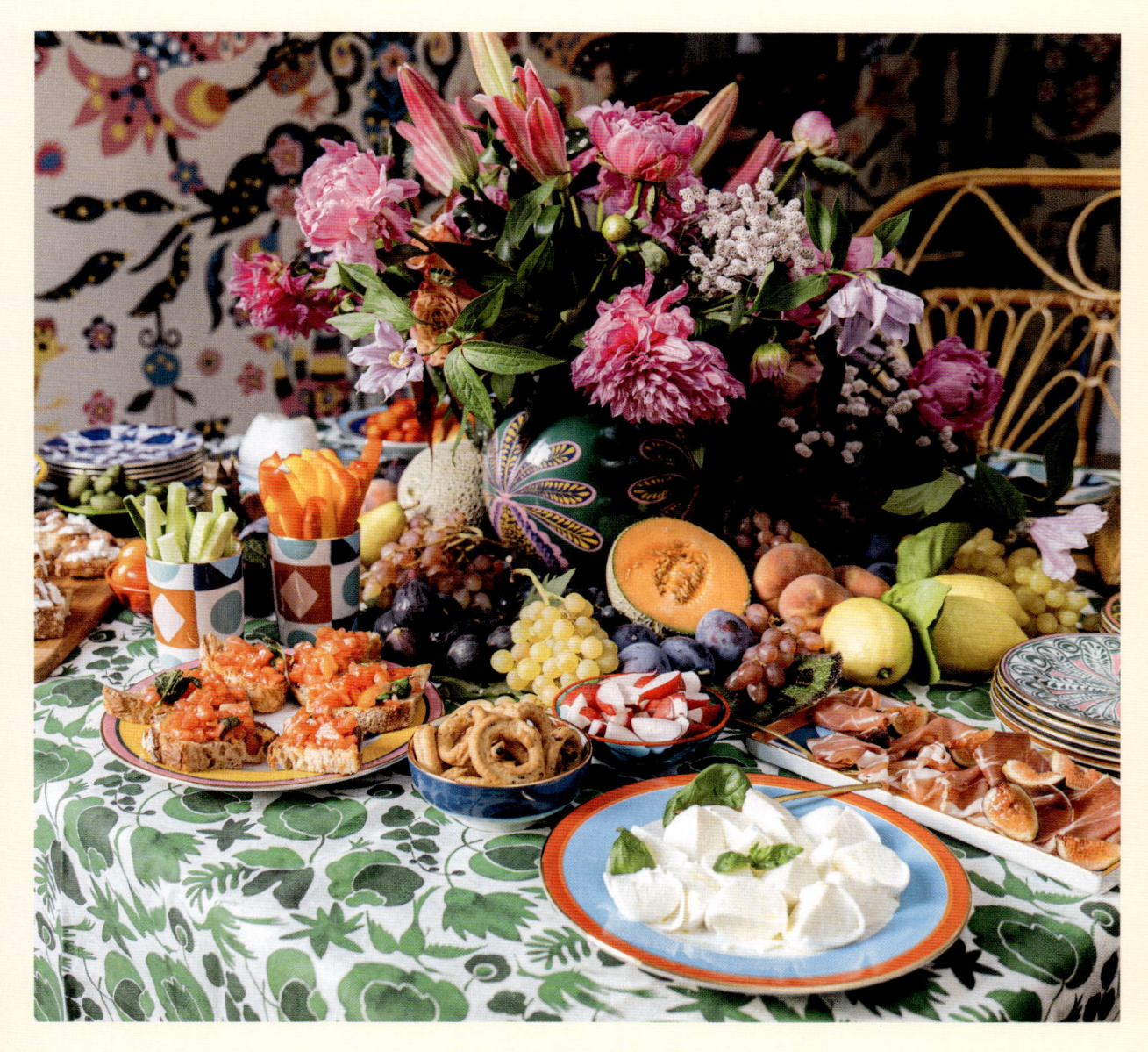

KITCHEN CONFIDENCE-IAL

Everything I learned from watching Italians doing their thing in the kitchen

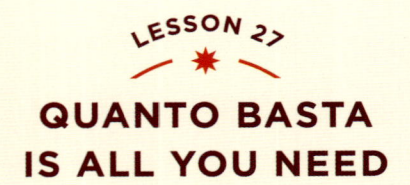

LESSON 27

QUANTO BASTA IS ALL YOU NEED

Italian cooking can be summed up by "QB", two letters taught to me by Tano, my first and only cooking teacher, in a class I took at his restaurant Tano Passami L'olio in Milan. It stands for *quanto basta*, a common qualifier among Italian chefs that means "as much as necessary." In Italy, no one tells you to "start with three tablespoons of oil in your pan," but rather to "start with as much oil as necessary."

At the start of each of our twelve classes, Tano would distribute copies of recipes in which the entire page was filled with ingredients and a crooked column of QBs. Italians love a handful of that, a fistful of this; they like to fill the water in the pan three fingers above the beans, with no idea of how many beans you actually need. "Cook it until it's done!" Tano would thunder at me with a happy shoulder shake. As an American, I like reliability. How on earth was I going to be able to guarantee a good outcome? In Italy there are no guarantees, just a willingness to try, to taste, to smell, and to allow in what wants to come through.

In the years since, and after being guided by the *zie* and other carefree, confident cooks, I've learned to prepare meals spontaneously, without the chokehold of any recipe or measurement. I just follow my heart and stomach.

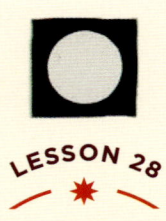

LESSON 28

KEEP IT SUPER SIMPLE

Once I was a guest at the home of Cristiana Ruella, who at the time was managing director of Dolce & Gabbana. When we arrived, she had walked in from the office minutes before in a skin-tight pencil skirt, silk blouse, and what looked like twenty-inch heels. As if it were the most effortless thing in the world, she waltzed up to her Poliform kitchen counter and showed me how to make a broccoli *pesto* in fifteen minutes.

Frozen broccoli was pulled from the freezer and dumped into boiling water, while a pan of hot oil simmered with four dried crumbled *peperoncino* and three garlic cloves (that had to be removed before the broccoli was satuéed and later smashed up with a wooden paddle). That was the first time I realized that Italians like to make sauces in the same exact time it takes to boil the water and cook the *tagliatelle*, so everything is completed at once.

If you put too many ingredients in one dish, an Italian will tell you it ruins the flavor. Then again, a tomato or a fava bean tastes so good in Italy, you don't need to add much to enhance it. The flavors are already so bright and zingy, they coax the purity of the ingredients forth.

ITALIAN LESSONS

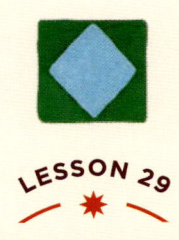

LESSON 29
EAT IT WHEN IT GROWS

In Italy, you would never, ever serve a mushroom in summer or sprinkle pomegranate seeds into a salad in the spring—out-of-season fruits and vegetables are no-nos. Actually, you can't even if you wanted to, because they simply aren't available. And of course, the highest-quality raw materials (fruits, vegetables, meats, fish, and herbs bursting with life force) are absolute requirements for every meal.

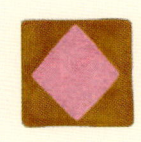

LESSON 30
REPEAT SO MANY TIMES YOU CAN DO IT BLINDFOLDED

The first time I ever met Andrea's grandmother, she was ninety-five years old. We went to her tiny fifty-person town, Mercatino Conca in Le Marche, to visit her. She jumped up from the lumpy couch and immediately began to make fresh *piadina* in honor of our arrival. Her eyes barely topped the kitchen counter. Her arms shot up and she whipped the whole thing up without even needing to see what she was doing.

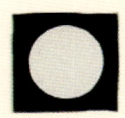

Yes, I did learn a few recipes by heart that I pull out when guests spontaneously show up at my apartment for dinner—from Cristiana's broccoli *risotto* to Maria Luisa's *peperonata*. I stashed all of my back-pocket recipes inside a banged-up notebook that I keep in my kitchen drawer.

LESSON 31
TREAT OLIVE OIL LIKE FINE WINE

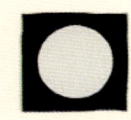

Olive oil is beyond food—it's a teleporter, it's a state of mind. Each one brings a whole bouquet, place, and experience to what you're eating. You use some for raw food, you use some to cook, you use some to dress a salad, and some—delicate as a petal—as a final flourish. At Tano Passami L'olio, where more than two hundred olive oils lined the restaurant walls, every single dish we made required a different olive oil. I could smell the grapes or the pepper in one, a tomatoey finish in another.

In America I had a fear of oil making me fat. Now, I dump raw olive oil on top of vegetables or a salad or pasta that I'm about to eat as if I'm filling up my car with gas. It's so good for you, I drink the stuff like water. I can't bear to have it in America if it has no flavor or scent.

LESSON 32
THERE ARE NO SECRETS

In Italy, there is complete generosity in sharing culinary wisdom. No one hoards a recipe. Once I realized this, I began to interview everyone and anyone who prepared something I liked. On my first trip to Pantelleria, I sat down in a six-table restaurant near the port and ate the best caper-olive-tomato pasta of my life. I walked into the tiny steaming kitchen to interview the cook on how he made it. He was delighted and shared with me every little detail while he stirred his sauce; the trick was, as in all Italian recipes, getting the right raw materials. The capers had to be from Pantelleria and packed in salt, the olives had to be *taggiasche*, and the purple onions had to be as sweet as apples.

Luckily, Esselunga, Italy's national supermarket chain, had all three when I was back in Milan! Now this is one of my go-to recipes for dinner parties.

MAMMA MILANO

LESSON 33
DON'T SWEAT THE FU*% UPS

Cooking in Italy is wrapped in patience, acceptance and, very often, imprecision. My mother-in-law would say, "Oh, the *tagliatelle* came out good today." Or it came out bad—*brutto,* literally "ugly." It was never the fault of the recipe because there was no recipe—it was whether or not she was aligned in the kitchen with the task. Sometimes she wasn't. There was real tolerance for this from all eaters. I came from a fear-based American mentality that everything has to be perfect to be great, but I saw that it didn't have to be flawless every time. No one was judging; everyone was eating.

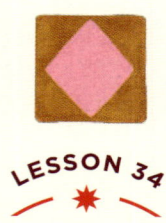

LESSON 34
LET COOKING FEED YOU CREATIVELY

At a certain point, I began to notice that making my own food became an enriching creative process. I would cook, write, and decorate my home (which I was always doing) all at the same time, and something started to brew and mix alchemically within me.

I learned that if you get blocked on one creative effort, you move on to another. So if I couldn't write, I would cook instead, which has a more reliable aspect to "creating." This would bring the joy factor up and put me into a state of pleasure flow, at which point I could sit back down and be receptive to writing. Later in my spiritual practice, I learned that there is a "creator state of consciousness"—another Divine Mother energetic—that can be tapped into for us to expand our creative faculties. Cooking was oil for that prolific machine.

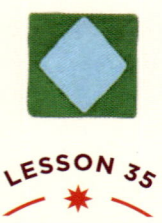

LESSON 35
DON'T SPEED THROUGH IT

Everyone sits down for every meal in Italy. There is no walking/eating, working/eating, driving/eating. There is no rush, ever. Not even in a restaurant. No one tries to kick you out of your seat so someone else can come for the next seating. This brings such a sense of relief to the proceedings, with no fear of the cut-off time, that everyone just melts into the scene and truly relaxes.

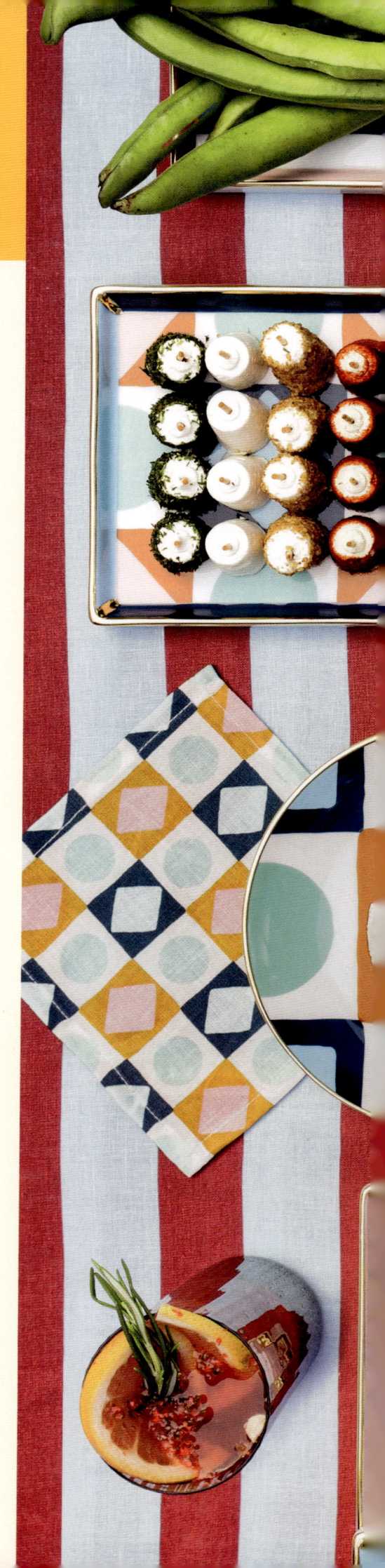

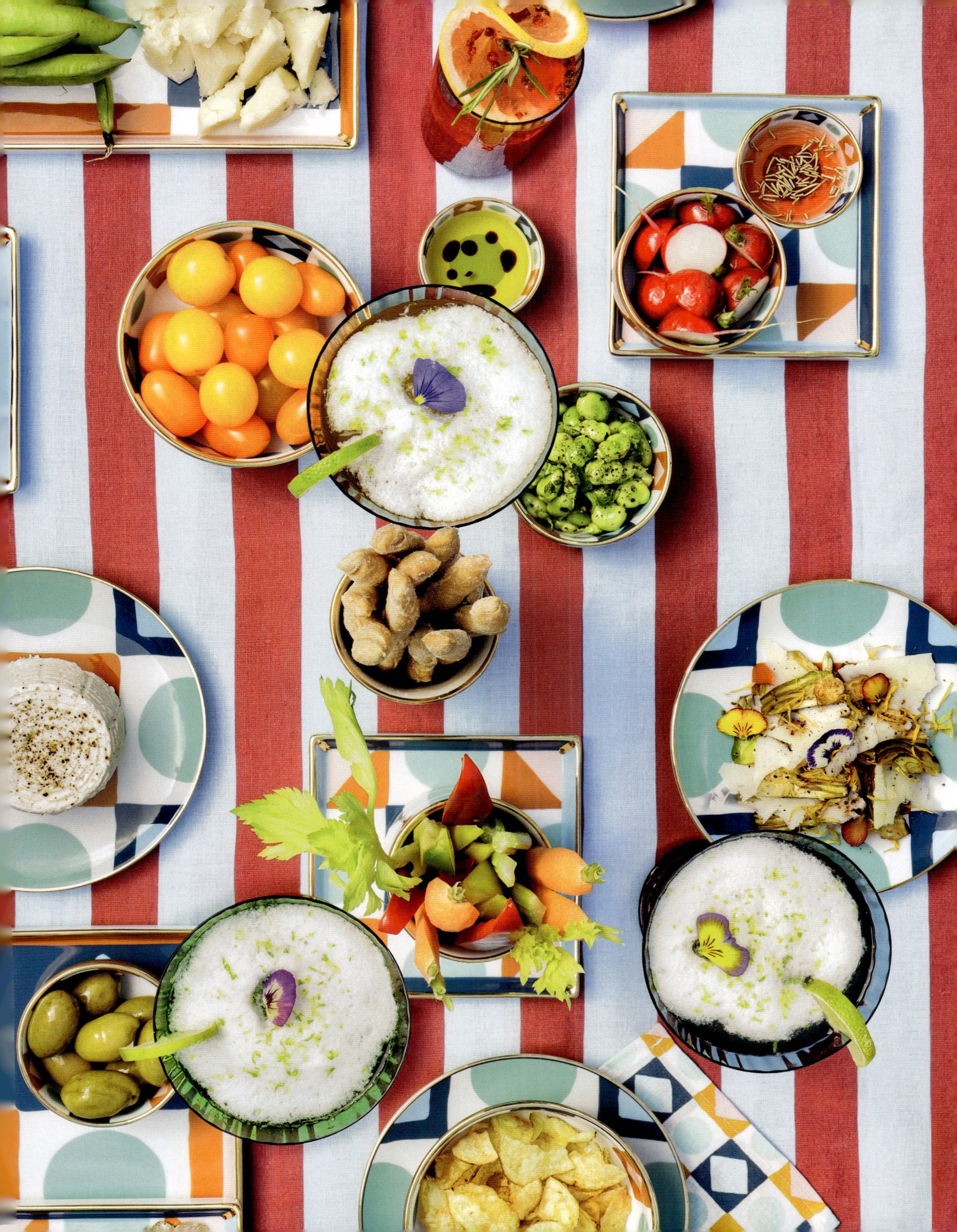

MAMMA MILANO

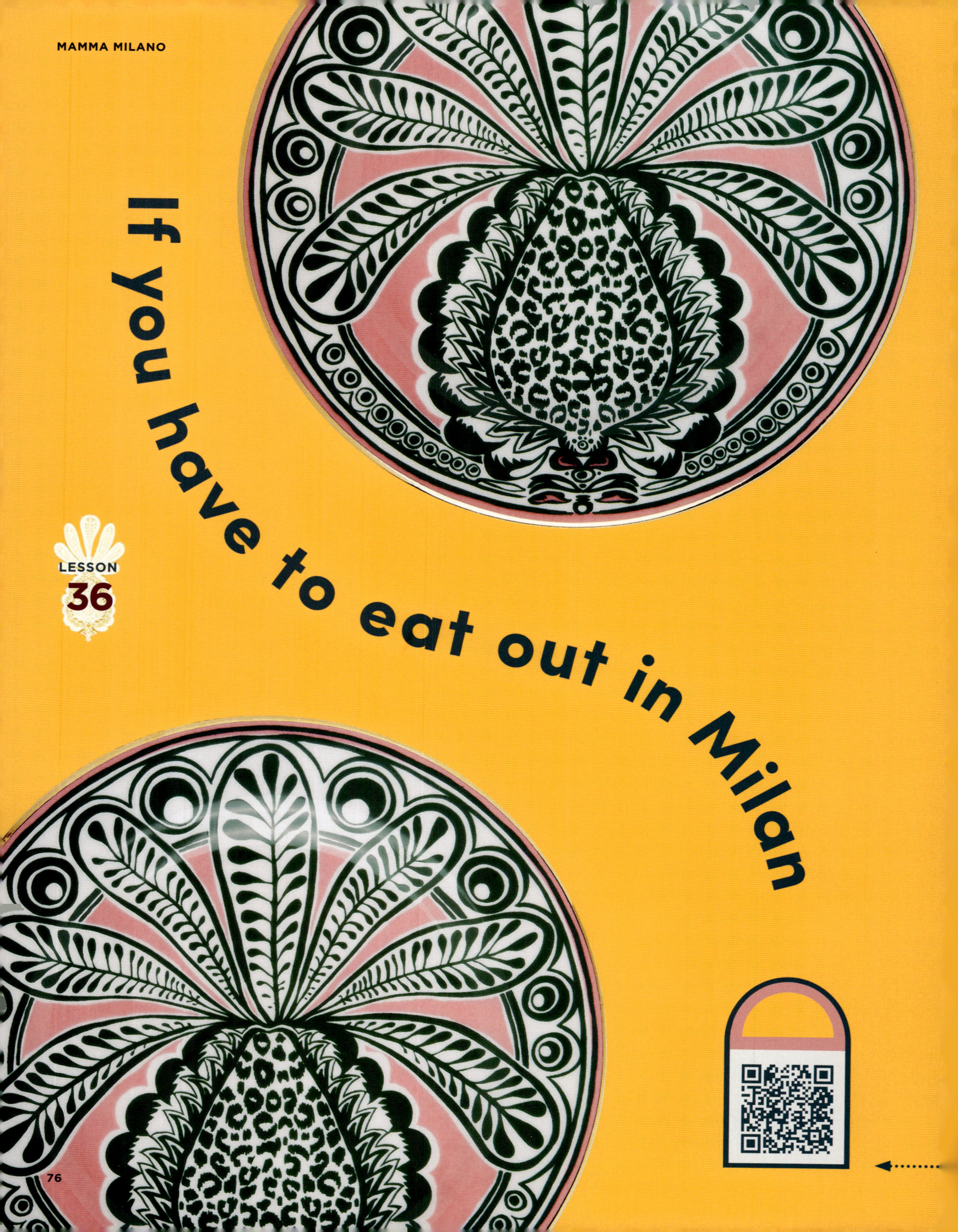

LESSON 36

If you have to eat out in Milan

Truthfully, it's not a very Milanese thing to eat out in restaurants. The real hotspots in town lie behind Fascist-era facades, up mid-century staircases, and inside beautifully appointed spaces in private homes. When I did go to restaurants in Milan, it would always be the same ones so that I could get that feeling like I was at home with people I knew. Also, the restaurant scene in Italy is nothing like it is in America—new places do not birth, explode, crash, and die the way they do in Manhattan or Los Angeles. They stick around for sixty years, never change the menu beyond the seasonal clock, and keep the same waiters for decades. But since everyone asks me, you can find my favorite Milanese spots, the friends in charge, and my go-to dishes, in our Milan Guide here.

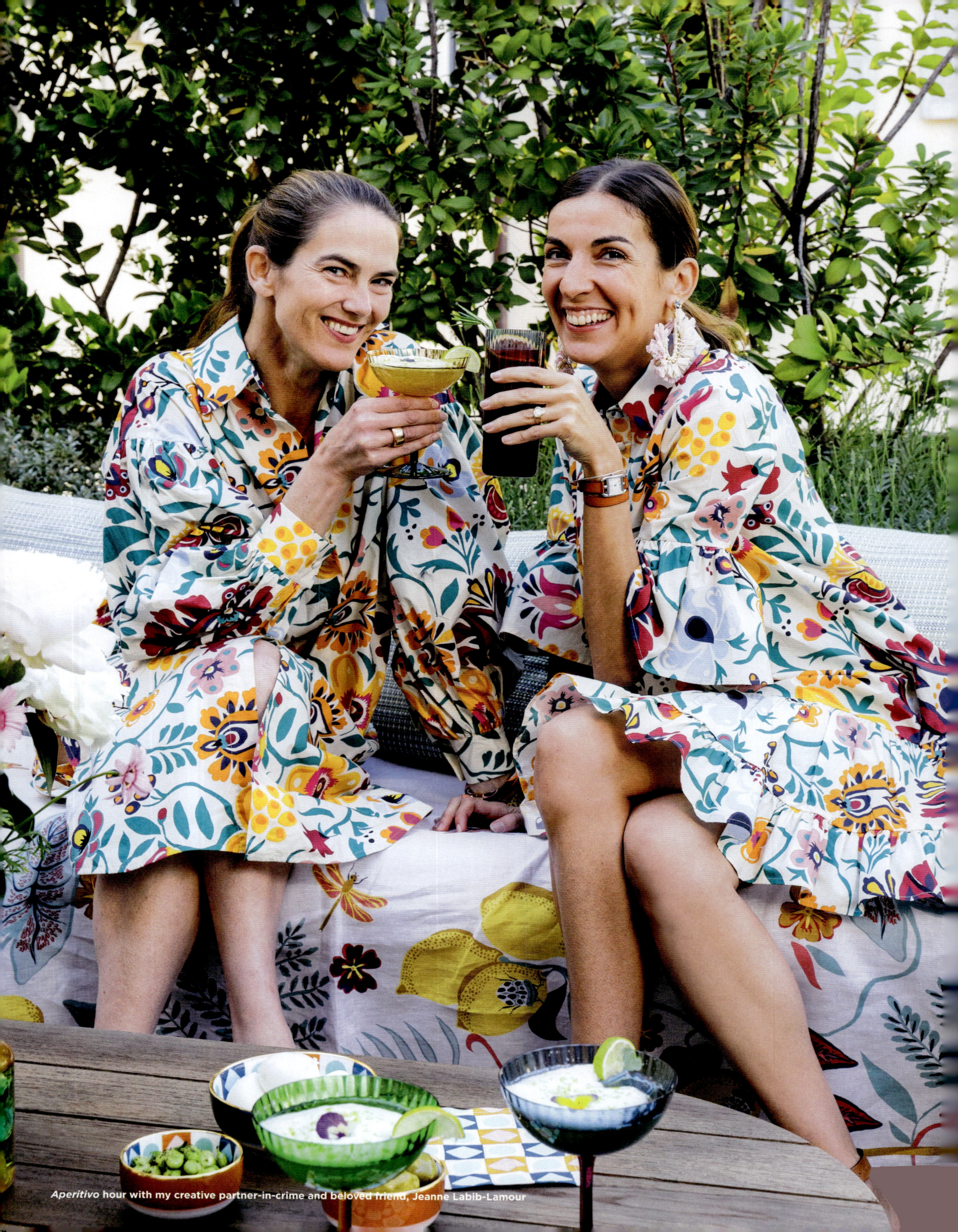

Aperitivo hour with my creative partner-in-crime and beloved friend, Jeanne Labib-Lamour.

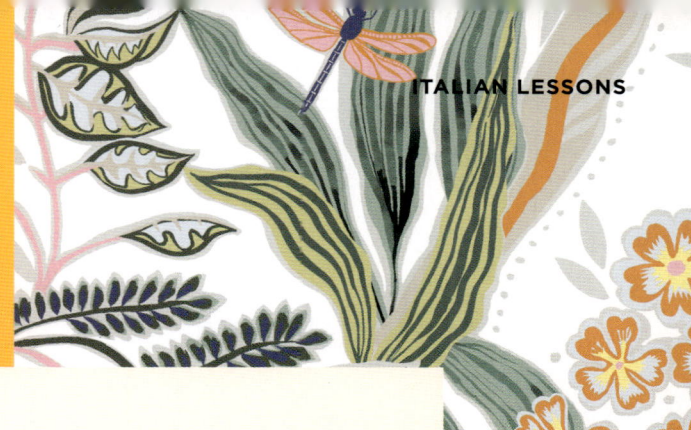

THE MORE, THE MERRIER

Learning how to cook was not just a nice thing to do, but a basic survival tool. The next step was learning how to invite other people into my home without a plan or a recipe.

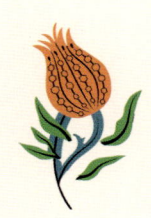

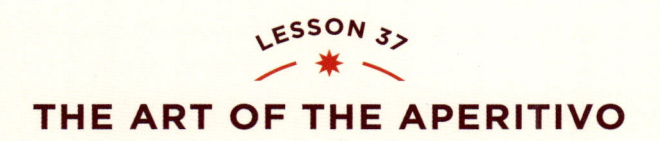

LESSON 37
THE ART OF THE APERITIVO

Aperitivo hour in Italy is a holy time. It lasts well over an hour and is always fortified with enough tasty treats to keep Americans like me from complaining about the late-night dinner time. The mark of an excellent Italian *aperitivo* is one that can be decided upon at the last minute (since no one likes a plan), and whipped up in less time than it takes to dry your wet hair.

A decent Italian kitchen pantry is always stocked with these essentials, so spontaneity is a cinch: awesome olives (always use the big, meaty ones); artisanal *taralli* crackers from Puglia; a towering hunk of eighteen-month aged Parmesan cheese that can hold ground like the Statue of Liberty inside your *frigo* all year round; a block of dry-aged meat (such as *bresaola*); a tasty vegetable submerged in a great olive oil (such as roasted artichoke or eggplant); crispy, artisanal-style potato chips; and a multi-grain, yummy seeded cracker.

These items last longer than most high-school romances, and because of their longevity, you can do what the Italians do and invite anyone over at any time without any prior grocery shopping.

The key element, like all things joyfully Italian, is the following mantra: the more the merrier! So be sure to stuff your cocktail table with as many tasty treats as possible, mix and match your printed napkins with your printed dishes, and always, always, always be willing and waiting for your friends to show up with unexpected guests. It's the best part of Italy's beautiful game.

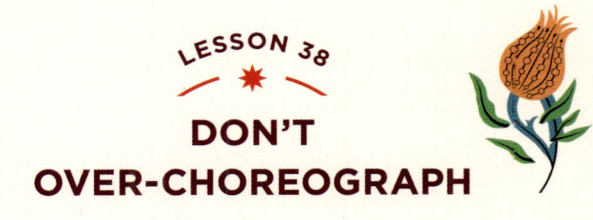

LESSON 38
DON'T OVER-CHOREOGRAPH

A healthy dose of serendipity does wonders for oiling up a rusty crowd, so you need to be flexible on format, timing, and attendees. Inevitably, half of your guests will be forty-five if not ninety minutes late. This is fine.

Also, it's practically guaranteed that one of them will bring another person to your house without any forewarning. These random extra people always end up spicing up the crowd stew. If you accept and embrace it, it boomerangs into something great. And, as I think I've mentioned before, don't plan your dinner too far in advance. No one can possibly know how they will feel about coming three weeks in advance.

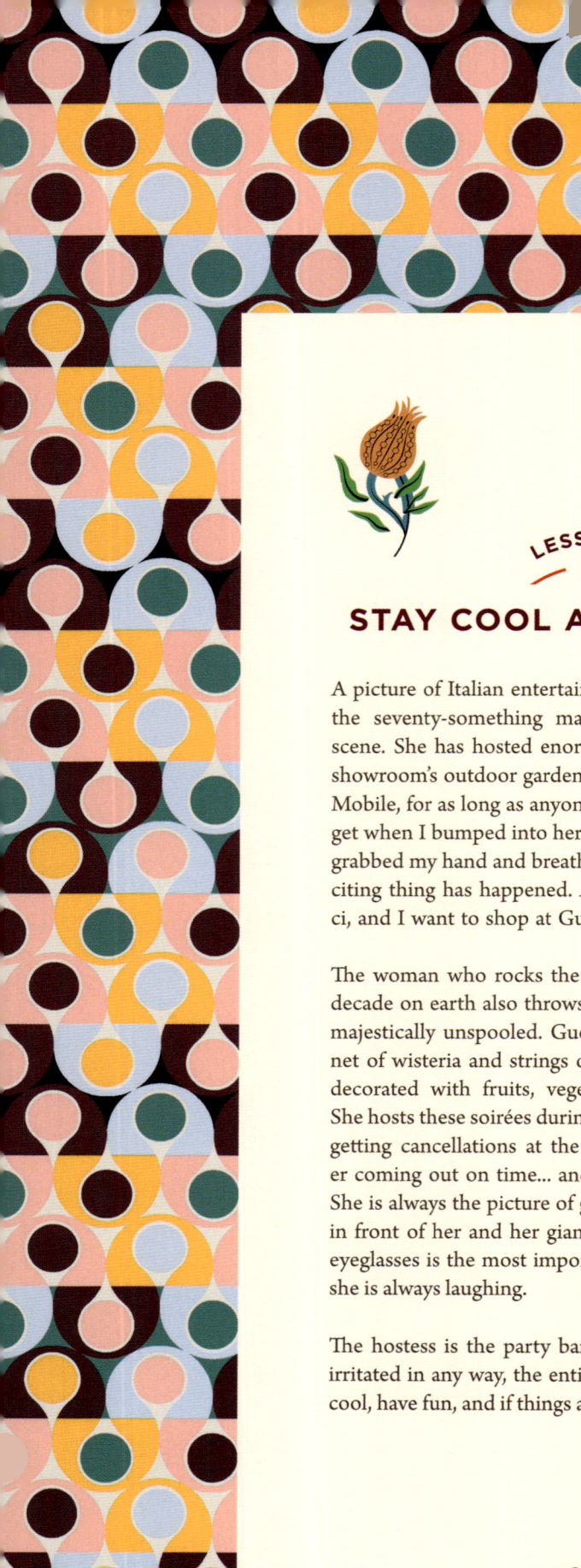

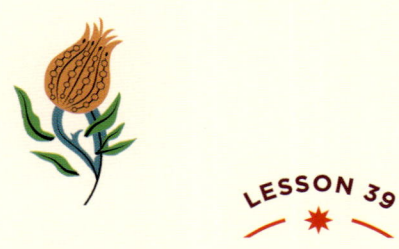

LESSON 39
STAY COOL AND HAVE FUN

A picture of Italian entertaining grace is Rossana Orlandi, the seventy-something matriarch of the Italian design scene. She has hosted enormous sit-down dinners in her showroom's outdoor garden every April for the Salone del Mobile, for as long as anyone can remember. I'll never forget when I bumped into her on the street in Milan and she grabbed my hand and breathlessly reported: "The most exciting thing has happened. Alessandro Michele is at Gucci, and I want to shop at Gucci again and get everything!"

The woman who rocks the Gucci runway in her seventh decade on earth also throws dinner parties that are just as majestically unspooled. Guests are always seated under a net of wisteria and strings of draped light bulbs, at tables decorated with fruits, vegetables, and lazy wildflowers. She hosts these soirées during Salone week, so she is always getting cancellations at the last minute, the food is never coming out on time... and Rossana could not care less. She is always the picture of grace and warmth. Whoever is in front of her and her giant, saucer-size, signature tinted eyeglasses is the most important person in the world, and she is always laughing.

The hostess is the party barometer—if she is stressed or irritated in any way, the entire party falls apart. Keep your cool, have fun, and if things are not perfect, just laugh.

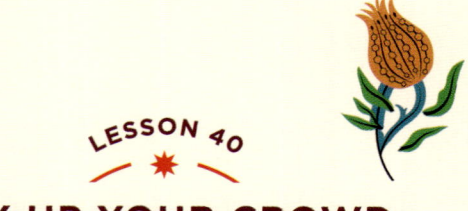

LESSON 40
MIX UP YOUR CROWD

At her dinners Rossana has a mix of big-name architects and furniture designers, journalists, friends, and Milanese locals. If you mingle people from different creative industries with old people, maybe add a finance guy, throw in a kid and dog, you've got an Italian guest list. Also, seated dinner parties are lovely for an intimate evening (I like eight, ten people max), but informal ones are way better. We all do better as butterflies.

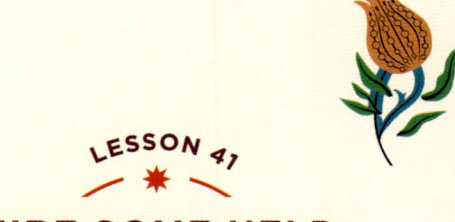

LESSON 41
HIRE SOME HELP

Most Italians have some kind of help in the house—this is not a bougie thing, it's cultural. You can cook to your heart's delight—which I do, and you should—but I learned that, in Italy, no guest wants to see a harried hostess carrying dishes back and forth and cleaning up the mounting mess. I actually use my sixty-eight-year-old door lady, who is thrilled to put her five decades of cooking experience to good use for a very reasonable rate. She's from Sardinia and does not know the meaning of light food. She prepares amazing *risotti*, *ossobuco*, veal cutlets, and pastas in my kitchen, and comes out for a reluctant bow afterwards.

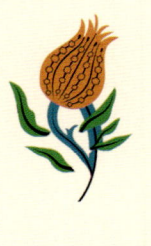

LESSON 42
...OR, PUT YOUR GUESTS TO WORK

When there isn't help, everyone joins in. But they need to be given roles. After being a guest at so many *casino* dinner operations—where everyone was in the kitchen—I began to assign duties and ask for opinions from my own guests. Most of the people coming to my house were way better cooks, with far more talented grandmothers, so I decided to put them to work co-creating the meal. One time I sent Carlo Clavarino, a very fancy-pants aristocrat (who always

ITALIAN LESSONS

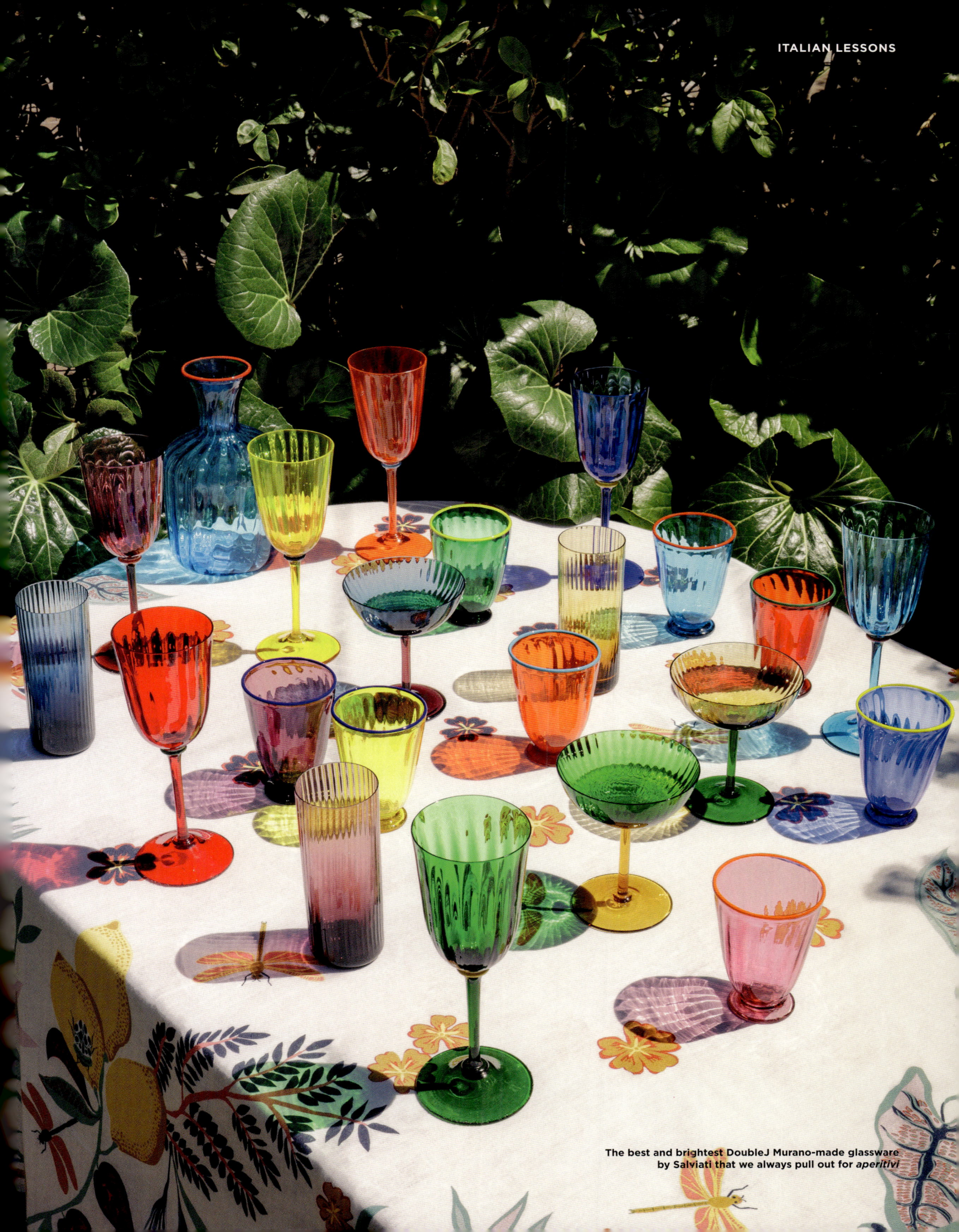

The best and brightest DoubleJ Murano-made glassware by Salviati that we always pull out for *aperitivi*

MAMMA MILANO

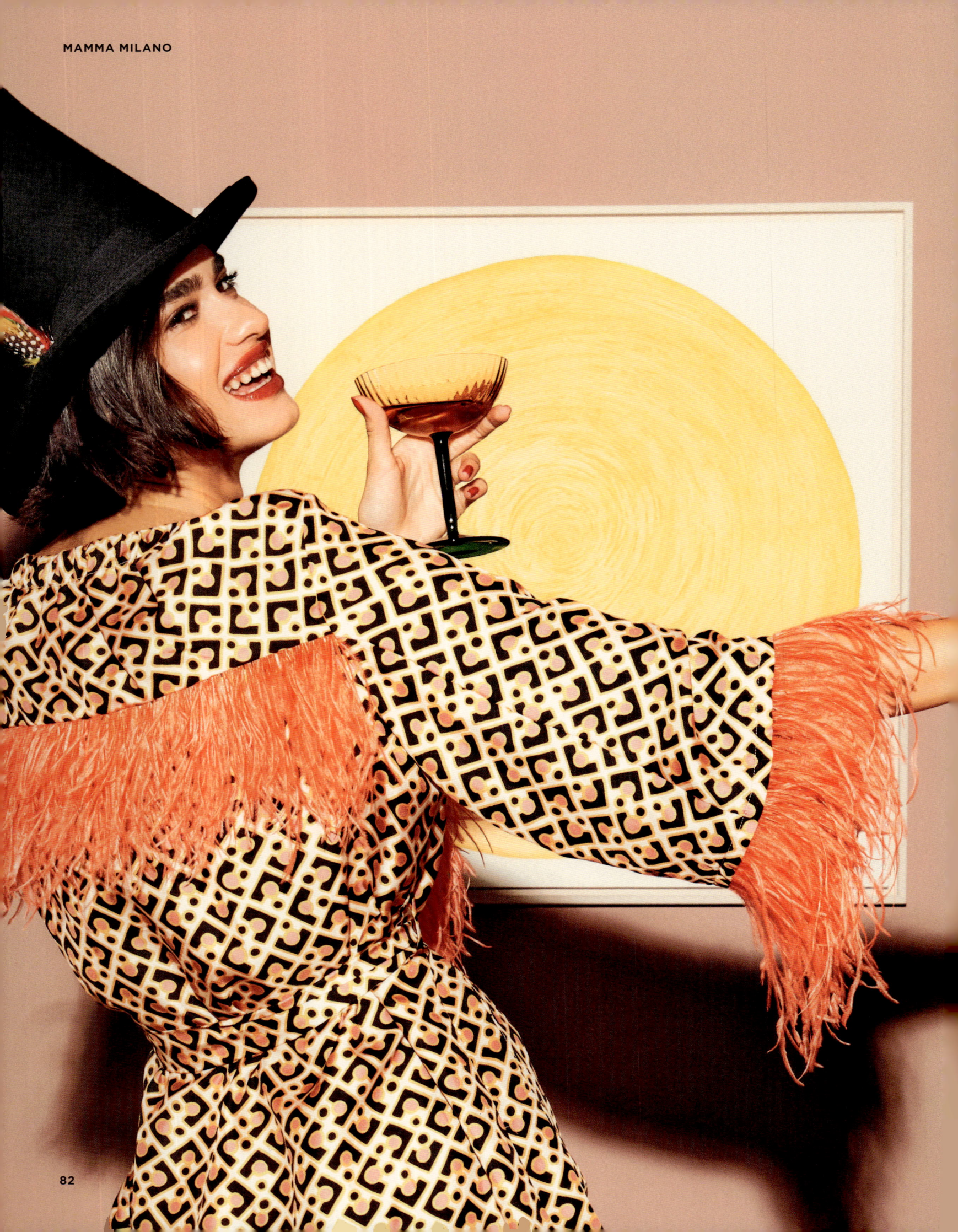

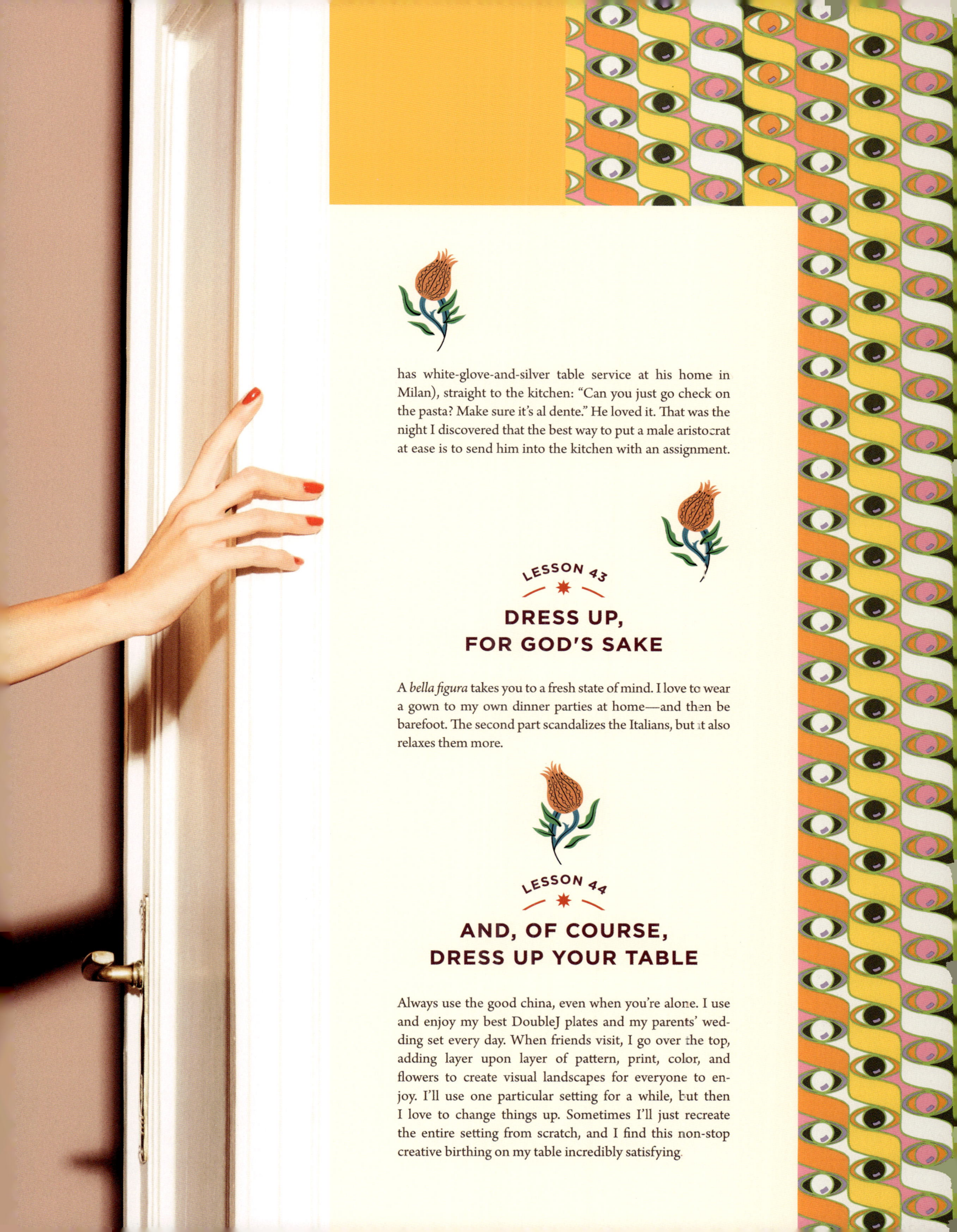

has white-glove-and-silver table service at his home in Milan), straight to the kitchen: "Can you just go check on the pasta? Make sure it's al dente." He loved it. That was the night I discovered that the best way to put a male aristocrat at ease is to send him into the kitchen with an assignment.

LESSON 43

DRESS UP, FOR GOD'S SAKE

A *bella figura* takes you to a fresh state of mind. I love to wear a gown to my own dinner parties at home—and then be barefoot. The second part scandalizes the Italians, but it also relaxes them more.

LESSON 44

AND, OF COURSE, DRESS UP YOUR TABLE

Always use the good china, even when you're alone. I use and enjoy my best DoubleJ plates and my parents' wedding set every day. When friends visit, I go over the top, adding layer upon layer of pattern, print, color, and flowers to create visual landscapes for everyone to enjoy. I'll use one particular setting for a while, but then I love to change things up. Sometimes I'll just recreate the entire setting from scratch, and I find this non-stop creative birthing on my table incredibly satisfying.

INTERMEZZO

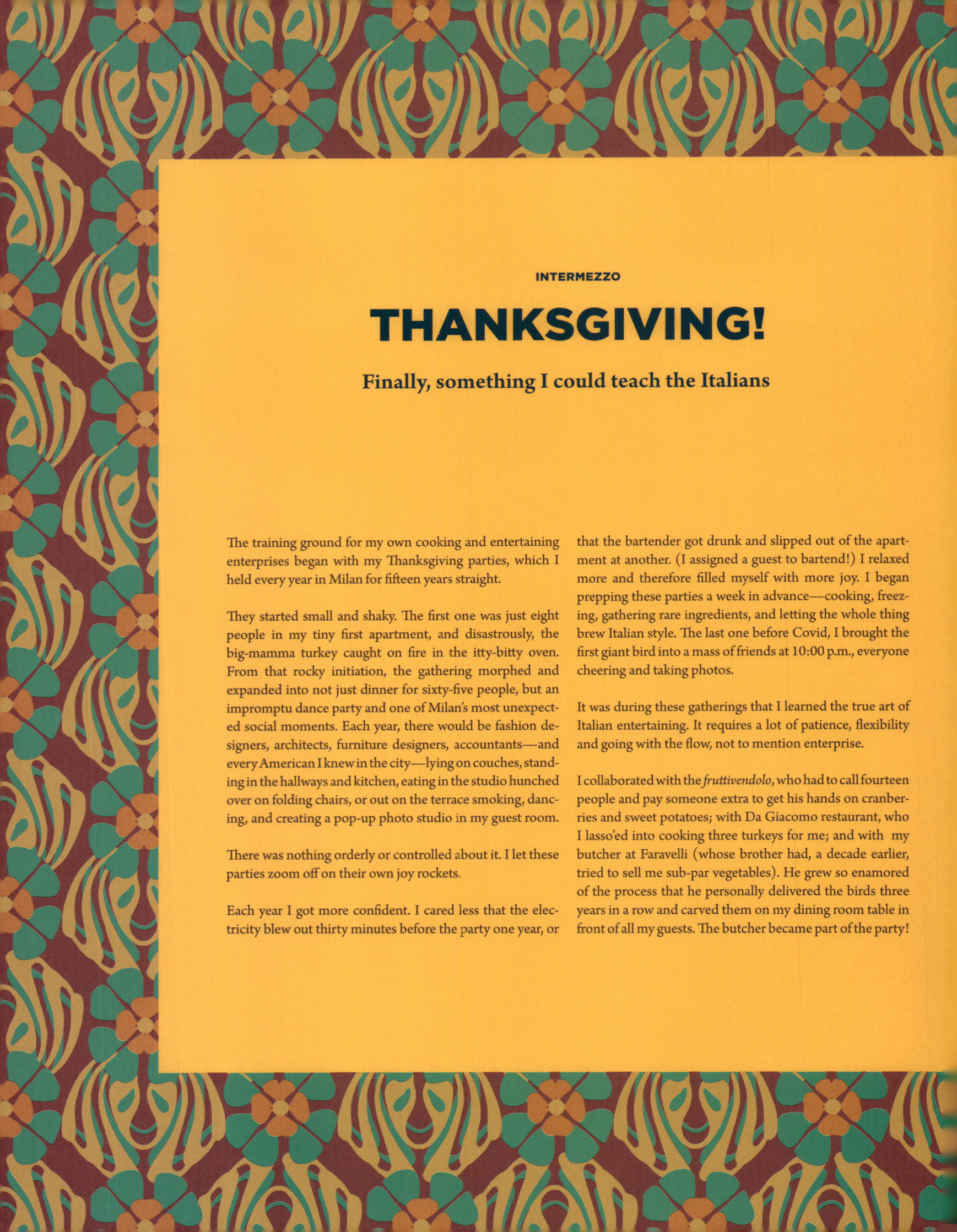

THANKSGIVING!

Finally, something I could teach the Italians

The training ground for my own cooking and entertaining enterprises began with my Thanksgiving parties, which I held every year in Milan for fifteen years straight.

They started small and shaky. The first one was just eight people in my tiny first apartment, and disastrously, the big-mamma turkey caught on fire in the itty-bitty oven. From that rocky initiation, the gathering morphed and expanded into not just dinner for sixty-five people, but an impromptu dance party and one of Milan's most unexpected social moments. Each year, there would be fashion designers, architects, furniture designers, accountants—and every American I knew in the city—lying on couches, standing in the hallways and kitchen, eating in the studio hunched over on folding chairs, or out on the terrace smoking, dancing, and creating a pop-up photo studio in my guest room.

There was nothing orderly or controlled about it. I let these parties zoom off on their own joy rockets.

Each year I got more confident. I cared less that the electricity blew out thirty minutes before the party one year, or that the bartender got drunk and slipped out of the apartment at another. (I assigned a guest to bartend!) I relaxed more and therefore filled myself with more joy. I began prepping these parties a week in advance—cooking, freezing, gathering rare ingredients, and letting the whole thing brew Italian style. The last one before Covid, I brought the first giant bird into a mass of friends at 10:00 p.m., everyone cheering and taking photos.

It was during these gatherings that I learned the true art of Italian entertaining. It requires a lot of patience, flexibility and going with the flow, not to mention enterprise.

I collaborated with the *fruttivendolo*, who had to call fourteen people and pay someone extra to get his hands on cranberries and sweet potatoes; with Da Giacomo restaurant, who I lasso'ed into cooking three turkeys for me; and with my butcher at Faravelli (whose brother had, a decade earlier, tried to sell me sub-par vegetables). He grew so enamored of the process that he personally delivered the birds three years in a row and carved them on my dining room table in front of all my guests. The butcher became part of the party!

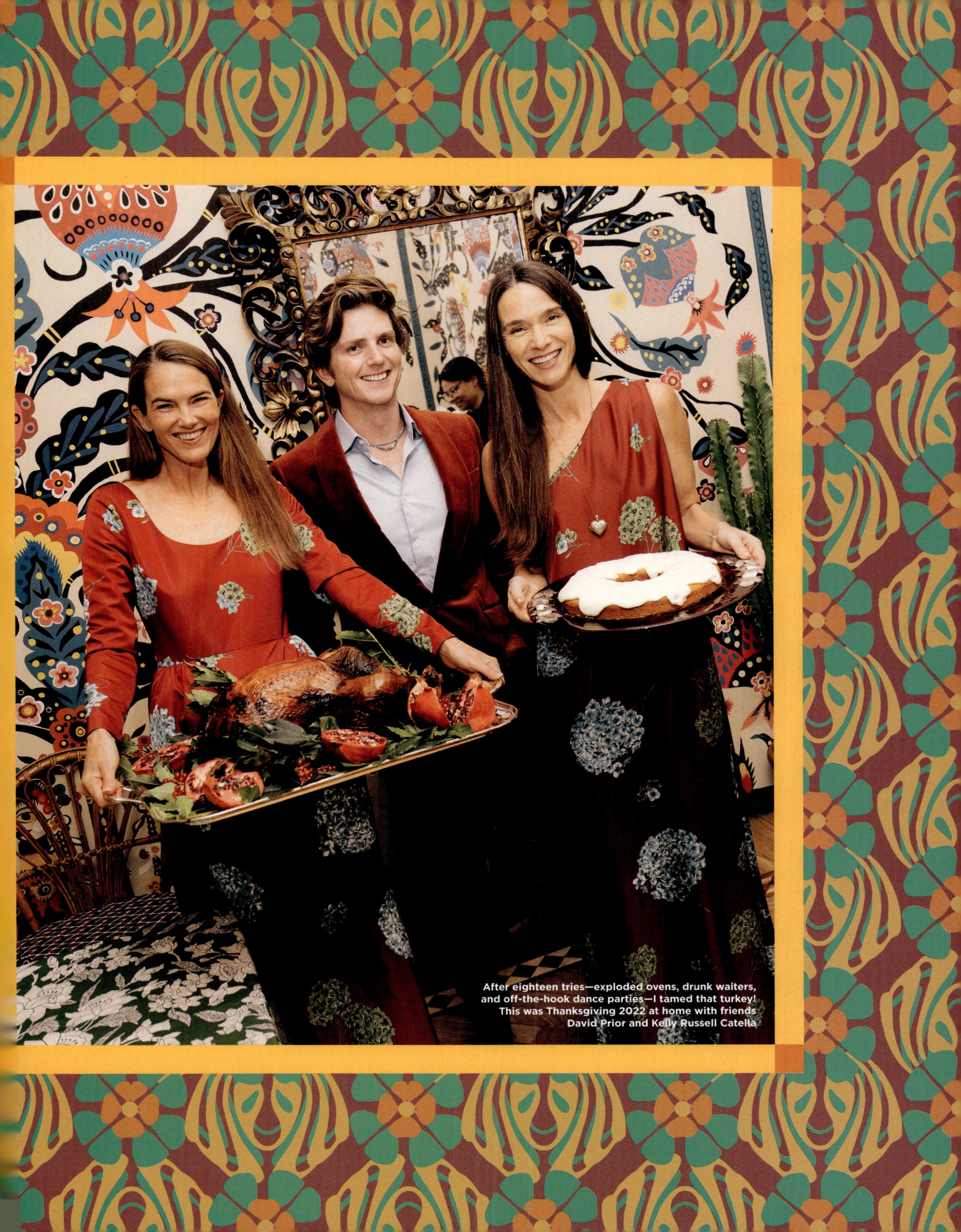

After eighteen tries—exploded ovens, drunk waiters, and off-the-hook dance parties—I tamed that turkey! This was Thanksgiving 2022 at home with friends David Prior and Kelly Russell Catella

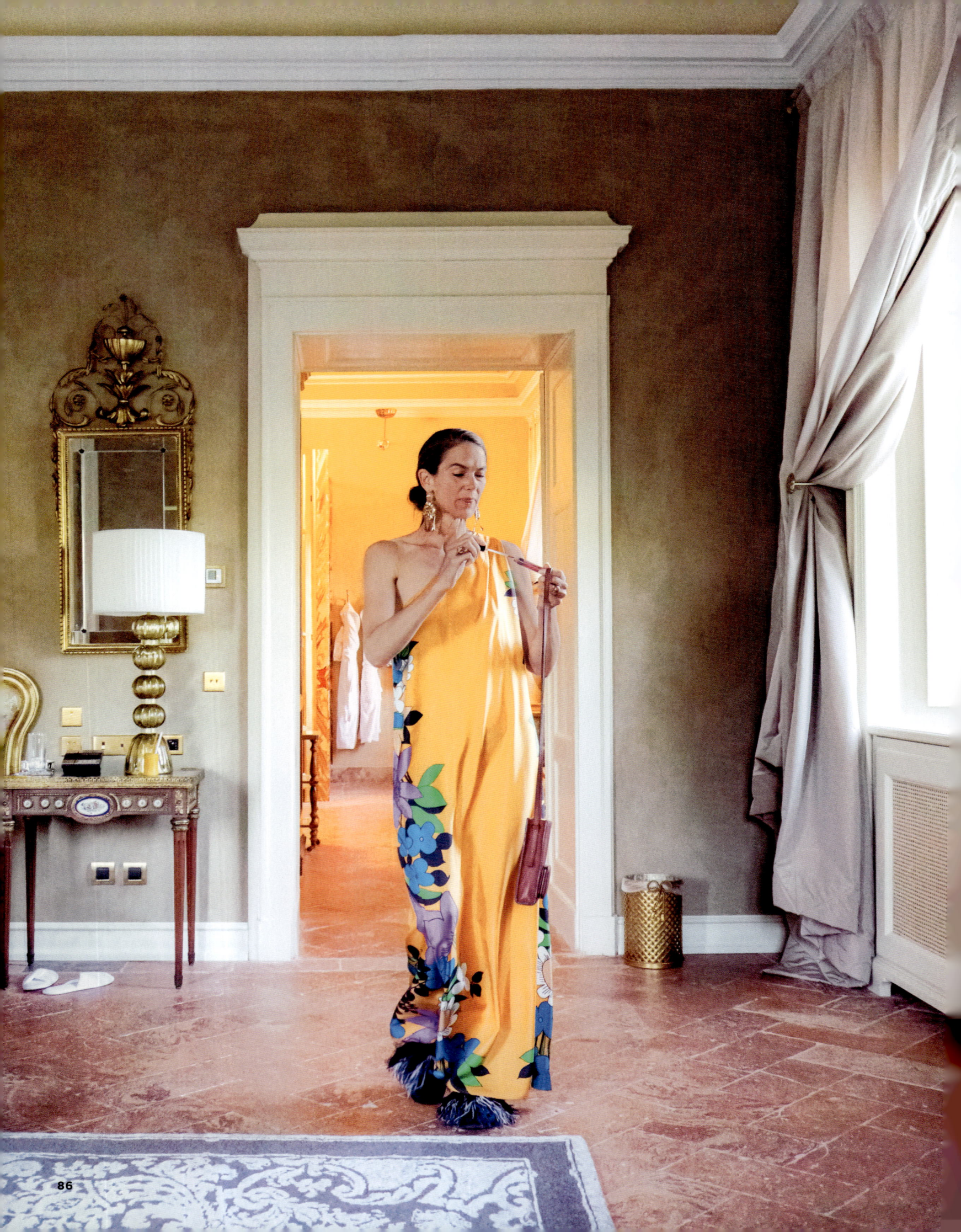

LESSON 45

CIAO, BELLA

Italians' innate sense of beauty and style plugs them into a higher plane of existence

Italians are possibly the world's greatest aesthetes. They are nuts about beauty—in things and in people. And no wonder—the country is spilling over with it, with its gilded, frescoed churches and manicured ribbons of Tuscan roads; its clusters of pastel *palazzi* in tiny seaside towns; and confetti-colored, tiered gardens that tumble into the country's spectacular lakes. "Oh my God, it's so beautiful!" they'll cry, whether it's a business deal that's going well or your taxi driver swooning over how elegant you look in your Marni dress and Chloe sandals. (Another reason why flirting doesn't feel like a lascivious tongue-wag—it's a genuine response to being visually dazzled.)

Italians are so obsessed with beauty that it's a barometer by which everything in their lives is measured. Italy is the only country I know where aesthetic judgments are also moral ones. *Bello* and *brutto* (beautiful and ugly) are used to mean "good" and "bad." The weather is never bad, it is *ugly*. It is not nice to see you, it is *beautiful* to see you. My first years in Milan, just to be clear, were terrifically *ugly*. I had an on-going, *unattractive* headache, and many *super-ugly* days, despite the fact that I went to so many *gorgeous* parties and had such a *beautiful,* burgeoning journalism career.

It is hardly surprising, then, that Italians place a lot of importance on appearance. Absolutely everyone in Italy has a sense of style. When I first moved to Milan, I would watch in wonder as women in Ray-Bans wearing full, giant Prada skirts, perfectly starched Aspesi shirts, and kitten heels glided by on their bicycles. Men, too, would leisurely bike home from work in trim, double-breasted jackets with silk pocket squares, polka-dot ties, and shiny Cordovan shoes without socks. Not a helmet nor bike short was in sight.

Looking astonishingly dapper, Milan's *carabinieri* (police officers) have a magenta stripe running up the side of their cornflower-blue pants (plus they carry swords!). The delivery boys for Esselunga, heaving big bags of groceries, each wear a ridiculously well-cut pair of pants and slip-on suede moccasins. Even the nuns have style. I recently saw one hurrying off to church in Corso Italia with a sensible but stylish Mandarina Duck khaki purse that was an exact match for the light shade of her springtime habit.

Italian children, too, are attuned to appearance very early on. One time in Portofino, some well-dressed young girls were wandering around our *aperitivo* tables in the *piazza*. "I love your sandals," I cooed to the youngest, who was wearing a simple navy A-line linen dress and classic navy-blue sandals with two thick, sturdy vintage straps. She was having an old-Celine moment and didn't even know it. She looked up at me with big, pure blue eyes, not yet old enough for compliments. Her older sister butted in next to her, flashing her look-at-me pink polka-dots. "She looks like a friar," the seven-year-old informed me with a scowl. Andrea explained that I'd offended her: "Why have you noticed her plain friar sister and not her in the beautiful pink ruffles?"

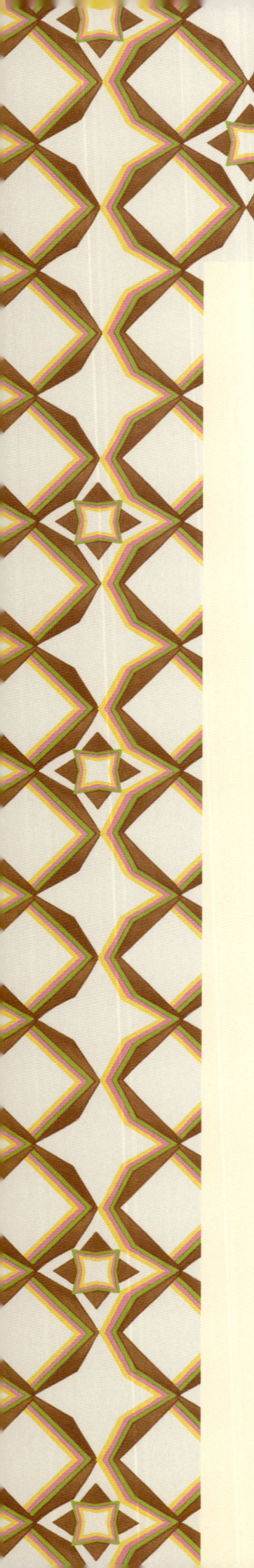

Caring so much about beauty and beautiful pink ruffles may seem superficial. But in nature, high-frequency patterns and codes—known to the ancients as sacred geometry—are the building blocks of everything that we consider beautiful. Our eyes, minds, and bodies respond with openness and receptivity to visual harmony unfolding before us in shapes and colors, in part because they are symbolic of our own natural inner realm. Beauty is a state of grace. Sacred geometry underpins nearly every Renaissance painting, not to mention the glorious churches and cathedrals shooting majestically up from Italy's rich soil. Every great spiritual practice recognizes the inherent value of gorgeousness—it is the visual manifestation of an inner consonance. The Italians, often even without knowing it, are just naturally attuned to this galactic coordination.

I've always been a beauty lover. From a very young age, I was jumping into my mother's closet to stroke her late '70s wardrobe, pulling on my grandmother's neck roped with shiny objects, and fascinated by friends' mothers who poured themselves into tight Gloria Vanderbilt jeans and silky blouses. Although my mom had my hair cut into a no-nonsense, fierce bowl cut until I was six, and dressed me frequently in my brothers' denim or corduroy hand-me-downs, deep down I knew I was a dress girl. I couldn't wait for fashion sovereignty, and when I had it, I went full in.

This love for fashion and ornamentation was an early and life-long obsession—but I didn't realize there was actually something deeper going. I knew that the sight of an embellished cape or a magically printed 1970s gown sent a jolt up my spine and calmed my nervous system with a feel-good blanket. Later, I learned that beauty is actually vibrating on a very high energetic level and that, since I was an epic empath, I would drink it in and get buzzed. For many years, I over-indulged in this, consuming beauty through the traditional lens of unconscious shopping. But then I began to realize that beauty did not need to be bought, owned, and dragged home to become a prisoner inside my closet. Like all sacred objects, it just needed to be acknowledged and worshipped—and, eventually, produced and revered within myself.

The beauty of Italy is opulent, wildly abundant, and above all, free to everyone with their eyes and hearts open. As my consciousness developed, I realized it was a higher force that I could literally suck into my cells, by sitting inside a church or at the Prada fashion show. Doing this more and more helped me cultivate beauty within myself and without, especially within my company. It began an expansion of and transformation within me.

Here's how beauty swirled up through Mamma Milano's style portal and poured into the rest of my life...

◦◊• PHRASEBOOK •◊◦

BELLO! BELLISSIMO! STUPENDO! STUPENDISSIMO! GORGISSIMO! SPAZIALE!

Italians are full of superlatives to express how beautiful it all is. Add an -issimo to the end of any word, and it inflates the meaning tenfold.

ITALIAN LESSONS

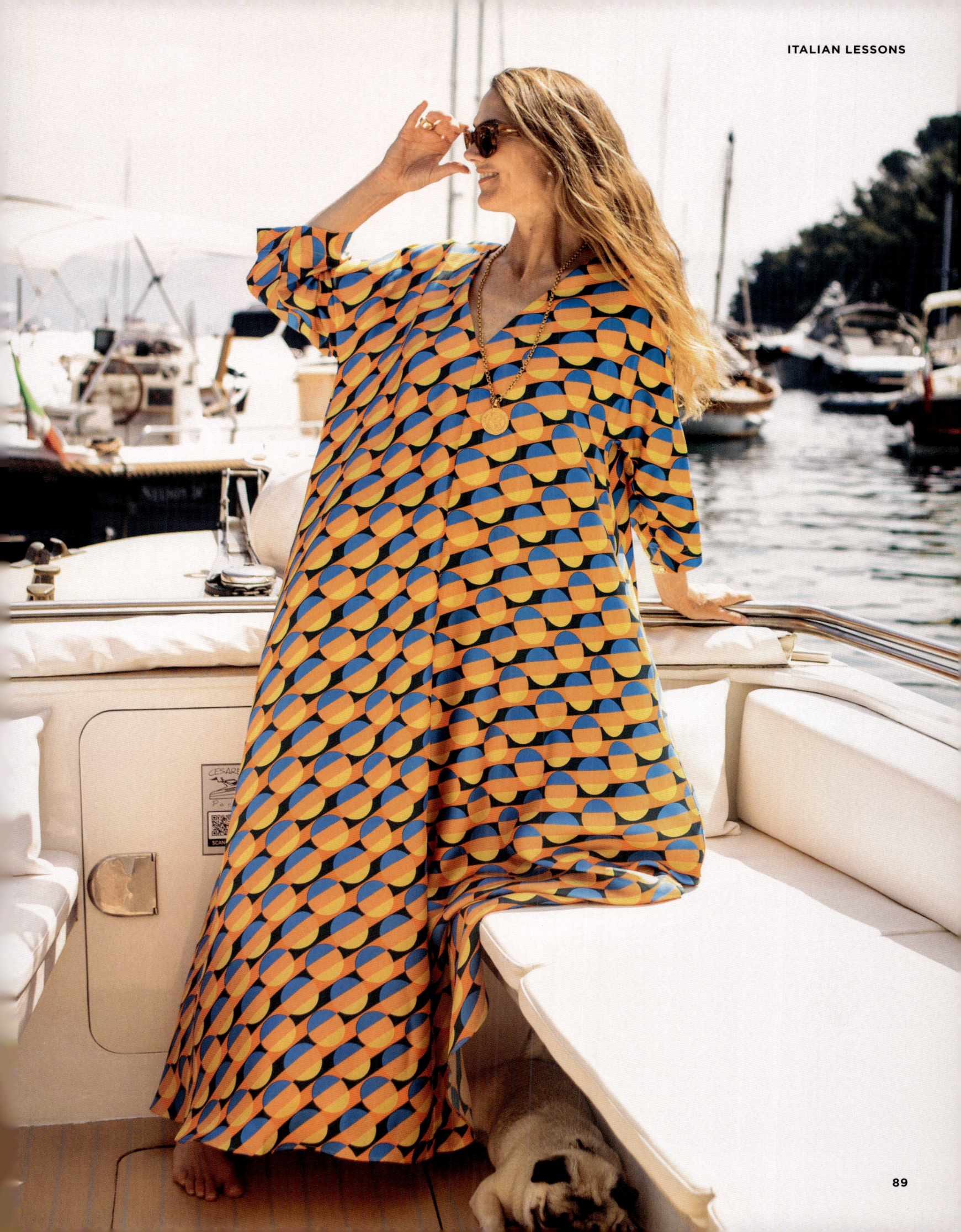

MAMMA MILANO

A FEW THINGS I LEARNED FROM THE GIANTS OF ITALIAN FASHION

GIORGIO ARMANI
HOW TO KEEP A RAZOR-SHARP FOCUS ON YOUR VISION

VALENTINO
HOW TO ENJOY THE GOOD LIFE AND ALL ITS FABULOUS TRAPPINGS

ANGELA MISSONI
HOW YOU TO TREAT YOUR CREATIONS AS A FAMILY AFFAIR

MIUCCIA PRADA
HOW TO FEARLESSLY MIX PRINTS, COLORS, AND HIGH & LOW

ROSSELLA JARDINI (MOSCHINO)
HOW TO GET DRESSED WITH STYLE AND FLAIR

DONATELLA VERSACE
HOW TO THROW A BANGING PARTY

LESSON 46
MAINTAIN A *BELLA FIGURA*

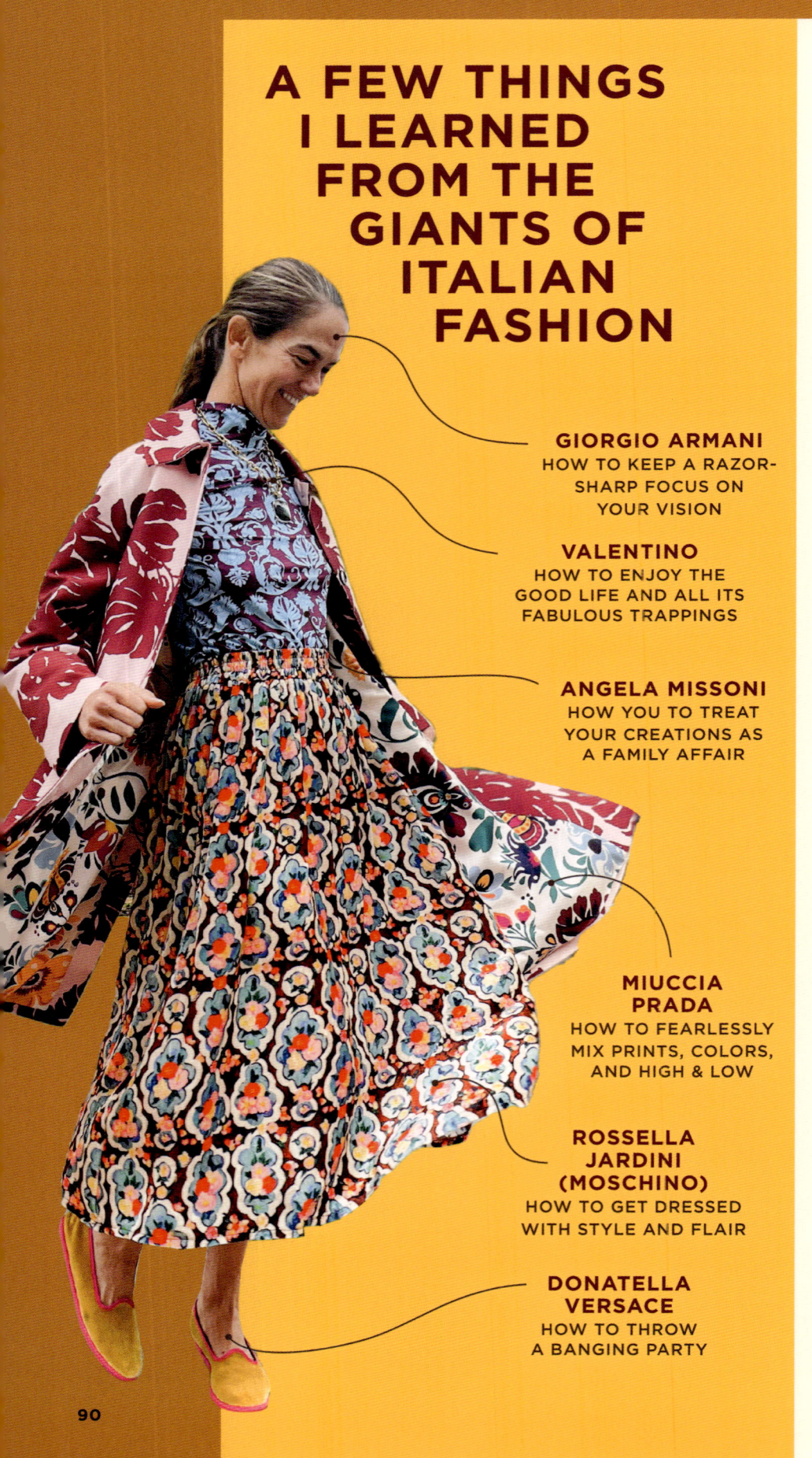

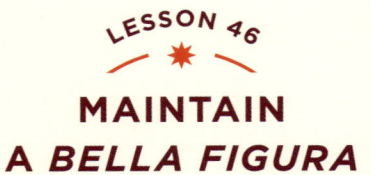

In Italy, you will often hear the phrase *bella figura*. This is sort of an extension of the *bello–brutto* axis of judgement. The *figura* is how you come across—it's literally your face, but it's all about making a good impression. The opposite, *brutta figura*, means ugly face, but really it means you've embarrassed yourself, by making a social or cultural faux pas, or by looking sloppy or ridiculous. For instance, a person who cares about a *bella figura* wouldn't wear sweatpants or flip-flops in public. So *figura* is also about dignity.

I come from Los Angeles, the birthplace of workout-wear-worn-everywhere. When I moved to Milan in 2001, there wasn't a sweatsuit in sight. You didn't even see a tennis shoe walking down Via Montenapoleone. Jeans were very rare (this was before the birth and explosion of the D&G second label from Dolce & Gabbana, which transformed Milanese streets around 2005). If you found a pair of shorts wandering the city, they most certainly belonged to a tourist.

Although jeans and tennis shoes came and soiled these perfect shores, there is still a resolute dedication to dressing properly. You don't have to be fancy, but you do need to be well-put together. A good shoe. A collar. No sloppiness. Even the T-shirts in Italy look tailored. During the summer my husband always wore a jacket, or at the very least a collared shirt with tailored shorts. A slim, muscular, tanned man—like a mahogany Weimaraner in tight navy Bermudas, tight white shirt tucked in, and white leather Hogan platform tennis shoes and no socks—is a uniquely Italian look.

I came to see in Italy that putting care into your appearance is a matter of self-respect. It's about lifting your own energy and that of others by striving to create something beautiful. Now when I return to LA, I look around and wonder, "What the hell is everyone doing in their yoga pants all day long?" I'm always in a skirt!

Of course, with Covid, people relished the all-day comfort of pyjamas. But it is important to rise out of the slob ashes and let yourself become ornamented and regaled in beauty, as an outward symbol of the magnificence that you constantly (not just for Instagram party photos) possess within.

LESSON 47

FOLLOW YOUR OWN BEAUTY ANTENNA

I was deeply impressed and a little intimidated by Milanese style when I arrived. I had worked at Calvin Klein, but mostly my wardrobe was filled with cheap clothes and some wacky vintage pieces I'd picked up at the Chelsea Flea. I wasn't particularly sophisticated in my dressing, but I did have an eye for print, pattern, and embellishment. My eye got refined and recalibrated after sitting through five hundred fashion shows and going on hundreds of photo shoots during my years as a fashion journalist. But it was studying the real women of Milan that taught me the most.

The majority of Italians follow certain rules in "dressing well"—they are not as willing to be as weird with fashion as an Anglo Saxon might be.

That said, there were several women in Milan whose eccentricity amused and inspired me. I spent hours in former Karl Lagerfeld muse Anna Piaggi's dark, dusty apartment, interviewing her about the towers of wacky clothes that she considered living beings; I watched as Anna dello Russo transformed herself from the mannish, minimalist editor of *Uomo Vogue* I first met in 2003 into a street style, walking-runway peacock. I marveled at design gallerist Nina Yashar's flair in turban and feathers, and I sat mesmerized in front of Manuela Pavesi, Miuccia Prada's best friend and muse, who glittered like a galaxy during our coffee interview at Cova.

These women had fashion balls. They had a deep inner knowing of who they were and how they wished to express themselves creatively. I could feel their freedom and I bathed happily in it.

It was similar to the energy at Miuccia Prada when I first moved to Milan in 2001. At that time, Prada was epic and Miuccia was queen of the Milan scene; her odd color palette, eye-busting patterns, and opulent embroideries nodded to Italian rules of elegance and formality, as well as smashing them to smithereens.

I'd never seen anything like it. And yet, her work always had a strong vintage influence, so I felt a kinship with my own collecting compulsion that was seeding and growing back home in my own closet—everything from five-dollar dresses plucked from the bottom of dirty bins to vintage Valentino couture that I had nabbed in the back of some tiny Italian shop. During my first decade in Italy, I would walk into the Prada shop as a weekend ritual, literally to just sniff in Miuccia's magical, original fragrance and leave.

Risky, playful, but deeply considered. All of these women in my early years in Milan were light-bearers for me. They made me feel accepted as I waltzed around Milan's elegant streets in my vintage clothes, startling the well-heeled locals.

They all showed me that style is a deeply personal tonic that can only be brewed within you.

ABBONDANZA

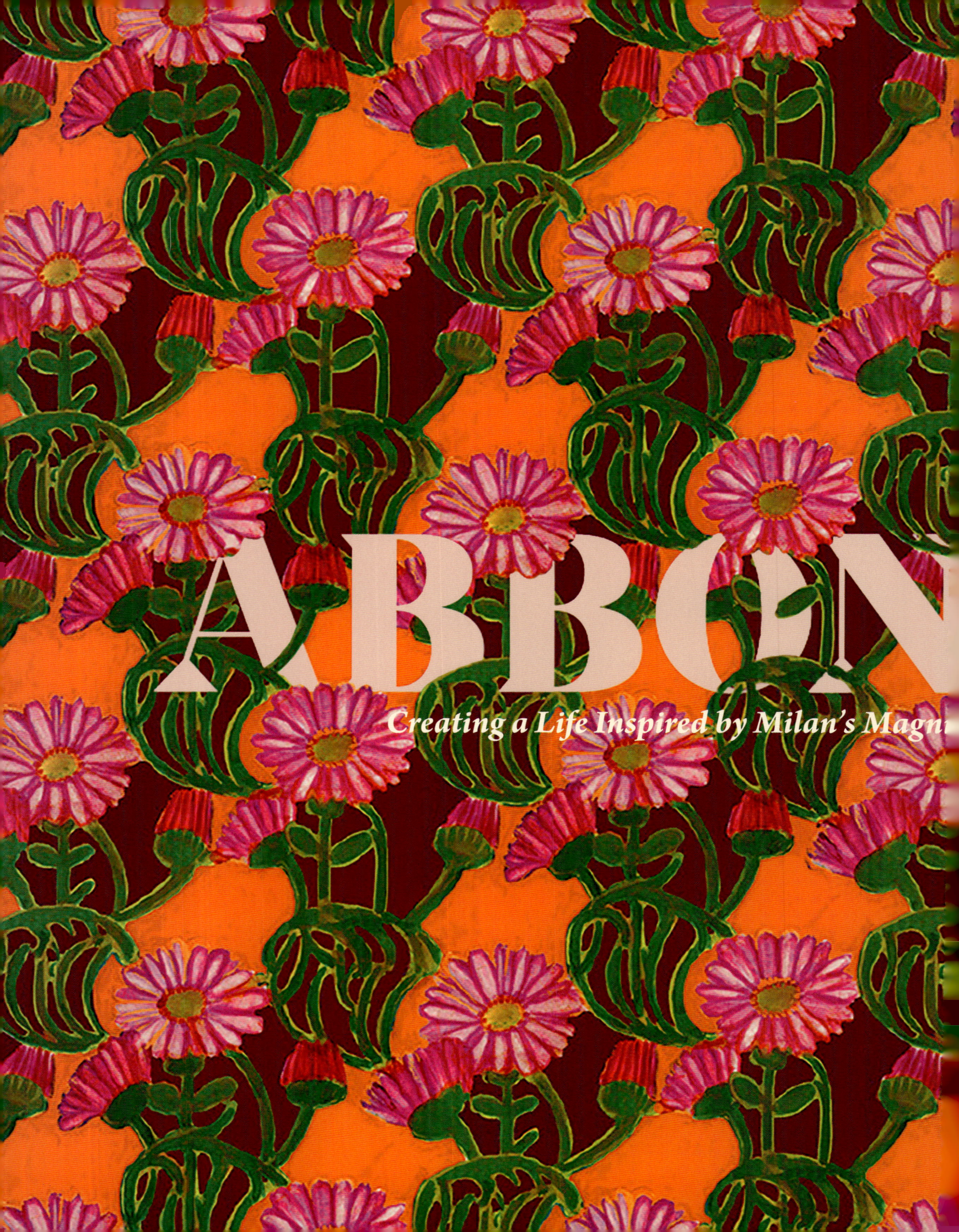

Creating a Life Inspired by Milan's Magn

DANZA

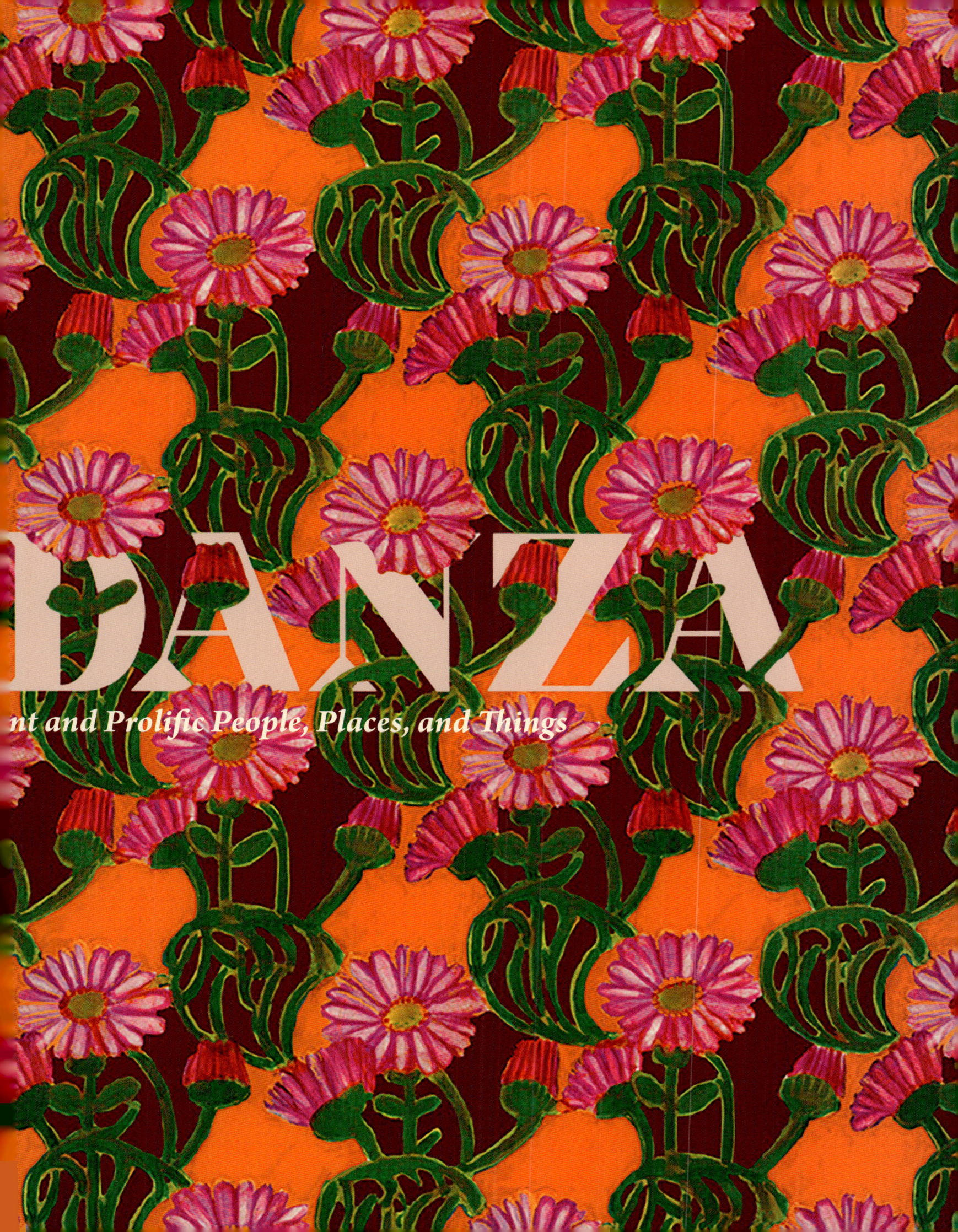

nt and Prolific People, Places, and Things

MAMMA MILANO

JOINING CREATION NATION

During my first decade in Milan, I was learning lessons the hard way: kicking, screaming, and occasionally crying. But once I exhausted my ego's puny resources and realized that it was futile to fight an entire country's invisible laws, I surrendered to the chaos.

Instead of complaining, white-knuckling, or fighting to change everything, I allowed things to unfold the way the Big Mamma Boss wanted them to.

When I loosened my grip I did not find myself in a prison of panic, but rather wrapped in the cushiony, coddling arms of Mamma Milano. She began to nurture and nourish me with more generosity than I had ever known.

The lessons I'd learned over the last few years—relaxing, accepting, connecting, feasting, playing, and flirting with life (and everyone in it)—became milk from the Mother that recalibrated my brain chemistry, mutated my thoughts, and cleared my energy field. This nutrient brew fertilized my inner soil, putting me in a creator state of consciousness. It birthed a new energetic field in me.

I had splashed down into—and was happily bobbing along on—Italy's creative wellspring.

Creativity is a divine feminine force. Once you clear away fear, judgment, and punishment (of yourself and others), you can cultivate a safe, sacred space for the seeds of creativity to root and surge into being. Italy, with its Edens of abundance (food, beauty, sunshine, and laughter), had always operated according to this natural law. But I, Jennifer Jane Martin, had not.

Now Mamma Milano and I were attuned to the same frequency. Not only did this energetic match make me a happier person—like an exiled, naughty child finally welcomed to the dinner table—it also allowed me to plug into the wild, powerful energy grid of creativity that spun and buzzed across the country.

I began magnetizing Milan's creative people around me, supercharged by their souped-up genius.

Later, I would activate my own creative channels and give birth to prolific projects in ways I'd never known.

THE CREATIVE HEARTBEAT OF MILAN

After my first scrambled years in Milan, my job at *Harper's Bazaar* started spouting like a city street fountain. I found myself jumping on (or into) the boats, homes, villas, and breakfast tables of global fashion designers nearly every week to interview them for feature stories and to style shoots.

The flow dropped me inside Giorgio Armani's monolithic, monochrome closet at his home in Milan and his sleek, dark green yacht in La Spezia, into Donatella Versace's glittering gold living room, and Diego Della Valle's hidden Capri villa compound. I wrangled every member of the ginormous Ferragamo family for a portrait on their Tuscan estate, and helped script Dolce & Gabbana in the roles of Batman and Robin to Naomi Campbell's Catwoman for a photo shoot. It was exciting to drop into the glamorous worlds of these big-name designers, but also inspiring to see the passion they had for their work and vision. With my new lens, I could see how rigorously they approached their craft, and how Italian that fixation really was.

The exact same force that drove Armani's army of beige minimalism across the globe also inspired a no-name fourth-generation shoemaker to obsess over the stitching no one sees on a single handmade sole, or pushed an aproned shopkeeper to fill his tiny storefront with nothing but mushrooms of every size and shape. No matter what they are creating or how many people see it, the Italians seem to be united in their love of beauty, obsession with quality, and a tendency towards high-standard specializations.

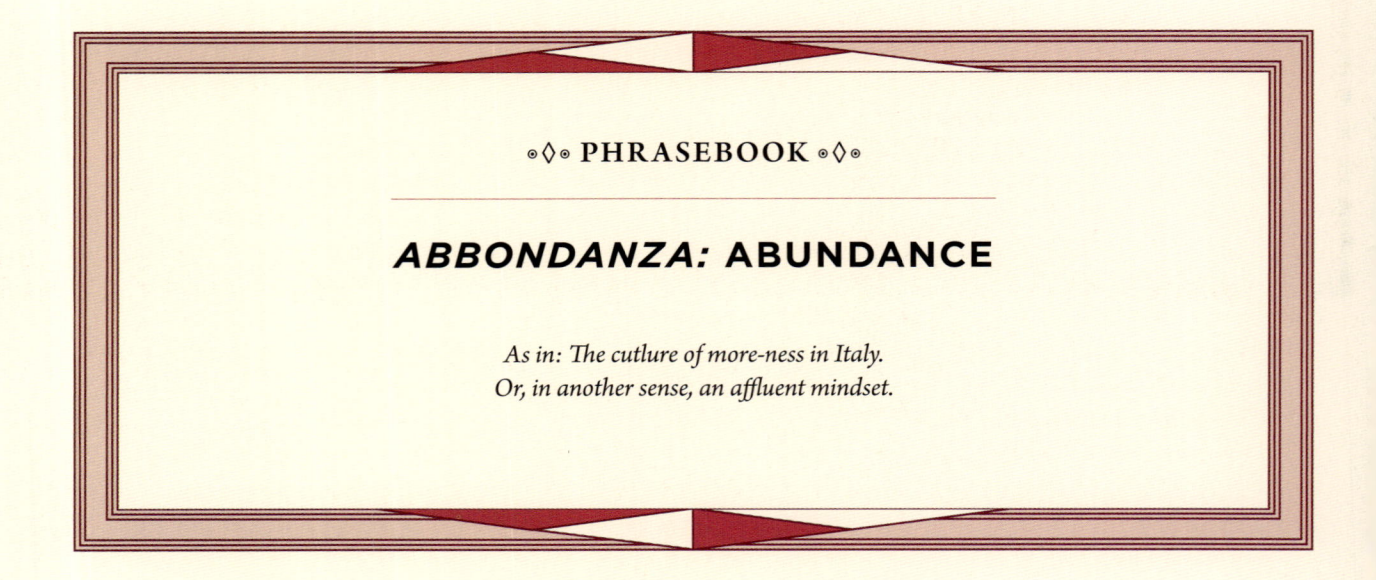

◦◊• PHRASEBOOK •◊◦

ABBONDANZA: ABUNDANCE

*As in: The cutlure of more-ness in Italy.
Or, in another sense, an affluent mindset.*

MILAN FASHION WEEK—THE JOURNALIST YEARS

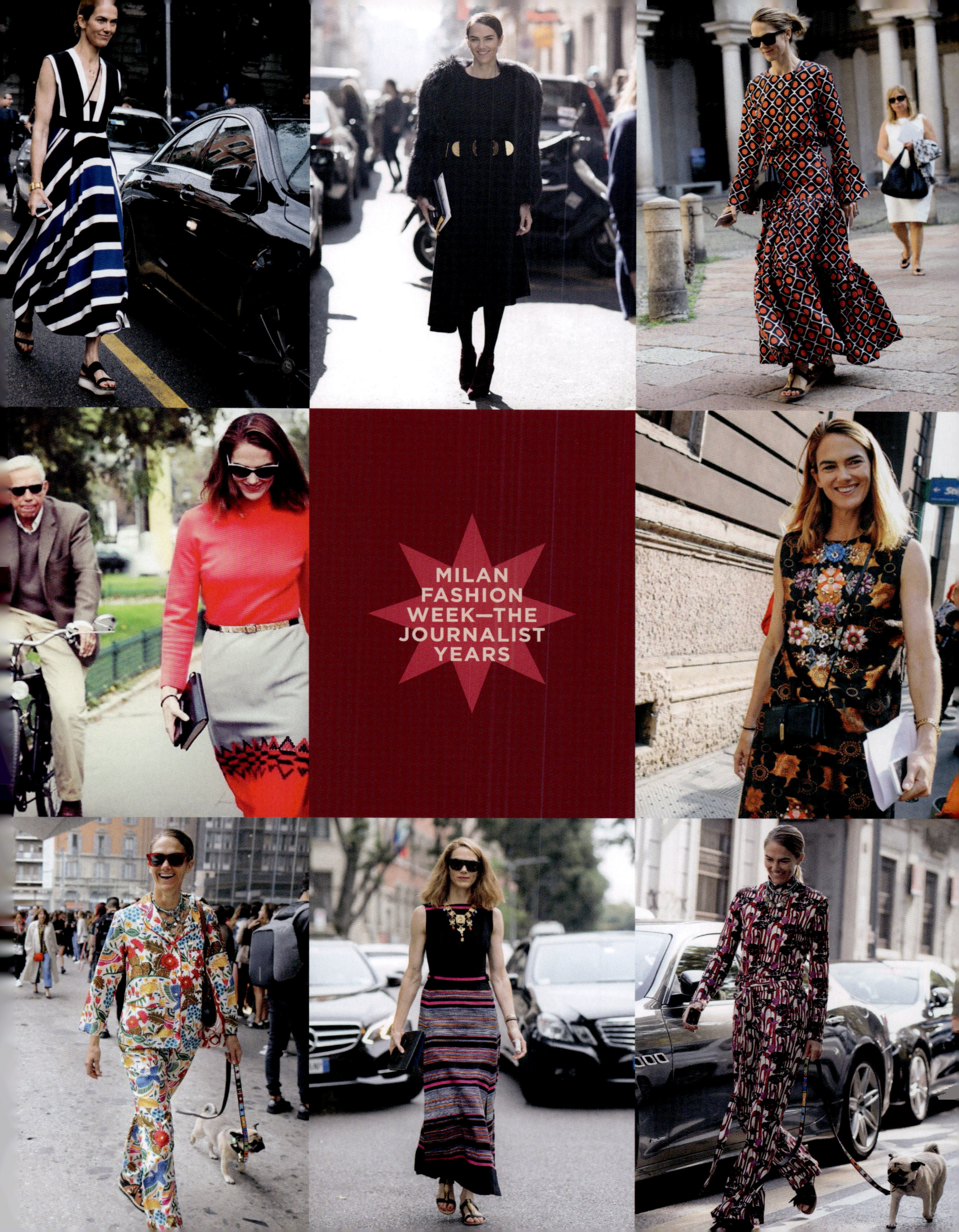

MEETING
MILAN'S MASTER CREATORS

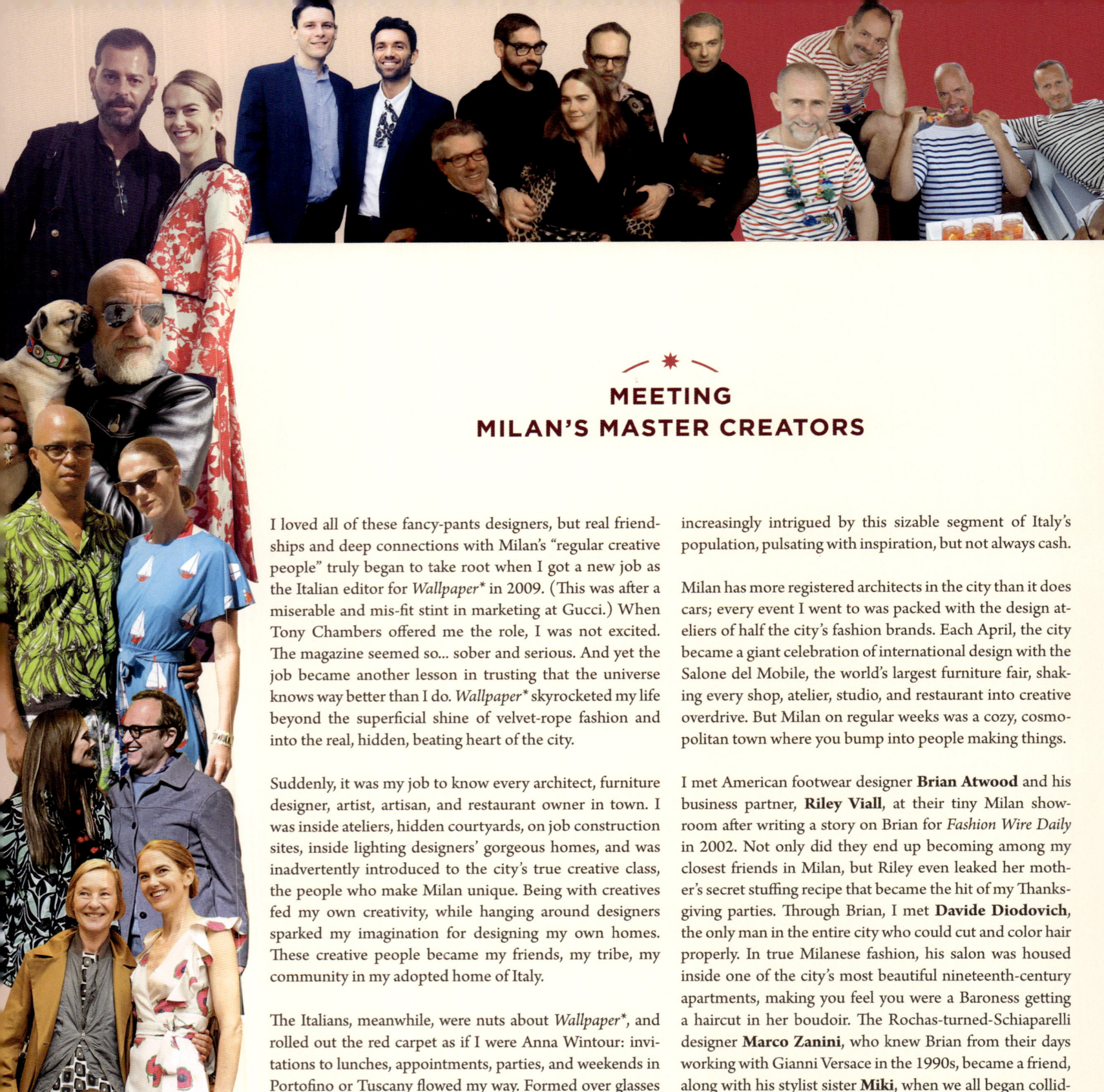

I loved all of these fancy-pants designers, but real friendships and deep connections with Milan's "regular creative people" truly began to take root when I got a new job as the Italian editor for *Wallpaper** in 2009. (This was after a miserable and mis-fit stint in marketing at Gucci.) When Tony Chambers offered me the role, I was not excited. The magazine seemed so... sober and serious. And yet the job became another lesson in trusting that the universe knows way better than I do. *Wallpaper** skyrocketed my life beyond the superficial shine of velvet-rope fashion and into the real, hidden, beating heart of the city.

Suddenly, it was my job to know every architect, furniture designer, artist, artisan, and restaurant owner in town. I was inside ateliers, hidden courtyards, on job construction sites, inside lighting designers' gorgeous homes, and was inadvertently introduced to the city's true creative class, the people who make Milan unique. Being with creatives fed my own creativity, while hanging around designers sparked my imagination for designing my own homes. These creative people became my friends, my tribe, my community in my adopted home of Italy.

The Italians, meanwhile, were nuts about *Wallpaper**, and rolled out the red carpet as if I were Anna Wintour: invitations to lunches, appointments, parties, and weekends in Portofino or Tuscany flowed my way. Formed over glasses of *prosecco* and bowls of *pesto*, these relationships bewitched me with the spell of Italy's pulsating colors, elegant shapes, and tender traditions, changing everything for me.

Fortunately, my editors were less after the big-ticket advertisers (such as at the fashion magazines I'd been toiling at) than they were the cool creatives. My very first feature was about nearly forty best-in-class furniture designers, restaurant owners, shop owners, architects, and gallery owners, many of whom were not household names. It was the perfect introduction to the city's creative heartbeat. I grew increasingly intrigued by this sizable segment of Italy's population, pulsating with inspiration, but not always cash.

Milan has more registered architects in the city than it does cars; every event I went to was packed with the design ateliers of half the city's fashion brands. Each April, the city became a giant celebration of international design with the Salone del Mobile, the world's largest furniture fair, shaking every shop, atelier, studio, and restaurant into creative overdrive. But Milan on regular weeks was a cozy, cosmopolitan town where you bump into people making things.

I met American footwear designer **Brian Atwood** and his business partner, **Riley Viall**, at their tiny Milan showroom after writing a story on Brian for *Fashion Wire Daily* in 2002. Not only did they end up becoming among my closest friends in Milan, but Riley even leaked her mother's secret stuffing recipe that became the hit of my Thanksgiving parties. Through Brian, I met **Davide Diodovich**, the only man in the entire city who could cut and color hair properly. In true Milanese fashion, his salon was housed inside one of the city's most beautiful nineteenth-century apartments, making you feel you were a Baroness getting a haircut in her boudoir. The Rochas-turned-Schiaparelli designer **Marco Zanini**, who knew Brian from their days working with Gianni Versace in the 1990s, became a friend, along with his stylist sister **Miki**, when we all began colliding at Cucchi with **Lawrence Steele** and **Francesco Risso**.

The very first fashion review I ever wrote in 2002 was on **Neil Barrett**'s show in a glorious courtyard in Milan. Little did I know that he and his boyfriend/business partner, **Carlo Barone**, would become dear friends and epic Milanese party throwers. I met **Massimo Giorgetti** of MSGM and **Dean and Dan Caten** of Dsquared[2] the same way—interviewing them—but ended up hanging out with them in Neil's dining room. Designer **Ennio Capasa** and his business partner-brother, **Carlo**, were not only the first

ABBONDANZA

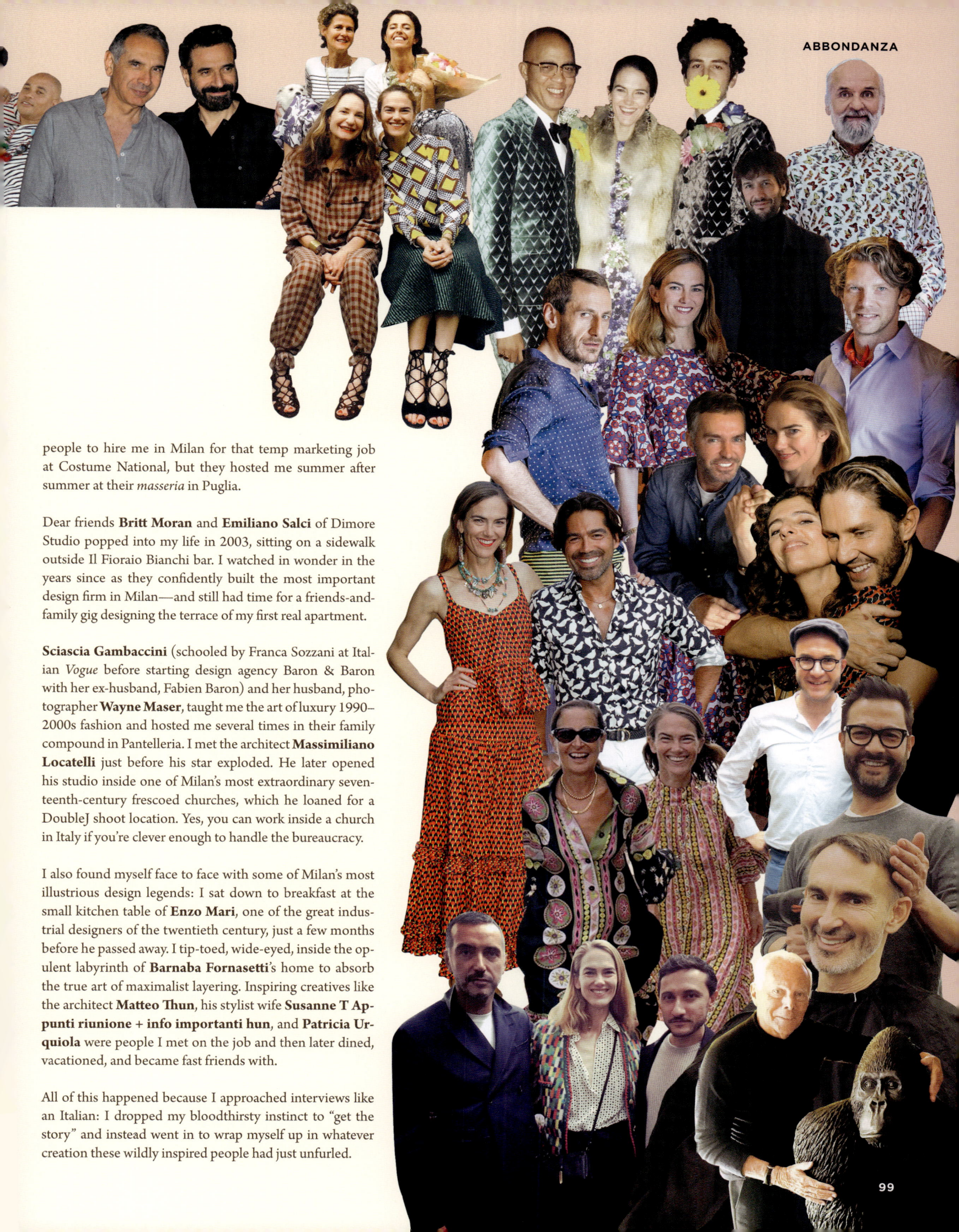

people to hire me in Milan for that temp marketing job at Costume National, but they hosted me summer after summer at their *masseria* in Puglia.

Dear friends **Britt Moran** and **Emiliano Salci** of Dimore Studio popped into my life in 2003, sitting on a sidewalk outside Il Fioraio Bianchi bar. I watched in wonder in the years since as they confidently built the most important design firm in Milan—and still had time for a friends-and-family gig designing the terrace of my first real apartment.

Sciascia Gambaccini (schooled by Franca Sozzani at Italian *Vogue* before starting design agency Baron & Baron with her ex-husband, Fabien Baron) and her husband, photographer **Wayne Maser**, taught me the art of luxury 1990–2000s fashion and hosted me several times in their family compound in Pantelleria. I met the architect **Massimiliano Locatelli** just before his star exploded. He later opened his studio inside one of Milan's most extraordinary seventeenth-century frescoed churches, which he loaned for a DoubleJ shoot location. Yes, you can work inside a church in Italy if you're clever enough to handle the bureaucracy.

I also found myself face to face with some of Milan's most illustrious design legends: I sat down to breakfast at the small kitchen table of **Enzo Mari**, one of the great industrial designers of the twentieth century, just a few months before he passed away. I tip-toed, wide-eyed, inside the opulent labyrinth of **Barnaba Fornasetti**'s home to absorb the true art of maximalist layering. Inspiring creatives like the architect **Matteo Thun**, his stylist wife **Susanne T Appunti riunione + info importanti hun**, and **Patricia Urquiola** were people I met on the job and then later dined, vacationed, and became fast friends with.

All of this happened because I approached interviews like an Italian: I dropped my bloodthirsty instinct to "get the story" and instead went in to wrap myself up in whatever creation these wildly inspired people had just unfurled.

CO-CREATING WITH MILAN'S MAGIC MAKERS

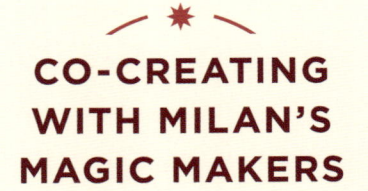

When creative people hang around together, sparks of inspiration fly. It was around this time that I discovered the vibrancy and the originality that can swirl out of the alchemy of two (or more) creative people coming together: inspirations merge and ideas expand, with the result being bigger and better than what you could ever do on your own. Co-creating with my friends became one of my favorite hobbies, allowing my own imaginative instincts to emerge, and laying the foundation for the stream of collaborations I later did with La DoubleJ.

"Beauty seeks beauty." Fabio Zambernardi, the design director of Prada, told me this after sending the most over-the-top, banging bouquet of flowers I'd ever seen before one of my Thanksgiving dinners. My heart exploded when I saw them. How had he known exactly what would pop my rocks off? Fabio himself was co-creating with a florist that brought him the city's strangest, most wonderful blooms.

"The secret is having someone who knows you and that you can have a conversation with," he said. "I merely told him what you were like."

I began to realize that these creatives in Milan understood me in a way no one ever had. I'd found my tribe, my family, my fellow weirdos. They were activated by my enthusiasm, I was expanded by their energetic presence, and I began to realize that I never feel as good as I do when in the company of artists, designers, photographers, and makers of all kinds. Luckily, Milan is bubbling over with them.

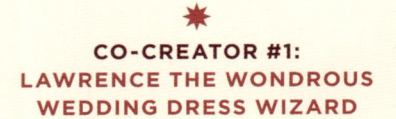

CO-CREATOR #1: LAWRENCE THE WONDROUS WEDDING DRESS WIZARD

My first co-creative concoction was my wedding dress. Stepping into vintage boutique Didier Ludot between shows during Couture Week in Paris in 2005, there on the racks was a beautiful yet demure 1960s vintage Balmain haute couture column dress, in a pale celery green with intricate beading and brocade. It might have been full length for a woman of that era, but it was 4 inches too short for me. I bought it anyway and brought it home to show my friend Lawrence Steele, an American designer who had spent years at Prada and Moschino before launching his own label. We'd met a few years earlier at a Neil Barrett fashion show in Milan but weren't super close. Still, I felt like I wanted a slice of his supernatural talent.

I invited Lawrence to coffee (of course) and asked if he could help me vamp it up for wedding day splendor.

He shot out an unequivocal yes! We spent a month on the floor of his apartment in Milan with his sixty-something tailor Tina taking in, pulling out, and making gown-glorious additions. Lawrence cut right into the prissy neckline, giving me a dramatic *V* shape; he slashed off the mumsy backflaps, added two satin backstraps, and sliced into the back of the dress to add a train of pale celery lace that circled in front to lower the hem length. He took me to Jacassi, the secret vintage lair frequented by all Milanese fashion designers, to paw through hundreds of pieces of lace until we found one that was the exact shade of the dress.

I wore the dress with a pair of antique Buccellati earrings, loaned by Andrea Buccellati himself. I met him at a dinner and, in typical Italian fashion, he thought I should borrow these magnificent jewels from his historical family business.

ABBONDANZA

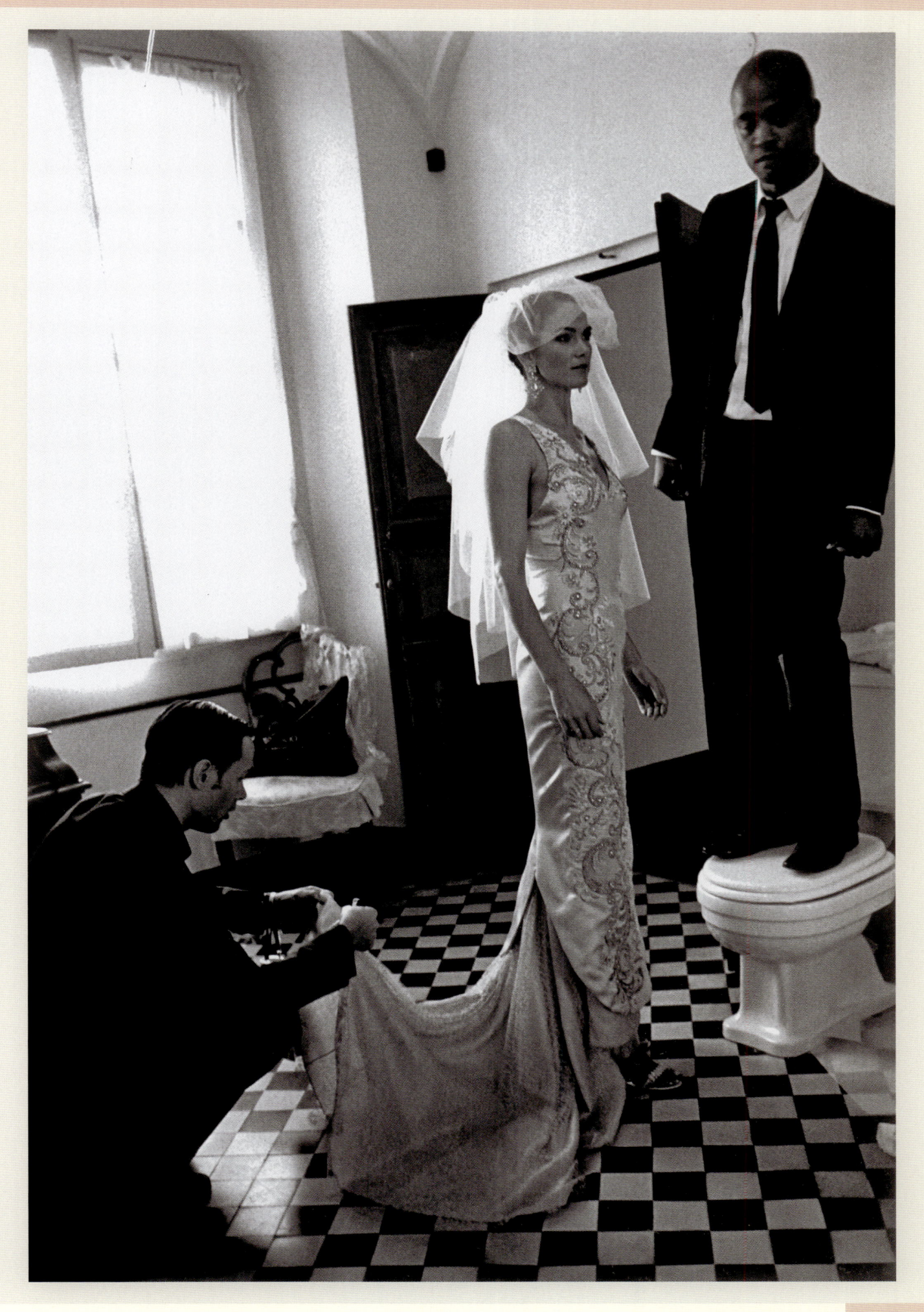

In my vintage Balmain wedding gown with magician-designer Lawrence Steele (right)

MAMMA MILANO

★

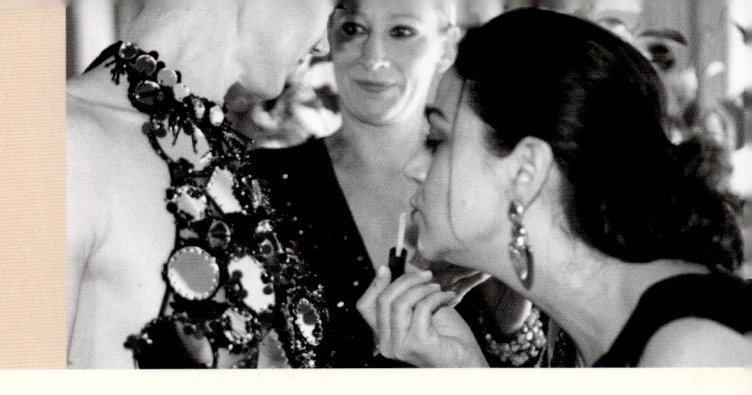

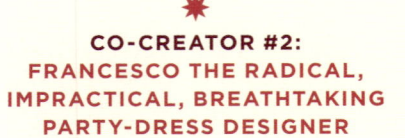

**CO-CREATOR #2:
FRANCESCO THE RADICAL,
IMPRACTICAL, BREATHTAKING
PARTY-DRESS DESIGNER**

I met Francesco Risso—now the big-name creative director of Marni—at Pasticceria Cucchi while he was a young fashion assistant. Over Aperol spritzes one evening, I told him I'd been invited to Brian Atwood's birthday party in Mykonos with a themed dress code: the Greek Gatsby. I was completely stumped. What did that even mean?

"I know *exactly* what it means!" Francesco cried. In the following days he proceeded to hand-sew a crinkled, gold lamé draped toga gown with a crown of gold feathers. In it, I really did embody Greek Gatsby.

Francesco became a dear friend whose creative waters were always rushing. He was wide-eyed, playful, totally impractical, and in love with creating beautiful things. He was also wildly generous with his talent.

Later, when he was working at Prada, he offered to design my fortieth birthday dress while juggling his real job of making runway and red-carpet gowns for celebrities.

We did fittings in his apartment in Milan, then he'd take the pieces back to the office to be sewn up in a sort of Paco-Rabanne-meets-Queen-Victoria mash-up. The halter top was made from huge pieces of mirrored embroidery and was paired with a feather-trimmed lace hoop skirt that was shorter in the front and long in the back.

Francesco showed up to the black-tie party—held in a gilded eighteen-century Roman villa—in a Comme des Garçons black suit covered in giant roses and a natty fisherman's hat, after we'd spent the day racing through Rome with fifty people on mopeds. He, this, all of it… was very, very Italian.

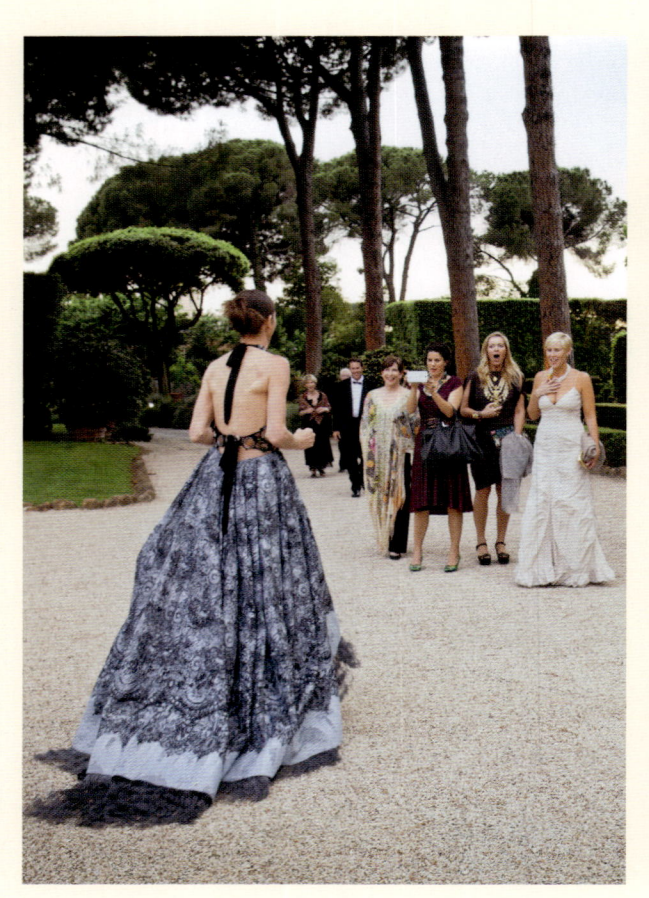

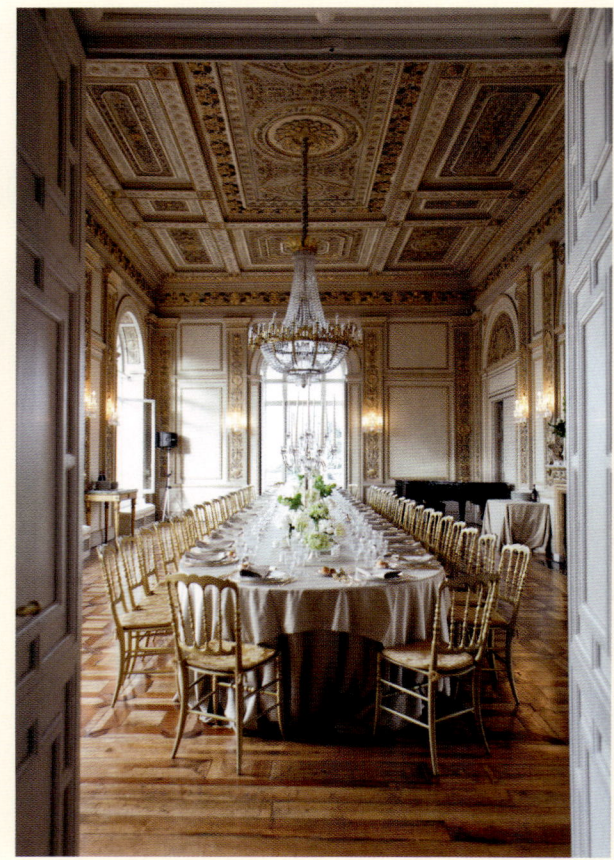

ABBONDANZA

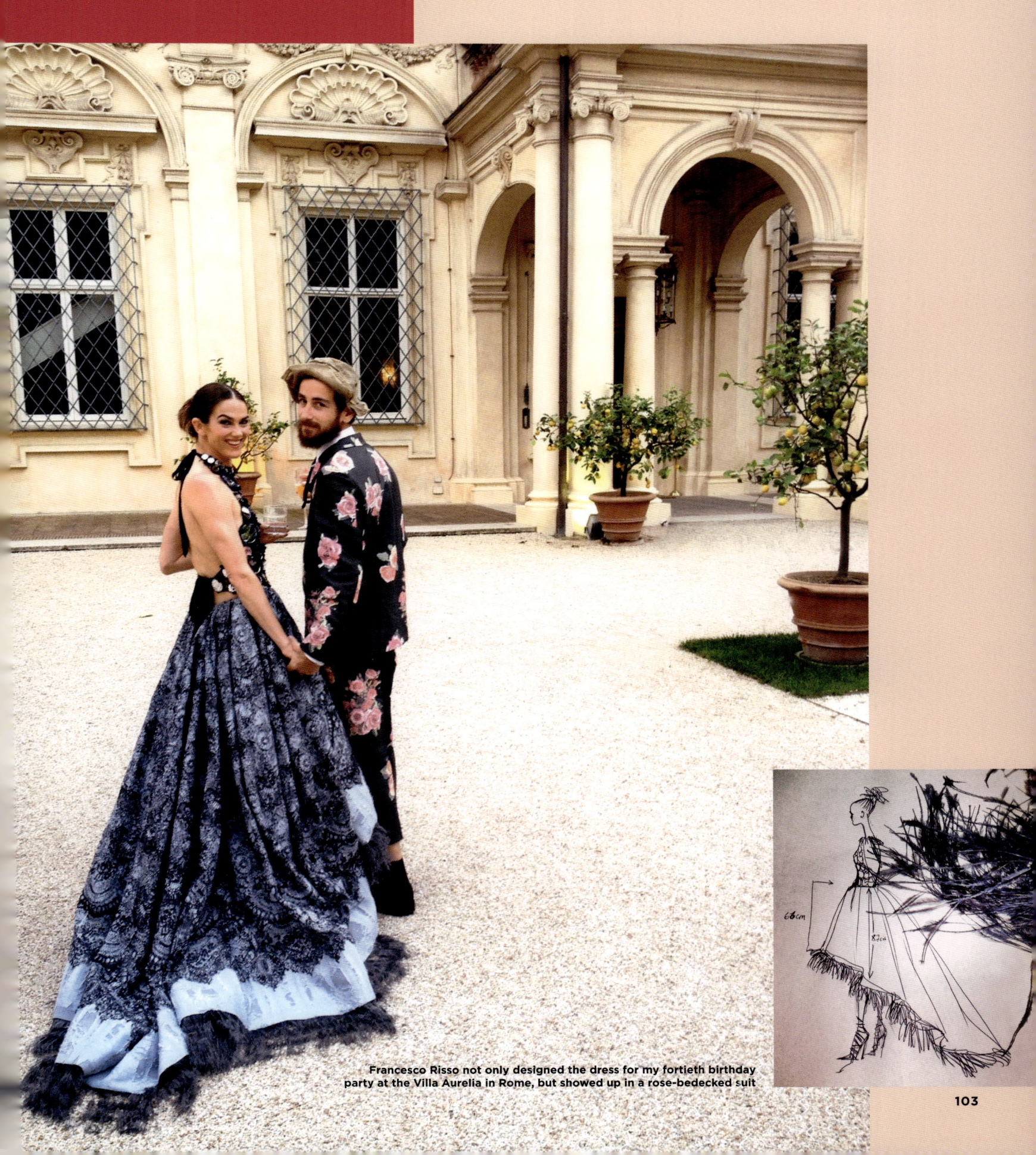

Francesco Risso not only designed the dress for my fortieth birthday party at the Villa Aurelia in Rome, but showed up in a rose-bedecked suit

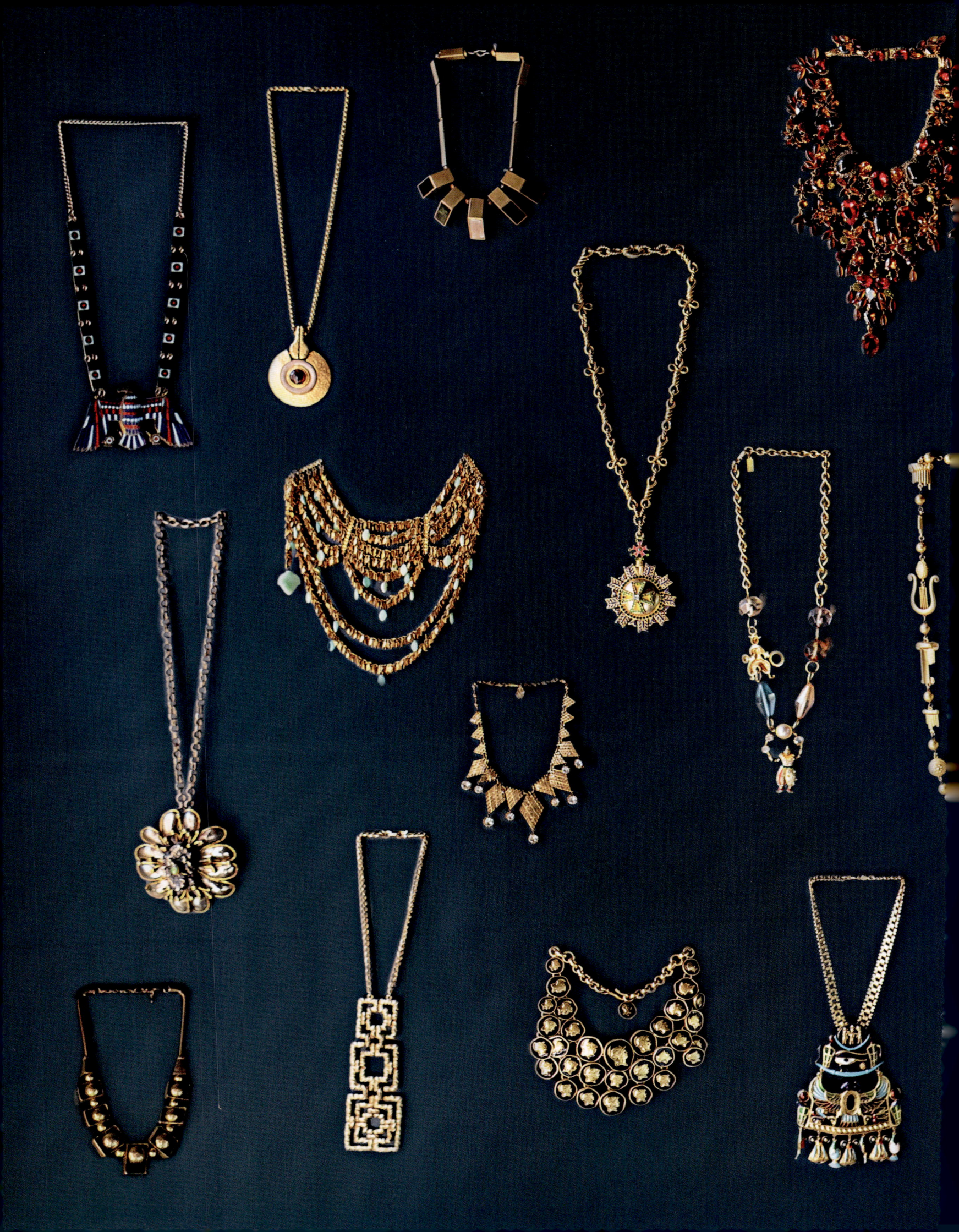

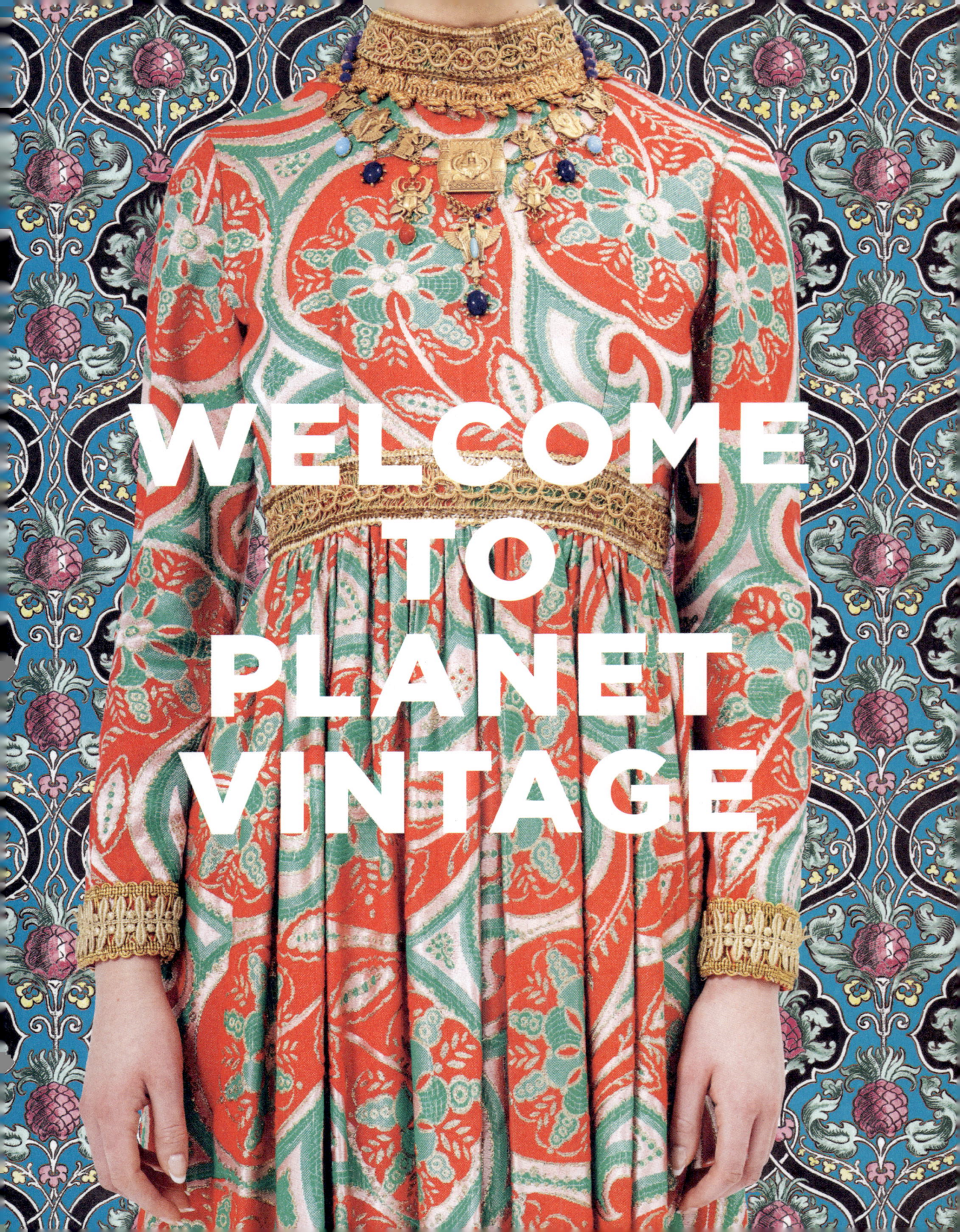

WELCOME TO PLANET VINTAGE

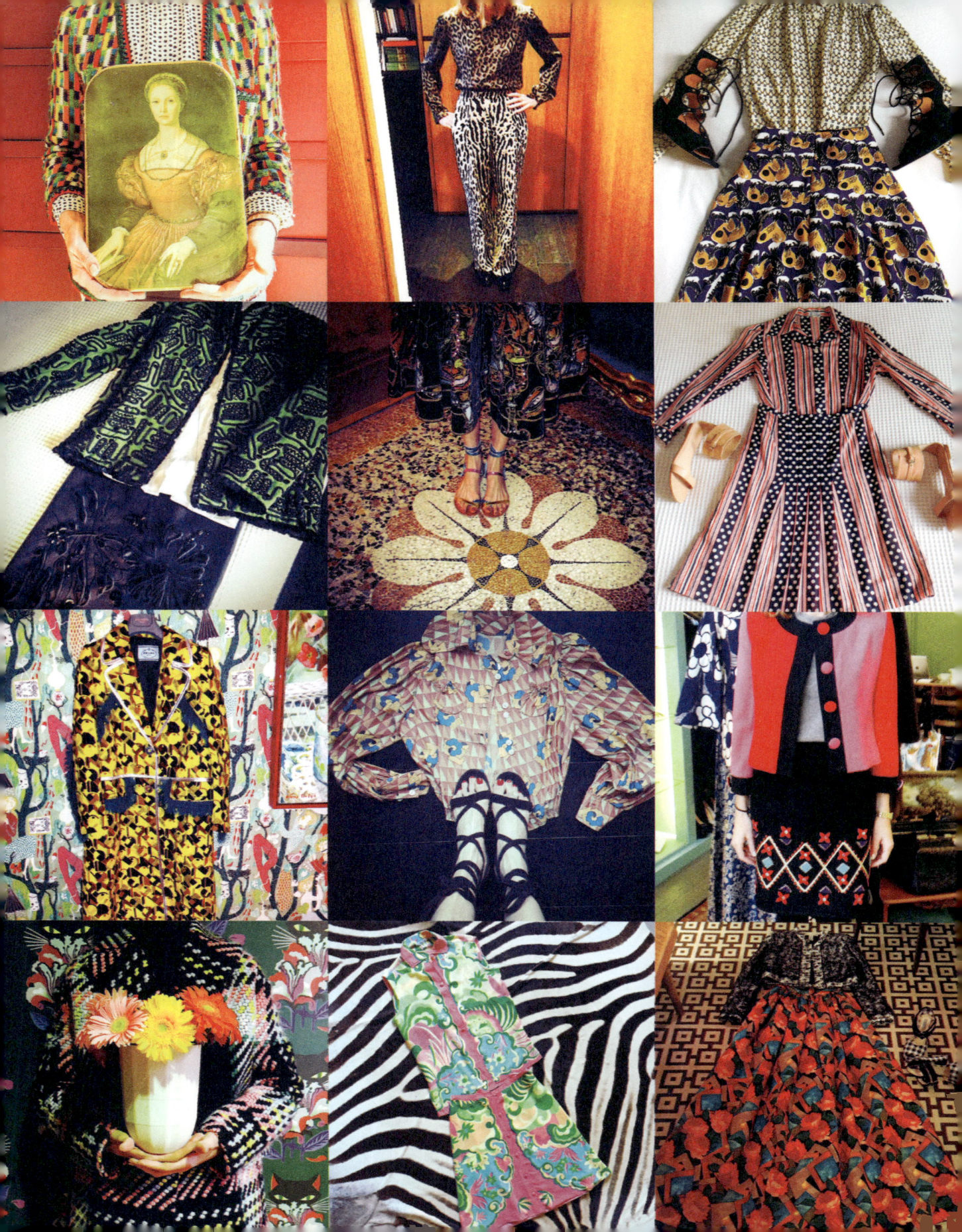

DIVING FOR VINTAGE TREASURES

My most opulent playground for early creative pursuits was planet vintage. I first touched down on its alien terrain in the late 1990s in New York. I was fashion-obsessed but did not have a lot of money, so I spent my weekends combing the stalls of the Chelsea Flea—where I discovered delicate 1940s gowns, eye-popping print dresses, and outrageous furs from the 1970s. I could not believe the bounty, the beauty, the exquisiteness of this treasure trove. Everything was under a hundred dollars at that time so I stocked up, but mostly I just wanted to be around those clothes.

My first purchase was a black A-line faux-fur coat from the 1960s with an enormous real fox collar. When I moved to Italy, I took my brightly patterned 1970s polyester dresses, 1950s printed house dresses, and my funny coat, and wore them on the streets of Milan.

I got weird looks from the stylish Milanese women, because vintage was still an underground pursuit used almost exclusively by fashion designers as a creative resource, not for the public.

Although I was baptized in America, my finishing school in vintage happened in Italy. My sensibilities and my sensory skills became more refined, refracted as they were through the chic taste lens that only Italy has.

For this upgrade I have to thank Spanish-born, Florence-based designer Álvaro González, who was just as obsessed with vintage as I was. An accessories designer at Jimmy Choo, he became my vintage buddy—we went to vintage fairs throughout Italy in sleepy towns every weekend we possibly could. Scouting with a designer was fascinating and educational. It trained my eye as I watched what he found interesting for his research, and sometimes it was nothing more than the cut of a sleeve on an otherwise useless ten-euro dress. Yes, a handbag designer cared about sleeves.

For about a decade in Italy, I visited hundreds of fairs, every local town's market, and teeny church sales, and I befriended many dealers who later became sourcing partners when I launched LaDoubleJ. I didn't spend much money on my vintage collection, but I bought like crazy. Some of my pieces were valuable, collectible items. I prized the hunt and the ability to score incredible deals in dusty back rooms of no-name shops in Italy or at some fancy *signora*'s house that was being cleared out. Most vintage collectors wrapped their pieces in tissue in the closet and waited for the big exhibit. I wore every single piece I ever bought. All of them.

This scandalized my friend Enrico Quinto, a vintage expert I met in Rome who has a warehouse dedicated to his museum-worthy collection. I always felt that, to explore the beauty of these clothes, they're not just to be looked at but really experienced. I wore a black chinoiserie, vintage haute couture Valentino cocktail dress to my interview with Tom Ford in London, and he jumped off his couch with a friendly, "Wow, nice to meet you—you look spectacular!" We got on like a *palazzo* on fire. And that's the power of clothing—disarming someone with unexpected beauty.

Shopping for vintage has always been an emotional experience for me. It's not logical, scientific or sensical. It's extremely intuitive and creates a physical sensation in my body: I take whatever makes my heart leap or stomach jump. I would glide my hands over the clothes, instinctually passing over black pieces and stopping right in front of a fantastic pattern.

All the prints that I've ever been attracted to speak to me with their distinctive personalities. They dance, scream, shout with joy—and I hear every syllable of it.

Later, in my energy practice, I learned that color has a high energetic frequency, so patterns, colors, and especially rich threads or beaded embroideries were literally vibrating. My ability to turn my brain off and be led by feeling only was a precursor to my spiritual journey.

Soon, I started connecting almost psychically with my vintage experience. Sometimes I'd arrive at a giant fair and say, *Spirit, take me where I need to be*. The next thing I knew, I'd turn a corner and be in front of a dealer with the most incredible Roberta di Camerino collection.

I never had an agenda. I went for the pure joy and the thrill of finding a perfect little golden nugget at the bottom of a bin.

I also began to notice that I was being drawn to the energy and life force in these clothes. Finding myself in the right place at the right time was divine alignment in action.

For almost a decade of my life in Milan, I wore vintage almost every day. I mixed it with new clothes and—crucially—also had an amazing tailor who made house calls and came over weekly to help me alter the items I bought.

Fernanda was a tiny woman with sparkling eyes and magic hands, who never saw a garment that she couldn't rework into my twenty-first-century silhouette. She was a co-creator; together we breathed new life into old things and allowed them to see another light of day in a completely different era.

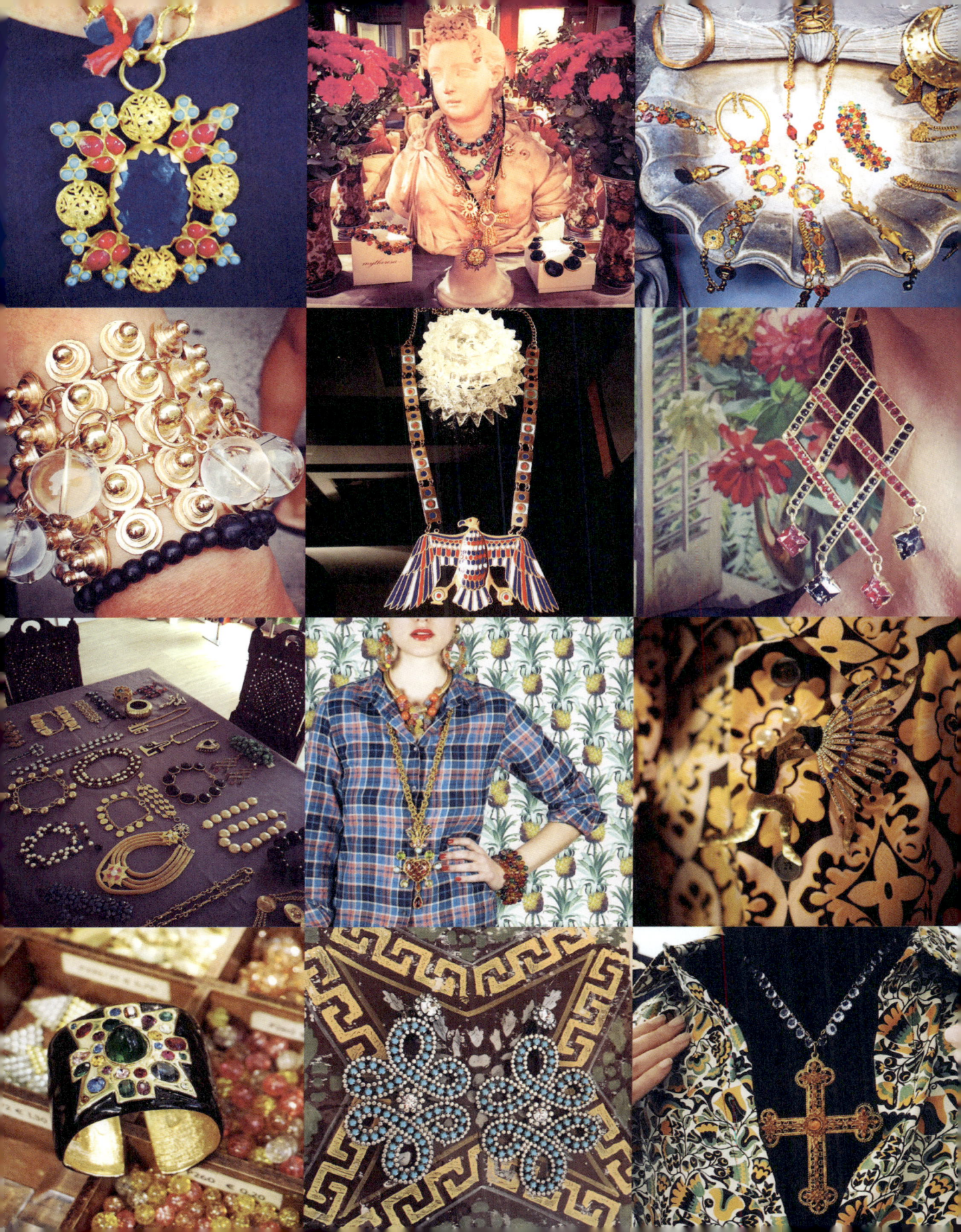

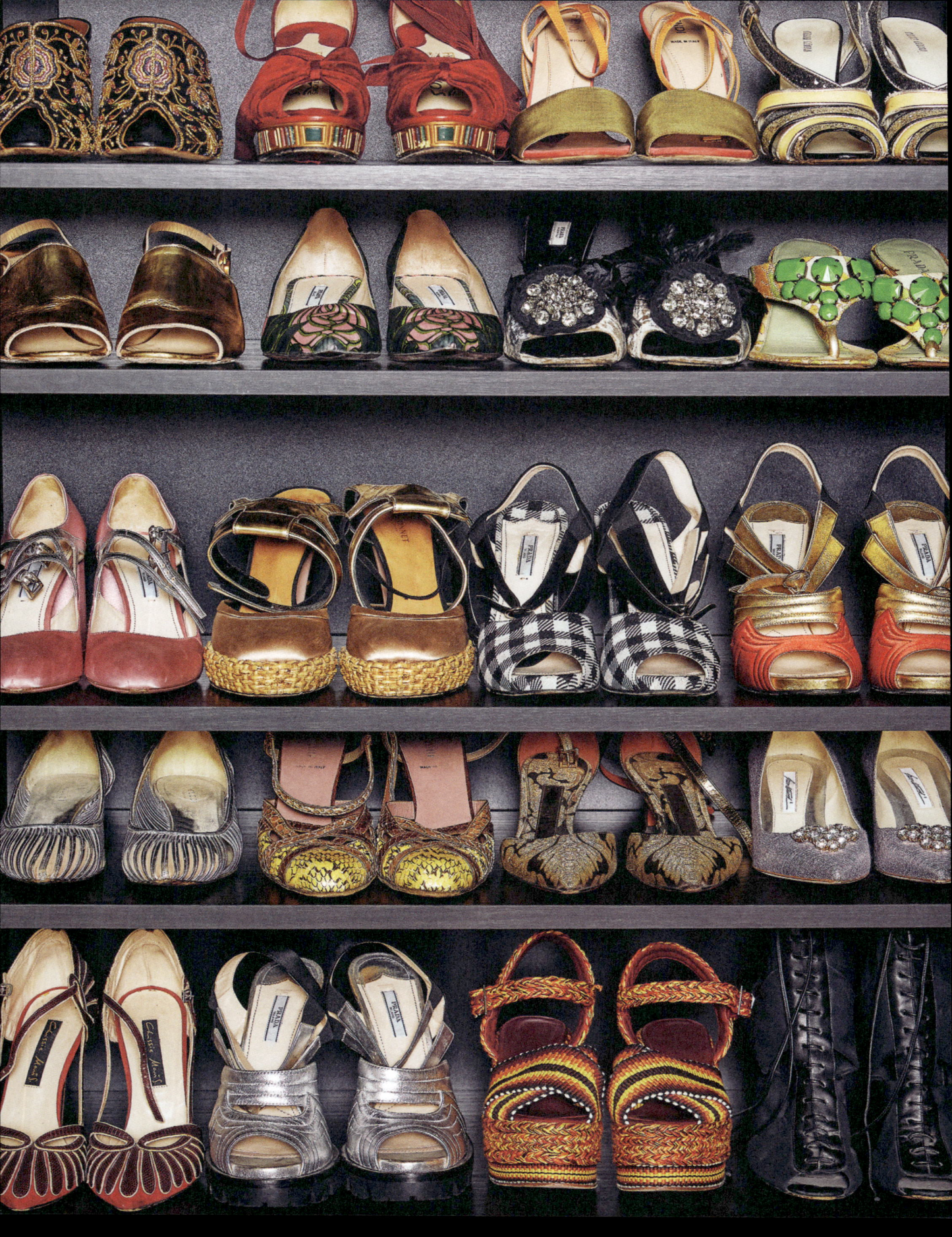

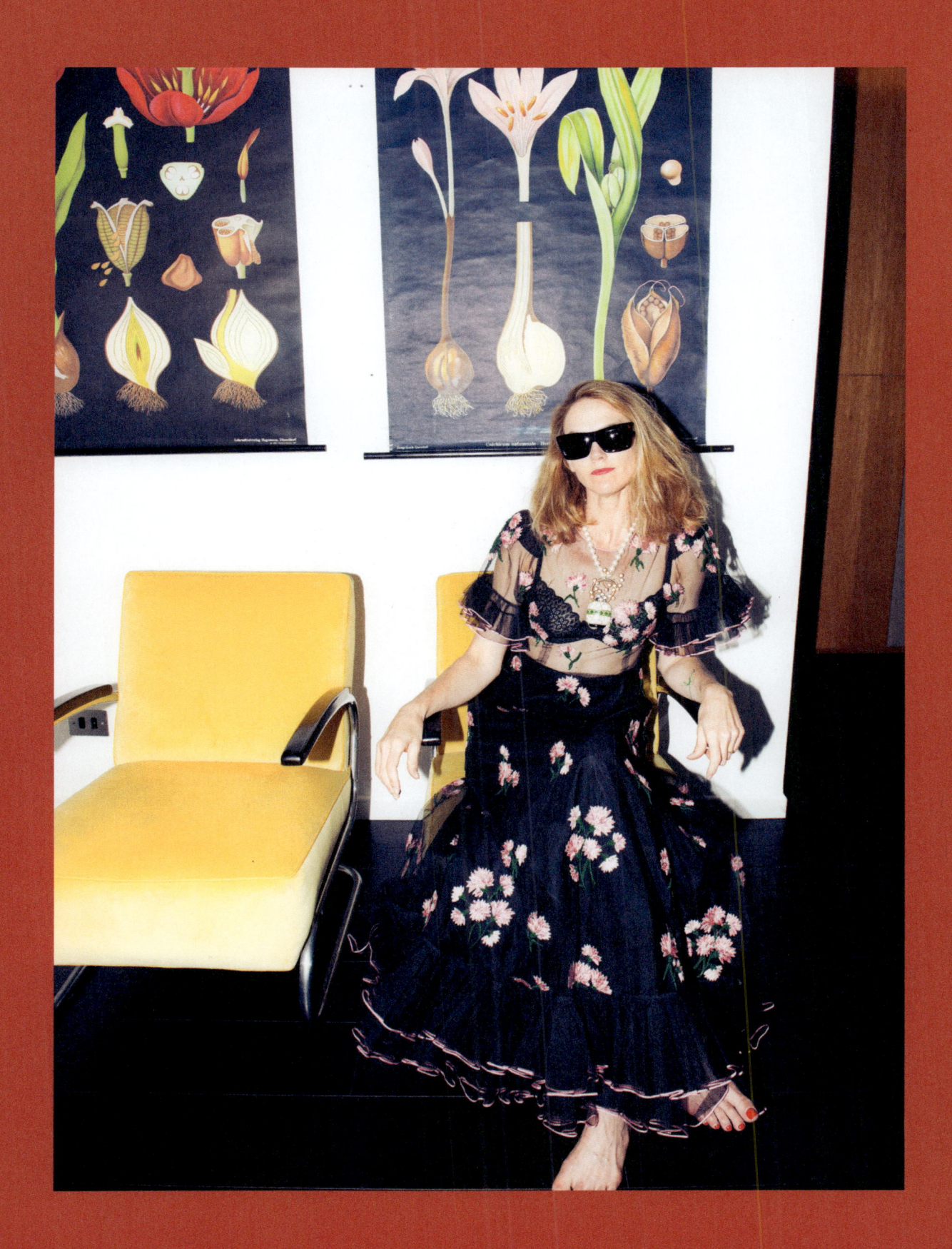

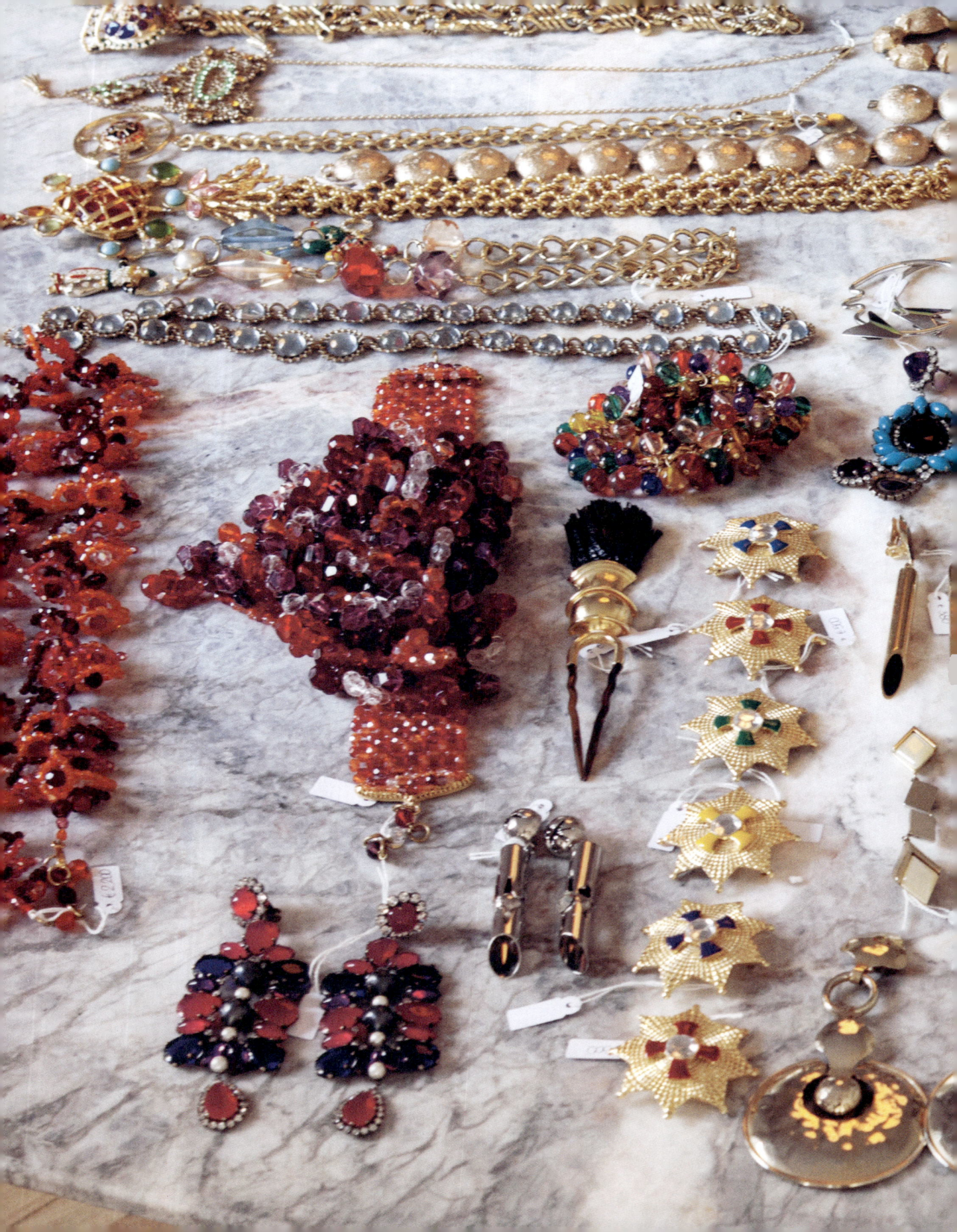

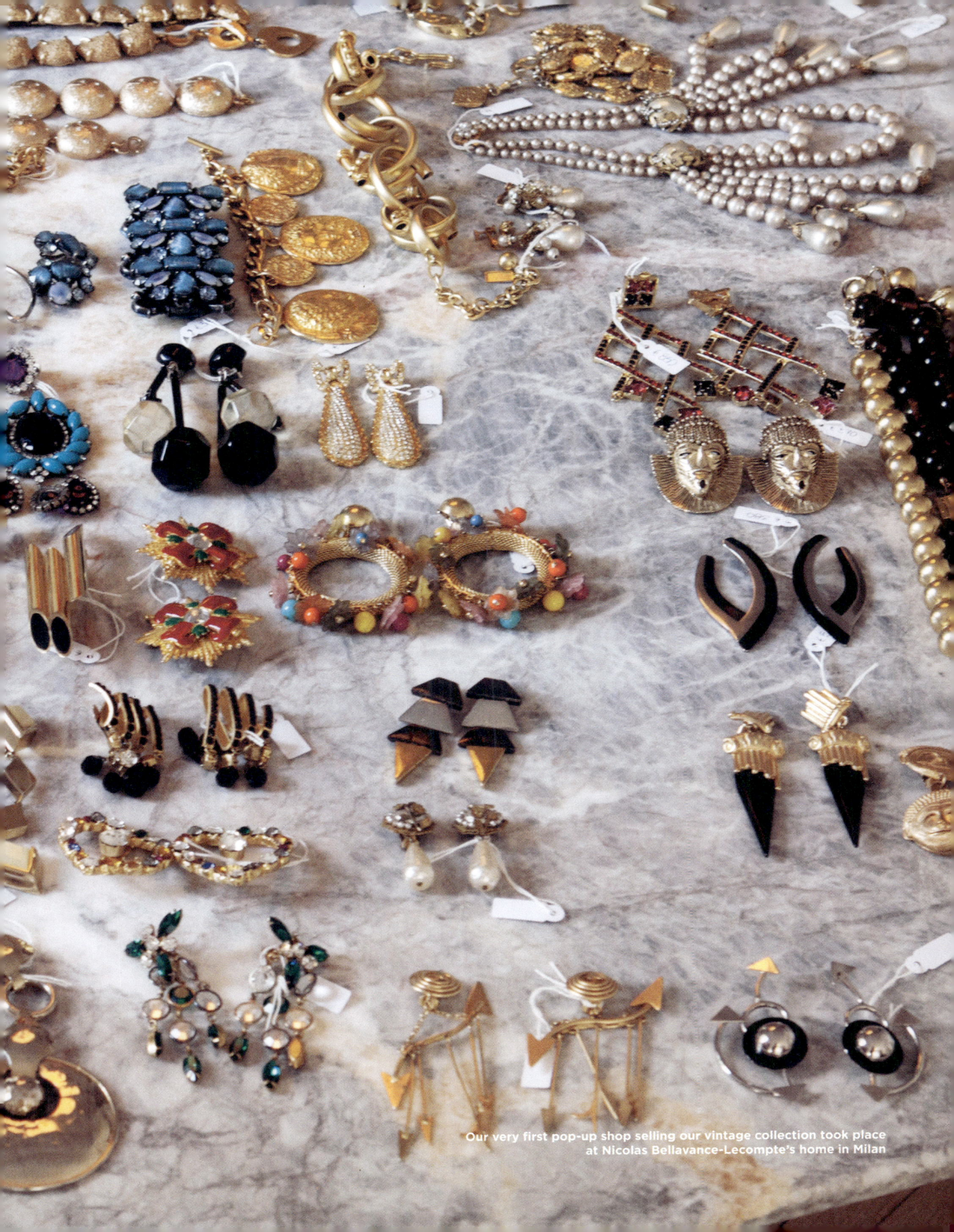

Our very first pop-up shop selling our vintage collection took place at Nicolas Bellavance-Lecompte's home in Milan

LA DOUBLEJ'S FIRST GODPARENT: DEANNA FARNETI CERA

Deanna Farneti Cera is a 4' 11" sassypants, intellectual Italian fashionista with a clipped American accent who ensures nobody ever bosses her around. She was also the world's foremost authority on costume jewelry, having authored more than ten books and curating the first-ever exhibit on fashion jewelry in 1991 in Milan and London. I discovered Deanna through a Milanese friend who was wearing a stunning 1940s necklace, and couldn't wait to visit her.

The global HQ for the world's preeminent vintage jewelry expert turned out to be a small ground-floor apartment behind a dark courtyard near Porta Romana. Most of her prized pieces—including vintage Chanel, Yves Saint Laurent, Versace, Valentino, as well as mountains of shimmering Coppola & Toppo, Miriam Haskell, and Ugo Correani—were shoved into tiny drawers in dark closets. The real good stuff, she said, "is hidden under my mattress."

Over a three-year period, I got an advanced degree in costume jewelry from Deanna. She knew the maker or designer of all jewelry produced from the 1890s to the 1990s, studied the hand of each, the embellishment or weight they used, what kind of metals and tecÿiques were possible.

She knew the office politics and the fashion catfights from fifty years ago; she knew the gossip behind every historical designer, who had talent and who didn't. She would not let me leave her until I sat down and got schooled in some important aspect of this history, usually by shouting at the top of her lungs. "Half of what Chanel produced after the 1980s was made in China!" she would scream at me, furious at the insult to her craft.

Every time I visited, I found a new drawer and a new cache of information that I would file into my brain or take back to the office to feed LaDoubleJ. Deanna could authenticate things that were not even logoed. (Logos only started in fashion and in fashion jewelry in the 1960s.) She was extremely passionate, extremely intelligent, and the most fun vintage resource I ever had. She was also fiercely, proudly Italian, and luckily one of several midwives and godmothers who arrived out of nowhere to nurse and nurture LaDoubleJ.

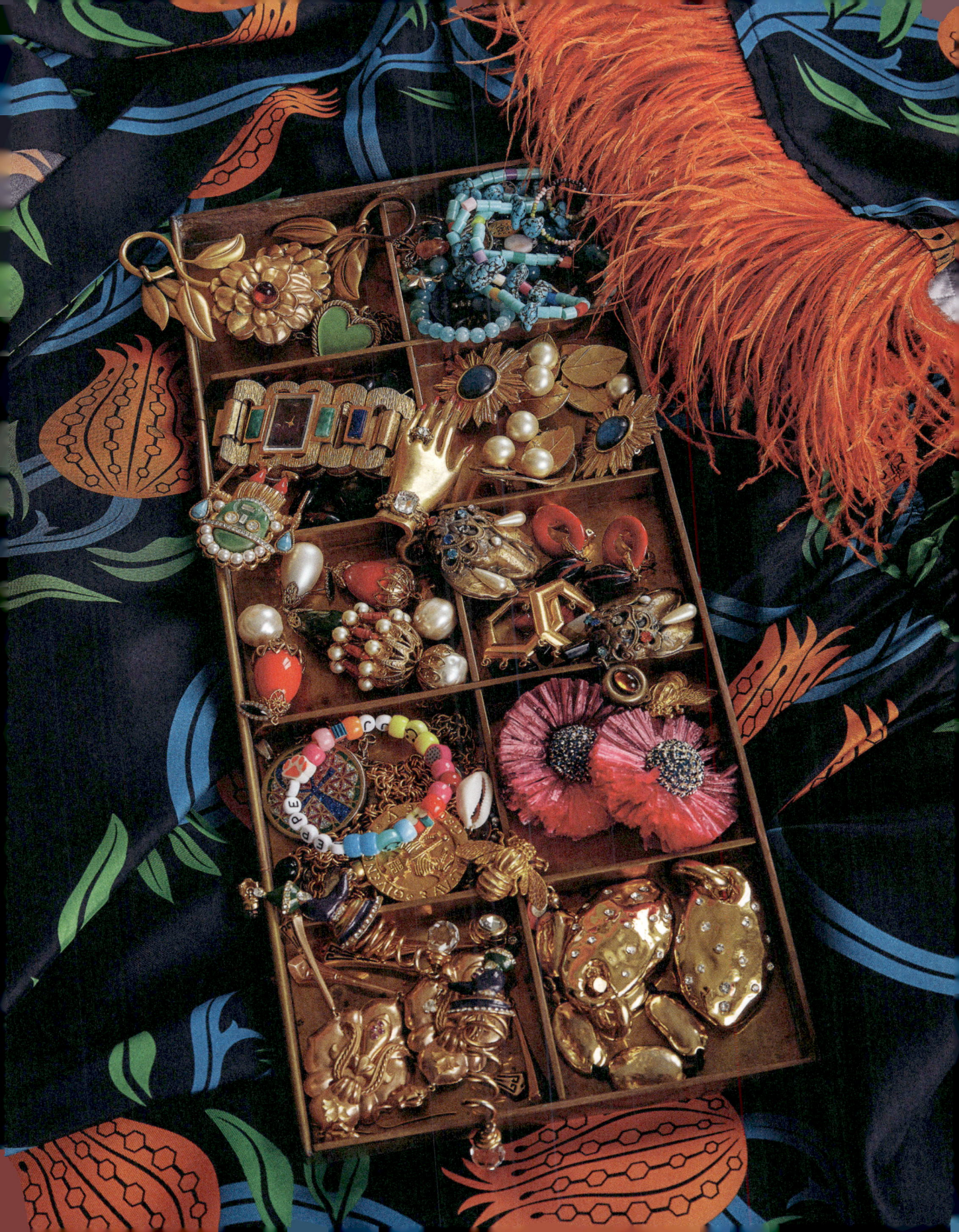

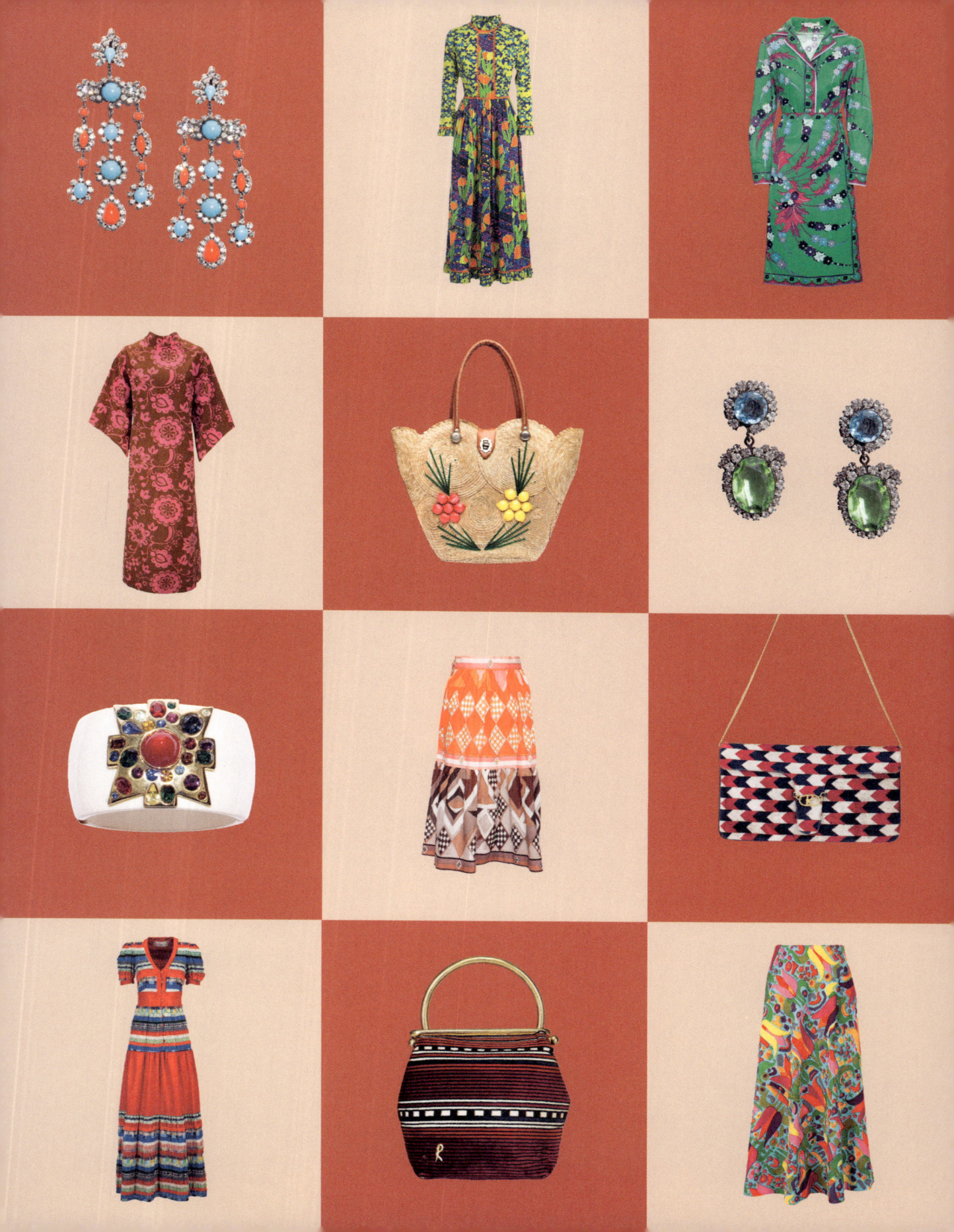

MY FOLLOW-YOUR-JOY CRUMBS VINTAGE RULEBOOK

People always ask for my tips on vintage: how to do it, where to do it, what to look for, and how not to get completely overwhelmed by the process. This is what I tell them:

✹ **Listen to your stomach.** Finding great vintage does not require as much brain capacity as it does gut work. See what sparks in your belly. For me, the vibrating color and pattern draw my eye in a heap of seemingly dead clothes. The silhouette is almost always secondary.

✹ **Look for prints and embroideries.** I never buy anything all black or all white—they don't age well. I also always look for embellishment like sequins, beads, and thread work, especially anything embroidered in Hong Kong in the 1960s, when the quality was fabulous.

✹ **Are you a hunter or a gatherer?** Decide if you are the kind of person who draws pleasure from sifting through junk bins for three hours. If so, it is worthwhile to do the scrounging and scouring the minute a giant fair or flea market opens up. Pasadena's Rose Bowl, Miami's Lincoln Road market and Los Angeles' Fairfax High School are still great resources for this; so are Italian charity church sales. If you don't enjoy that, then go to well-curated vintage shops that have done the legwork for you. I like William Vintage in London, Decades and Sielian vintage in LA, Madame Pauline and Cavalli & Nastri in Milan. Whenever you travel to a new city, or even a small town in Italy, always ask the locals when they have a market. Show up early.

✹ **Drop all expectations.** This is a spontaneous, not scientific, exercise. If you say, "I need a white dress," you will come home with pottery. The vintage gods always reward you when you go with wide-eyed wonder and keep an open mind.

✸ **Be realistic.** Unless you have a Fernanda the tailor in your life, do not buy anything that doesn't currently fit you. Or, find a Fernanda who shares your passion and can patiently handle the work involved.

✸ **Find the value.** The best deals these days are on intricate thread or bead embroideries that today are outrageously expensive to produce. You can still find pieces with incredible workmanship on them that make you feel like you're wearing a sculpture.

✸ **Clean it.** Don't just dry-clean your recently purchased pieces. Try cleansing them by putting them in the freezer for twenty-four hours, or by covering jewelry with rock salt overnight. You'll be glad you did.

✸ **Create relationships with dealers you like.** Negotiate, of course, but always be kind, charming, and respectful when you do so. Exchange phone numbers and let them know if you're ever in the market for something specific.

Little did I realize that as I honed my eye on vintage—the dazzling fabrics and dancing embellishments, the bezel of a ring, and clasp of a brooch, not to mention all of the vanishing tecÿiques of craftsmanship that had so thoughtfully shaped these beauties— I was experiencing a major shift inside. I was getting busy and brewing up something of my own.

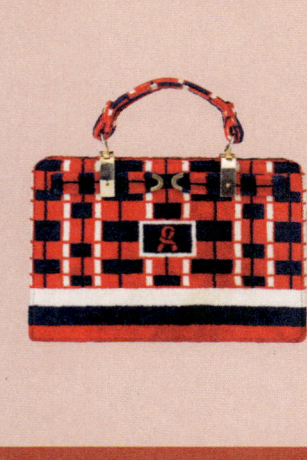

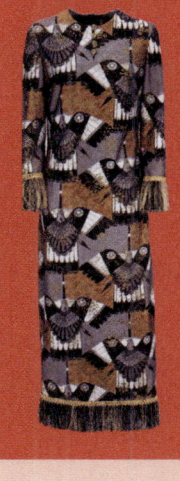

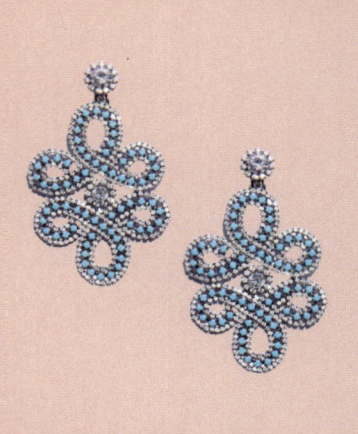

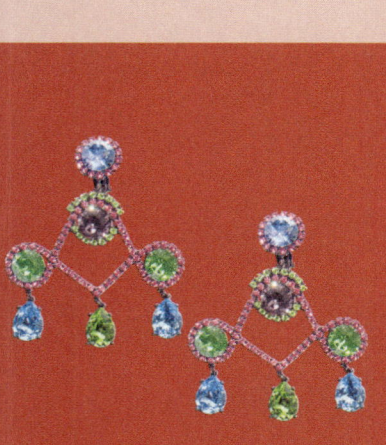

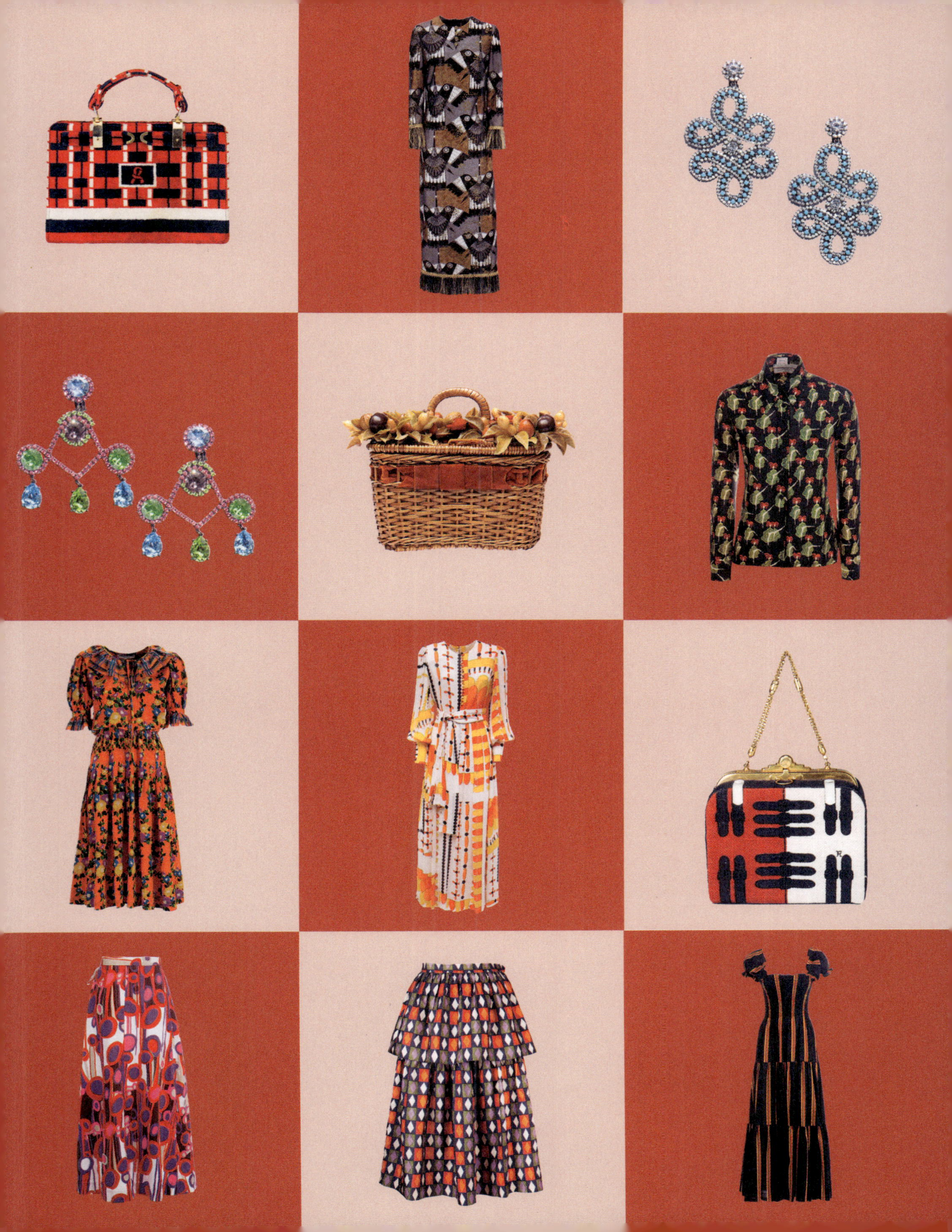

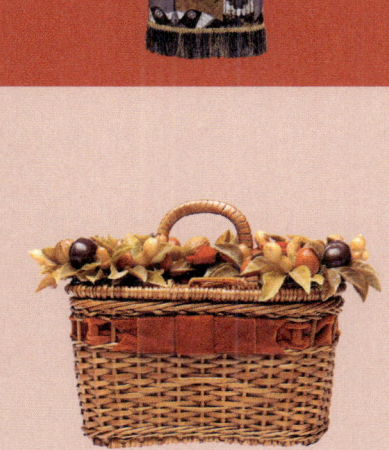

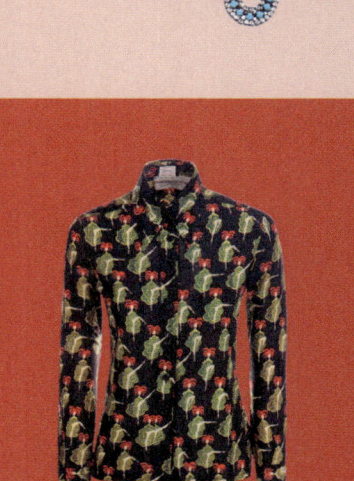

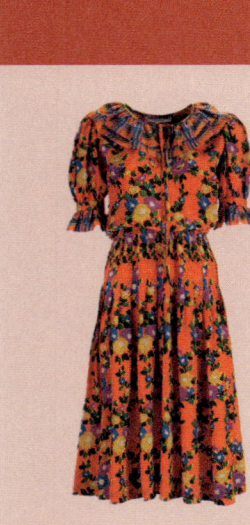

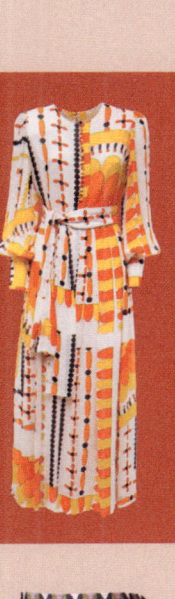

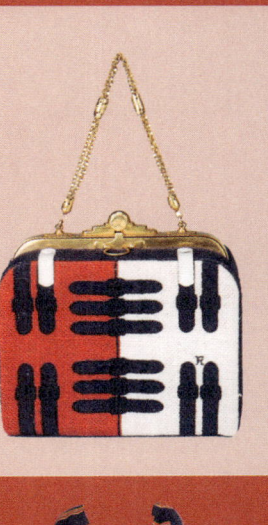

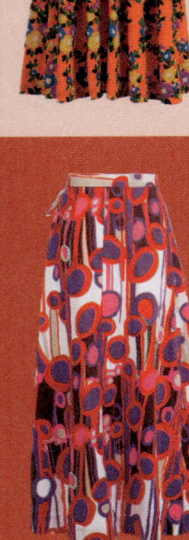

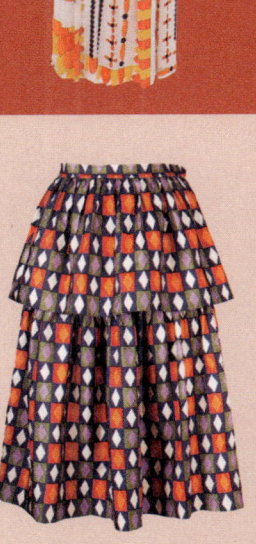

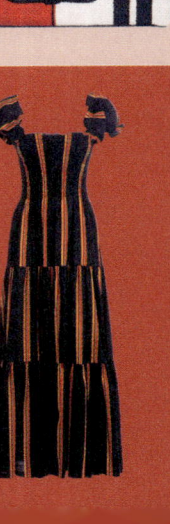

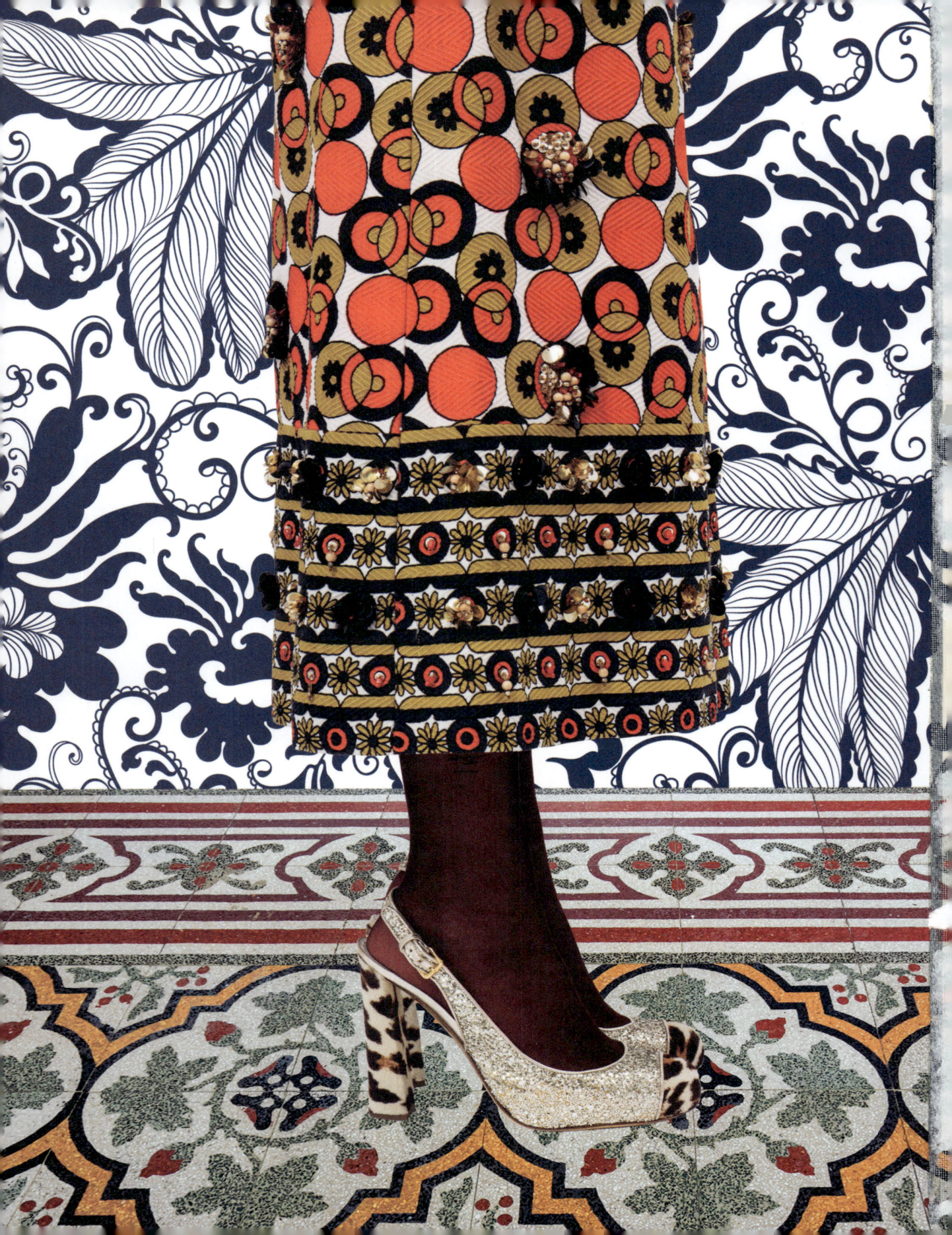

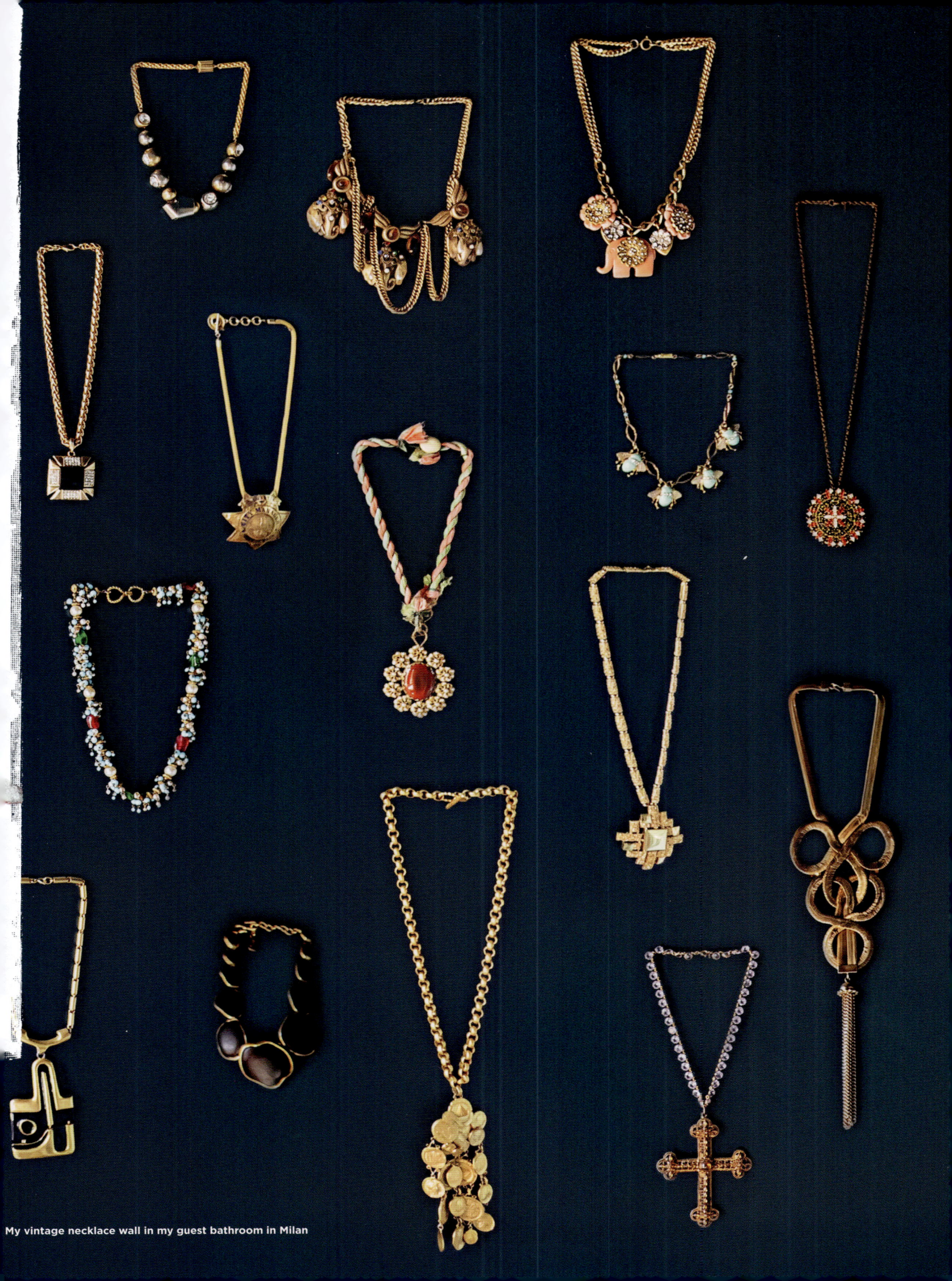

My vintage necklace wall in my guest bathroom in Milan

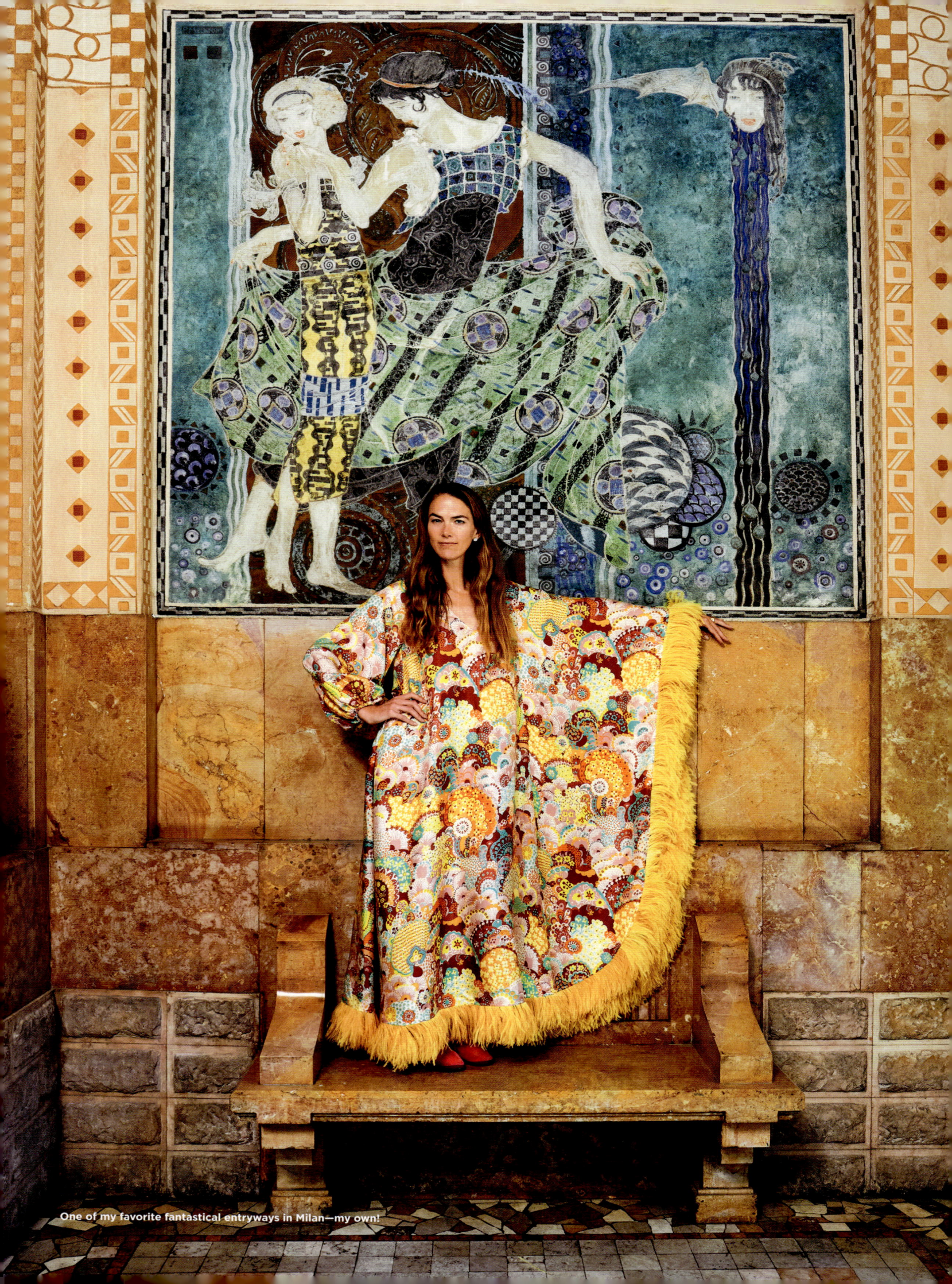

One of my favorite fantastical entryways in Milan—my own!

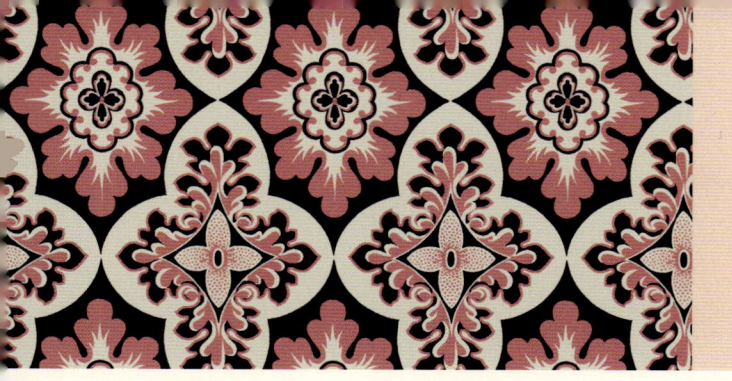

THE KEYS TO MILAN'S KINGDOM

Once I was floating, bobbing, and splashing in Italy's wild creative waters (rather than drowning in them), I became more receptive to Mamma Milano's energy codes. I grew happier and easier to be around. The scales of criticism and negativity fell away and I began to see the city with new eyes: she was truly *gorgissima*.

Milan is not a brazen, bare-chested beauty. She doesn't stun you with her flashy facades, like Rome or Venice can. She is a quieter, more mysterious muse that reveals herself slowly, peeling away the layers as she sees fit. This is so very Divine Mother of her—enigmatic, unpredictable, and Sphinx-like. Her luscious gardens, stunning courtyards, gilded and mosaiced doorways, marbled lobbies, and high-ceilinged homes are stashed away behind a door, a gate, or a wall. They require patience to find, slowing down to see, and friends to unlock them with keys.

Milan needed to be romanced, she needed to be courted. Once I began looking for her, listening and waiting, her beauty began to look for me.

On my fiftieth trip to Milan's train station, I finally stopped rushing and looked up at the most spectacular, 200-foot-high ceiling and almost fell over in awe. All of that hulking gray architecture I'd determinedly driven past in my Cinquecento were Fascist-era masterpieces. Where I used to dismiss the plainness of 1960s-era buildings, I suddenly became aware of every brass, marble, and wood inlaid detail in meticulous doorways and curved-desk lobbies lit by original 1970s Azucena fixtures. Beneath my feet, floors in apartments and shops suddenly appeared as jigsaw marble intarsias or wood herringbones. I spotted the magnificence of intricately hand-wrought doorknobs, the wedding-cake moldings atop soaring walls. Had they always been there? Yes, they had. I just hadn't taken the time to truly see.

At this point in my journey, doors flung themselves open to me with the easy energetic force of being in harmony rather than in opposition. There was beauty everywhere—once my heart softened enough to let my eyes open and receive the training that this design capital was willing to offer. I saw deeply, I appreciated fully, I revered humbly... and then my heart officially opened for business.

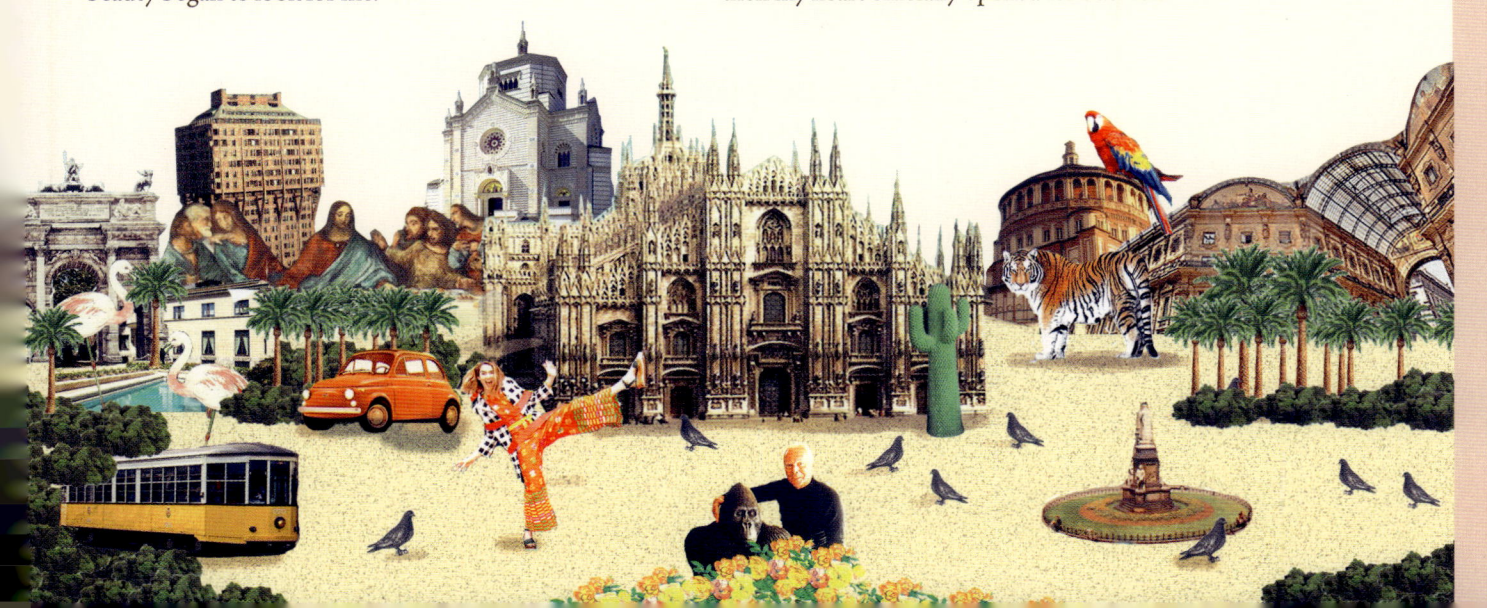

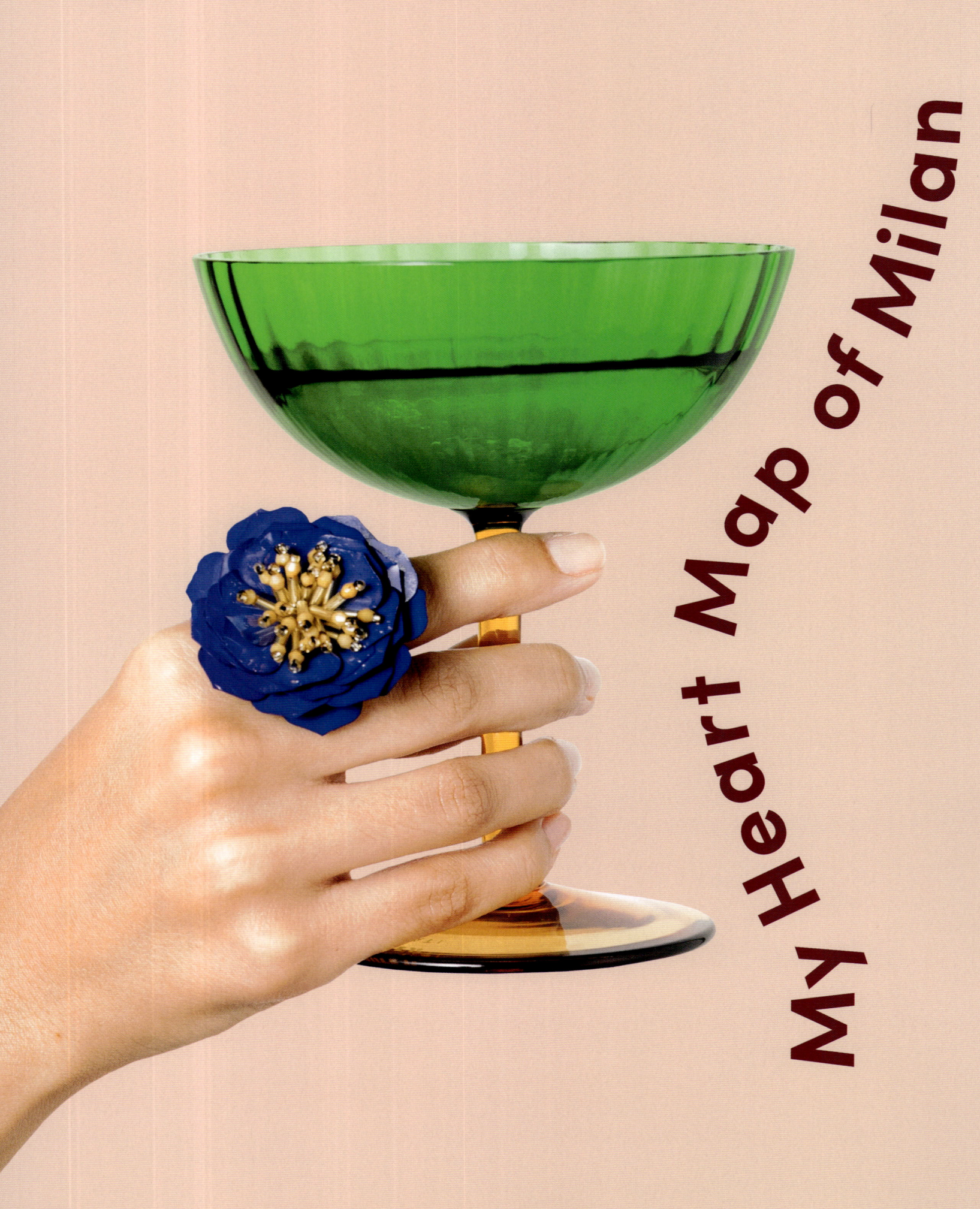

MAMMA MILANO

My Heart Map of Milan

Here are a few of the places—private *palazzi* and house museums, courtyards, and domed ceilings—whose beauty Mamma Milano sings to me like a siren any time I wander the city. **CASA GALIMBERTI** I discovered this building after my first Gucci fashion show in 2002, and its painted Liberty façade is sensational. **BAR BASSO** Powerfully evocative of the 1970s Milan design scene, this bar is a zoo during Salone del Mobile. I only ever meet creative people here. **MUSEO BAGATTI VALSECCHI** This is a replica of a Milanese Renaissance home, complete with tapestried walls and rows of armor. I did several shoots here, including portraits of jeweler Giampiero Bodino. **LA CASA DEGLI ATELLANI AND MUSEO VIGNA DI LEONARDO** Not only is this where Leonardo da Vinci slept while painting *The Last Supper*, there's a gorgeous hidden garden, too. La DoubleJ curated a space here for a *Cabana* event. **CASA MUSEO BOSCHI DI STEFANO** This is one of my favorite mid-century home museums, with a great art and furniture collection. **PALAZZO CLERICI** I nearly fainted the first time I saw a fashion show here: every wall and ceiling is covered in a bonkers amount of gold. **VILLA NECCHI** This is the most exquisite 1930s home museum in all of Milan. We hosted Andrea's birthday party here one year. **TORRE VELASCA** I had a view of this 1950s skyscraper—a radical early example of Italian modern architecture, by BBPR—from our Via San Barnaba home. I once got to visit the top-floor apartment with a wrap-around balcony. **THE DUOMO** I love walking to the roof for the views, but it's actually the marble and mosaic floor that makes me vibrate. **PALAZZO CRESPI** This private giant *palazzo*, with a private park in the backyard, suddenly became the venue for fashion brands and magazines to host dinner parties, and I ended up being a repeated guest. It never gets old. **PASTICCERIA CUCCHI** This is my Happiness Headquarters, as you know. **CIVICO PLANETARIA** Tucked unassumingly inside the Giardini Pubblici, this planetarium was designed by Piero Portaluppi, Milan's coolest mid-century architect, who also did the Villa Necchi. **VILLA CICOGNA** Alessandro Michele had an incredible dinner in this decadently frescoed private *palazzo* on Corso Monforte. **ROTONDA DELLA BESANA** Marni had their flower market here, and I used to jog in circles around it. **PARCO GIARDINO DELLA GUASTALLA** Pepper's first park was small but had a huge fountain that looked like an eighteenth-century swimming pool. **BAR LUCE, PRADA FOUNDATION** This was designed by Wes Anderson to look like a typical Milanese café. **LA SCALA** Nothing is more opulent, or makes you feel more instantly fancy-pants, than an evening inside Milan's red velvet–lined historic opera house. **CHURCH HOPPING** I'm a big church hopper and go only when there is no priest. I sit down and write. I am attracted only to those with crazy frescoed ceilings, which are huge creative vortex points for me. There's Chiesa di Santa Maria della Passione, Sant' Antonio Abate, Basilica di Santa Maria presso San Satiro and, my favorite, Chiesa di San Maurizio al Monastero Maggiore. **CIMITERO MONUMENTALE** The first time I went to Milan's biggest cemetery, I connected energetically to all the statues of the incredible dead creative people. It was very powerful. **EMANUELA SETTI CARRARO DALLA CHIESA** During a fashion show, I realized that Milan's ten-year-olds were studying in the most gorgeous spot in town. **MILAN'S OTHERWORLDLY STATUES** A lot of the buildings have statues that look like mythical guardians: half-human, half-animal beasts, angels, and other creatures. They're tucked all over the city and I loved discovering them. There's one that's right near La Scala, around the corner, that is really amazing. And there's one that was near my home on Via San Barnaba.

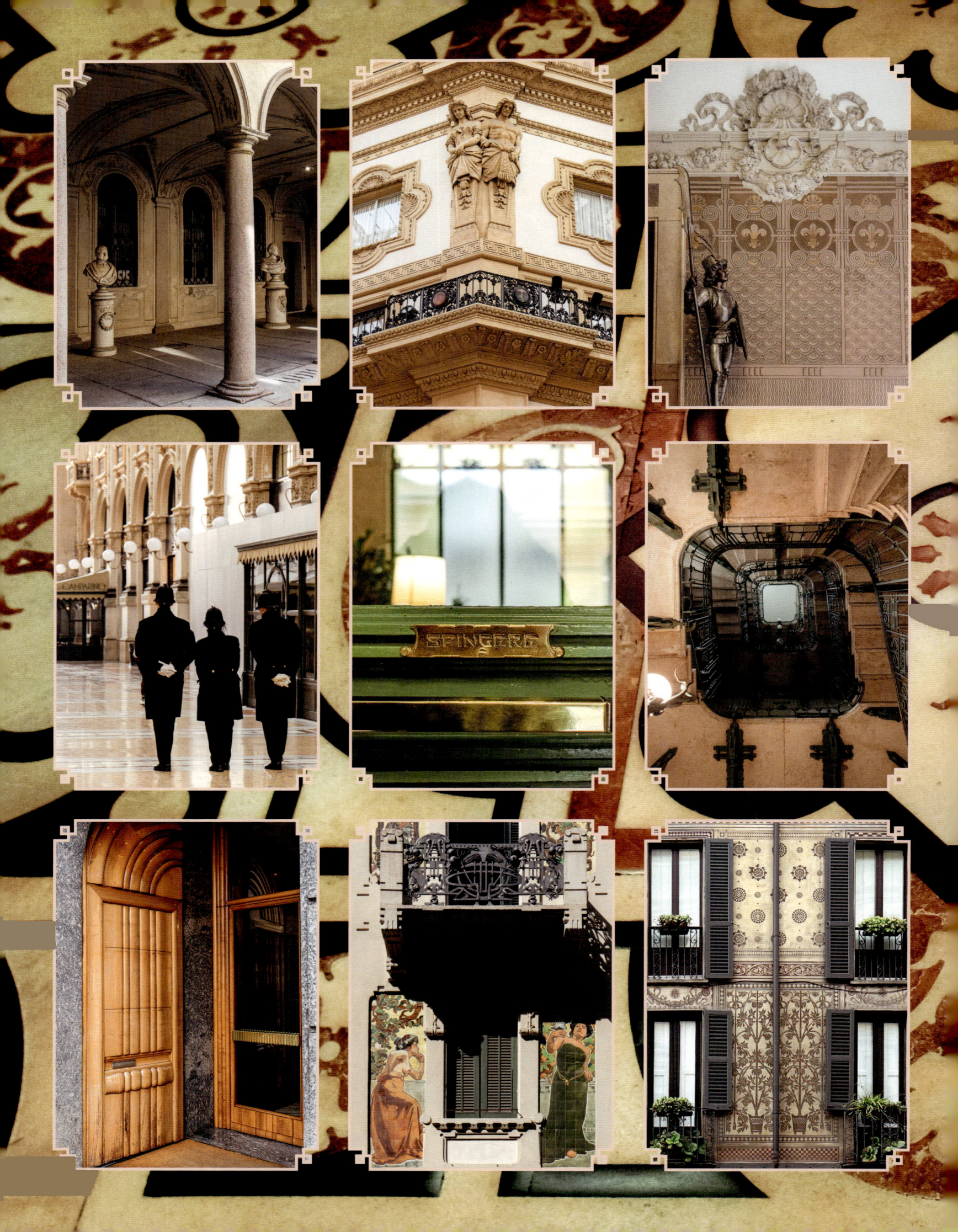

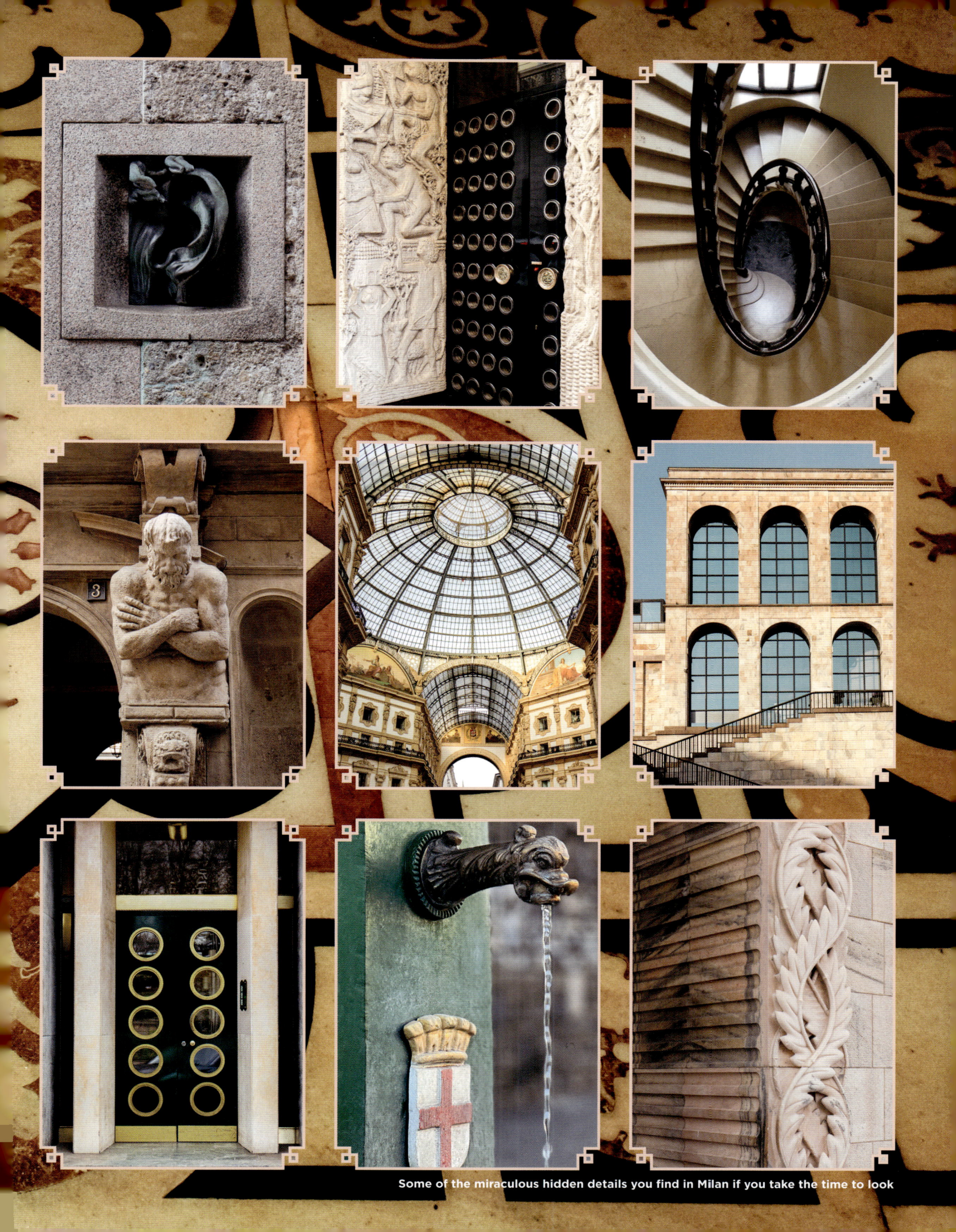

Some of the miraculous hidden details you find in Milan if you take the time to look

BELL

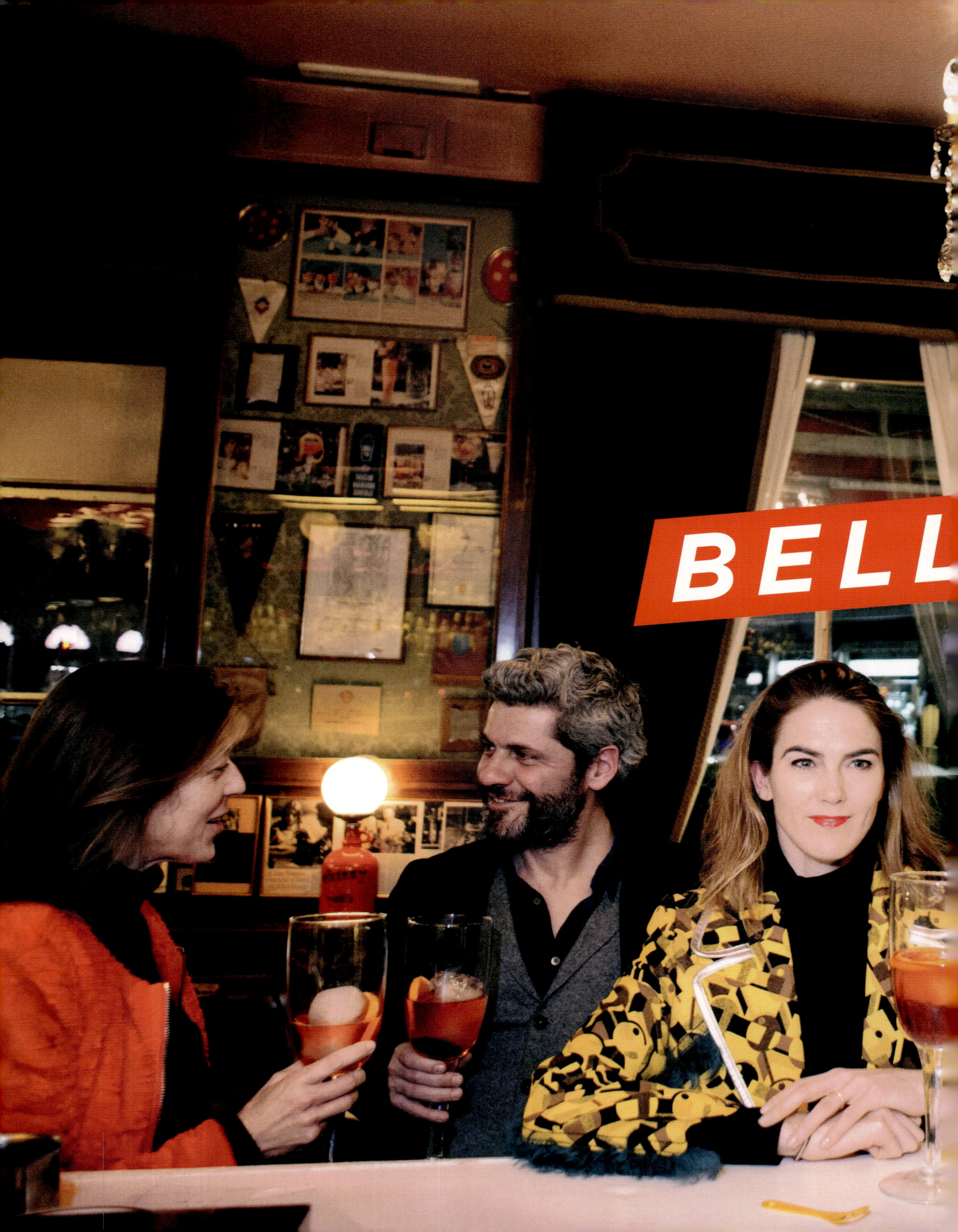

O BAR BASSO!

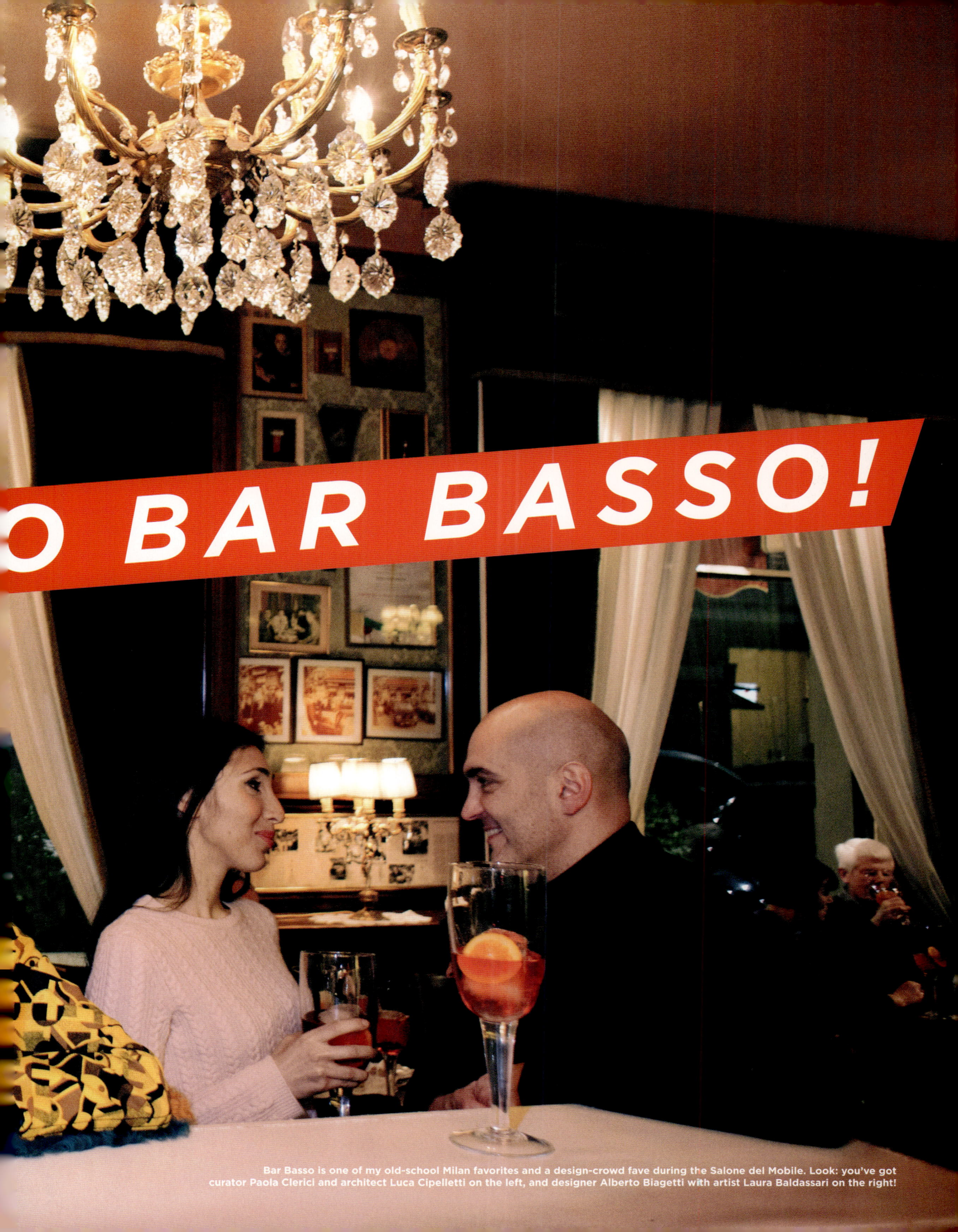

Bar Basso is one of my old-school Milan favorites and a design-crowd fave during the Salone del Mobile. Look: you've got curator Paola Clerici and architect Luca Cipelletti on the left, and designer Alberto Biagetti with artist Laura Baldassari on the right!

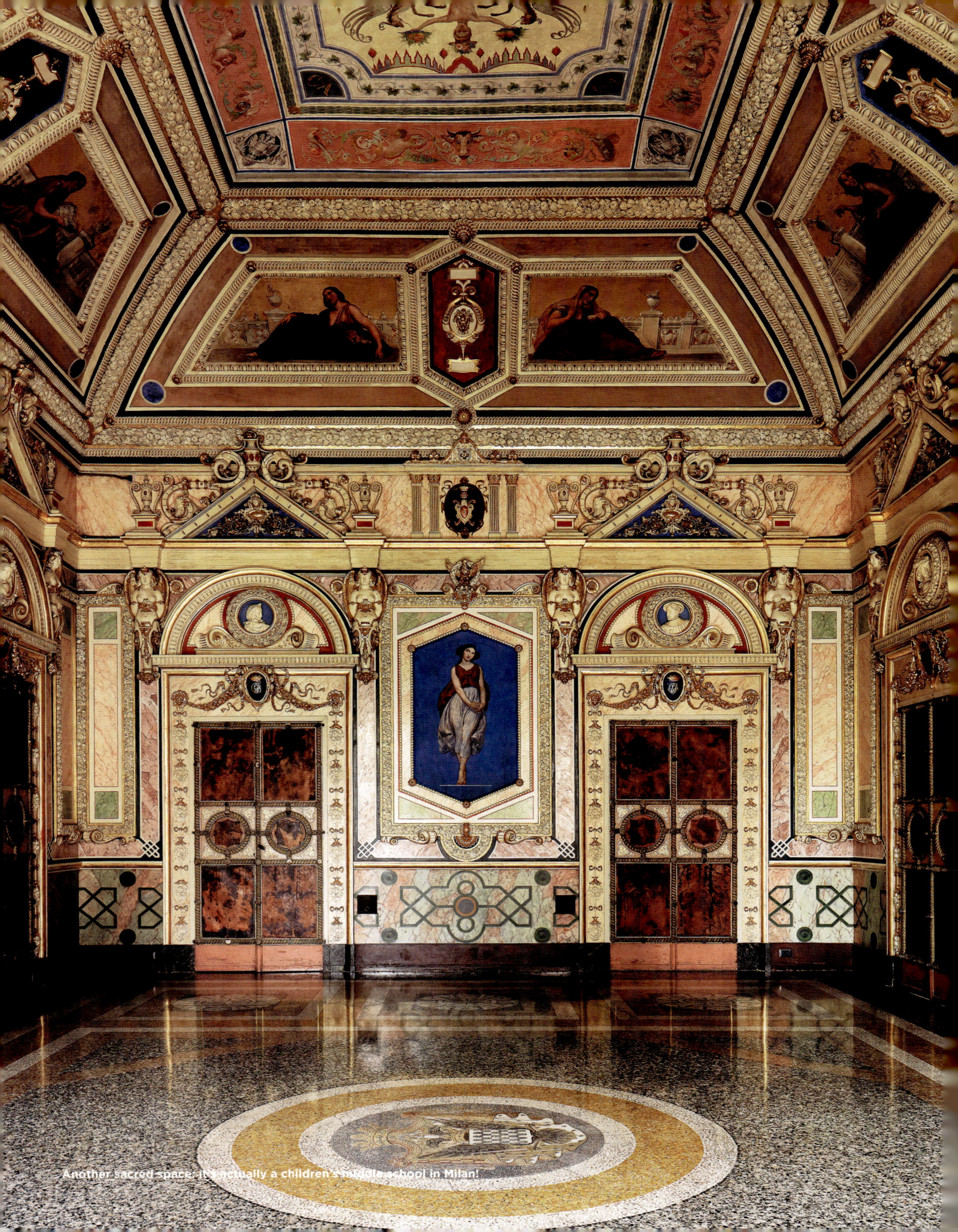

Another sacred space: it's actually a children's middle school in Milan!

FINDING SACRED SPACES FOR SWIRLING UP MY OWN CREATIONS

I was initially attracted to the churches in Milan and Sicily for their visual splendor—the soaring height of the wavy structures, the gloriously painted ceilings, the marvelous stucco work, the gilded walls, the intricately intarsia-cut marbled floors that fit together like a puzzle, the gleaming jeweled altars. But soon I began to get strange sensations in empty churches. Something was waking up. Coming into the quiet when the priest and congregation were long gone, I would sit, gaze at, and internalize the beauty, then close my eyes and finally go deep into my soul.

Sometimes I would meditate, sometimes I'd creatively pray, and other times I would whip out my computer and write like crazy in front of Jesus Christ. The creative channels were wide open in these churches.

Later I learned that most of these churches were built on the Earth's energetic leylines and were literally power seats. Additionally, Italy's Renaissance master craftsmen were all experts on sacred geometry, working with lines, proportions, patterns, and colors to evoke the divine. These were the world's original art galleries; all the creativity that existed on the planet was being funneled into these churches.

Whenever I sat there, the sacred visuals would swap out whatever gunk I had in my head, sink into my skin, and drill through my heart like a handheld Bosch hardware set. I began communing with the energy of the original creators, feeling lighter, more inspired and empowered to create my own inner and outer temples. My creative wayshowers became the Baroque artists of the fifteenth and sixteenth centuries.

PHRASEBOOK

SCOMODITÀ: INCONVENIENCE OR DISCOMFORT

Usage: As in, you have to work at it!

Italy requires a bit of elbow grease and effort to dig under its surface and get to the good stuff. It's like great vintage and it's like the city of Milan itself: the prize is not presented to you on a perfectly edited rack. (Take, for instance, the interior at left, which I randomly walked into during fashion week, only to discover it was the school of my best friend's kid!) You have to jump into the dark, dig around, pry her open, and eventually Italy's shiny pearls will pop out into your hands.

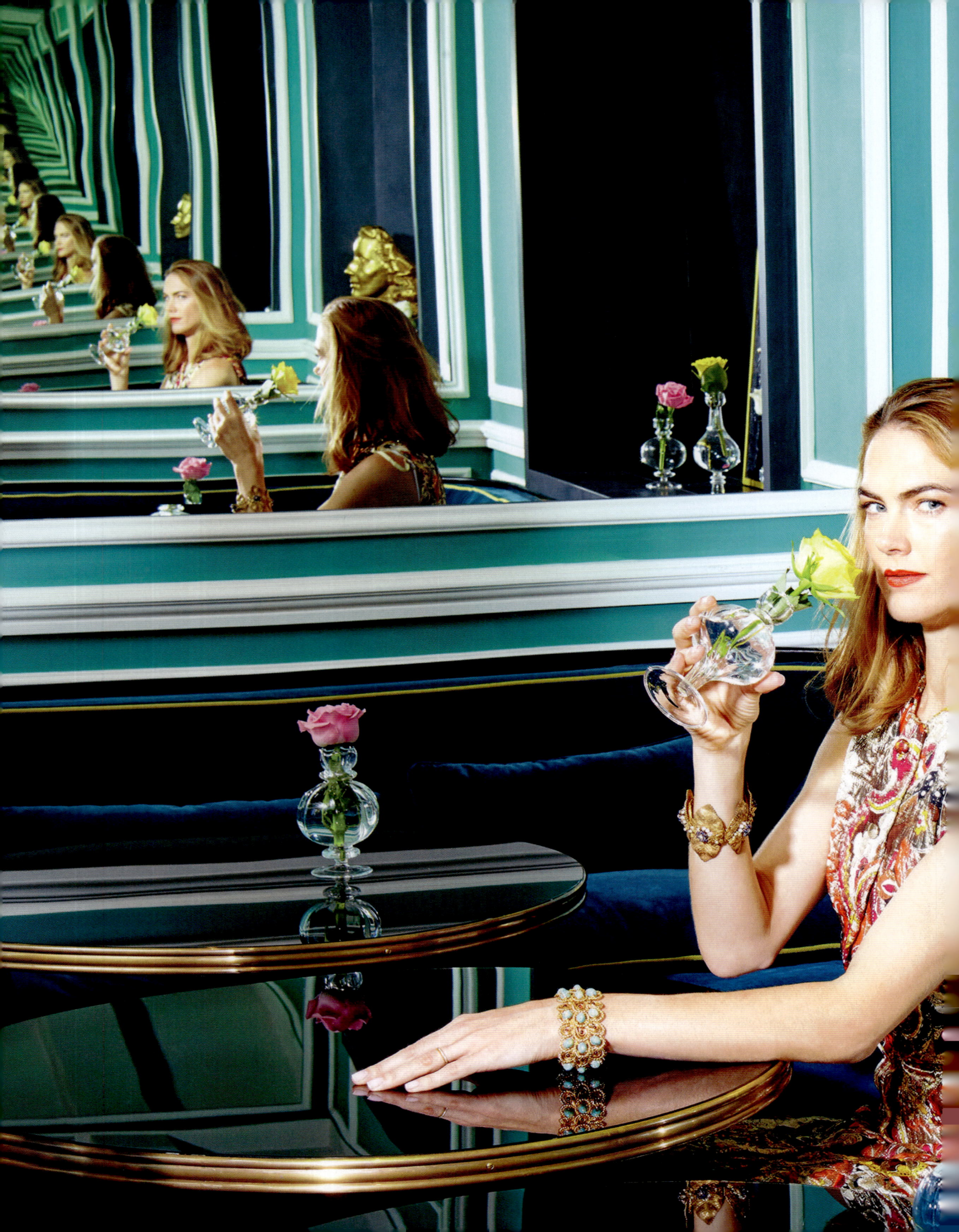

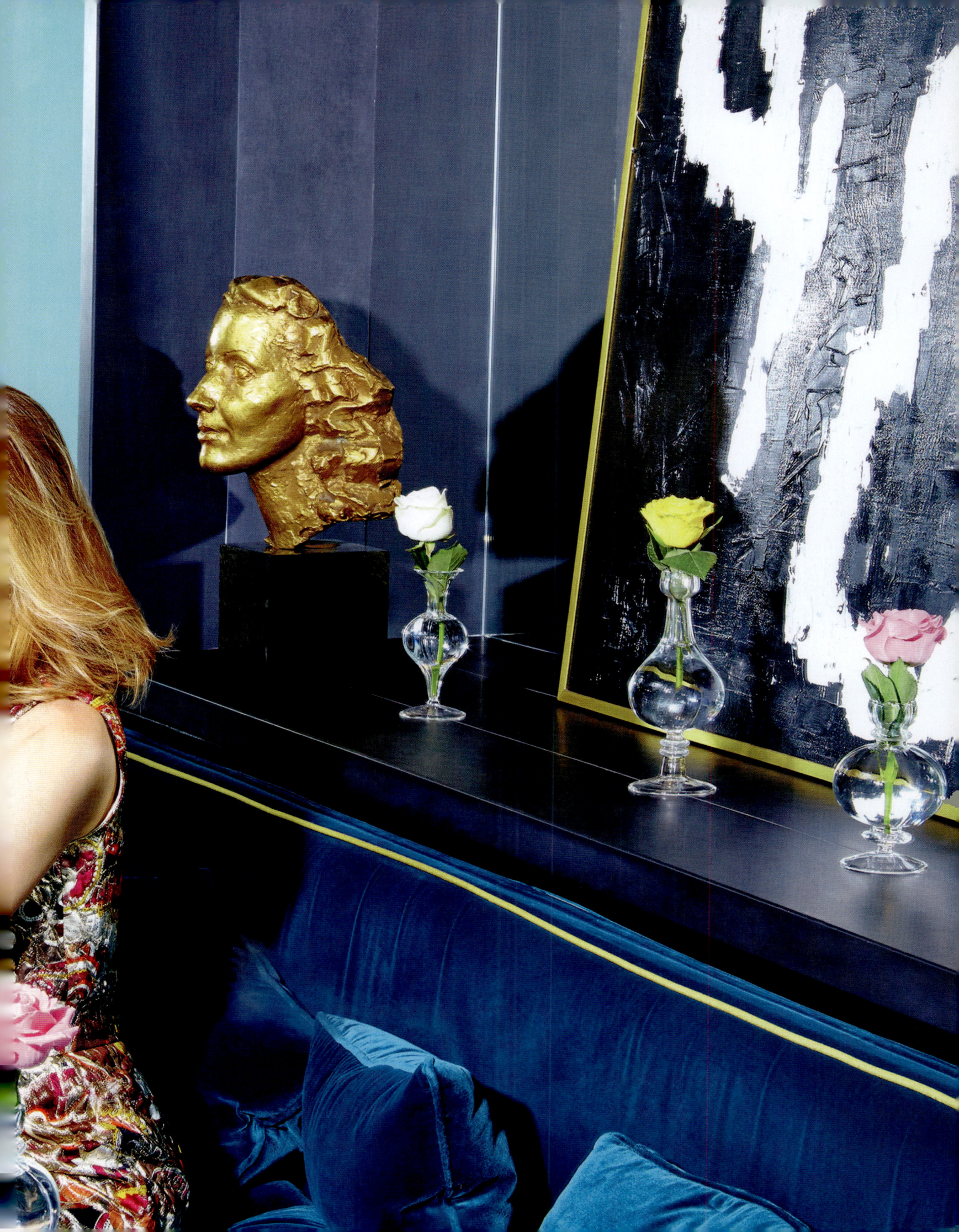

MAMMA MILANO

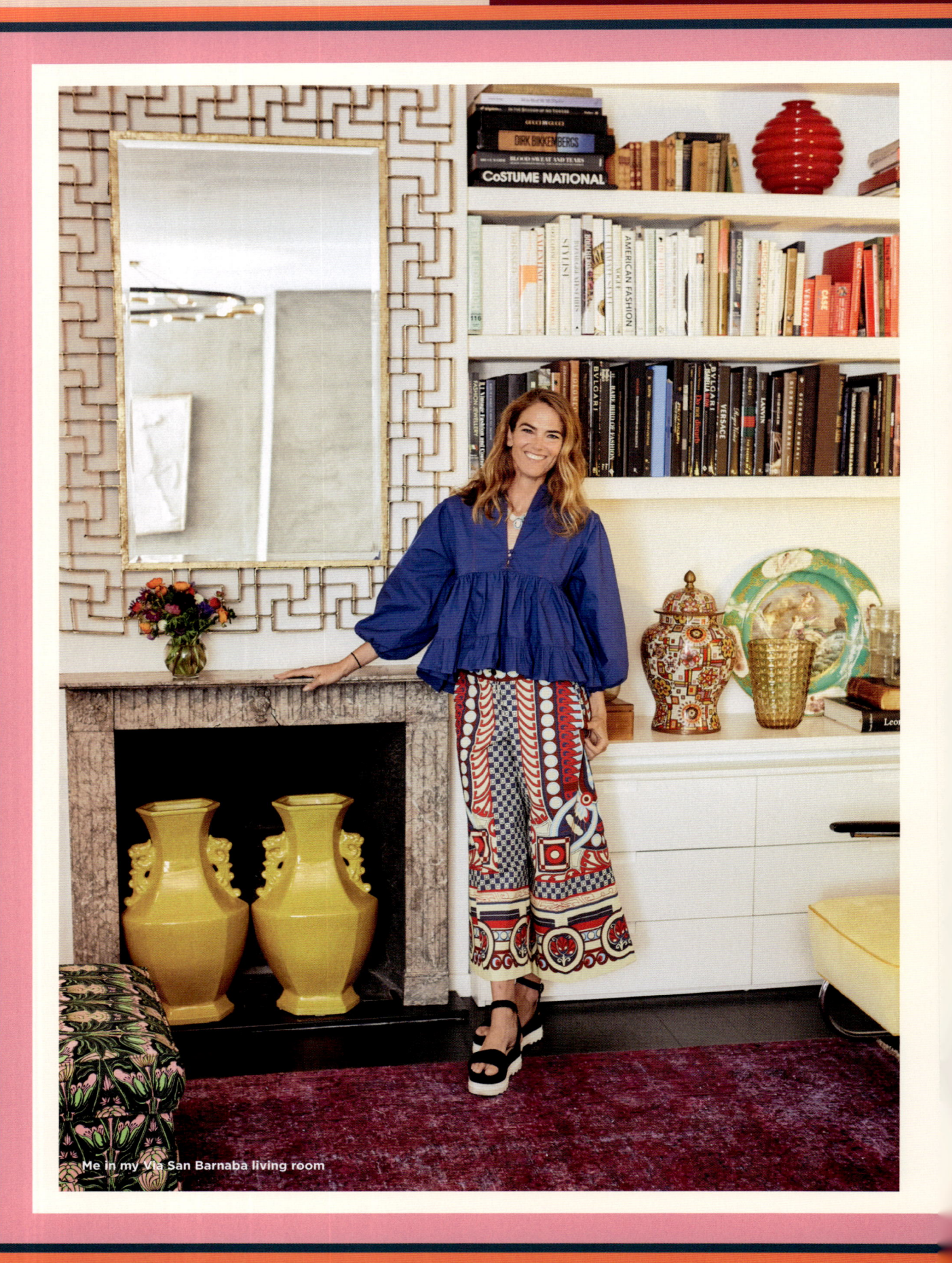

Me in my Via San Barnaba living room

118

ABBONDANZA

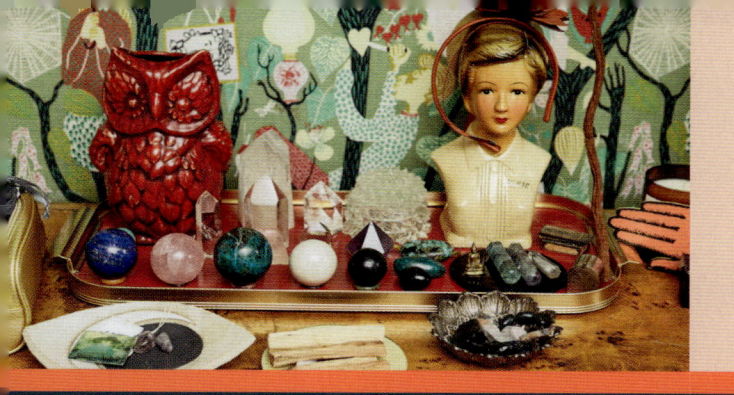

CREATING MY FIRST HOME: VIA SAN BARNABA

Dining in and drifting around gorgeous 500-year-old Milanese palaces, 1930s design gems, and quirky 1960s apartments had me dreaming of building my own creative container.

My search for a dream home lasted through two years of walking into ninety-three ho-hum properties shown by no fewer than thirty-two different realtors (so Italian!). Andrea and I finally landed on a wonderful apartment behind Milan's courthouse. It had a fabulous terrace with views of two buildings that sum up Milan's design excellence and its polarities: the 1958 modernist Torre Velasca and the fourteenth-century Duomo. We bought the apartment thinking there was very little to do, but suddenly walls came down, floors got ripped up, and bathrooms and kitchen were erased and rebuilt.

The architect was a blue-eyed Italian with brilliant ideas for dividing the space and designing all of the built-in oak furniture, which was later painstakingly crafted by two eighty-five-year-old men who worked by hand out of an old farmhouse in Pavia. But our young *architetto* had little sense of operations, coordination, organization, or even grade-school note-taking—he tended to scribble meeting notes on his hand. So, I assumed the role of project manager, clients' representative, budget enforcer, appointment keeper, and all-around mood enhancer.

I learned that demanding something be done, or offering more money for it to be done on time (which is what my mother helpfully suggested by phone from Los Angeles one day), would insult an Italian. The only way to get the construction workers, plumber, electrician, glass cutter, stone cutter, and carpenters to work in harmony was to throw away the schedule and flirt like mad (see page 37). Halfway through the renovation, I turned on the coquettish charm. And it worked.

In Italy, architects are usually doubly charged with furnishings, which is probably why most new Milanese interiors resemble slick design catalogs populated with Eero Saarinen tulip chairs and Eames lounge chairs—a cookie-cutter look I didn't want.

Without knowing anything about decorating, I became a decorator. I had an eye for vintage furniture, which I began to procure exactly as I collected clothes: I simply bought well-priced pieces that caught my fancy, not having a clue as to how I would use them. In a way, this was like an Italian picking the best tomatoes, basil, or ricotta, and then mixing it all together without much thought. Sometimes my random selections came together like a symphony—such as the enormous 1970s hula hoop-shaped chandelier I dug out of a dealer's dark basement storage, which I placed over a 1940s parchment-covered table from a Parma flea market.

But often, the randomness went nowhere. I re-did our entry and my writing studio no fewer than ten times. When the sweet Sicilian painter arrived for the sixth time in two years, I sighed and simply said, "Just

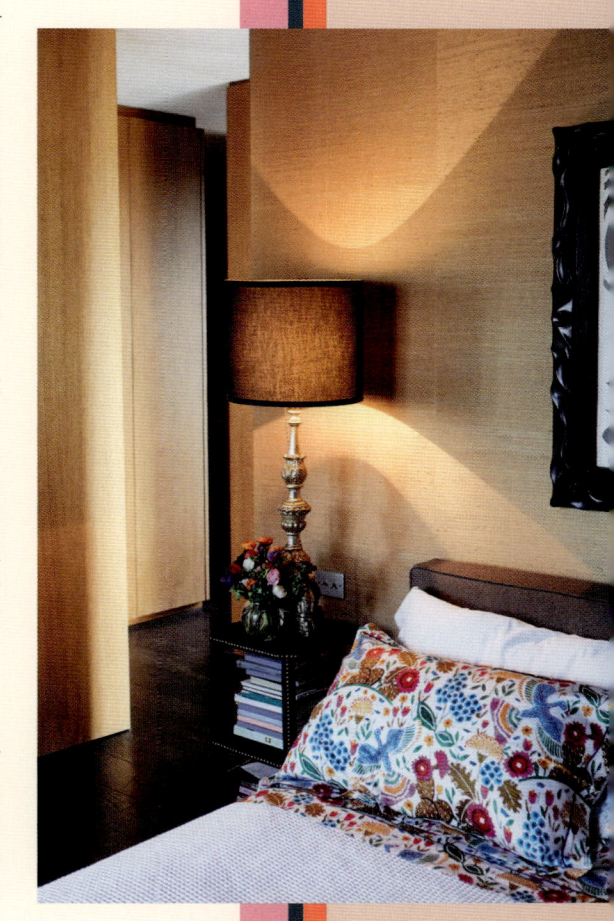

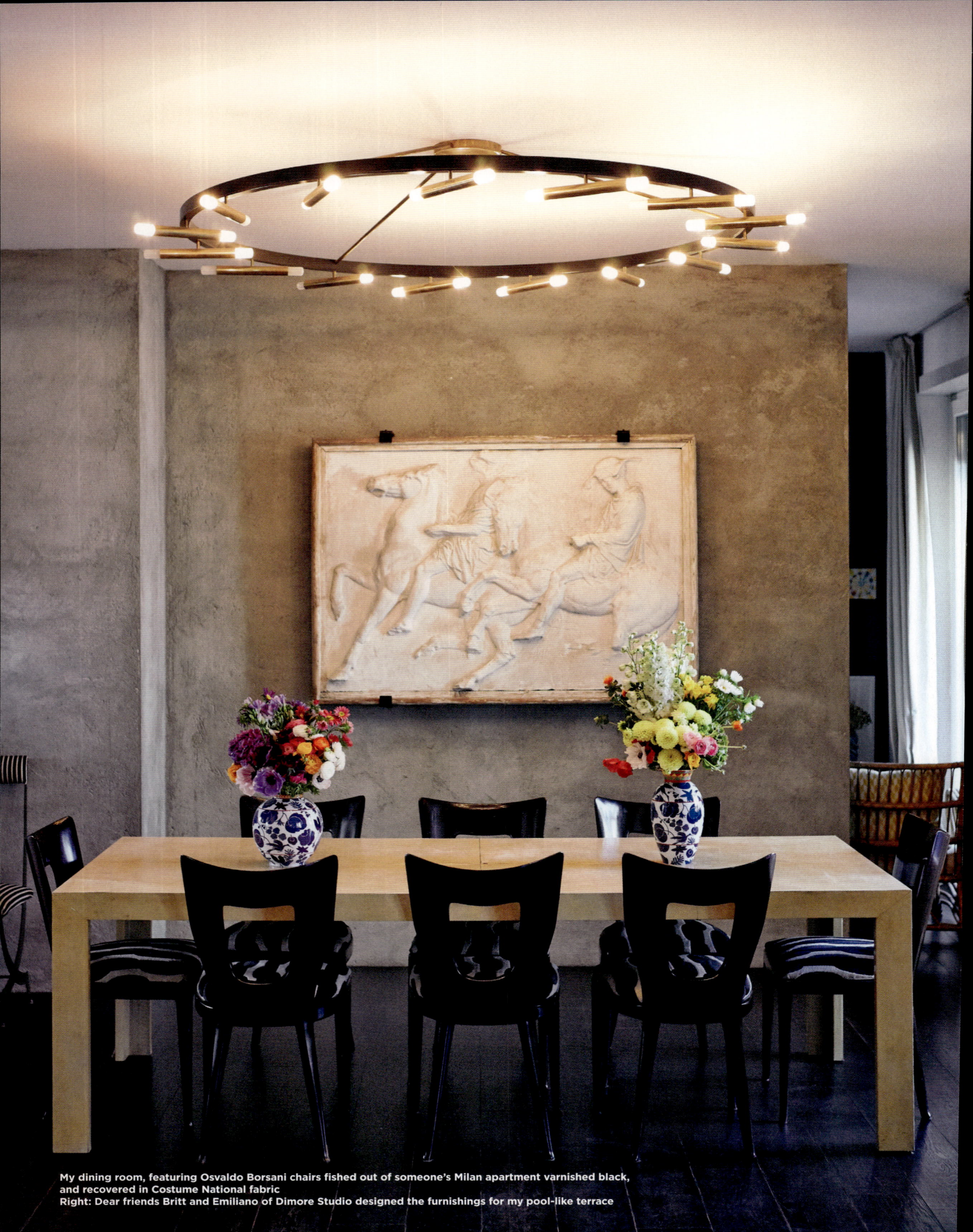

My dining room, featuring Osvaldo Borsani chairs fished out of someone's Milan apartment varnished black, and recovered in Costume National fabric
Right: Dear friends Britt and Emiliano of Dimore Studio designed the furnishings for my pool-like terrace

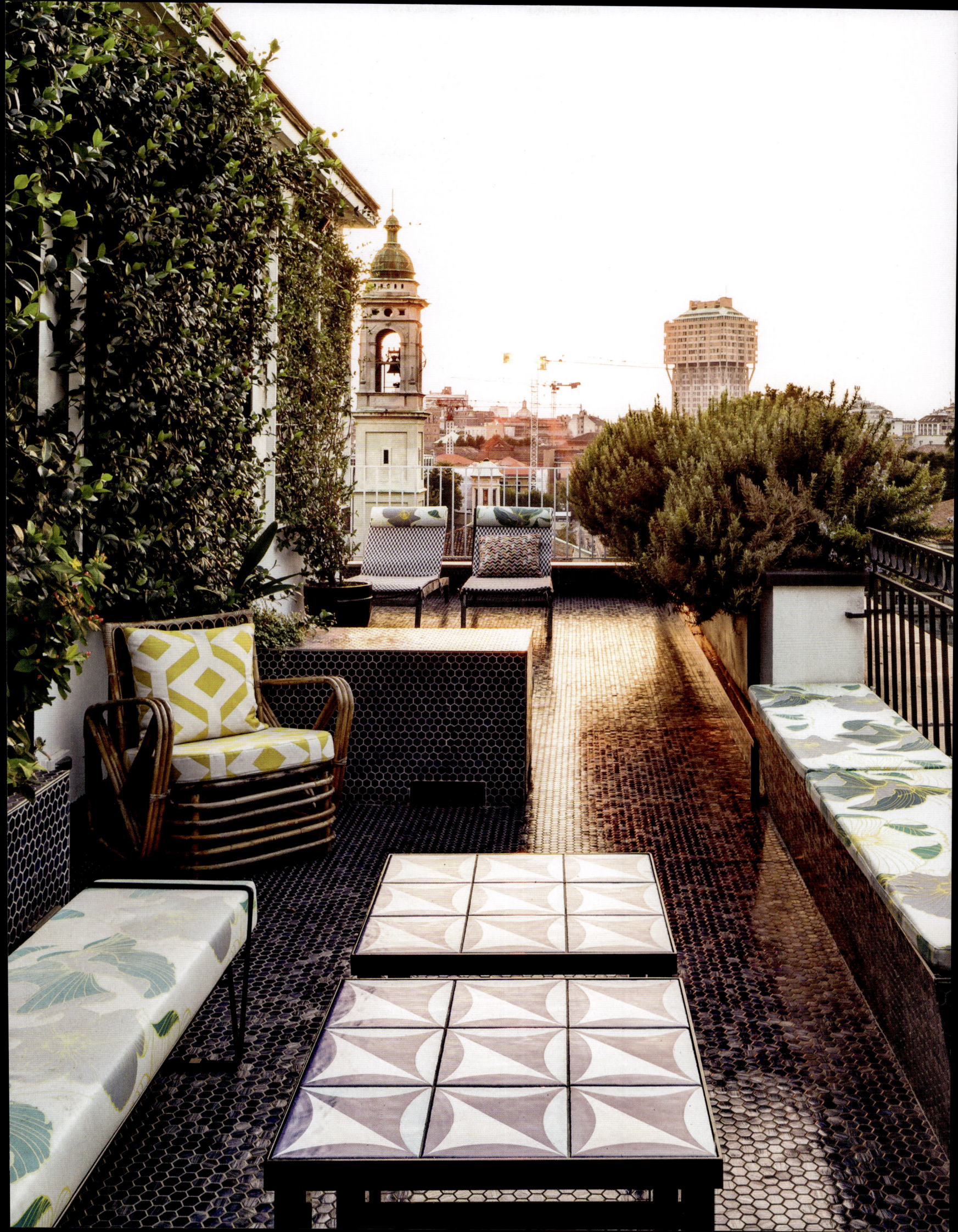

give me the color of the sea in Panarea." He beamed. "Signora, I am Sicilian!" he cried out with pride and clear comprehension. The next thing I knew, my walls got a home-brewed, shiny, lacquered shade of blue reflecting the sapphire-emerald sea around that special Sicilian island.

As a budding interior decorator, I employed my new Italian tool of Make Some Friends and Ask Them for Advice! I found eight vintage dealers in Milan that I liked and would visit on rotation every weekend. I would drop in, spend a couple hours talking to them, and ideas would bubble forth. I befriended shop owners like sisters Elena and Patrizia from Il Valore Aggiunto and Raimondo Garau, who would sigh every time I came into his shop with another outlandish idea. When I'd profess my need to buy one of his vintage tables, he'd clap back: "You don't need that, it doesn't work with your room!"

Only in Italy would a retailer stop you from buying something, and only in Italy would the same retailer be patient enough to sit down and teach you what does work.

Often these experts told me I was nuts, but sometimes I got an astonished look of approval—such as for a set of four rusted iron armchairs I fished out of the city's junkyard for 80 euro. I brought them to my auto-body shop, where the perplexed mechanics promptly told me that they definitely could not paint them the same red as my vintage Fiat Cinquecento. But I insisted, flirted a bit, and... they finally did.

"Do not try to decorate your house all at once. You have to live in the house first to feel her and understand what she needs." This was the greatest decorating lesson Raimondo ever gave me. But it was like putting me in a pot of boiling water. The American in me just wanted the job done. But Italy, as I've said, is the birthplace of patience, and I was learning it. So, I waited. I did the home itself in segments over a three-year period, and then later conquered the terrace. I got very hot and very bothered... But a couple of years later, the *casa* came out gleaming and dancing on the cover of *Elle Decor* US.

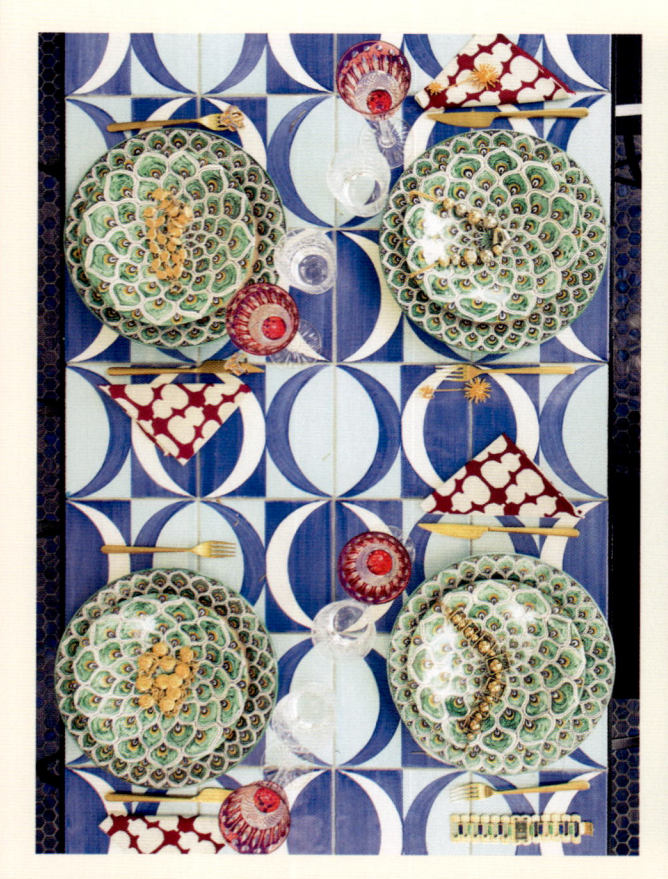

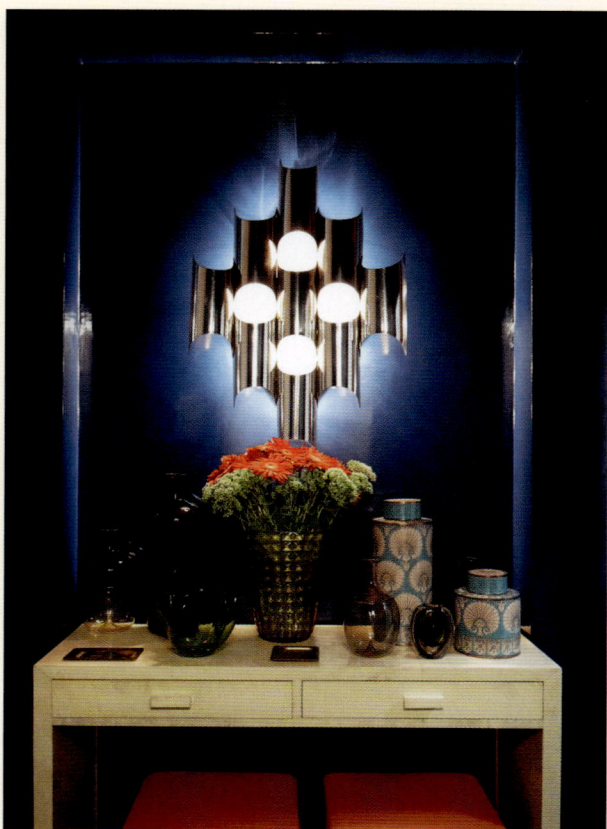

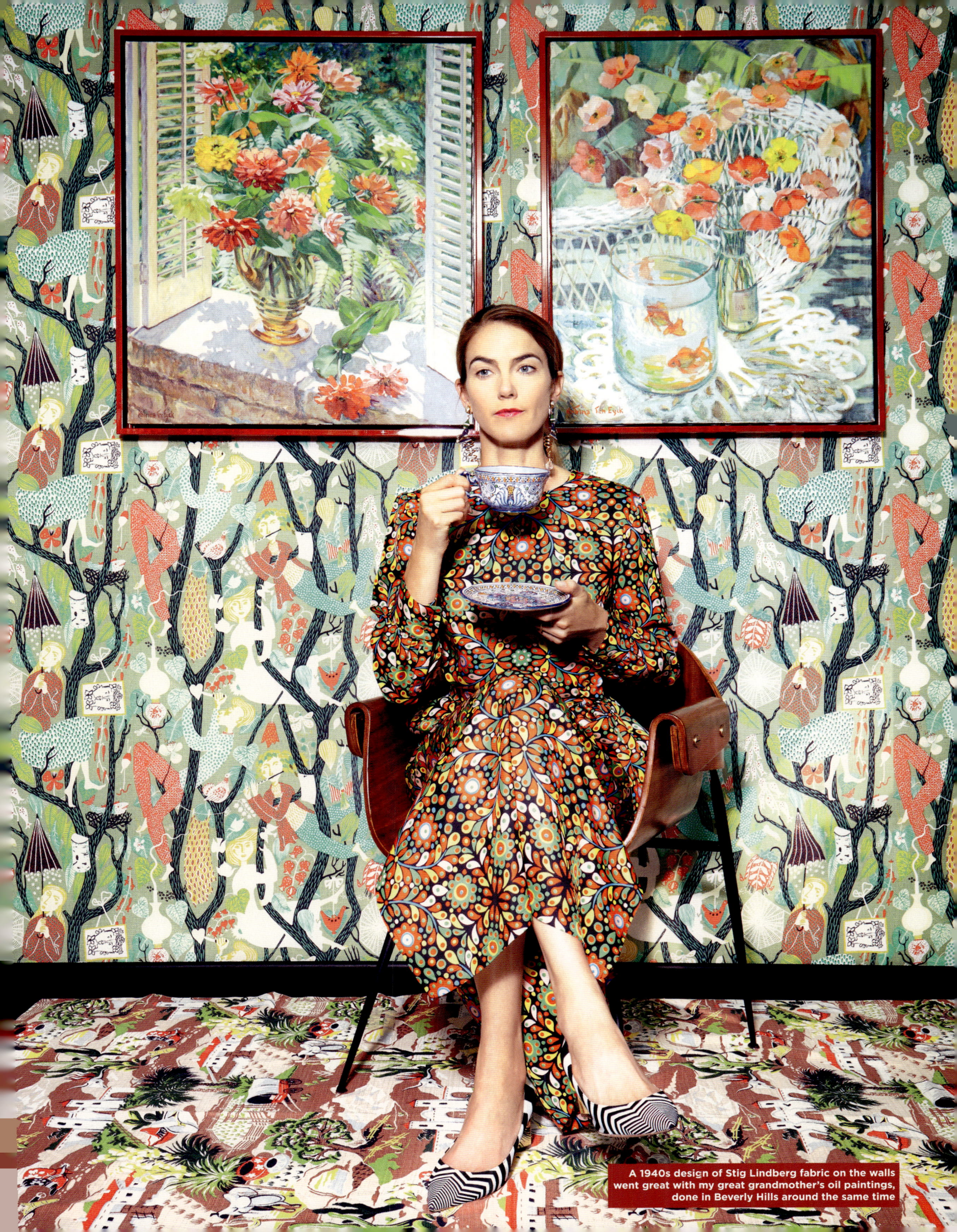

A 1940s design of Stig Lindberg fabric on the walls went great with my great grandmother's oil paintings, done in Beverly Hills around the same time

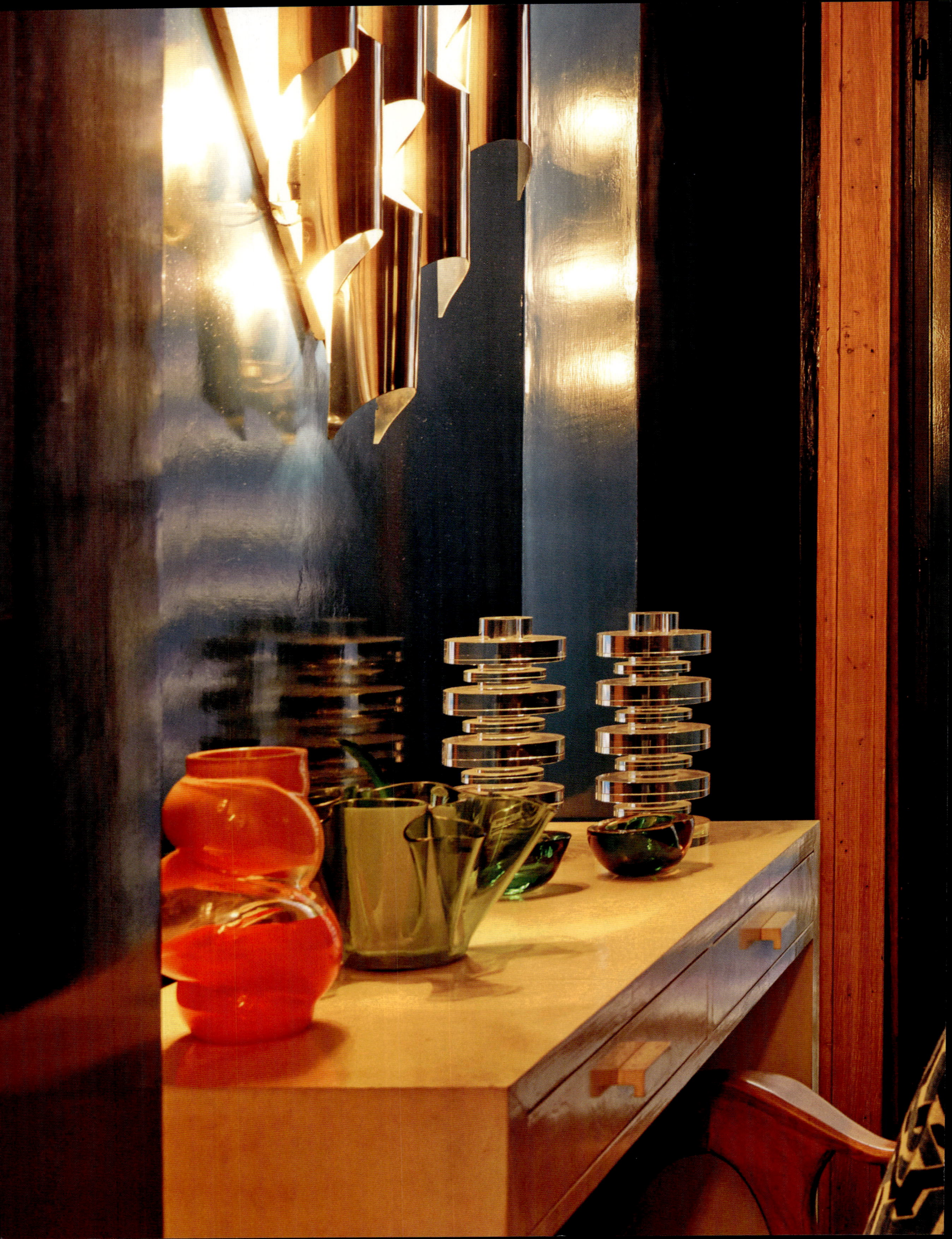

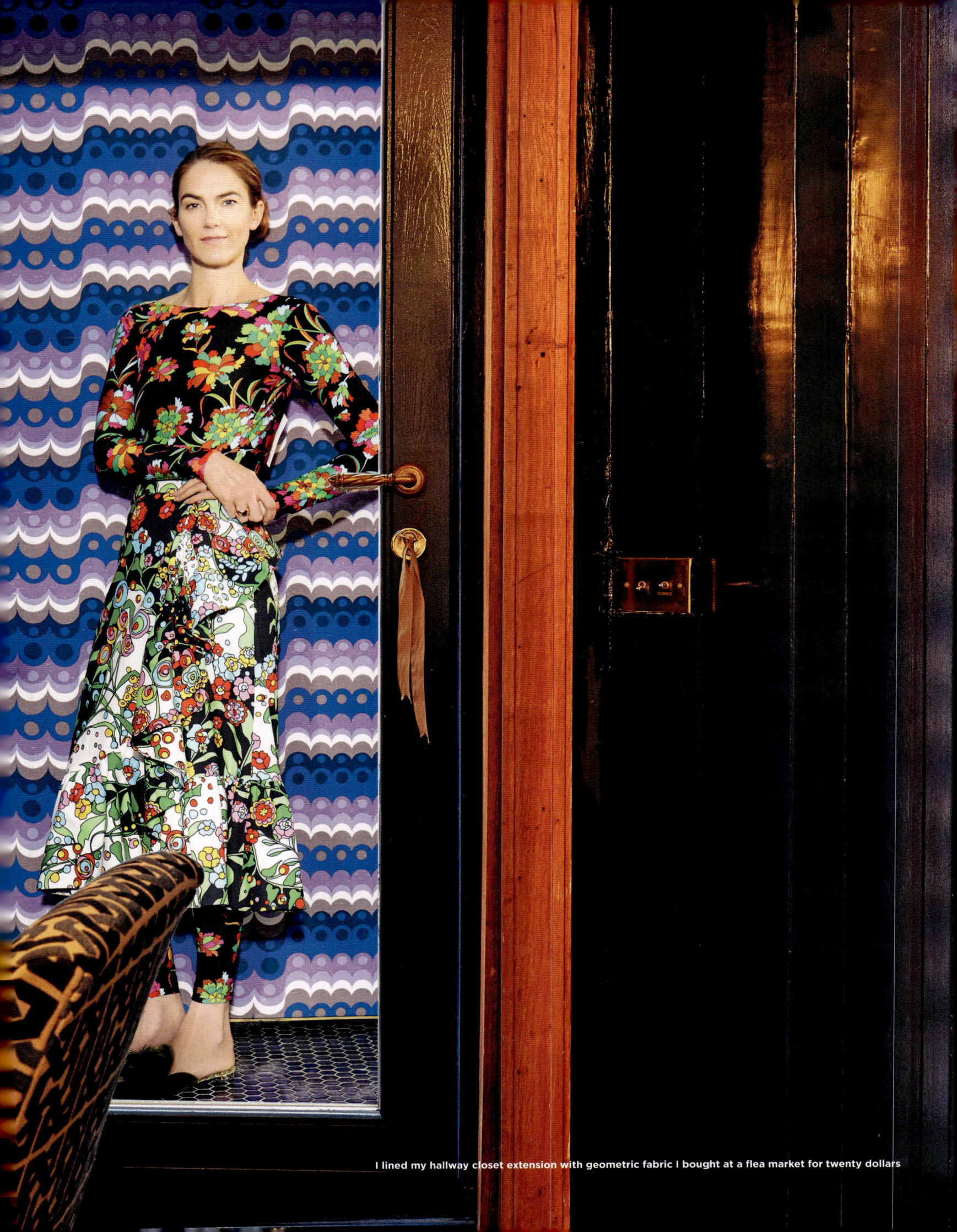

I lined my hallway closet extension with geometric fabric I bought at a flea market for twenty dollars

INTERMEZZO

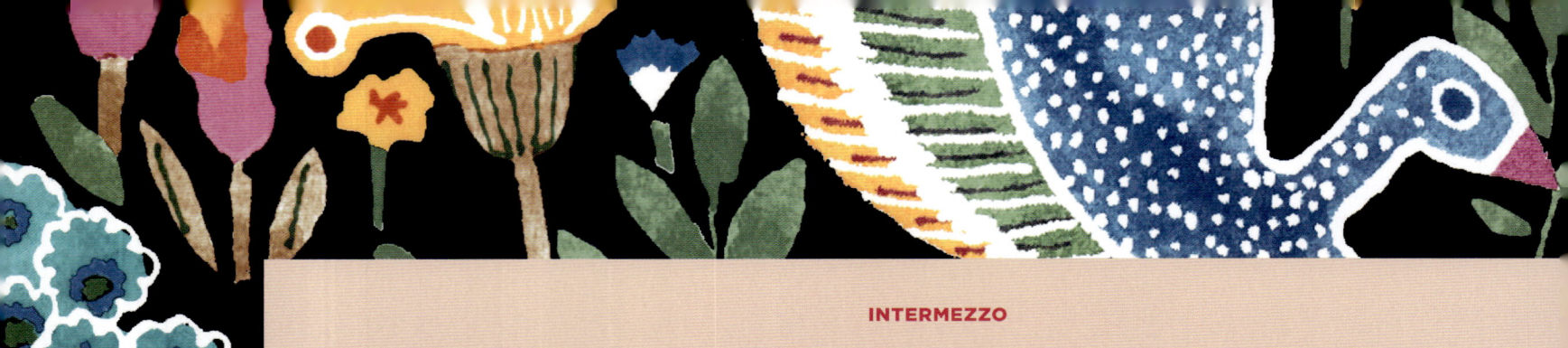

THE ROCKY ROAD TO CONCEPTION

After almost a decade living in Milan, I had labored over learning my Italian heart-opening lessons. But there were parts of myself that remained clenched and closed for business, like an Italian greengrocer in August. I realized this by falling into an unexpected pit of suffering, which unfortunately seems to be the way that most of us stubborn humans learn our greatest lessons. For six years I could not get pregnant—in a country that prizes children above all else. Like most thirty-five-year-old American women I knew dealing with infertility, I pushed and pulled, was poked and prodded, while insisting on reproducing... first by trying to control an unsexy sex schedule, and—when that didn't work—resorting to man-made babies via IVF.

I can do this!! I screamed to myself. And I did: I got pregnant through artificial means three times. And three times, I lost the fetus, which turned out to be chromosomally scrambled yet clawing on for dear life. One time, this hideous procedure actually took place during Milan Fashion Week—I raced out from the Armani show in my high heels and straight into a surgical gown. It never occurred to me that I could or should take time off work; right away, I would snap back to living the way I always had—running, writing, organizing, producing, socializing, photo-shooting, achieving, and striving. I couldn't give my heart, soul, or body the time and space they needed to let life spark.

The storming and razing of my womb was emotionally, psychologically, and physically destabilizing. I was raving crazy, raging mad, and in the dumps of depression for a very long time. Then, on the very day I received yet another no-go call from the gynecologist, a friend from college passed me the name of her energy healer. Just as with Italy, when I decided to surrender my fight, my bad-ass angels showed up big time. They led me to Elisabeth Manning, a bright spirit who lived across the world in Petaluma, California, and who connected with me each week on a Skype call.

During these energy healing sessions, I began to learn what real fertility means and how to cultivate it in my own life. From an energetic and emotional standpoint, whether you want to be a mother to a manuscript, a new business, a blog, a women's group, an epic dinner party, or three screaming infants in the back of a minivan, the creative brief is the same. We women are natural-born creators. New life can blossom in our hands, eyes, hearts, and stomachs, but it all starts from the womb, what yogic practitioners call the sacred second chakra energy point. It is here that we cultivate and practice self-love, self-worth, self-acceptance, and deep inner listening. The soil in this container is enriched with the exact same juicy nutrients that Mamma Milano was already feeding me—patience, tolerance, flexibility, feeling, intuition, and above all, receptivity.

In the end, my body said no to children. But from this energy work, I learned to surrender to the wisdom of the universe, no matter how unfair and awful it felt. I began to realize that every roadblock and pain point we endure has been ordered up from the divine cafeteria to feed key growth spurts in our lives. First it was Italy, now it was infertility. Most of it was painful, but none of it was by chance. All of it could be used to fertilize myself and grow my own sacred vessel.

There were so many other creations ready to be fed, incubated, baked, and given birth to. New life was waiting, I just didn't know what it was. I did something new—I opened myself to receive what wanted to come through.

Mamma Milano had put me exactly where I needed to be.

Pregnant with possibility

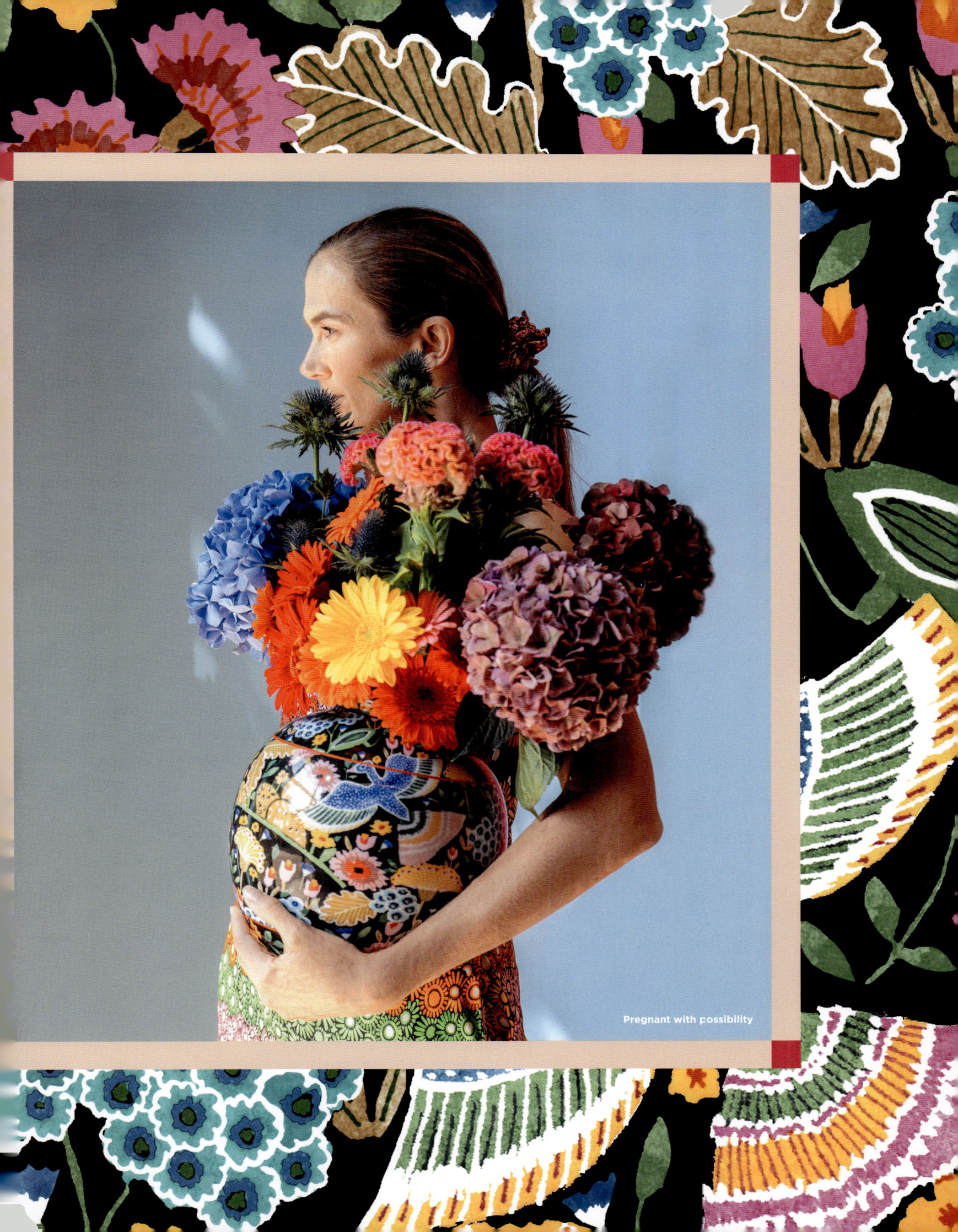

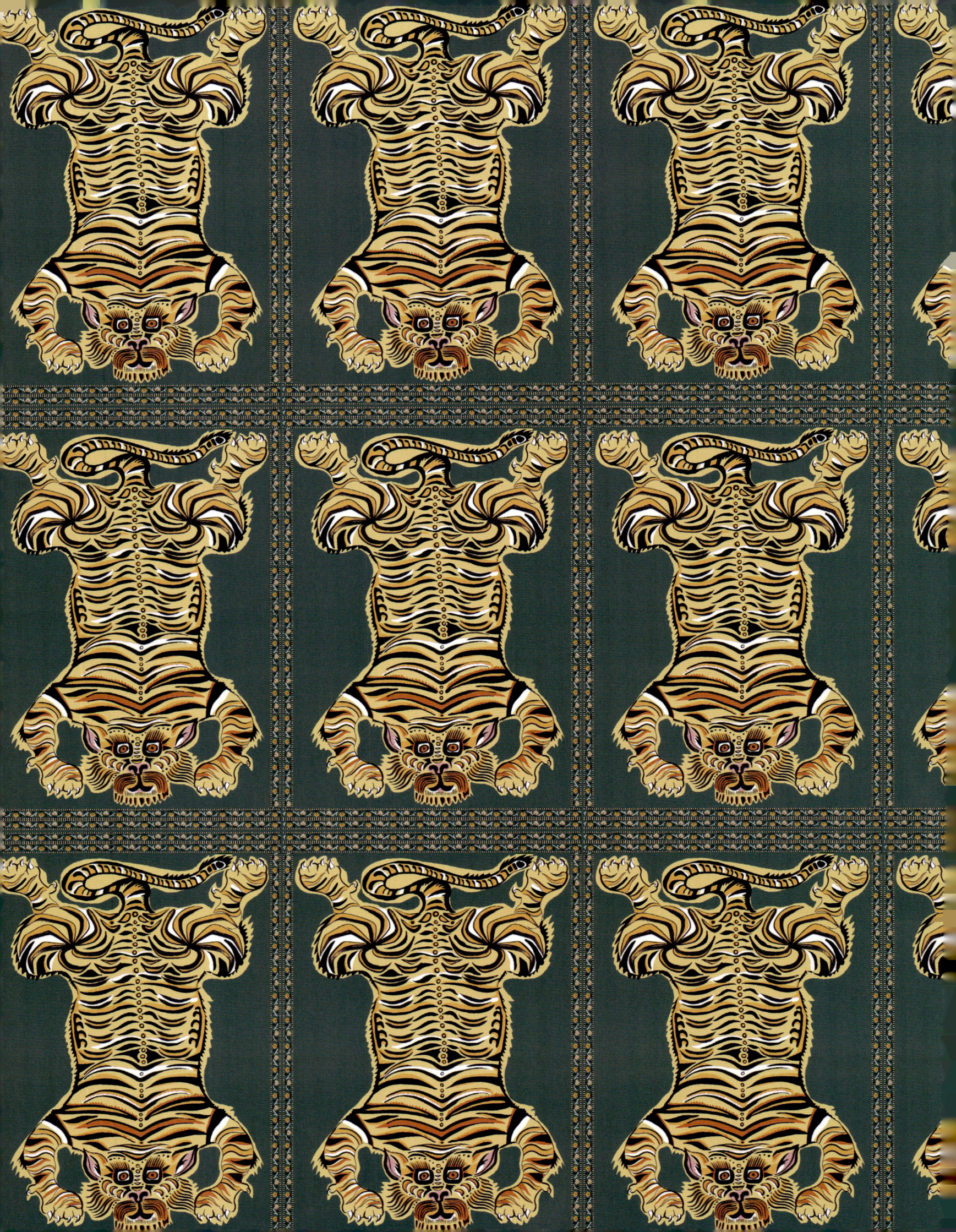

BORN TO BE WILD

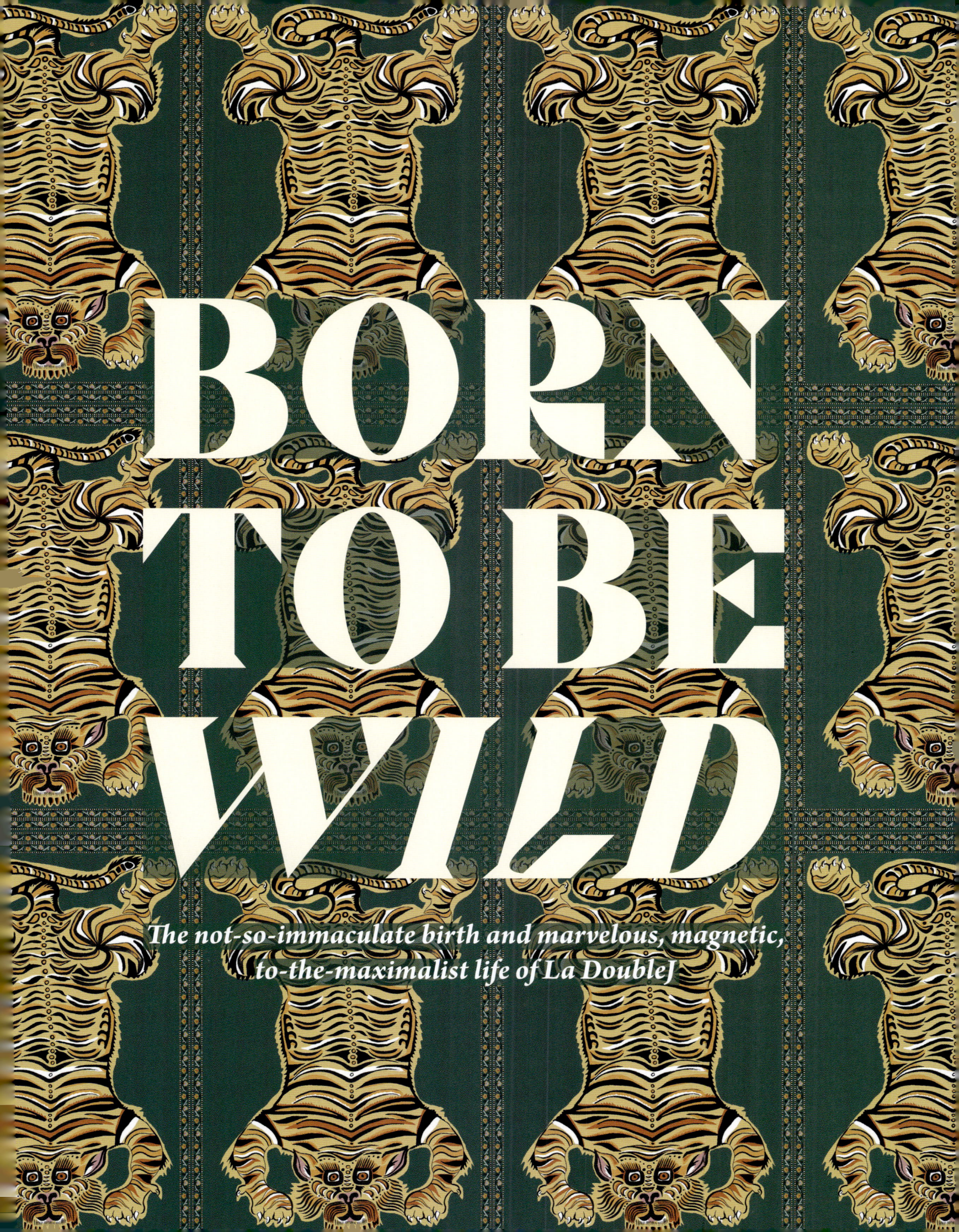

The not-so-immaculate birth and marvelous, magnetic, to-the-maximalist life of La DoubleJ

FLIPPING THE CREATIVE SWITCH

The kingdoms of Italian fashion and design I'd been traveling in for the last decade were miraculous, marvelous realms. Both their royalty and spirited, subversive citizens had opened my eyes to how a passion for beauty and craft, fueled by wild imagination and boundless vision, can be transformative. However, my job as a journalist had been largely to listen to other people's dreams and innovations, and to package them into digestible story nuggets for magazines—not really to create intuitively from my own wild gut.

Furthermore, this job had me permanently anchored inside the unhappy role of The Critic: is this awesome? Bad? Ugly? Gorgeous? Cool? Or totally lame? Looking back, I realize that this cloud of power was really fueled by toxic criticism and judgment. I was living in and contributing to the land of fear, but didn't really know it at the time.

Besides, by 2012 the glossy, privileged print media world that I'd worked so hard to scale was now cracking and crumbling, bleeding ad dollars and slashing staffs. The rise of speedy and slim digital platforms—Instagram was just catching on—and their bloggers and influencers meant that anyone could become a writer, photographer, or content producer with the flick of an iPhone.

On top of this, I didn't think I could bear to squeeze out yet another profile of Dolce & Gabbana or Armani, the industry's biggest luxury advertisers (as much as I loved them), or any of the other deep-pocketed designers that every magazine wanted me to lasso for their pages.

The creativity and freedom of those early years had faded. I was a little bored. My stomach itched for something new.

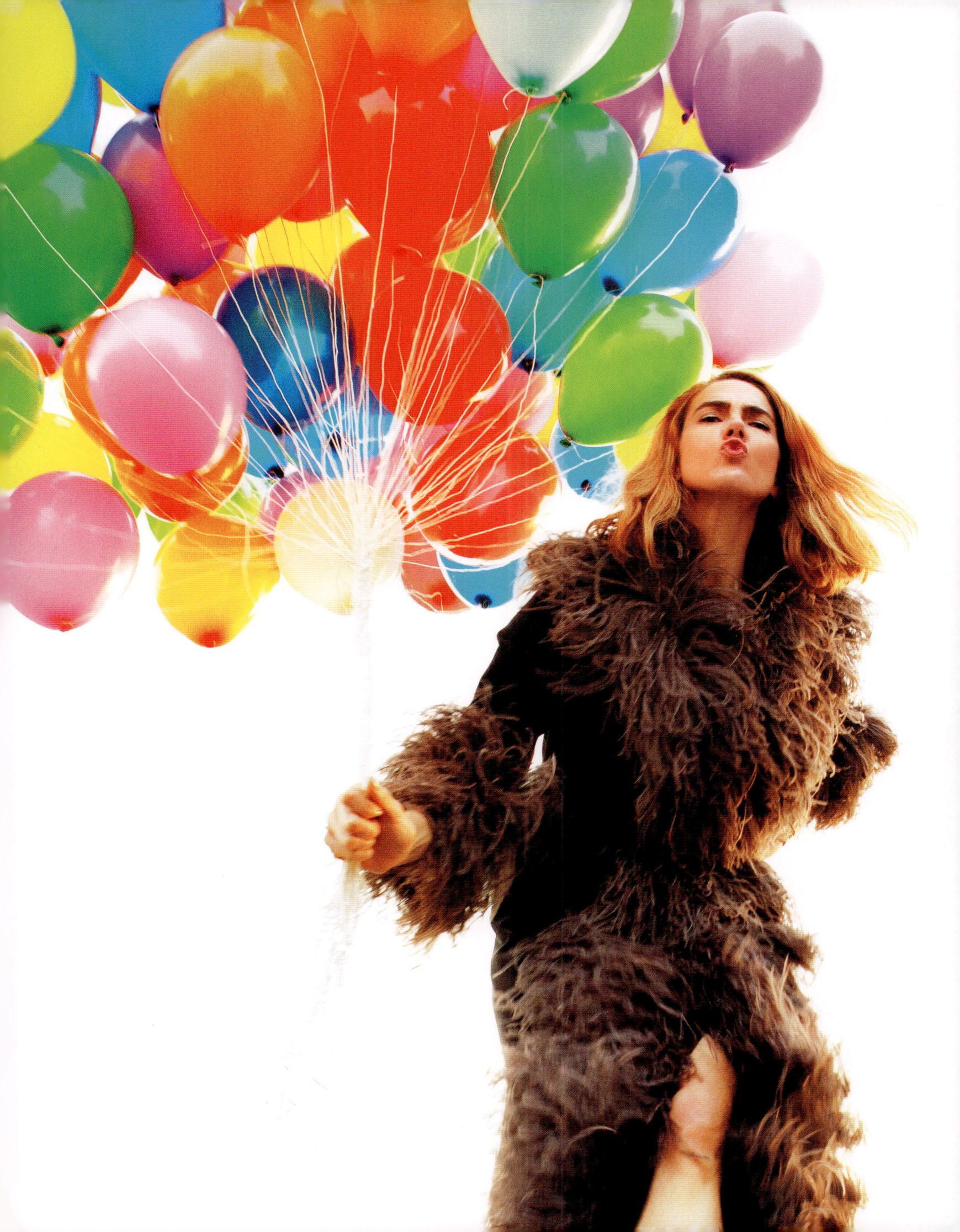

MAMMA MILANO

SEED #1

TURNING A PASSION INTO A PORTAL

"You know, you should really sell your vintage collection online."

With those words casually tossed off by my husband Andrea over dinner one evening, the first seed of La DoubleJ was planted. But it didn't take root, at least not at first. In fact, I brushed it away. Sell my vintage clothes on the internet? Andrea was at the time running The Level Group, an e-commerce company that built websites for big fashion brands, so he knew what that was about. To me, it just sounded like a logistical nightmare.

Yet over the next few days, after settling in the dark, loamy recesses of my consciousness, that seed began to germinate. Unfettered by practicality or logic, I sat back, closed my eyes, and allowed a dreamy download to come rushing forth:

Well, if I did want to sell all my vintage clothes online, which were currently busting out of my closets and basement... Maybe I could ask some of my vintage dealer friends if they wanted to pool some of their product too, to have a deeper selection but all curated according to my maximal sensibilities... If I do this, then it would have to look unimaginably delicious and totally different from all the dusty crapola vintage e-commerce drooping on dirty mannequins you see on every corner of the internet... Maybe I could ask all of the incredible creative women I've met and interviewed over the last fifteen years in Milan to be my models. That would be my chance to finally tell the stories of these legendary Italian ladies, fling open their homes, and do full-fledged glossy magazine features on each. I could show their closets, cupboards, tables, revealing how they dress themselves, decorate, and entertain! The whole website could be a shoppable magazine dedicated to Living Like an Italian...

Suddenly, a single small seed to sell my vintage closet had sprung into a jungle rippling around in my head.

Just by creating an open field—free from doubt, criticism, and cynicism—the embryonic idea was permitted to spin lawlessly into a whirl of possibility.

Then, of course, reality set in. I had no business plan. No inkling if anyone in the world was buying vintage besides me (especially the one-of-a-kind historic pieces I was selling, not last season's Prada). There were hardly any good models back then for merging e-commerce with an online magazine. No moneybags investor to foot the bill. And no staff. I was all alone.

But I stayed firm, pulling on the gifts, talents, and passions that I knew I had stashed in my pockets. My body fired up, my skin tingled, my heart glowed on, and I allowed myself to fall in love with this weird idea.

I felt no fear. I became fully ripe with my energy baby growing and spinning inside me.

133

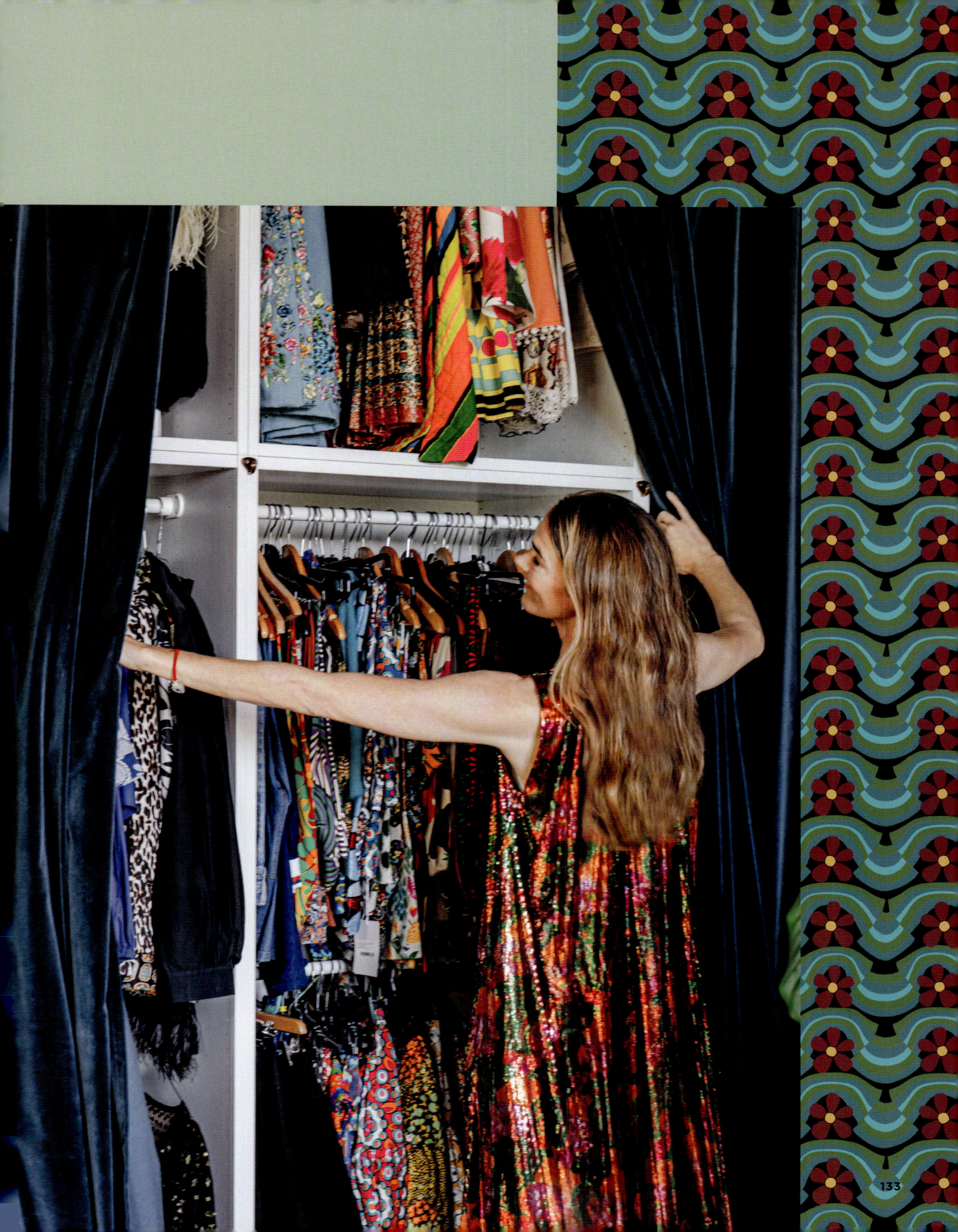

MAMMA MILANO

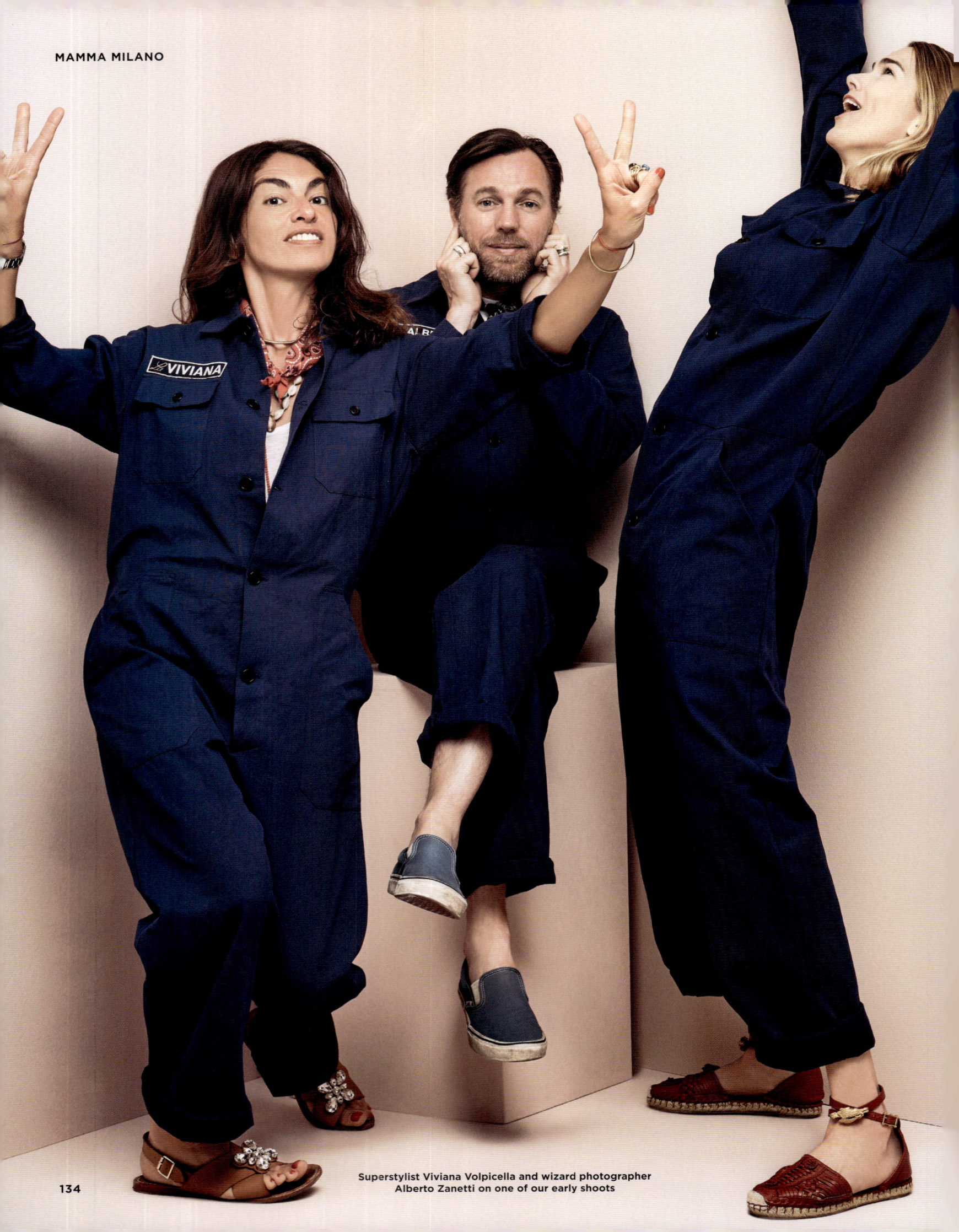

Superstylist Viviana Volpicella and wizard photographer Alberto Zanetti on one of our early shoots

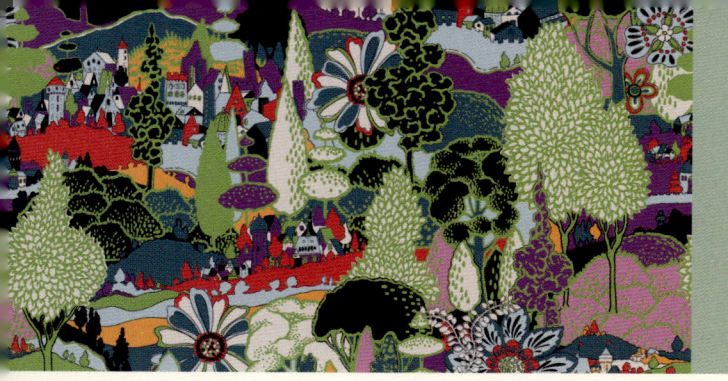

ENTER THE GODPARENTS

Starting a company was challenging to pull off in a country packed with centuries-old mom-and-pop ventures and tangles of red tape, and not exactly known for its entrepreneurial innovation; one in which, as I've said, there's an expectation that you need to be *un figlio di'*—the child of royalty or aristocracy or a billionaire industrialist—to make any impact. This is where my ballsy, American, I-can-do-or-be-anything approach came in handy. But this defiance had to be coated in a uniquely Italian glaze. It had taken years of persistent coaxing, flirting, vacationing, and long lunches to squeeze out the sustenance that this life form would require. My years of toiling in Milan had created an enormous sticky web of friends, colleagues, contacts, and collaborators.

So, I did what any Italian would do. I called everyone I knew, blew my enthusiasm into their ears, made the energy contagious, and invented ways for us to work together. Everything popped up and out of these relationships, including mutual backscratching for those who wanted a stage to flex and squeeze their creative juices to the max. I didn't realize how important this was to photographers, stylists, designers, and writers—how creative people working in fashion often feel strangled or deflated.

At this point, Andrea was rolling his eyes about where I'd run off with his little seed. But he agreed to consult on the business and his company, TLG, would build our website—thank the goddess.

Then I turned to Alberto Biagetti, a furniture-designer/art-director friend I'd met in Milan in 2001 when he was on the founding team of Yoox. Biagio, as I called him, was an imaginative Italian maverick, unfettered by the chains of logic. His heart was straight out of the Renaissance. He lit up at my challenge to whip up the most gorgeous, funny, and fabulous website ever. His company, Frank Studio—co-owned by TLG—didn't charge a fee for our first year.

A key godparent in all this was freelance stylist Viviana Volpicella, a Puglia-born, Milan-based firecracker with fabulous taste whom I'd met when she was star-stylist Anna Dello Russo's assistant years before. I needed someone to help me put together the photos for the website, and her face popped into my head one day while daydreaming at Cucchi. Viviana and I met in the back of a car between shows during Paris Fashion Week, where I proposed the idea. "I will be your fashion director!" she practically shouted.

From that moment on, she and I became a vortex of volcanic creative energy, a Mount Etna of ideas feeding off each other, and laughing our pants off the whole way.

Nothing I said to her was too weird. She took every idea I had—such as "Who Wore it Best? Vintage War" photo shoots using ourselves as models—and made it better, more brilliant, and more beautiful. She devoted herself to La DoubleJ as if it were her very own baby, showering her with her impeccable taste, styling shoots, wrangling women, and sketching my wacky ideas in rainbow markers. Together, we were totally seismic. This is the power that occurs when you co-create with your soul family.

Viviana brought in photographer Alberto Zanetti to take the portraits of our Milanese wonder women—divided into "Great Gorgeous Girls" for the younger creative set, and "Legendary Ladies" who held world records in style and entertaining but were also fierce creative powerhouses at work. They all fed into a column called "The School of Sciura" (using the Italian for "Supreme Milanese Housewife"), because they also knew the rules inside and out on how to be commanding domestic goddesses. Albi had been an assistant to photographer Pier Paolo Ferrari and art-world-darling Maurizio Cattelan on *Toilet Paper* magazine, so he was trained in visual humor and irreverence. He volunteered to work for free so long as I paid his assistants.

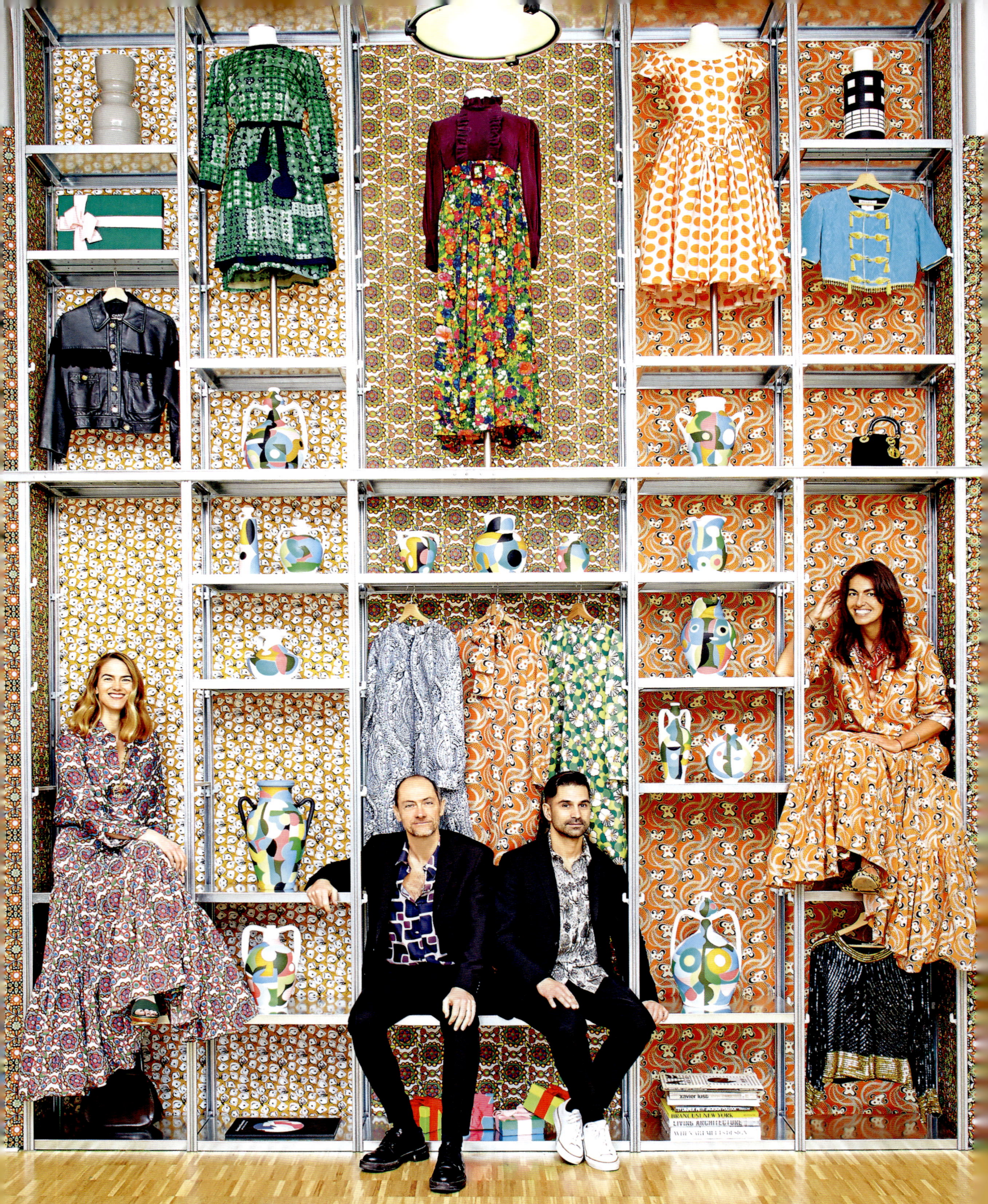

The DoubleJ "Wunderwall" designed by Luca Cipleletti, featuring our godparents
Andrea Ciccoli, Cristian Musardo, Viviana Volpicella, Laura and Alberto Biagetti, and Alberto Zanetti

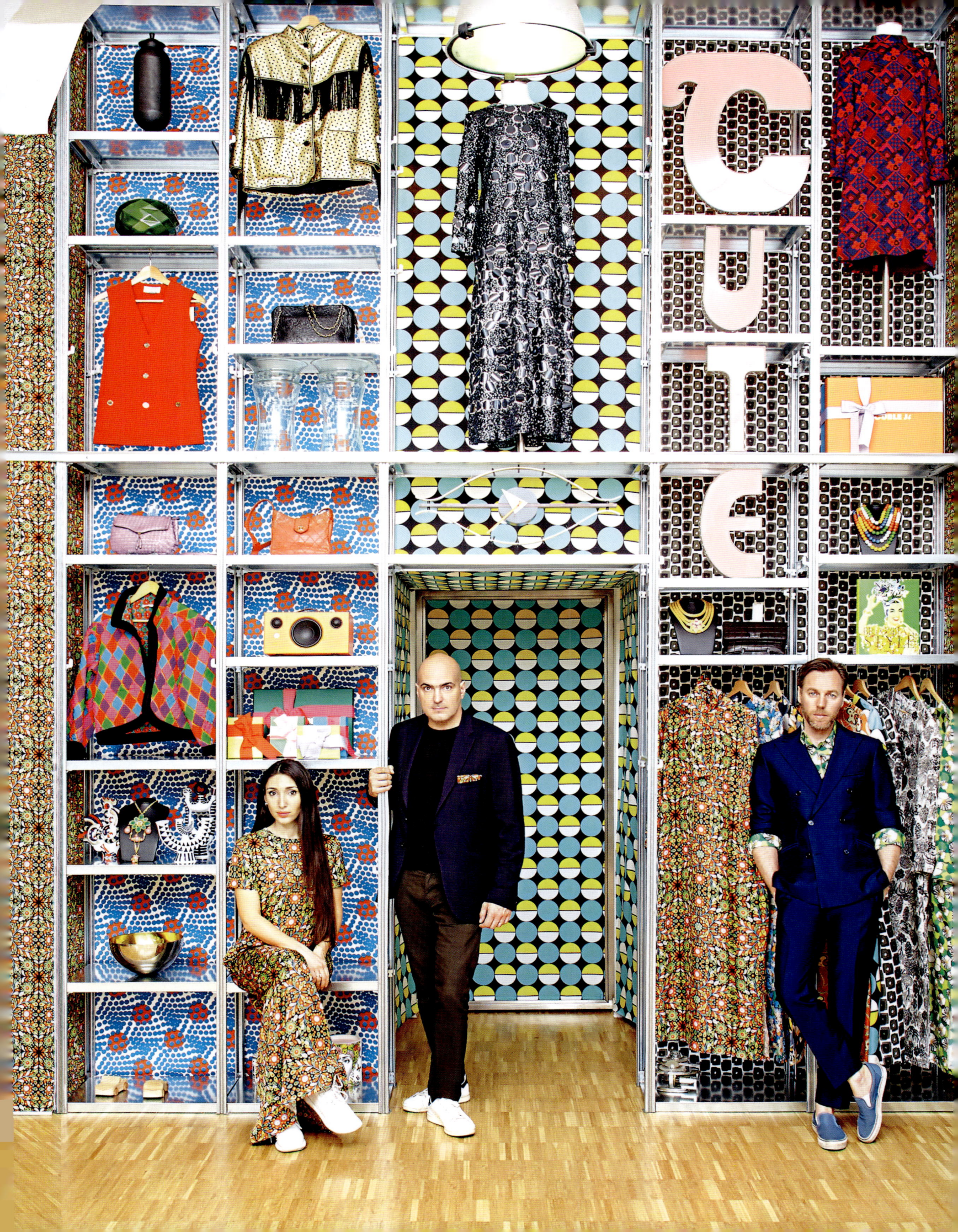

MAMMA MILANO

The portraits that Albi shot for the first two years of the company were eye-popping masterpieces, that made our e-commerce operation sing a wholly original tune. There was tough, turbaned design queen Nina Yashar, standing barefoot on her Carlo Molino–designed dining room table; design-gallery goddess Rossana Orlandi removing her signature sunglasses in public for the first time; and ex-Moschino creative director Rossella Jardini arriving at her Milanese abode in a bathrobe and gold jewelry, carrying her dog.

In all, we produced fifteen full-scale photo shoots in two months with the same quality photography, styling, and writing I had been doing for *Harper's Bazaar* and *Wallpaper**. All of it was completely shoppable and highly readable. We ran, we jumped, we laughed, we played, and together our trinity made magic.

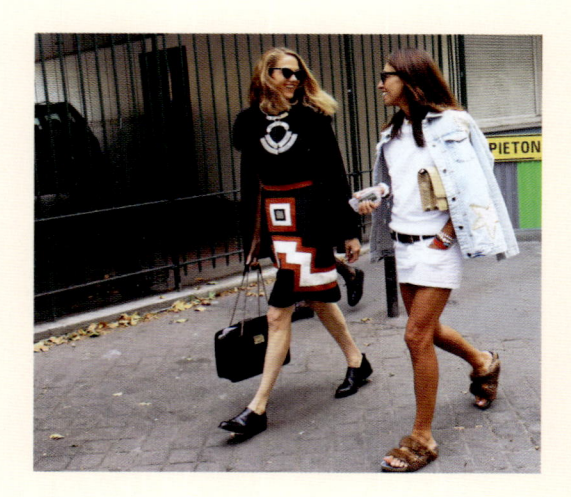

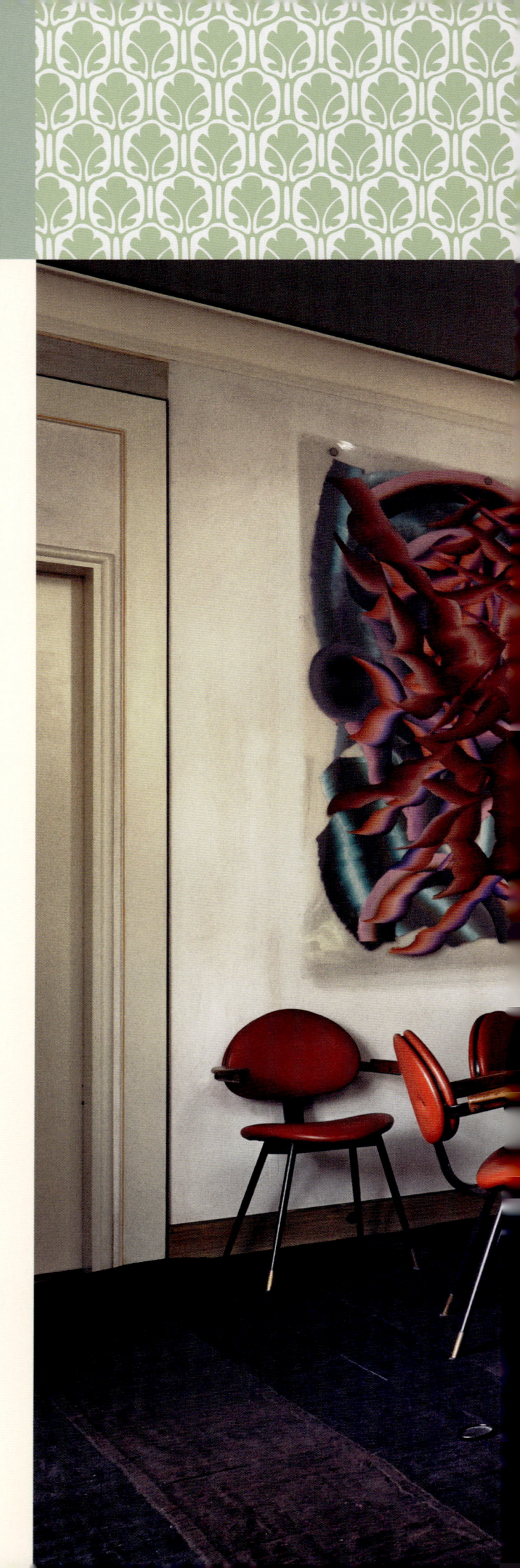

138

BORN TO BE WILD!

Gallerist Nina Yashar at home in Milan, barefoot on her dining-room table and wearing our vintage caftan
Opposite: the very day during Paris Fashion Week, in October 2014, when Viviana agreed to become Fashion Director of La DoubleJ

MAMMA MILANO

MILAN'S LEGENDARY LADIES

These women, photographed by Alberto Zanetti for La DoubleJ's launch, are fantastic and iconoclastic, some of Milan's brightest creative talents who inspired me as I finally gained access to Milan's closed-door kingdom. I watched them, learned from them, and celebrated them on our website as goddesses on both professional and domestic fronts.

▼ **PUPI SOLARI**
LEGENDARY MILANESE RETAILER FOR CHILDREN AND BRIDES

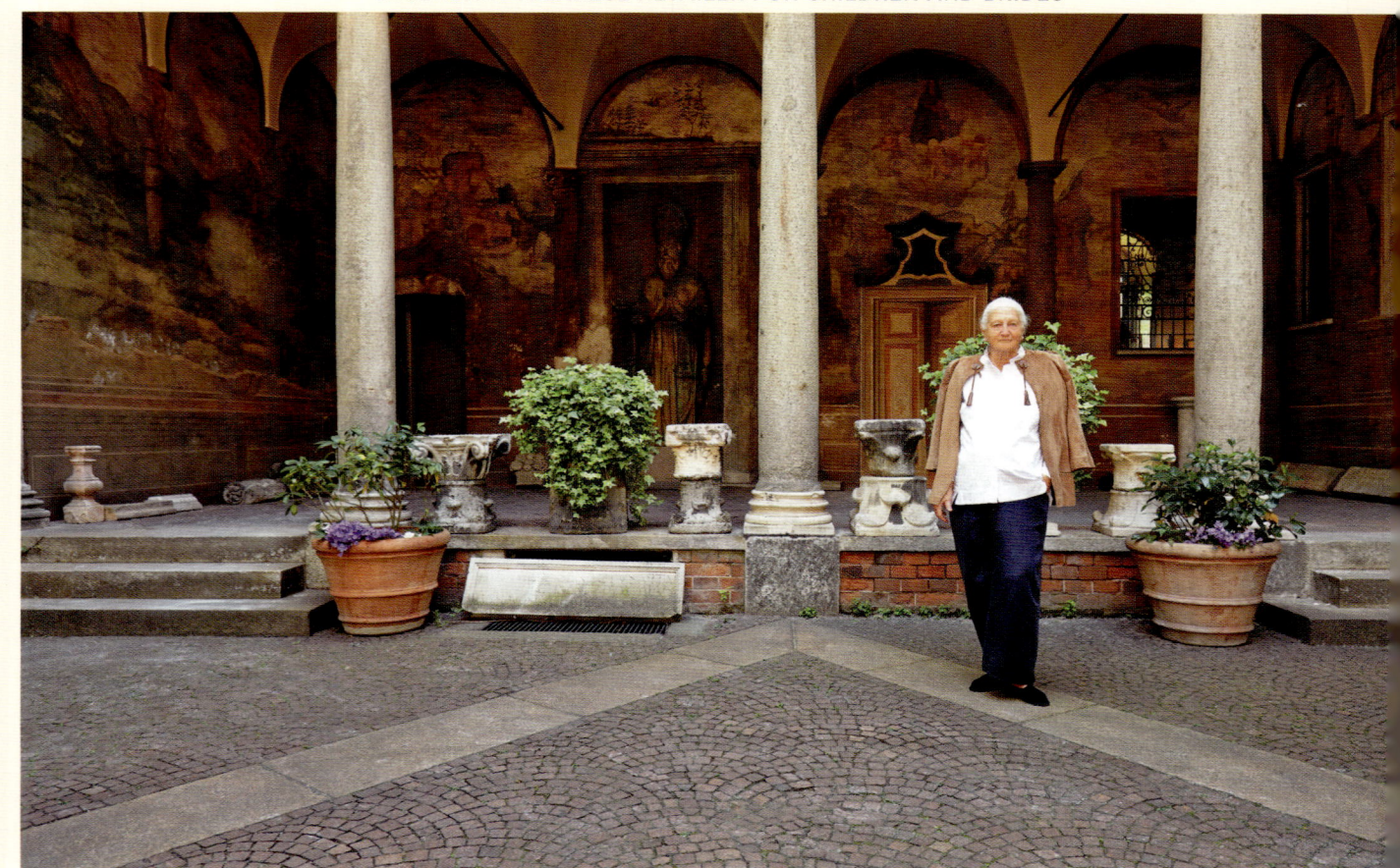

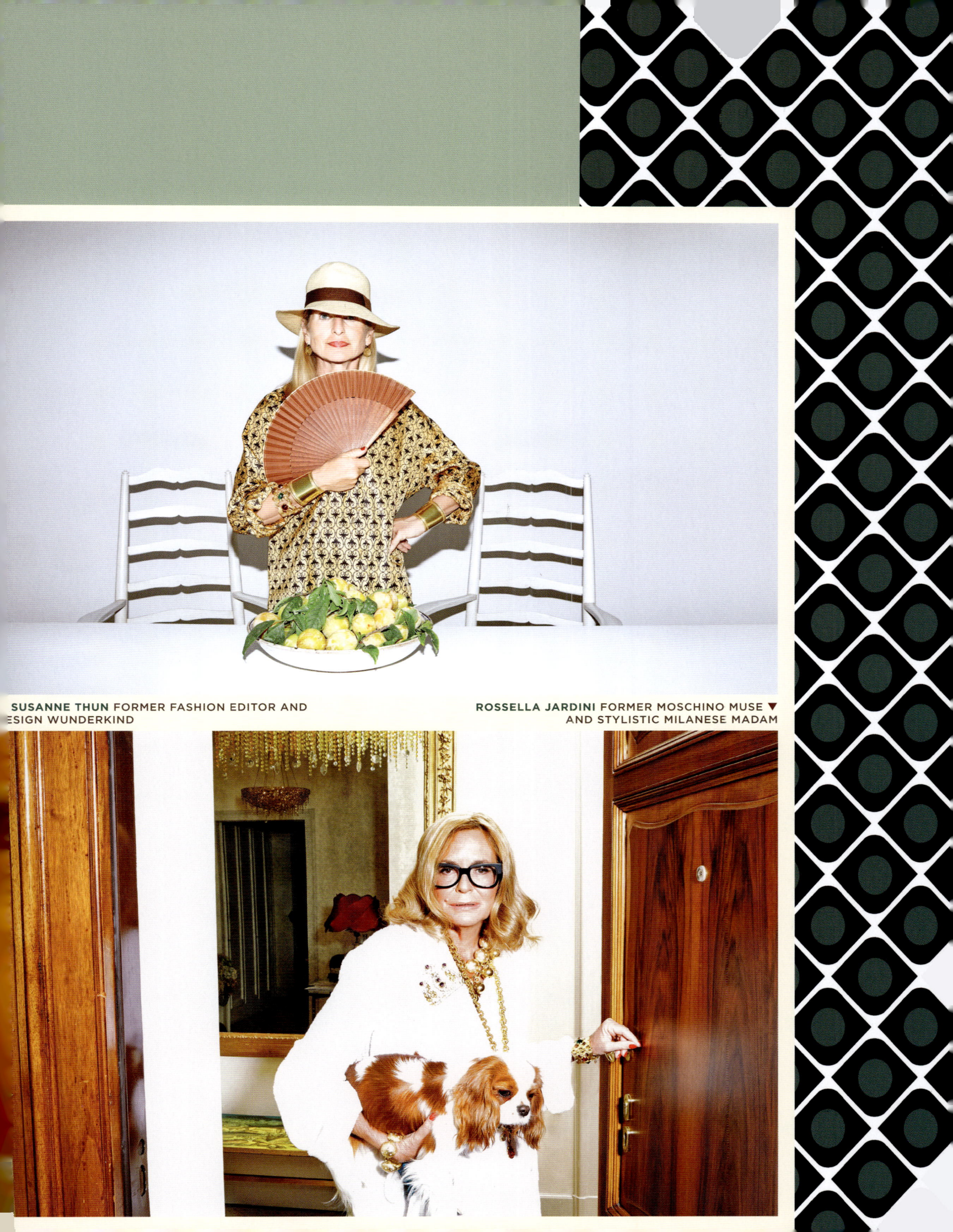

SUSANNE THUN FORMER FASHION EDITOR AND
ESIGN WUNDERKIND

ROSSELLA JARDINI FORMER MOSCHINO MUSE ▼
AND STYLISTIC MILANESE MADAM

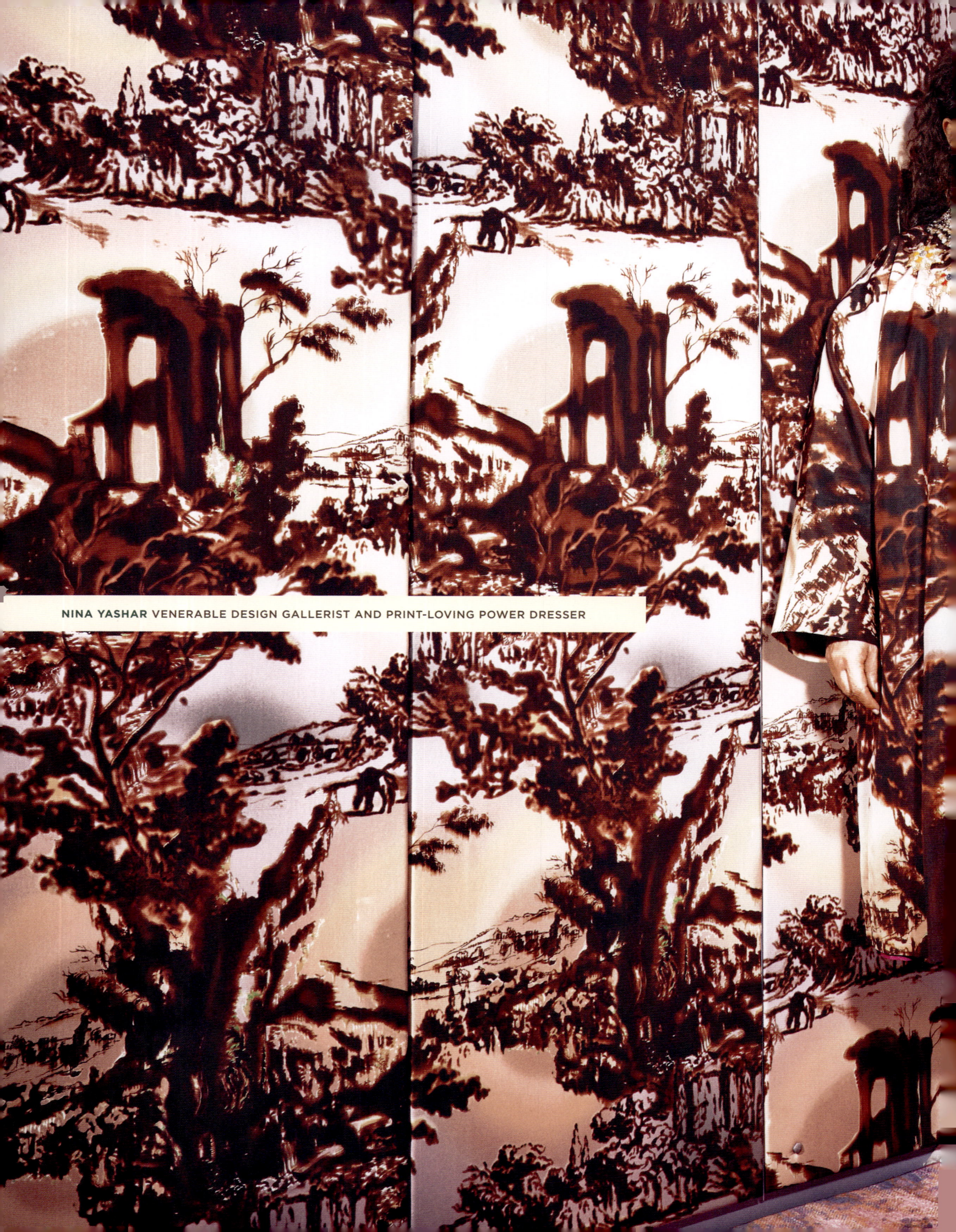

NINA YASHAR VENERABLE DESIGN GALLERIST AND PRINT-LOVING POWER DRESSER

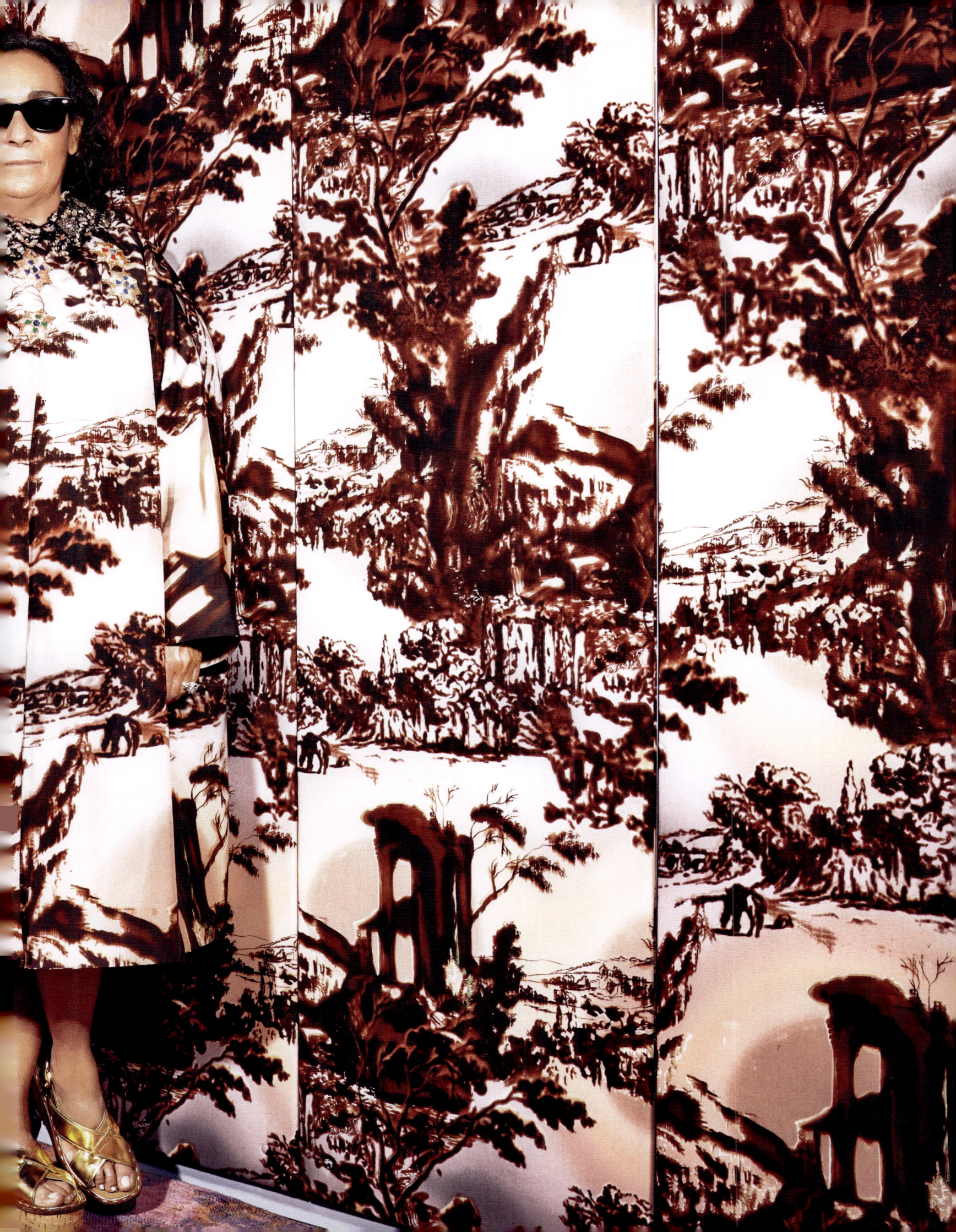

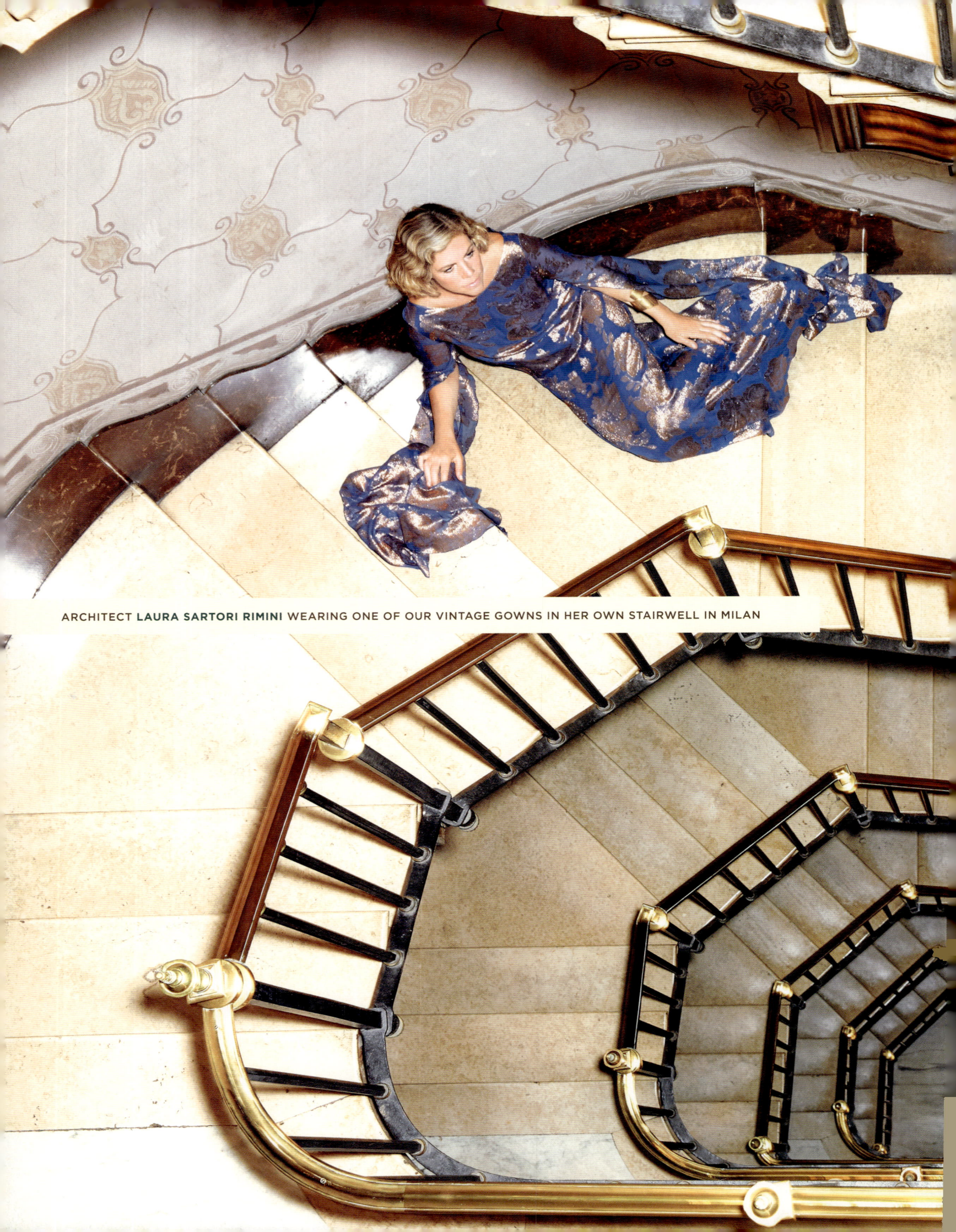

ARCHITECT **LAURA SARTORI RIMINI** WEARING ONE OF OUR VINTAGE GOWNS IN HER OWN STAIRWELL IN MILAN

THE SCHOOL OF *SCIURA* RULEBOOK

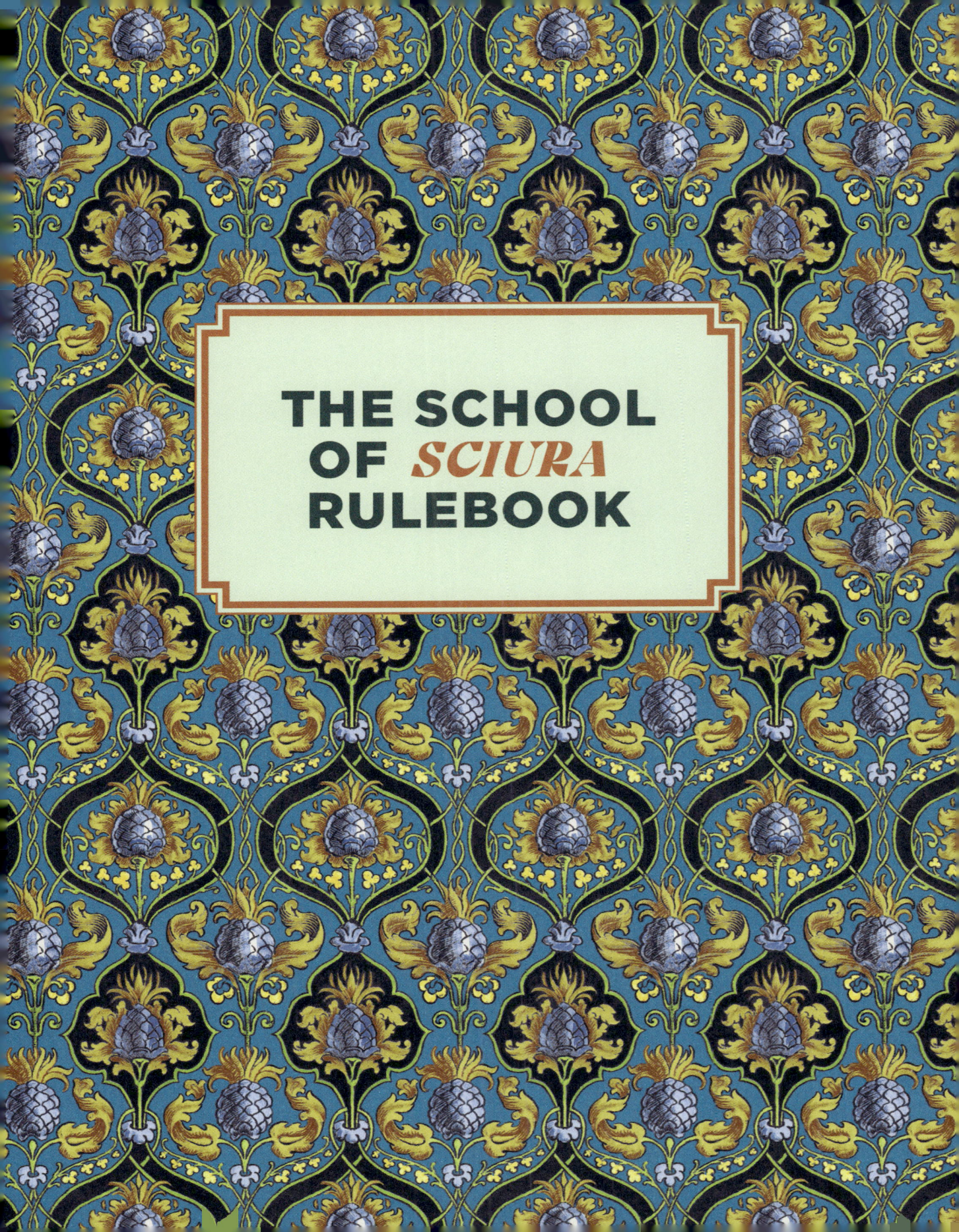

THE (UNTIL-NOW) UNWRITTEN RULES FOR NAVIGATING POLITE SOCIETY AND PROPER HOUSEHOLD MANAGEMENT IN MILAN

What the heck is a sciura?!

In Milan, there's a special word to describe the city's elite housewives: *sciure*. Immaculately groomed, beautifully dressed, impeccably behaved, none would ever disgrace themselves by appearing on a reality show. They don't even know what a reality show is.

Technically speaking, a Milanese *sciura* doesn't work. She's too busy managing her multiple homes in the city, country, mountains, and seaside, and sometimes on a boat, too. She's mastered the art of effortless entertaining, designing, dressing, and cooking—and overseeing a fleet of people to ensure that all of this meets her exacting standards. She is also deeply classic and a faithful servant to Milan's codes of moral, social, and aesthetic conduct.

How did I learn about these Milanese paragons of style and society? By being a guest in other people's homes. These occasions were a kind of finishing school for me, a Californian who never learned to set a five-course dinner table properly or iron a linen pillowcase, and always wears sandals "in town."

But many of the women I learned these civilizing rules from are not actually *sciure* at all. They are rule-breakers, who all have day jobs as some of Milan's brightest creative talents. What always interested me was the way these women so artfully borrow from both old and new worlds to create something fabulously current and wholly distinct. They have a total reverence for "The Rules" of household management and the art of Living Like an Italian, but they do it with their own unique packaging.

These were the same women who were featured as DoubleJ's original Legendary Ladies, shot in their gorgeous homes, wearing our vintage. Later, we distilled their sheafs of wisdom into a "School of Sciura Rulebook" on our website, sharing their insights and edicts for how to decorate, dress, set a table, throw a party, send thank yous, manage a staff, organize a closet, and age gracefully (never ever Botox!).

The Italians were quite shocked when our series of articles called attention to the *sciura* factor in their own closed circles. It was a word whispered in hush-hush tones—no one wanted to be one, but people used the word all the time. DoubleJ got the town talking. Journalists from the *Corriere della Sera* wrote about it—some even labeled *me* a *sciura*—and three years later, an Instagram account called @sciuraglam launched that now has over 280K followers. Frankly, I was honored.

So, what are these finely honed rules anyway?
LET'S TAKE A LOOK

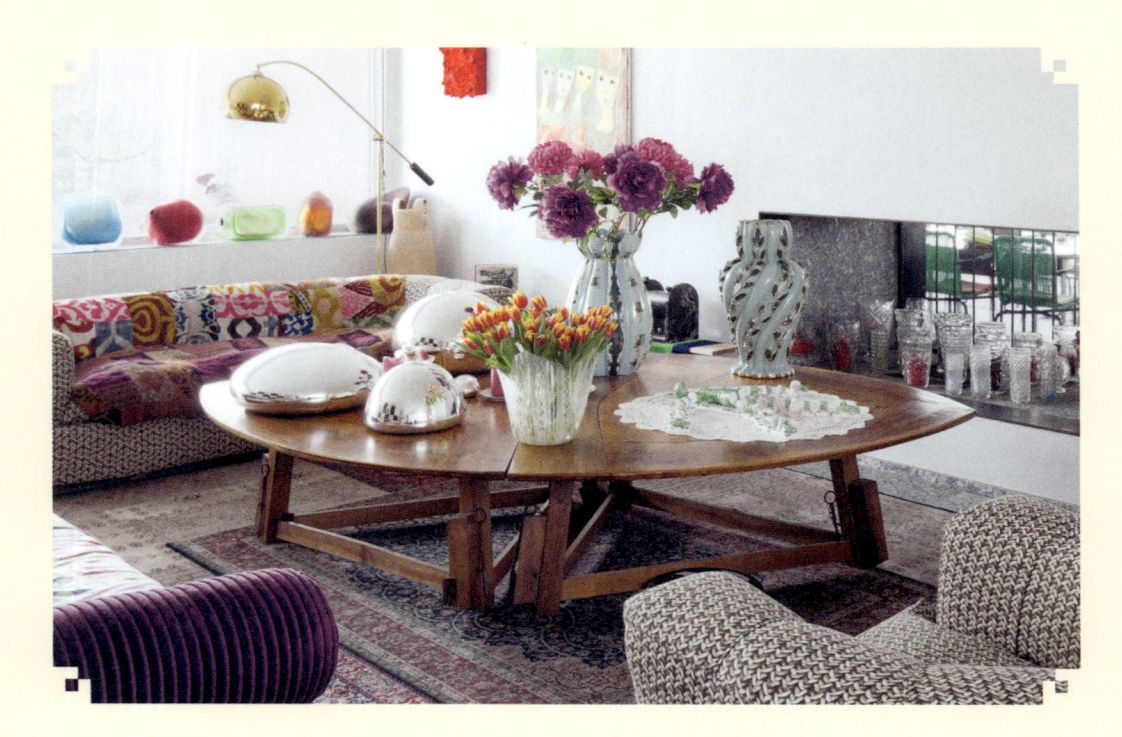

ANGELA MISSONI
MARVELOUS EPONYMOUS DESIGN MAVEN

The designer of her family's fashion house for over two decades, Angela Missoni's roles as grand matriarch and quintessential hostess never played second fiddle to her day job. The woman can balance a dinner party for fifty just as easily as she did her collections. Reigning from the family's country refuge outside Milan, Missoni entertains a nexus of cool creatives, fashion folk, and her beloved family.

"I never do a classic, serious table setting. I always mix things up with different colors and a variety of different objects so that every table has its own story. I like to make people laugh."

"Everyone is more relaxed when there is a buffet at a party—it allows more people to fit into a space and socialize."

"If you are short on time and even if there is nothing in the fridge, *risotto* will save you. You only need a bit of *zafferano* (saffron). And if you have any old veg lying around in the fridge, add that too."

"Most of my house is decorated with objects found in crappy second-hand shops. There are a few important and expensive pieces from Gio Ponti, Ettore Sottsass, and Franco Albini, but for the most part my house is filled with non-valuable items I love."

"I love all flowers and have a weekly supply of fresh ones dropped off at the house. The fun part is that I never know what I will get and let my friend make all the decisions."

"Once you pluck your eyebrows, they won't grow back. Let them be."

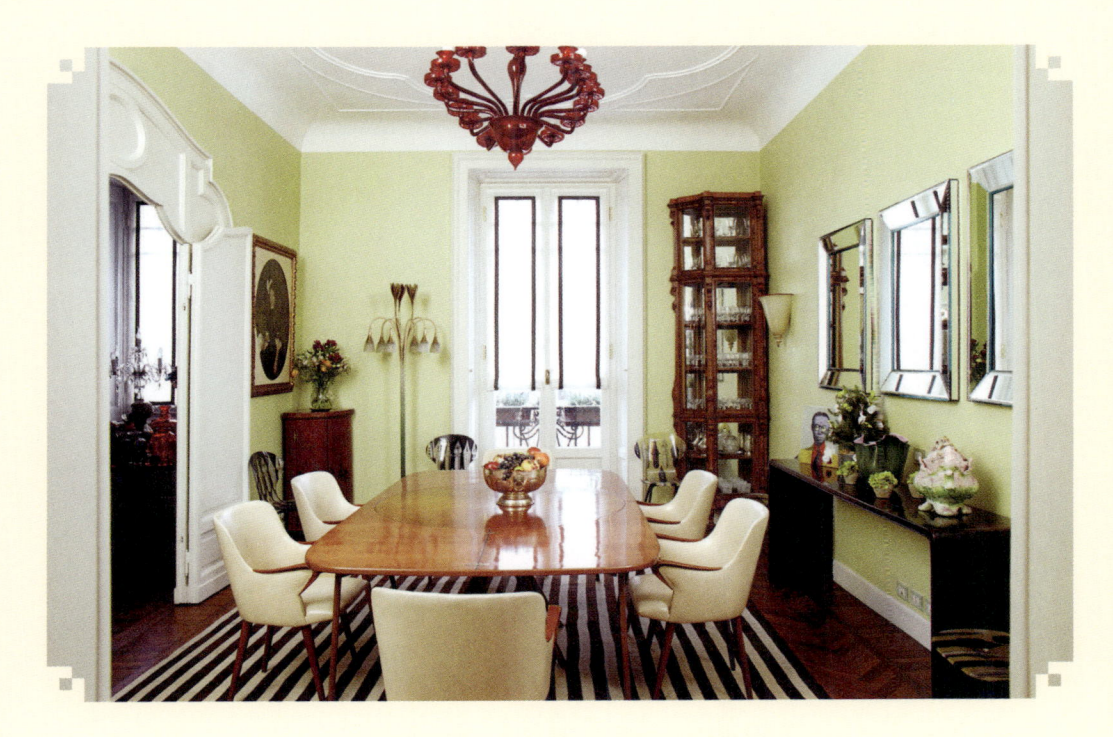

ROSSELLA JARDINI
FORMER MOSCHINO MUSE AND STYLISTIC MILANESE MADAM

Muse to the creative powerhouse Franco Moschino throughout the '80s and '90s, Rossella Jardini took over as creative director of Moschino upon his death and stayed several decades. Her mix of colors and materials in the home is unparalleled, and her butler is by her side for every whim and need.

"Flowers should be refreshed weekly. I send my maid to the flower market in Via San Marco each week. I like amaryllis in winter and peonies in the summer. Hydrangeas and white roses when nothing else works."

"If you're having more than twelve guests for dinner, enlist catering services."

"Set up house calls for as many appointments as possible. My veterinarian, manicurist, makeup artist, and hairstylist all come to my home."

"Walking the dogs, I wear velvet evening slippers by Charlotte Olympia or Alexander McQueen. And I bring along my Saint Laurent fringe bag."

"My maid irons my clothes and keeps my closets organized. When I travel, I tell her what I want to pack, then she folds and puts everything in my white Rimowa suitcase."

"Develop a tight rapport with a good tailor."

"A proper vacation can't take place in a hotel. I much prefer renting a home rather than staying in hotels. That way your dog can come. Anything more than a weekend you need a house."

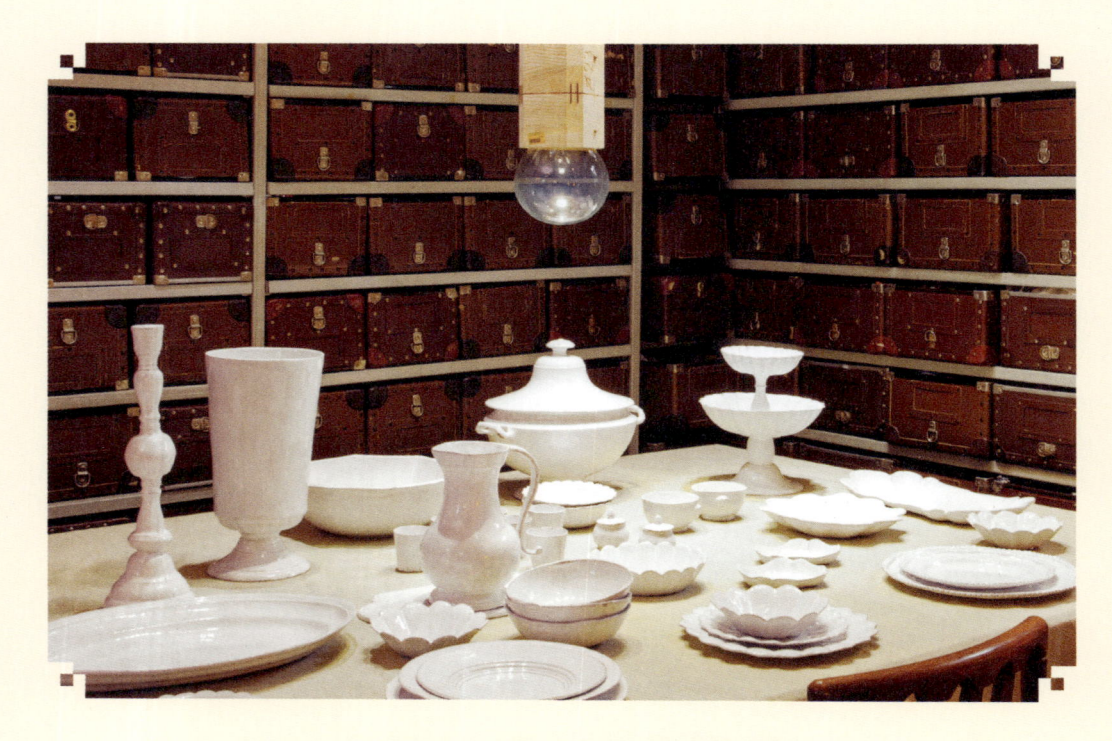

ROSSANA ORLANDI
MILAN'S PREMIER DRESSER AND DESIGN QUEEN

Rossana Orlandi is a counter-culture queen. She has built an empire as a design-world doyenne, doting for decades on the weird, the wonderful, the young, and the new at her eponymous Milan gallery. Surrounded by a formidable mix of dynamic creatives and design darlings, she rules the roost year-round in her trademark black-and-white style and enormous shades, and wry sense of humor.

"I hate doing dinners just for old people. I mix the old and the young as it's much more fun."

"I prepare everything except the food. I love to set up the table, clear it, and wash the dishes, but I don't know how to cook, so we prepare the food with our housekeeper."

"At home, the only thing I am nuts about are the closets—they must be organized. Everything is divided by type and then color. This is fundamental."

"I'm a maniac about ironing. Men's shirts are ironed but also the sheets. If the creases aren't right, I just assume they didn't do it at all. When I see wrinkles on my sheets, I go crazy."

"I wish people would age naturally. What I find embarrassing is when people come up to me and I have no idea who they are because everyone starts looking the same, with these huge lips and swollen cheeks."

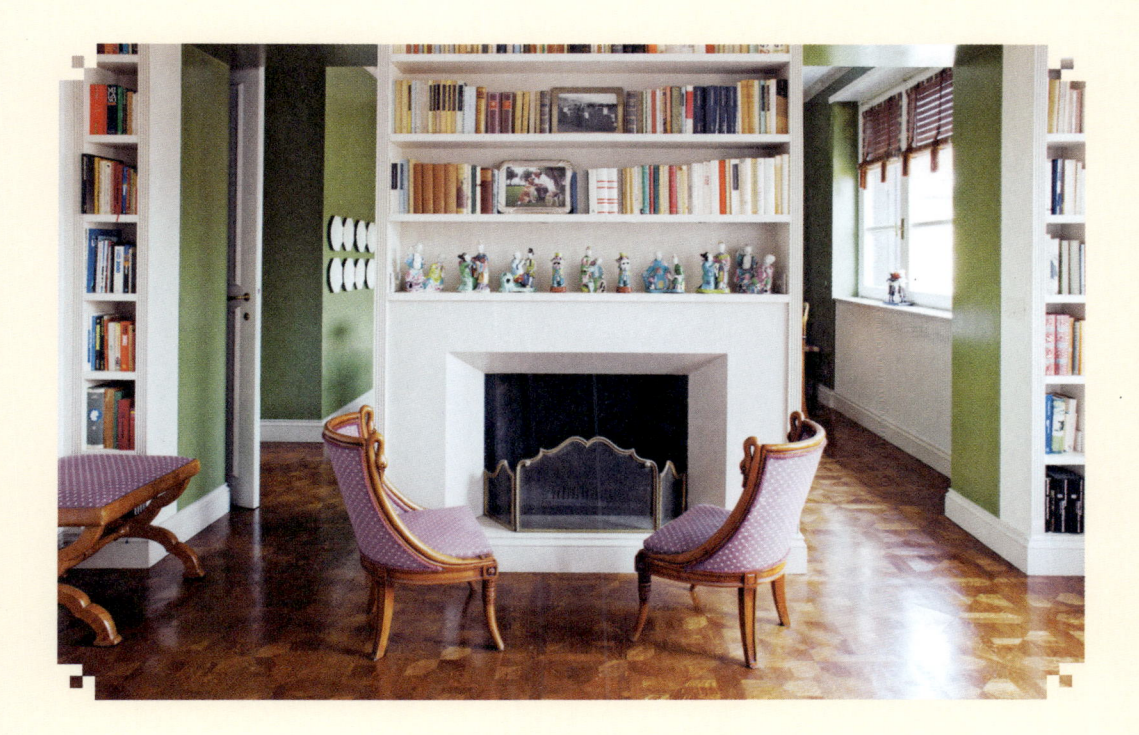

PUPI SOLARI
BUTTONING-UP THE CITY'S BEST DRESSED

Pupi Solari may hail from Genova, but she has long been a mainstay on the Milanese style scene. Her eponymous clothing empire, including her mecca for childrenswear, has become a pulpit from which Pupi dictates what brides, babies, and well-heeled Italians should wear, even into her 9th decade.

"Many women don't have the courage to dress *non moda*. Women go around naked these days! Their boobs are out. There's a continual provocation. Even the twelve- to thirteen-year-olds are going out like women twice their age. I hate that. They're afraid. I suggest to beautiful women to have the courage to go against fashion."

"I don't like sandals for the city, only for the seaside. Feet should be covered in the city."

"I love it when children look sporty. I don't like babies wearing formal jackets. I hate it! No polo shirt, no sweatshirt. They should not dress like miniature parents. At six years old they can finally have a jacket."

"I hate old people. They're always complaining and unhappy. I don't want to fall into a discussion about how my knee hurts. When I die, I will die. I'm not obsessed with age."

"Women should age gracefully. I don't use any creams, but I do like to use Tonico Spray Lentivo from the Farmacia Internazionale in Santa Margherita."

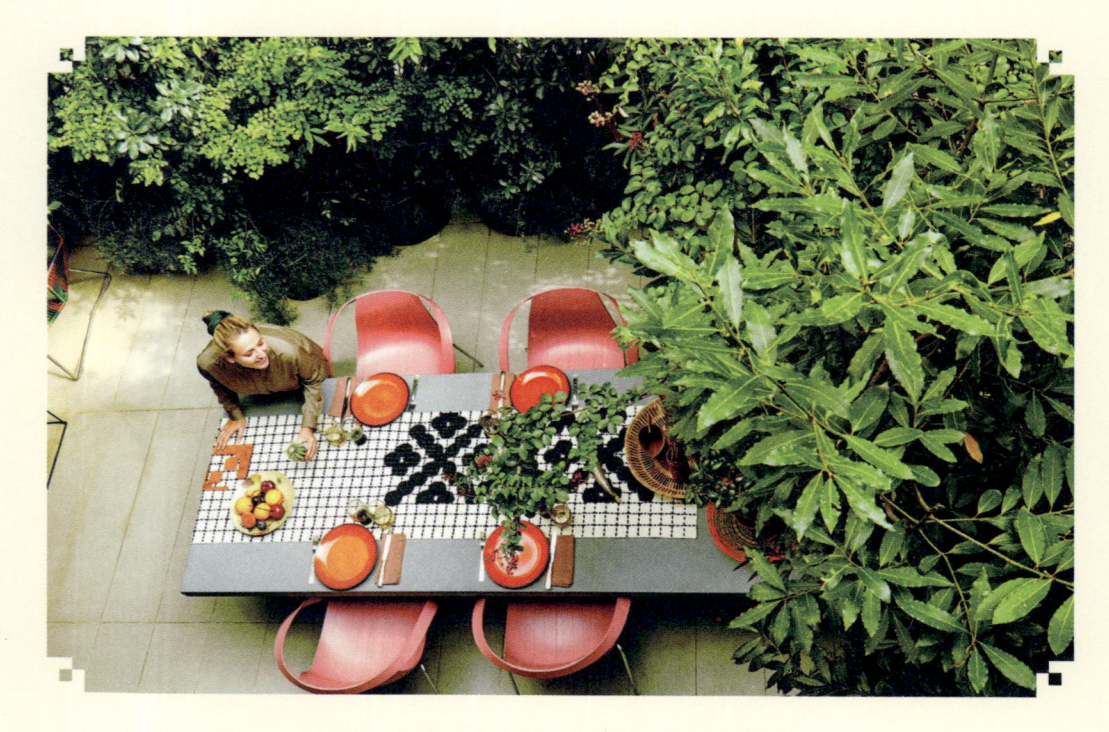

PATRICIA URQUIOLA
ARCHITECT AND FREEWHEELING FURNITURE DESIGNER

One of the few females who slips effortlessly into the male-dominated architecture field, Milan-based Patricia Urquiola takes the audacious approach to life. Everything from bold clothes to unscripted dinner parties gets her colorful, high-energy treatment. We adore her for her pure, unfiltered views, not to mention the homes, hotels, and furnishings she boldly designs.

"I cooked my whole life, but now my time is for work. So now I have a divine cook in the house who prepares everything."

"Never put a wine and a water glass from the same design family together. I mix vintage pieces with Kartell."

"I always put down a textile, but not a full tablecloth. I like it when it's in the middle of the table."

"I like having a lot of things on the table. I put a bunch of glasses on the end of the table just to make it more festive. I'll maybe add a straw bowl, a silver fish sculpture, and some fruit. Fruit always makes things better."

"My refrigerator is always full. I have a real fear of an empty fridge."

"You don't need to spend a lot of money on design for it to be good."

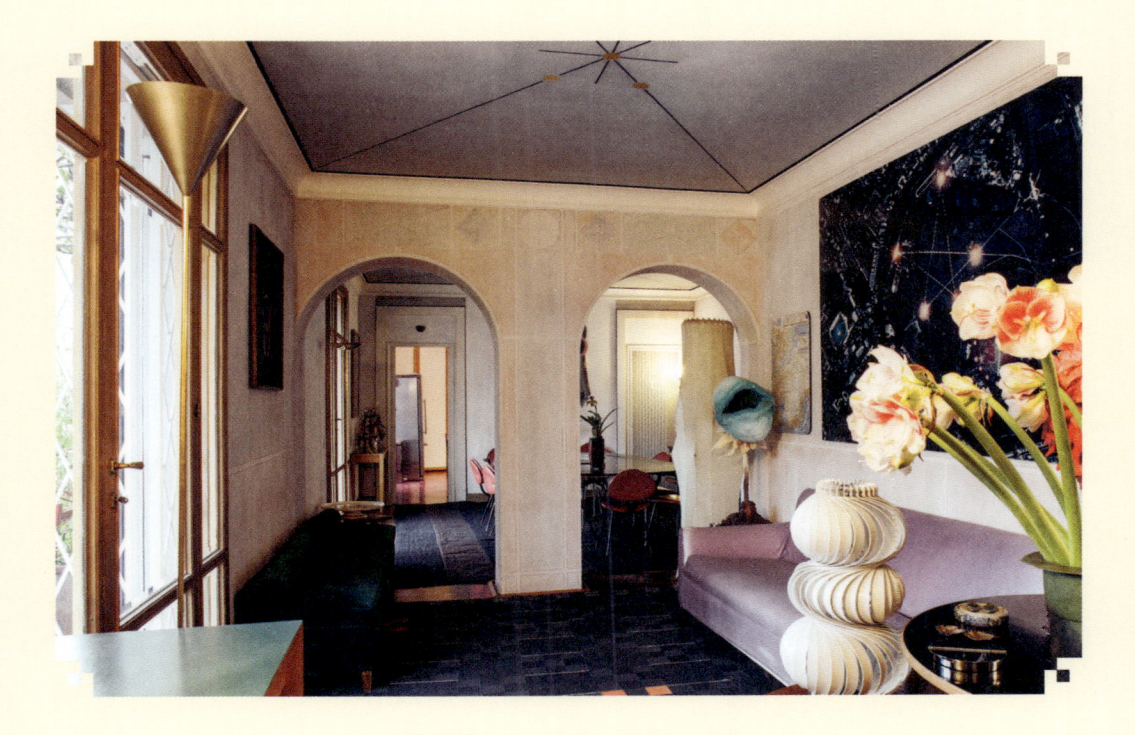

NINA YASHAR
DESIGN GALLERIST AND PRINT-LOVING POWER DRESSER

One of the most fiercely chic and radically independent dressers in the entire city, Nina Yashar is also owner of the globally esteemed design gallery Nilufar and its supermarket-size sister warehouse, Nilufar Depot. She may be the Queen of International Design, but she's also a stickler for perfectly hosted dinner parties and Prada-lined dressing rooms.

"Mix up your plates, especially for buffet dinners." Nina mixes traditional plates with modern flatware designed by Gio Ponti.

"For *aperitivo*, never serve drinks without an ample snack plate." She offers a *pinzimonio* (long, skinned vegetables placed in a tall jar) and cut up pieces of grana cheese.

"Try something chic in the powder room." She puts *huile de karité* oil from Paris's Sultan spa on her guest bath sink instead of lotion.

"A bottle of wine is an acceptable but boring hostess gift. I'll bring a little something from Prada. If not, I bring a book."

"I use turbans instead of going to the hairdresser." Nina's collection includes Prada, vintage prints, and fur turbans for winter.

"No jeans. Ever. The last time I wore them I was between eighteen and twenty years old."

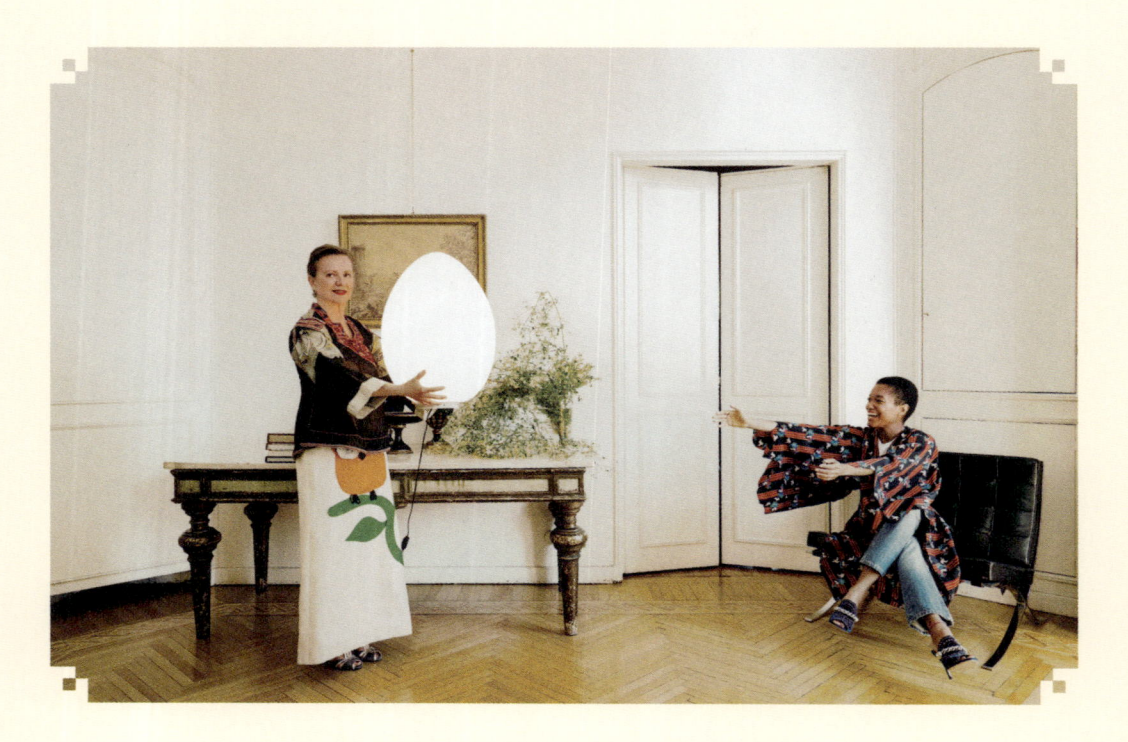

FRANCESCA TADDEI
TAMU McPHERSON'S ACADEMIC AND SUPREMELY STYLISH SUOCERA IS THE SOURCE OF ALL LOCAL WISDOM

Street-style photographer and Milan-based influencer Tamu McPherson is one of the most stylish girls in town. Guess where she gets her insider tips for true Italian style? From her supremely chic, former University of Bologna professor mother-in-law, Francesa Taddei, who is an encyclopedia of good taste.

Add mischief to the pomp and ceremony: "Francesca decorates her super formal table with pranks. There are ninety-six plates with vintage tablecloths and then a little plastic dish with a toad. Or a trick under the napkin like spiders and poop for the kids."

Upgrade your gifting game: "She's always bringing friends vintage objects, design objects, or jewelry from Oro & Incenso. Everything is extraordinary, like antique coral or glass. It's extremely personal and speaks to the person."

When in doubt, go formal. "She does full service, adding every plate and glass you can imagine."

Don't skimp on outerwear: "She taught me to always have proper coats. In New York you just have a parka, but here you have to have all of them—camel, black, blue coat—it's very specific."

Closets should look like a high-end boutique. "She is extremely organized. All of the hangers are white, from Ikea. Everything is color coded, folded, and handled immediately with the housekeeper or dry cleaner."

Jeans have only one purpose. Housework! "Francesca will only wear jeans to clean and tidy up, with a white shirt on."

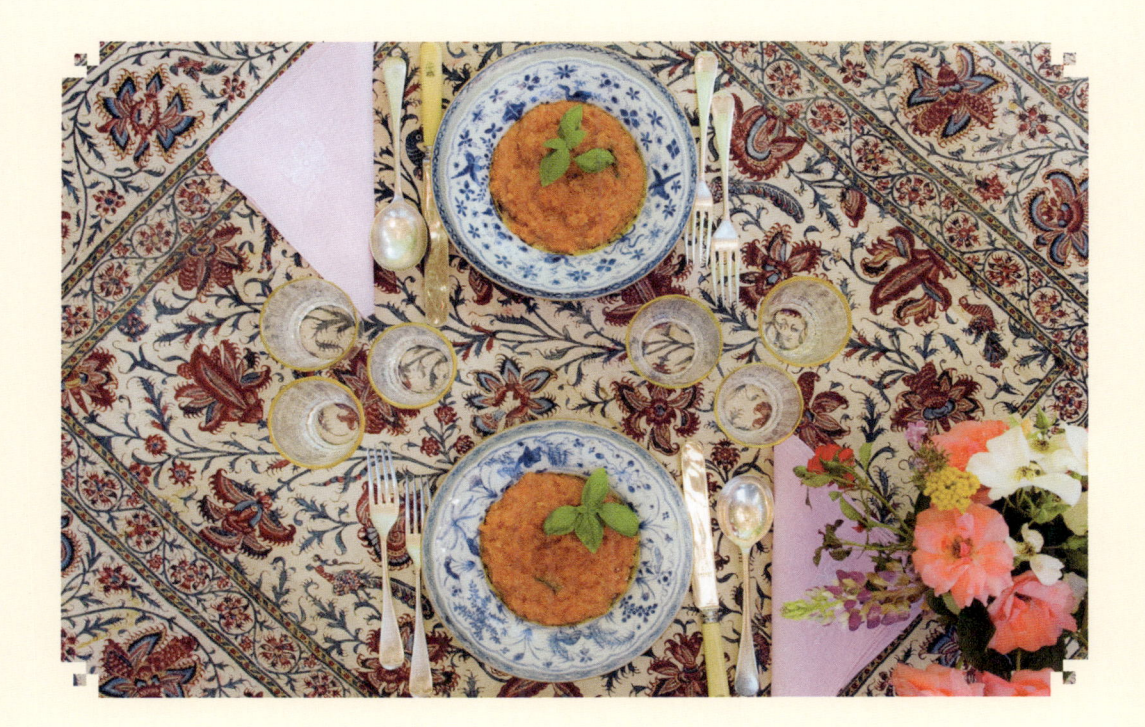

LAURA SARTORI RIMINI
ARCHITECTURAL DREAM WEAVER OF LAVISH, EXOTIC INTERIORS

Laura Sartori Rimini, known for perfectly recreating neo-classical and turn-of-the-century interiors, also has that magical Milanese combo of professional powerhouse and domestic goddess. She looks like a 1920s movie star, runs renovation worksites in her boots and jeans, and entertains at home.

"I prefer to invite people to dinner who do not know each other well. I think it's more interesting. Otherwise, you always see the same people and you say the same things. I think it's very nice to share new experiences."

"I always prepare the table. Even if it is just a midweek dinner for my family, there are fresh flowers, and in the evening there are candles."

"Having a proper meal together is important, it's a portion of time—half an hour, one hour—that the family talks. No cell phone at the table, no television in the dining room. We talk. We've done this since the children were very young."

"For stationery, pick something that will stand the test of time."

"At work, I'm always very simple with flat shoes, trousers, and never any jewels. As a woman on a building site, it's not so easy. The majority of people there are men—craftsmen, plumbers, electricians. It's difficult because people look at your blue eyes and stop following what you're telling them."

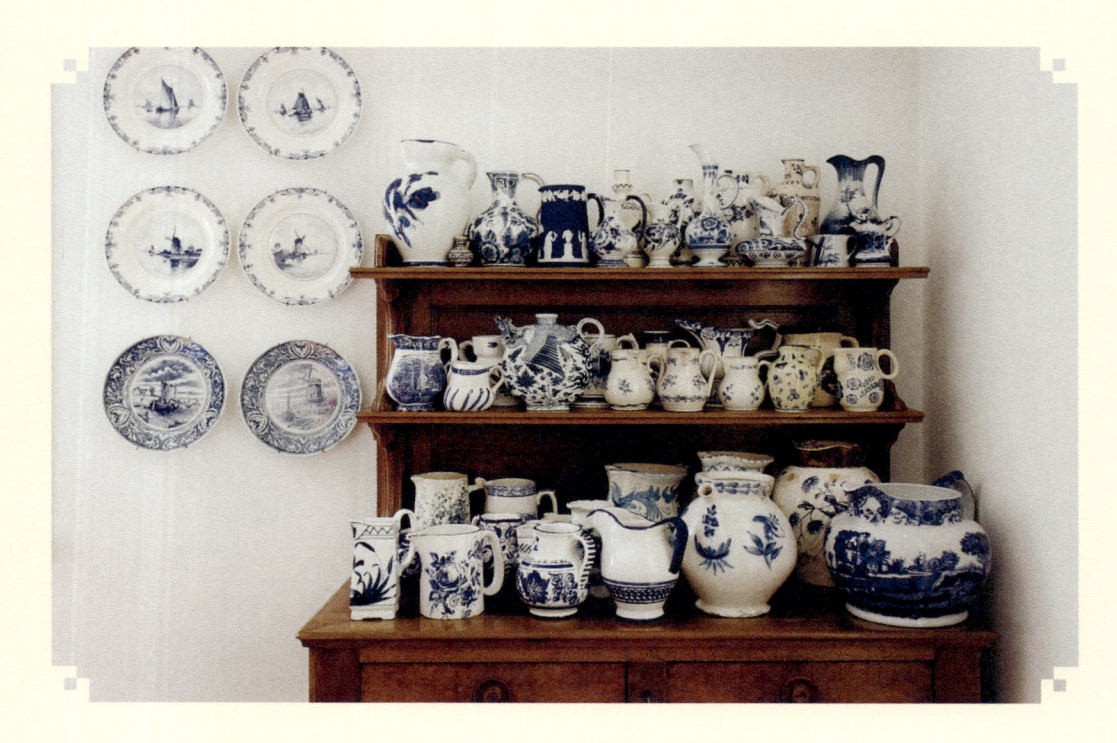

LAURA LUSUARDI
HIGH-OCTANE FASHION EXECUTIVE

Laura Lusuardi's sharp nose for style extends way beyond Max Mara's coat kingdom, where she's worked for decades. With her moccasin-clad feet firmly on the ground of the company's Reggio Emilia HQs, she rules with a quiet and a sharp wit. In between her high-octane work hours, she retires to her home near the factory, with a garden from which she pulls fresh herbs and vegetables.

"Always keep *prosciutto* in your fridge. This, coupled with a big hunk of *parmigiano*, means you're always ready for an *aperitivo*. I store the *prosciutto*—an entire leg that I slice myself—in a cotton kitchen towel to keep it fresher longer."

"We always drink sparking red wine made locally, but if you are having guests, serve *prosecco* with a bit of kir. It is a failsafe *aperitivo*."

"I sort all of my jewelry by color so that it is easier to match with my outfits."

"I have cupboards full of linens that I have bought on my travels, and they can take any table from flat to fabulous."

"I dress in a uniform—always a tunic top and trousers, and almost always in blue. It works well for me."

"Doing what you love keeps you beautiful. Work is my life, but I make sure to have a massage every Saturday, too."

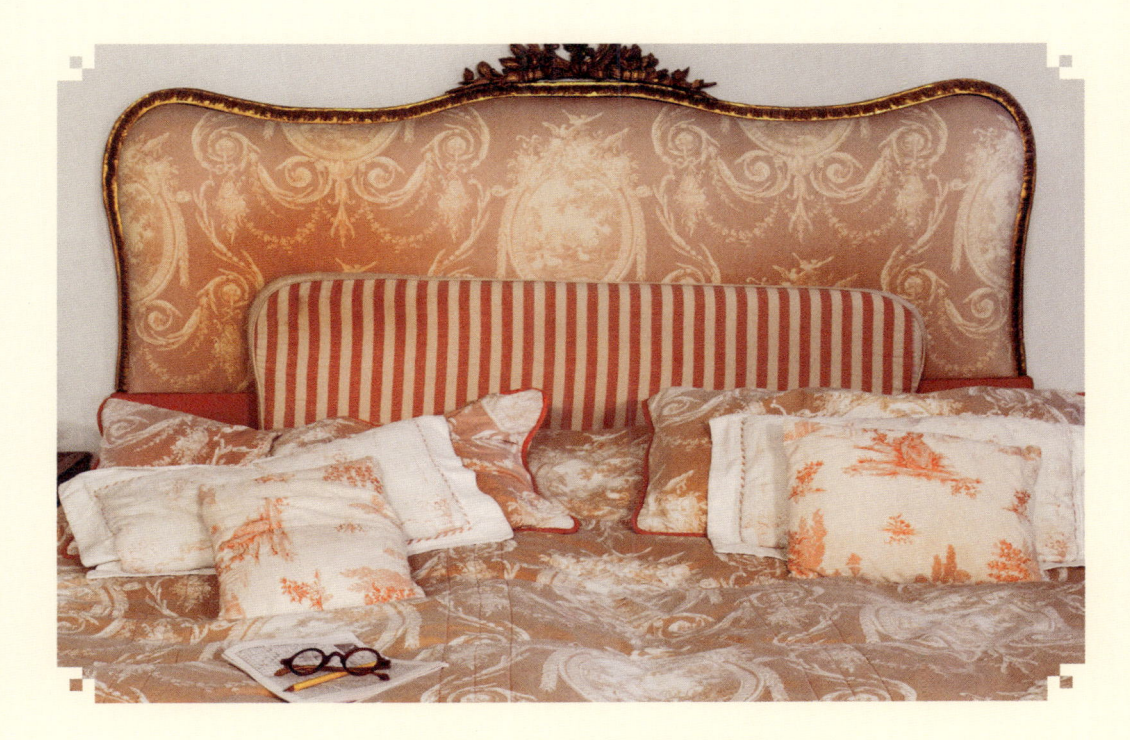

DONATA SARTORIO
RENOWNED FASHION JOURNALIST

With a Pilates-toned body and a vegan diet, fashion journalist Donata Sartorio is not your typical legendary lady of Milan. She's been a rebel at work for over four decades and still has time to write books and teach young fashion students. Plus, she's a stickler for The Rules.

"I do not want to hear *Ciao!* from the staff at a restaurant or store. You should never address someone casually unless you know them personally. Never give the *tu* to the cleaning lady, either."

"I like inviting people to dinner who have never met. I mix thirty-year-olds with eighty-year-olds—that's when something unexpected happens."

"Silver is something you need to clean regularly and use. You shouldn't put it away. It adds a certain elegance. All my silver comes from my family and my wedding gifts, and I use it daily."

"When I serve meals, I like to give people possibilities. I use two lazy Susans on the table with different olive oils, umeboshi vinegar, balsamic vinegar, algae, and sea salts so you can make your own flavors with the vegetables."

"The idea of searching for style—and not trends—is very Milanese. Women here are used to dressing in uniforms. There's a certain amount of formality, great culture, also a bit of humor."

"In Milan you can't go around with short shorts and Botox. There's still a classicism here."

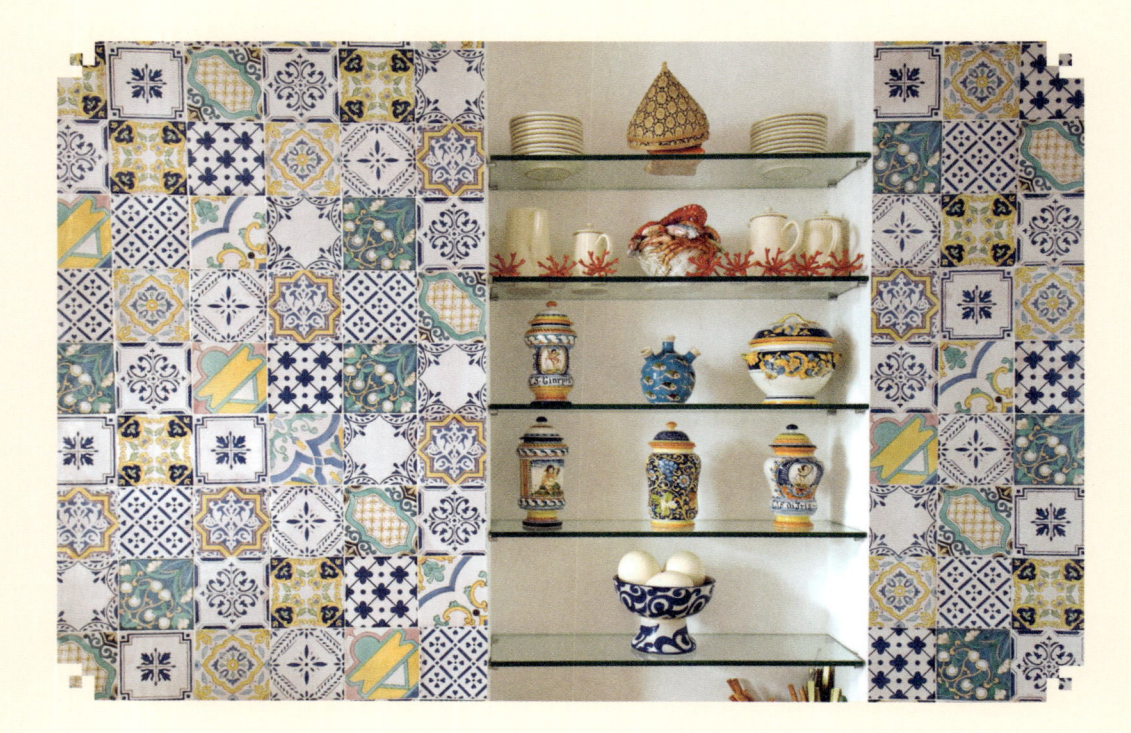

SUSANNE THUN
DESIGN WUNDERKIND AND MAGICAL HOST

The Austrian-born Susanne Thun does abundant Italian hospitality with laser-sharp precision, and the results are always glorious and perfect. A former fashion editor and ongoing creative partner to her architect husband, Thun marries beautiful design and her own unique taste—whether she's dressing herself, decorating a gorgeous home, or throwing a fabulous party.

"I always use a lace tablecloth; it makes me feel Italian."

"You never know when your next party may be, so always keep a big box of Hawaiian flower necklaces for your guests to dress up in."

"By the seaside, your silverware should change. I like to use bamboo."

"I love to have things properly ironed. I hate these people walking around all crumpled up."

"Normally staff uniforms are all gray. But in the summer, they wear dark blue Bermudas with a white T-shirt."

"Toes always stay covered in town. I don't like sandals in the city. I wear a sneaker, driving shoe, mules, or a loafer."

"Never put bags or hats on the bed. It's an old Italian superstition."

"I can't do makeup. I've never done it."

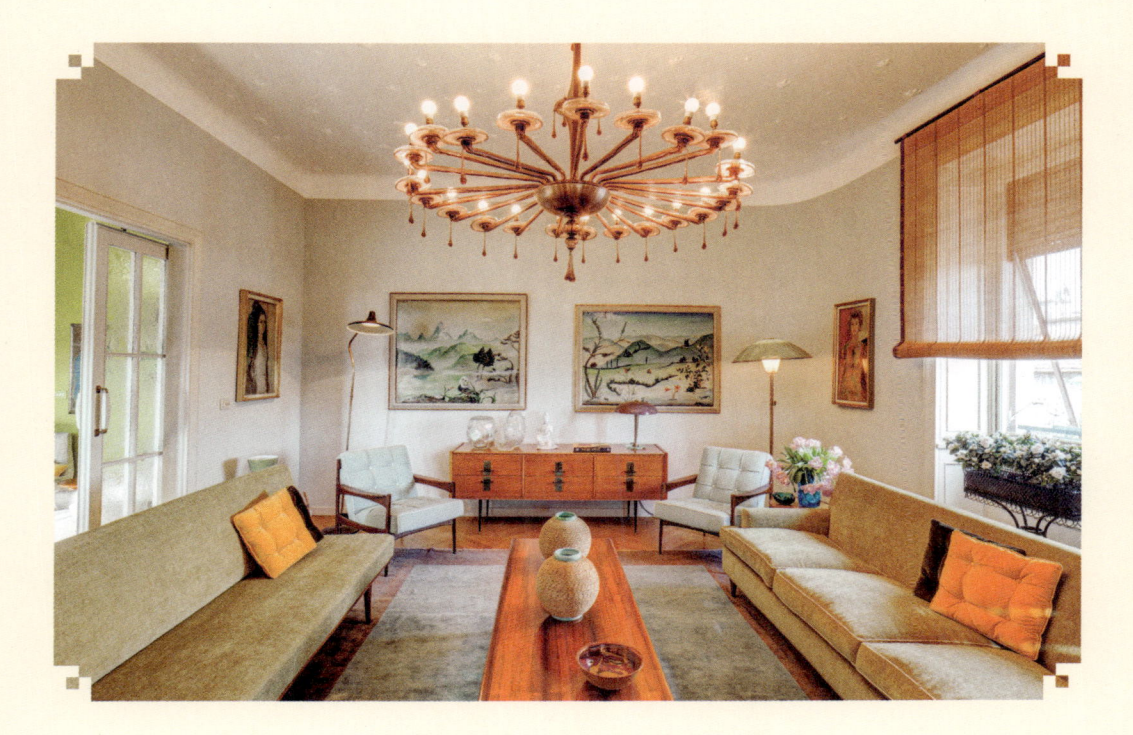

CHICHI MERONI
GRANDE DAME OF MILANESE STYLE

From Chichi Meroni's headquarters on Via Largo Augusto—where both her atelier and sprawling shopping destination, L'Arabesque, reside inside a sensational postwar building commissioned by her father—the endlessly chic designer sets the city's classic style agenda on everything from hard-to-find vintage clothing and furniture to bespoke wedding dresses and tabletops.

"I change table settings and plates each day even if I'm dining alone at home. If I don't do it for myself how am I supposed to do it for other people too?"

"I put the fork next to the plate, not on the napkin; this is how I was taught."

"I use only light linen bedsheets. I have old ones from my family. They're from my trousseau, which you inherit when you get married. But I also buy them, especially old ones, when I travel."

"I think that a woman, even if she has the most perfect body, should never dress like her daughter. You should dress to feel good about yourself, but you should never escape your age."

"Exercise clothes are for the gym only. I think it's horrific to go round in your exercise clothes or a tracksuit. You shouldn't wear it at home, either."

"All summer clothes are on an upper rack during winter. I have curtains between the parts of my wardrobe and exchange them every season."

"Please don't dye your hair peroxide blond unless you are twenty years old or look like Marilyn Monroe."

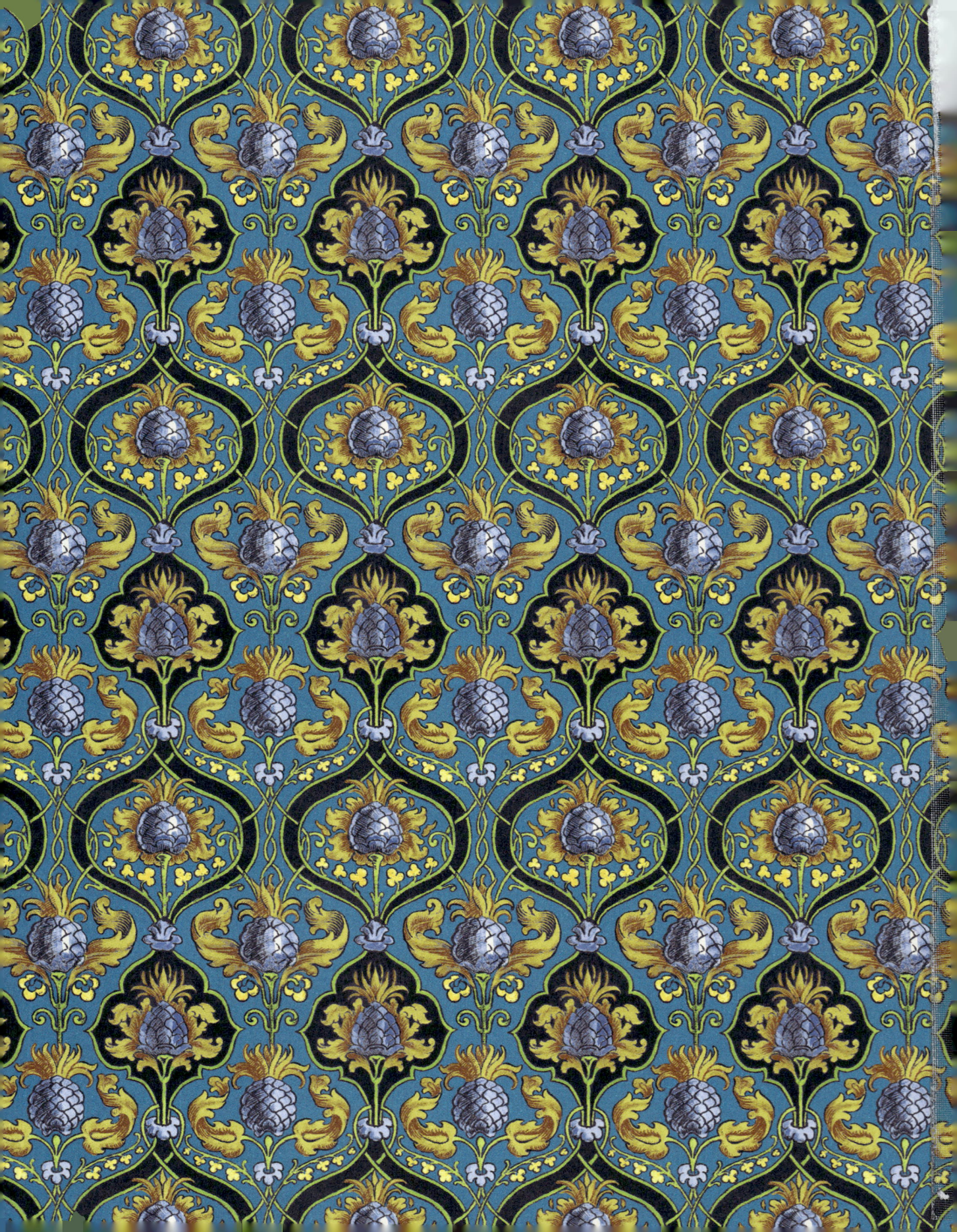

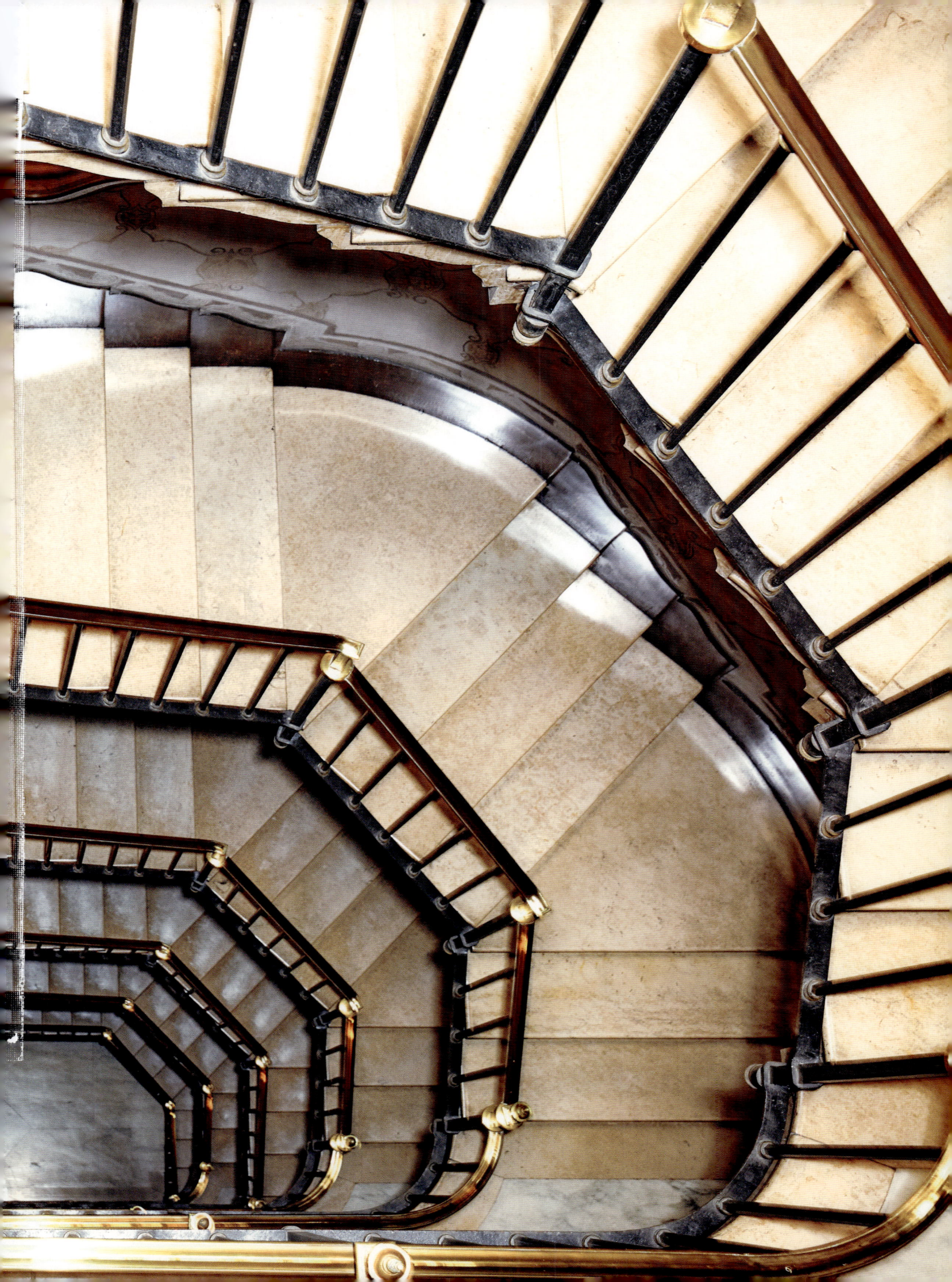

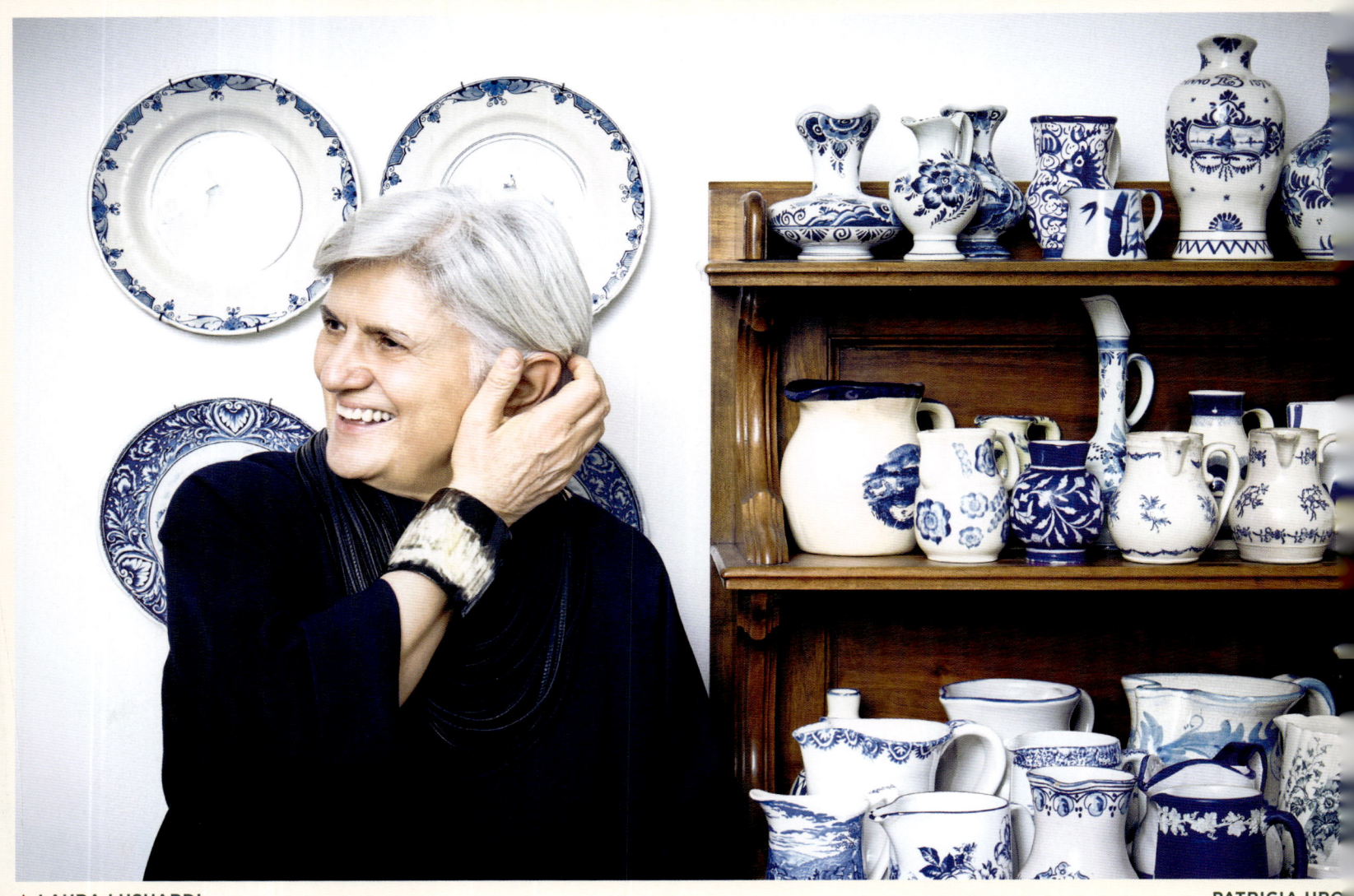

▲ LAURA LUSUARDI
HIGH-OCTANE FASHION EXECUTIVE FOR MAX MARA

PATRICIA URQ
ARCHITECT AND FREEWHEELING FURNITURE D

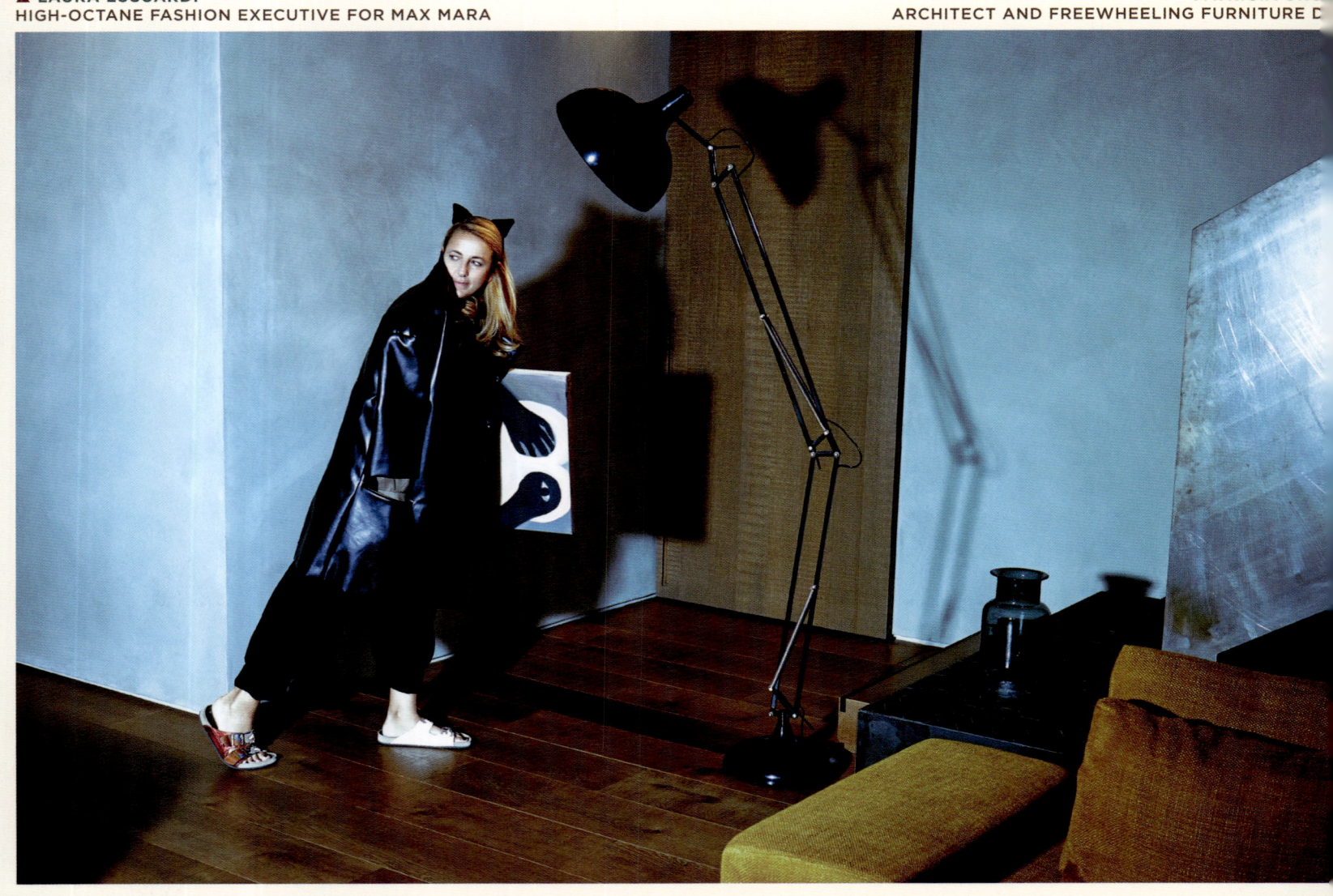

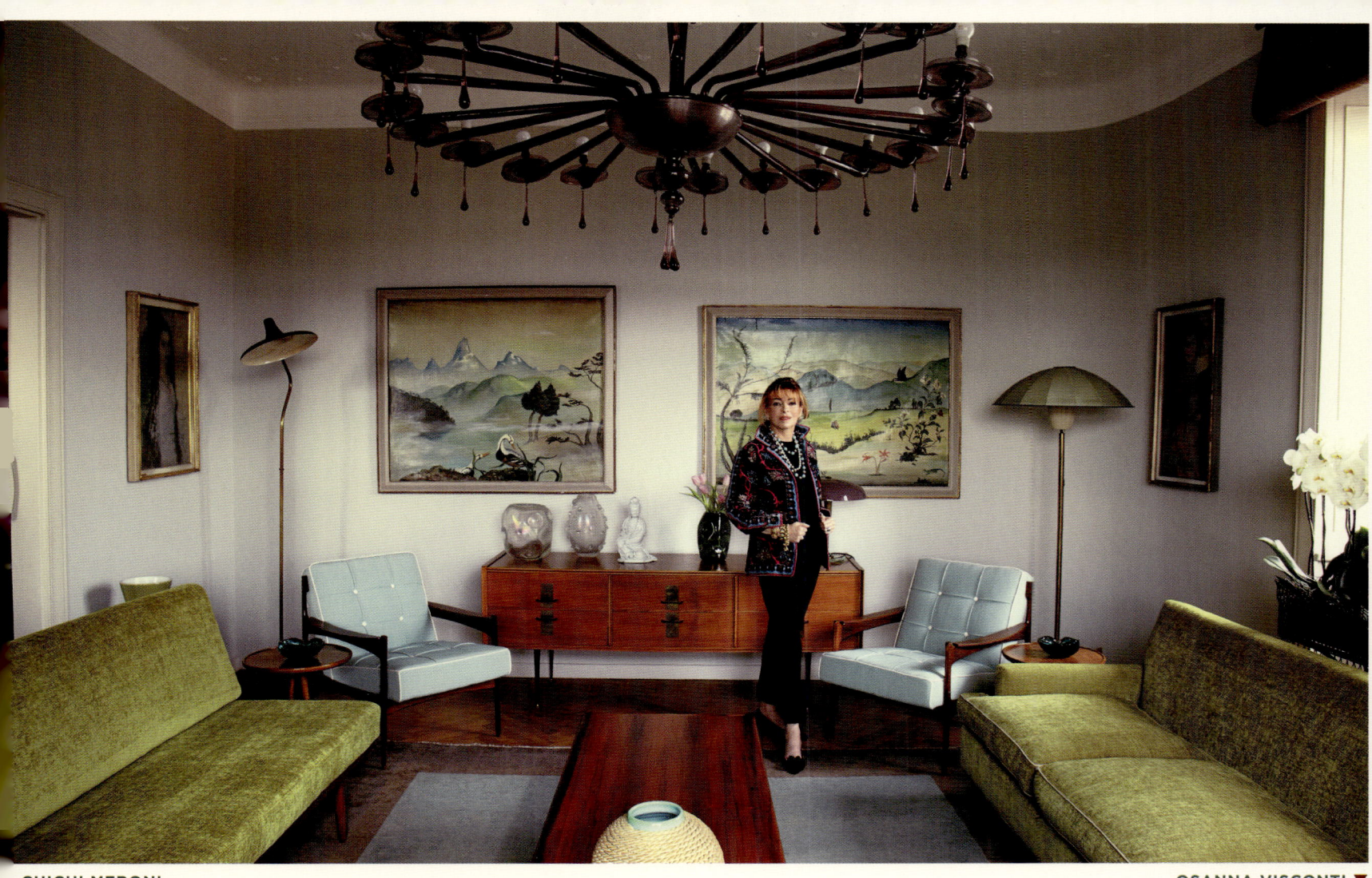

CHICHI MERONI
ESIGNER, RETAILER, AND GRANDE DAME OF MILANESE STYLE

OSANNA VISCONTI ▼
BOUNTIFUL BRONZEWORK AND JEWELRY DESIGNER

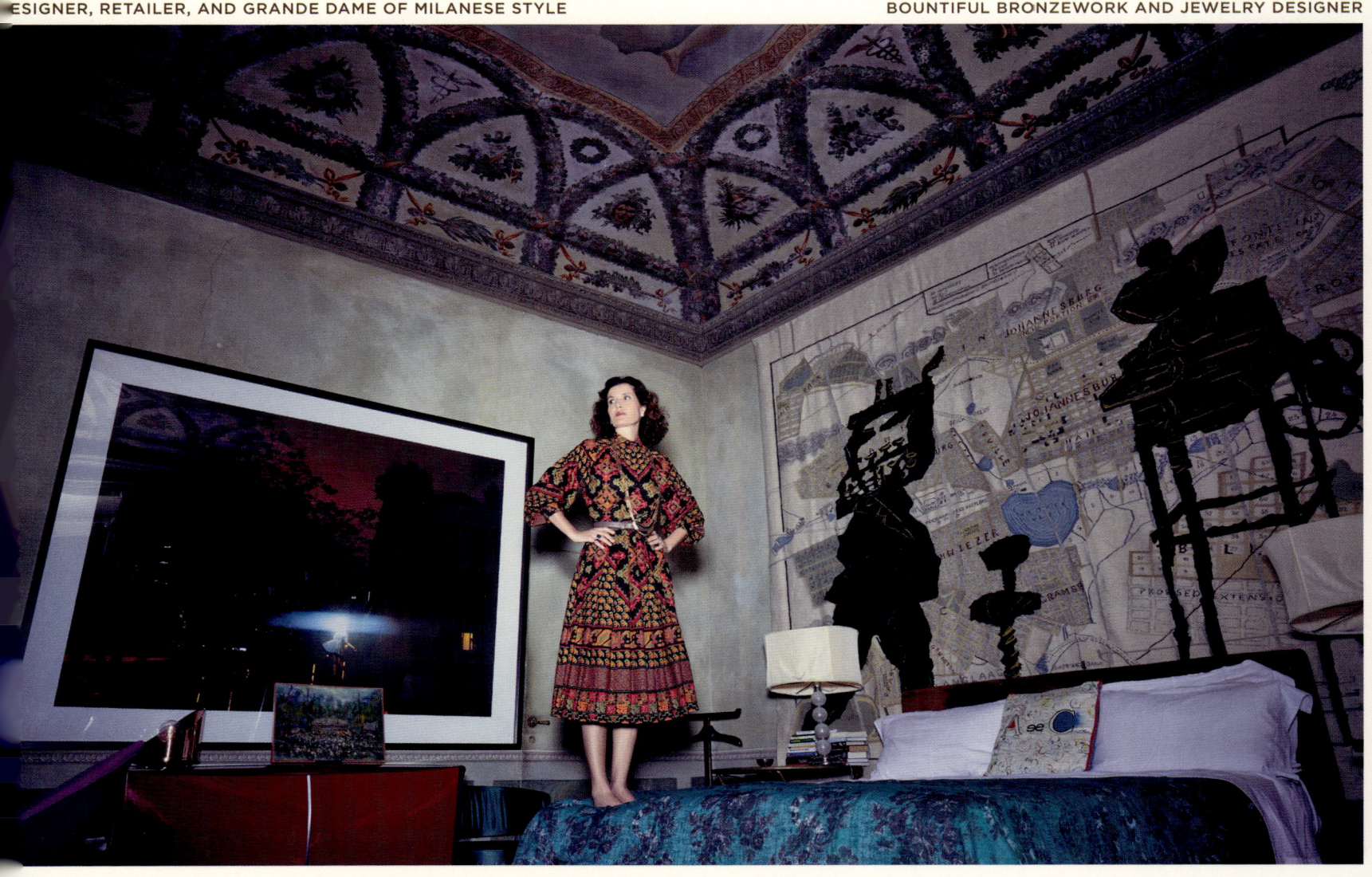

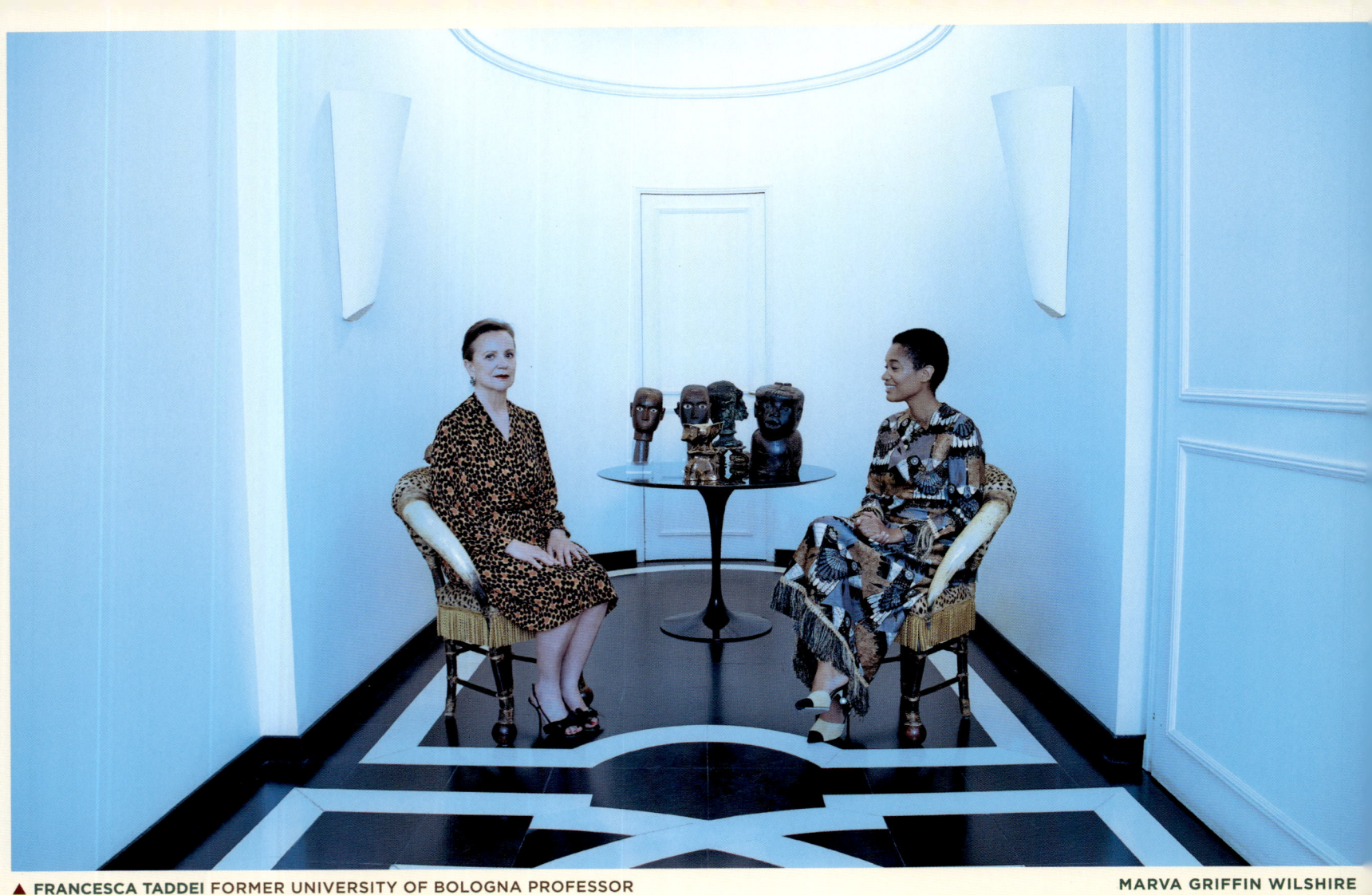

▲ **FRANCESCA TADDEI** FORMER UNIVERSITY OF BOLOGNA PROFESSOR
AND TAMU MCPHERSON'S SUPREMELY STYLISH *SUOCERA*

MARVA GRIFFIN WILSHIRE
VENERATED ICON OF MILAN'S SALONE DEL MOBIL

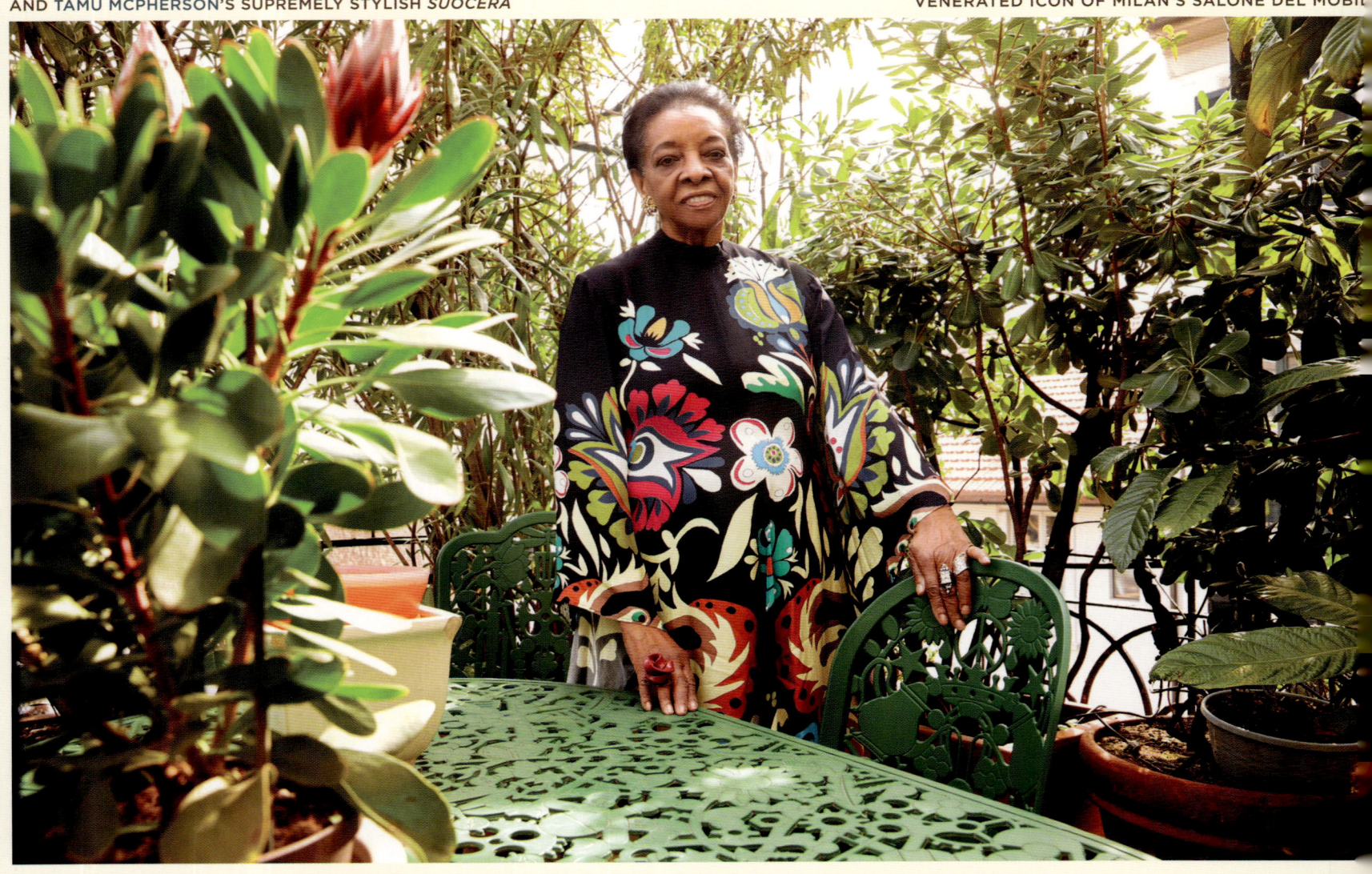

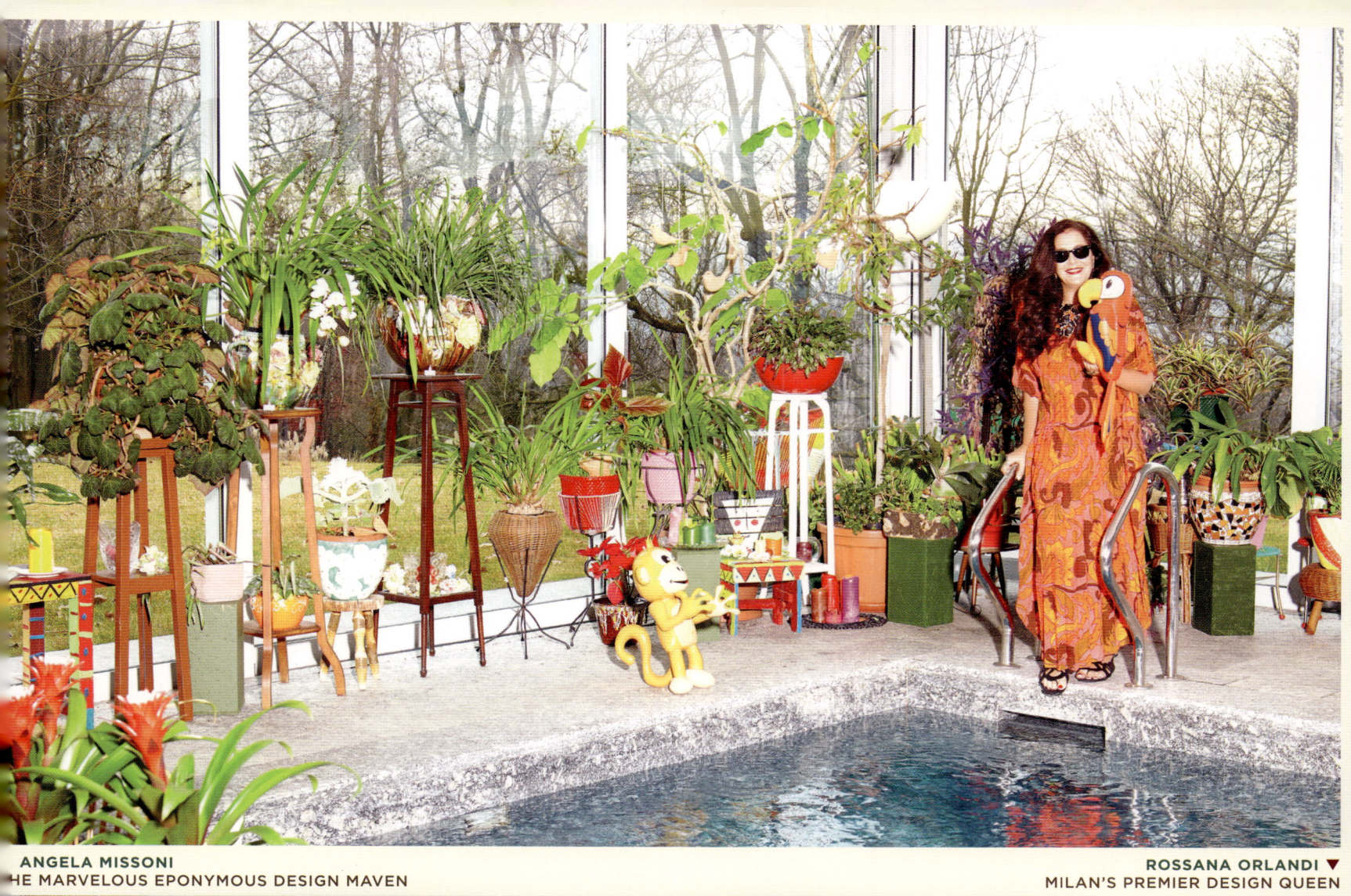

ANGELA MISSONI
THE MARVELOUS EPONYMOUS DESIGN MAVEN

ROSSANA ORLANDI ▼
MILAN'S PREMIER DESIGN QUEEN

MAMMA MILANO

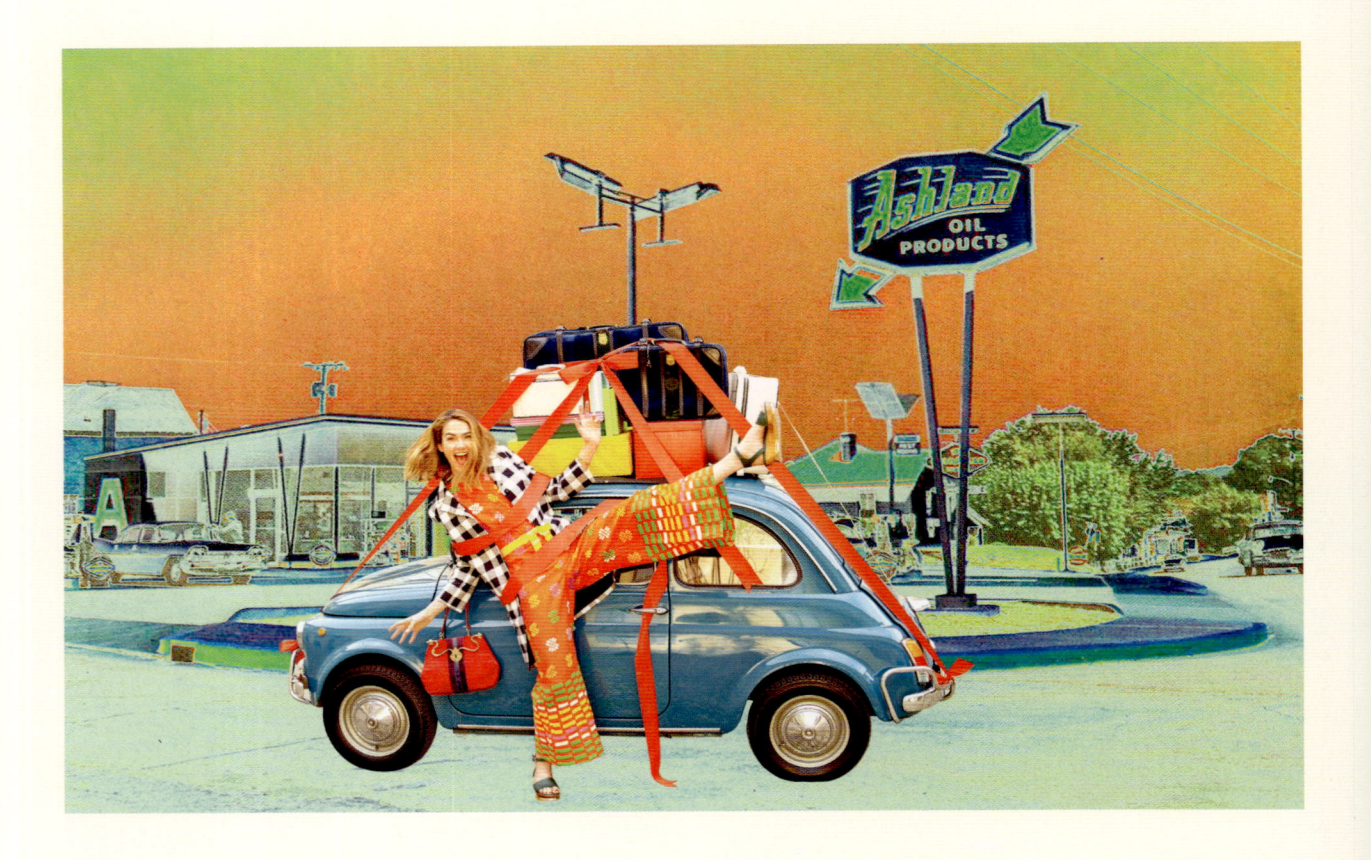

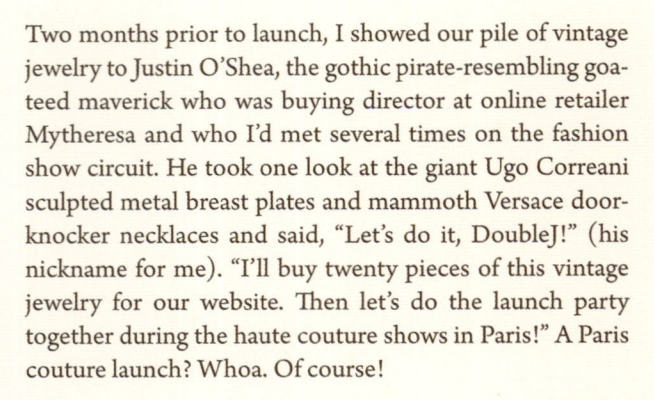

Two months prior to launch, I showed our pile of vintage jewelry to Justin O'Shea, the gothic pirate-resembling goateed maverick who was buying director at online retailer Mytheresa and who I'd met several times on the fashion show circuit. He took one look at the giant Ugo Correani sculpted metal breast plates and mammoth Versace doorknocker necklaces and said, "Let's do it, DoubleJ!" (his nickname for me). "I'll buy twenty pieces of this vintage jewelry for our website. Then let's do the launch party together during the haute couture shows in Paris!" A Paris couture launch? Whoa. Of course!

Everything else was up to me: photography, packaging, logistics, authentication, party planning. I called an old family friend in Los Angeles, Pamela Mullin, who had a majestic apartment on the Île Saint-Louis overlooking Notre-Dame. Might we be able to borrow the space for the evening? The answer? A magical yes.

La DoubleJ, our apple-cheeked babe, popped out wide-eyed and gurgling in 2015 as an online magazine selling vintage fashion and jewelry. There was, honestly, nothing on the internet like her. I had achieved it not through a rational business plan or desire to make money, but by channeling deeply the two things that drove me absolutely crazy with pleasure—eye-busting vintage, and those crazy Italians who had finally conquered my frosty heart. Then I swirled it up and served it in my own weird, wacky, multi-colored, maximalist package.

I sent the launch newsletter to every journalist I'd ever worked with and they all cheered, while many covered the news in their outlets. *New York* magazine called it the "best vintage website ever invented." *Vogue* said it "just might qualify as the best guide to insiders' Milan around." Franca Sozzani, the formidable editor-in-chief of *Vogue* Italia, invited me to her home in Milan to show her the website everyone had been talking about. A few months later, a Condé Nast publisher in Italy called to offer me the job of editor-in-chief of *Glamour* magazine. I was honored… but no. I knew that my old life was now behind me. I would not abandon my baby now.

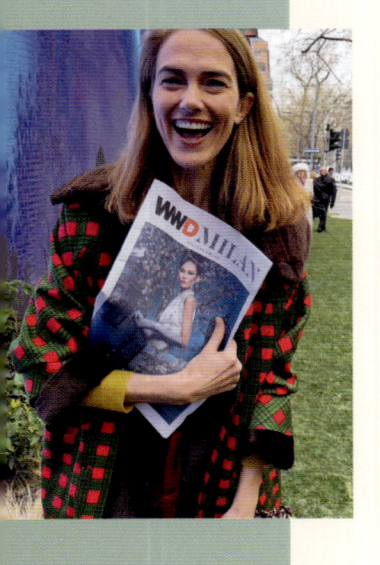

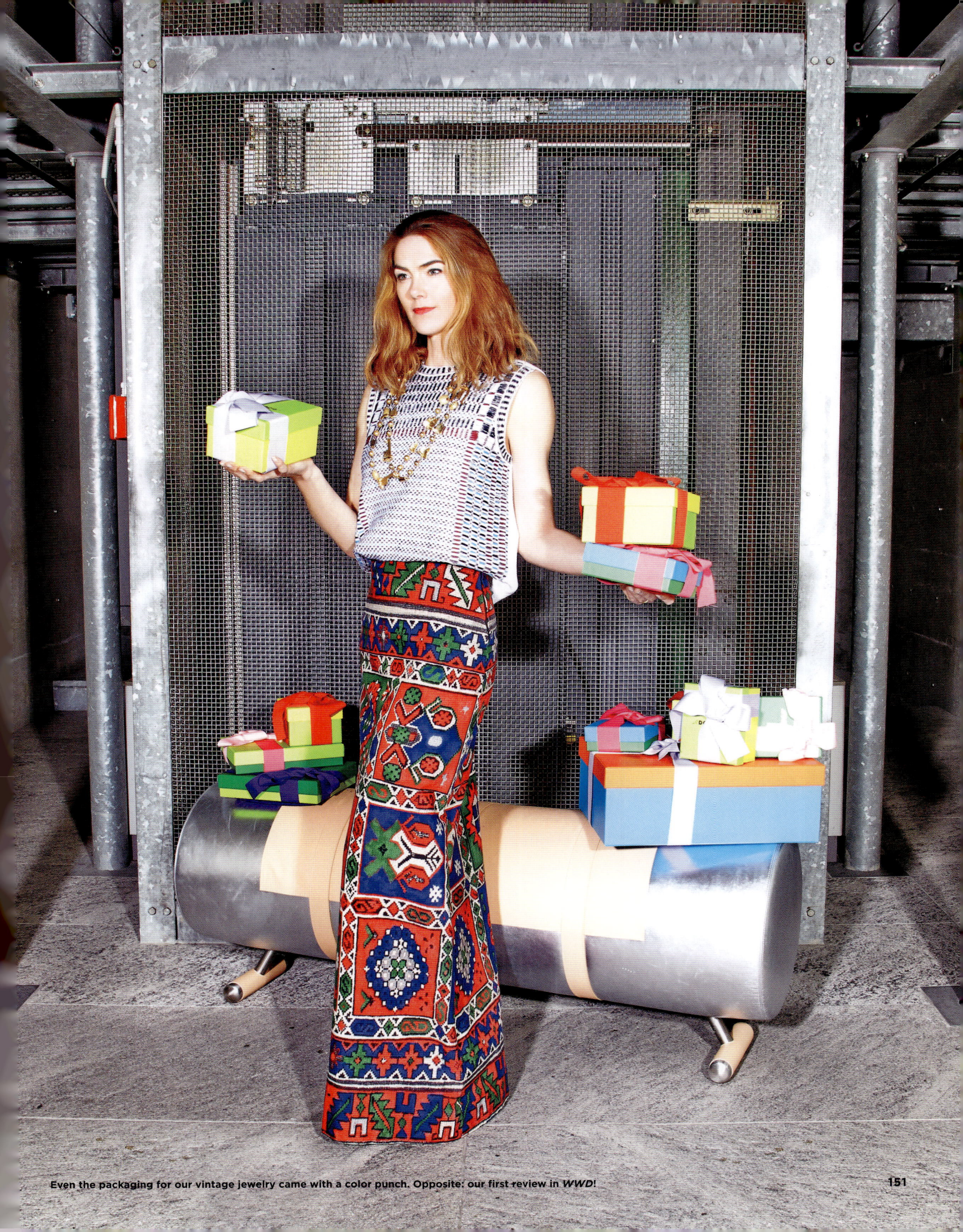

Even the packaging for our vintage jewelry came with a color punch. Opposite: our first review in *WWD*!

SCRAPPY BUT HAPPY: THE EARLY YEARS

From the very start, LaDoubleJ oozed joy. We were always smiling, joking, and screaming in delight in our tiny office, on our web pages, on Instagram, and in our laugh-tastic newsletters. We were not cool by fashion standards, but we were having fun, just like the Italians had taught me. Fashion people are often scowling, not because they're mean, but because they're scared or stressed out. I was often scared, too. I was frightened that my new venture wouldn't work out, that I'd fail, that I'd given up the keys to the kingdom, and would end up an irrelevant, self-exiled fool.

But the fear was blasted out by the joy I felt doing something that bubbled up from my belly and was truly authentic to me. I was sick of fashion parties, anyway. I *like* to smile in pictures. A smile welcomes people into your world, it opens doors, and it expands your universe.

I do think that the high-frequency vibration of the company—fueled by happiness and sheer guts—is our secret to continued success. Raise Your Vibration became a guiding light for me, and by extension, for the company itself. Certainly, it has brought guardian angels who have often dropped into our realm with uncanny timing.

For the first few months, I had just one full-time employee, Claire—a former Prada junior designer whose job it was to jump into my basement and sort and clean the vintage, plus handle the ordering, cataloguing, pricing, and photographing. It was up to me, then, to wear a zillion other hats, from CEO, creative director, and editor in chief on down to trash collector. I oversaw the website's design and implementation, the production of every photo shoot, the interview and writing of every single feature, the selection of every vintage piece, and the lasso-ing of a wild bunch of a dozen or so freelancers.

My London-based editor, Zoe Wolff, bundled and made my words better, and then we hired a full-time copy genius named Meredith, an American with sass in her pants and happiness spilling out of every cell of her skin. After a year in business, we had four full-time employees.

Everyone who launches a start-up struggles with the chaos that inevitably abounds without systems, structure, top-level management trained in the new venture and, of course, without heaps of cash. Andrea and I both plugged modest amounts of our savings into an account to cover overheads, and DoubleJ operated on a dental-floss budget for years. I'll never forget what Andrea told me, in our kitchen where I was working towards my unofficial MBA each night: *"Any business that doesn't become profitable after two years in operation never does."* These words felt prophetic. I did not want my baby to ever feel her stomach rumbling, so I became exceptionally frugal. I pinched every penny spent, and at the same time grew resourceful in finding new ways of doing things cheaply. Having no money forced me to think bigger and create better.

cobblestone streets or in front of its beautiful doorways for free. Nicolas Bellavance Lecomte, now the founder of Nomad design shows, shared his beautiful apartment for our first vintage pop-up shop during the 2015 Salone del Mobile (he showed his design work too, so it was a two-fer).

The limited budget was an ongoing activator for my creativity. In lieu of an expensive fashion show in 2018, we threw a dance party inside Milan's nineteenth-century Galleria.

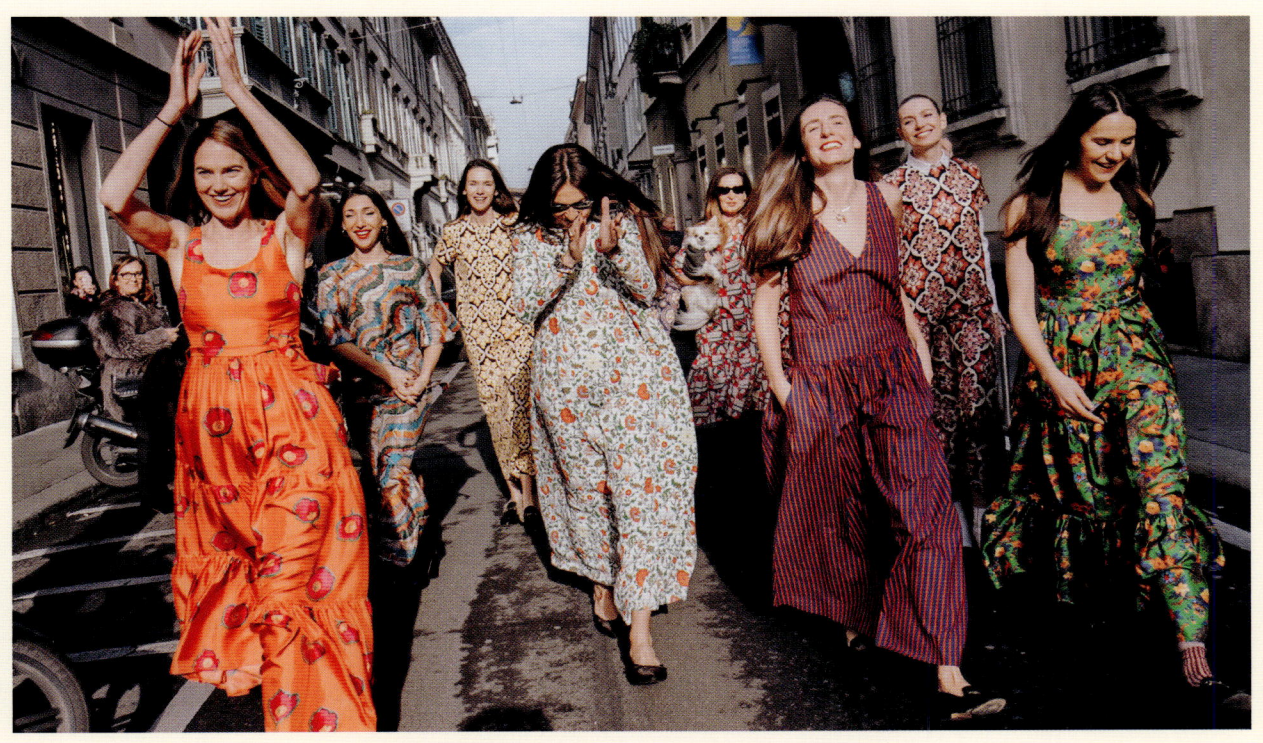

Storming the streets of Milan with our favorite girl gang

We were a lean, mean, happy machine. We may not have had the money for gloss, glamour, or fancy parties, but it turned out we didn't need it.

Andrea loaned us a small office in his Naviglio headquarters (which I papered in a Miu Miu cat print gifted to me years before by Fabio Zambernardi), and the use of a shared space with his other companies. Giulia Molteni gave us two used white Molteni office tables to work on.

For the e-comm photo shoots, we skipped hiring hair and makeup stylists and expensive models, instead using illustrated faces drawn by Liselotte Watkins, a Swedish artist who I'd met at Cucchi. We applied the faces like stickers onto the bodies of cheaper models, shot on Milan's

Who knew you could nab a public space in Milan for free as long as you had the patience to fill out the paperwork? Joy became the fuel of the business and our creativity, in turn allowing the company to keep spinning and expanding on its axis. I never once thought about making a big profit. I just hoped we could pay everyone enough to keep DoubleJ doing her unique backflips. This is what propelled me forward—what she needed in order to do her very best.

In this way, I was feeling very motherly. I was finally following my instincts completely. My gut and heart told me what to do. I acted out of love—love for her, for her potential, and her unique energetic imprint.

By year two, we were turning a 300-euro profit. We made it.

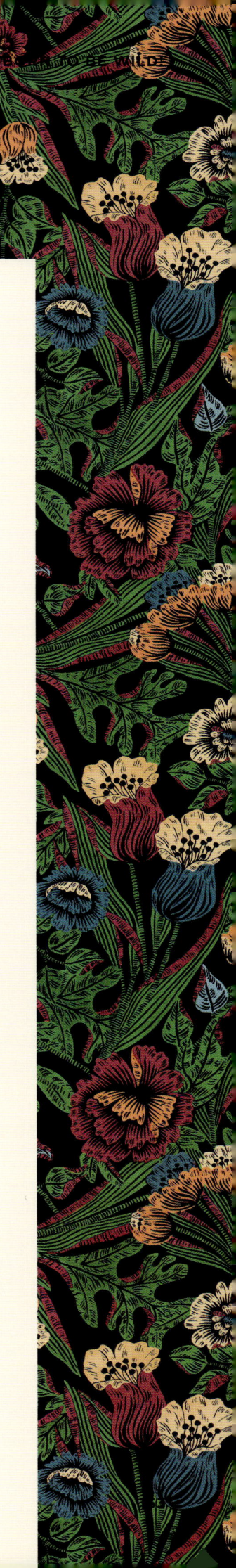

HAVE NO MONEY FOR MODELS?

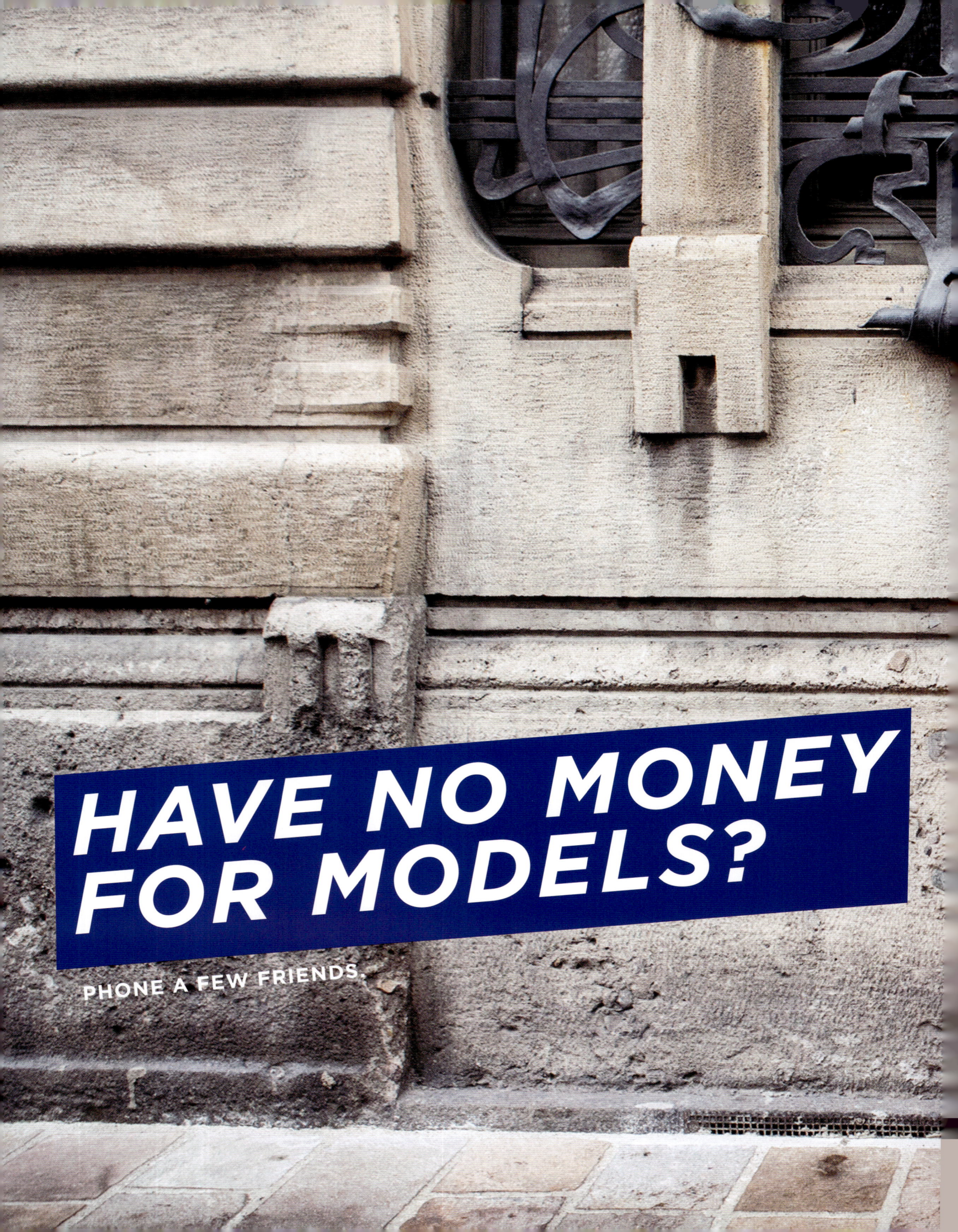

PHONE A FEW FRIENDS.

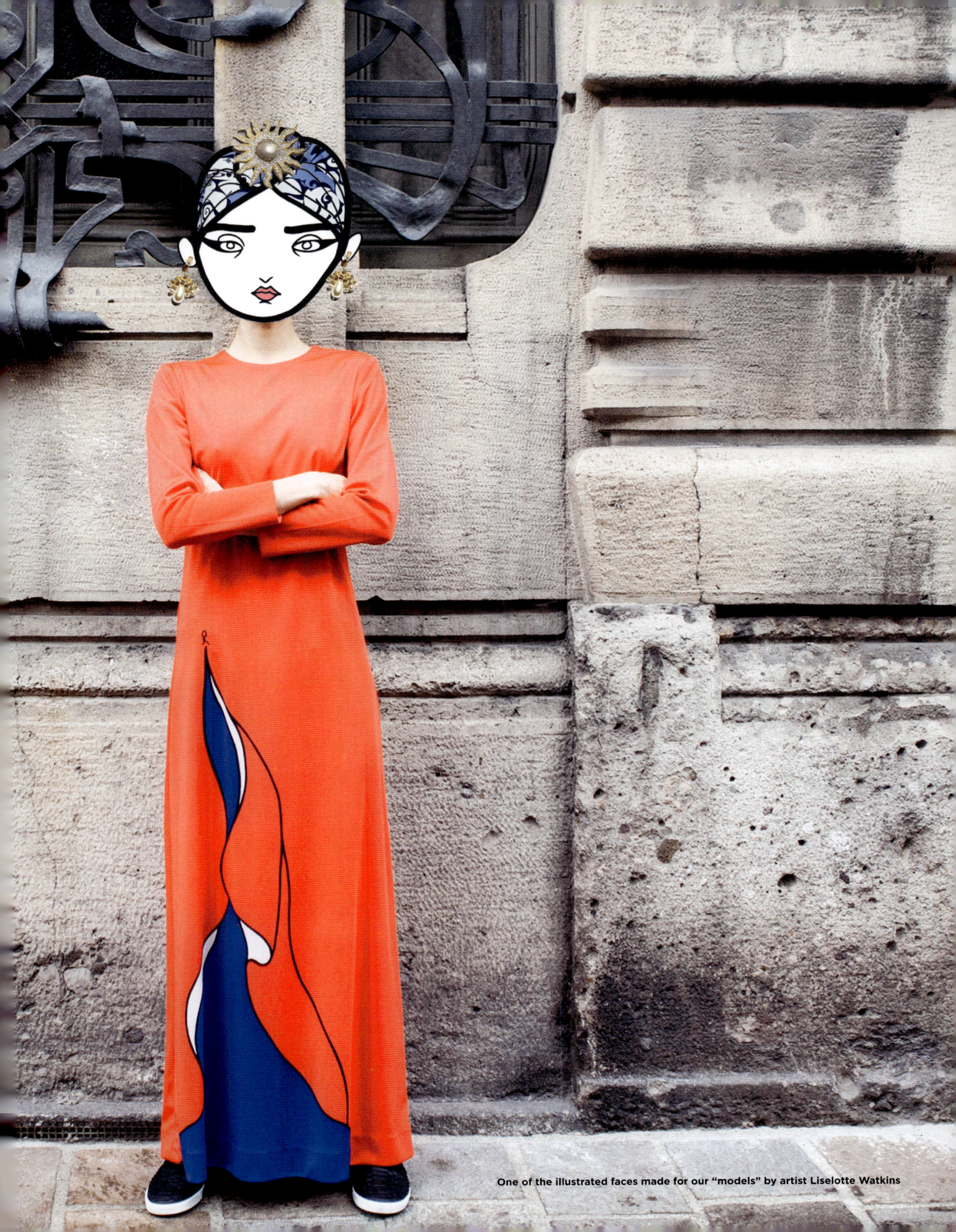

One of the illustrated faces made for our "models" by artist Liselotte Watkins

MAMMA MILANO

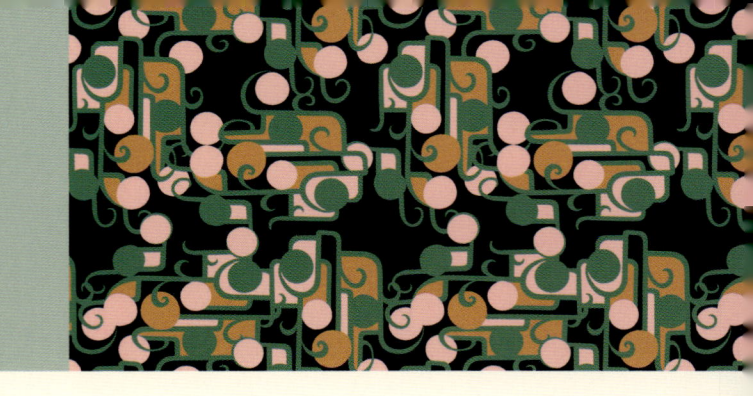

GREAT GORGEOUS GIRLS

From the beginning, we used the real creative women of Milan as our models, not only to sell our collection of clothing but to offer a glimpse into the lives of those I had met and loved, but didn't have a chance to write about in the big magazines. I jumped into the ateliers, showrooms, offices, and homes of architects, photographers, fashion designers, and stylists—all of whom we christened our "Great Gorgeous Girls."

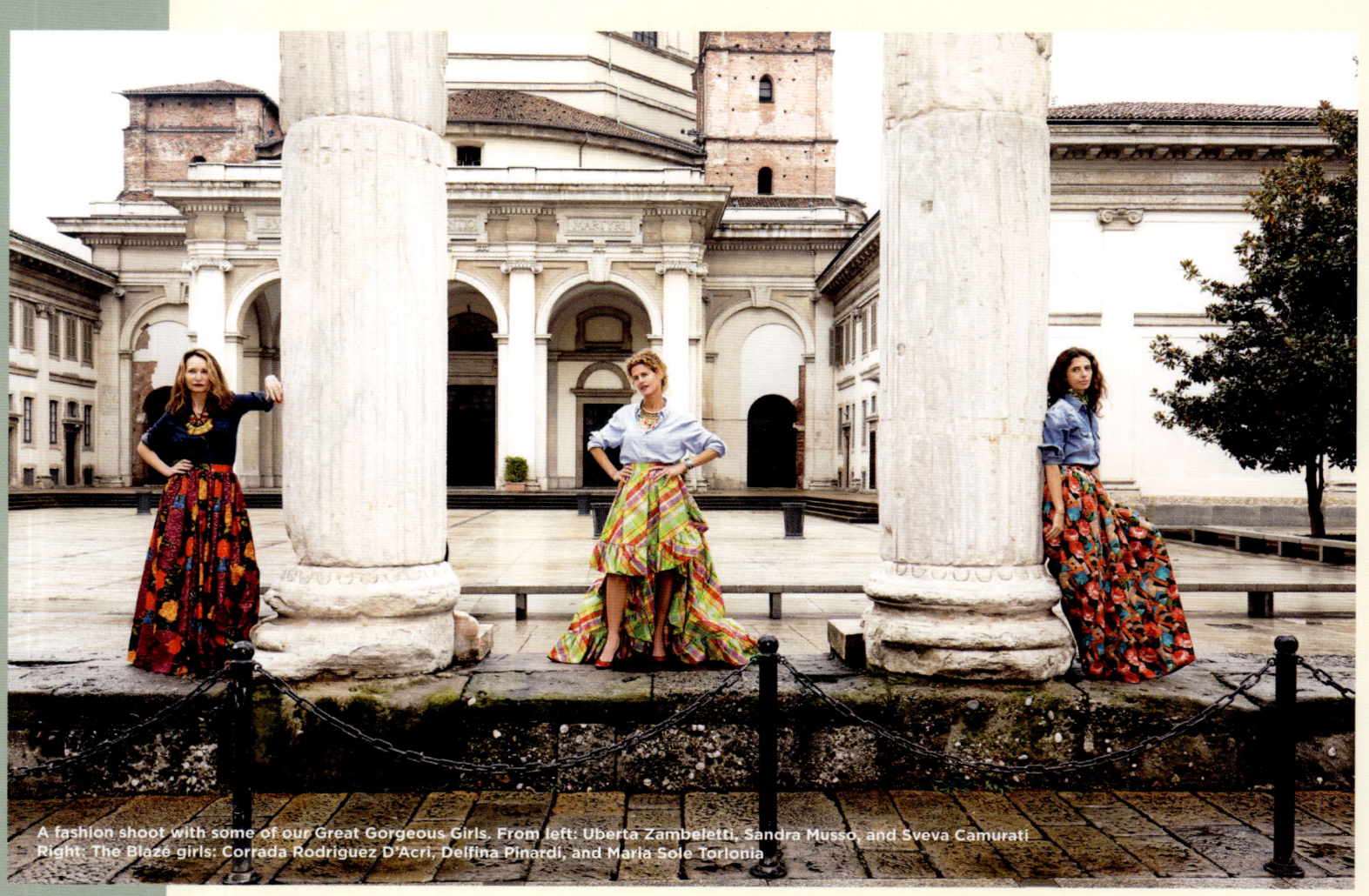

A fashion shoot with some of our Great Gorgeous Girls. From left: Uberta Zambeletti, Sandra Musso, and Sveva Camurati
Right: The Blaze girls: Corrada Rodriguez D'Acri, Delfina Pinardi, and Maria Sole Torlonia

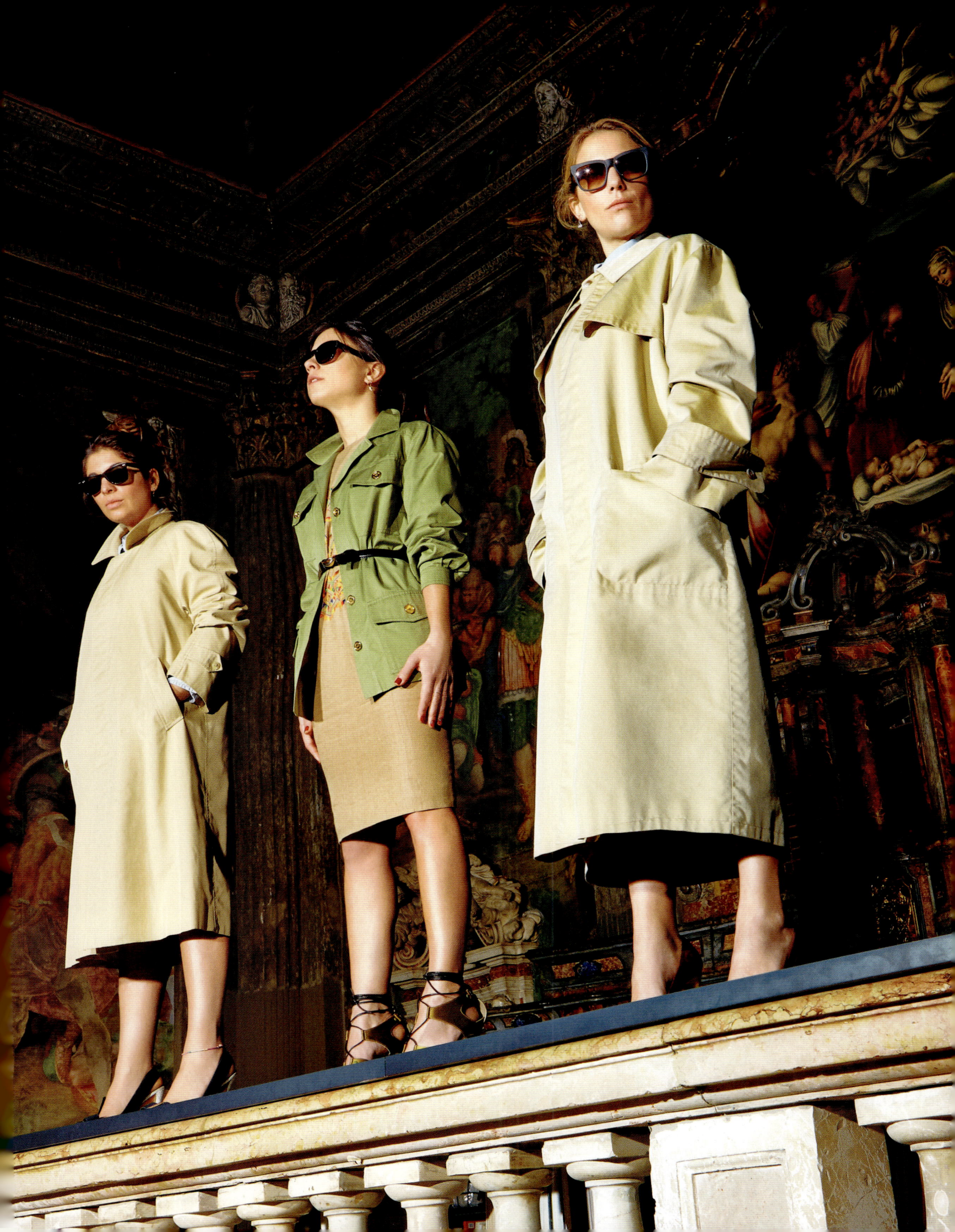

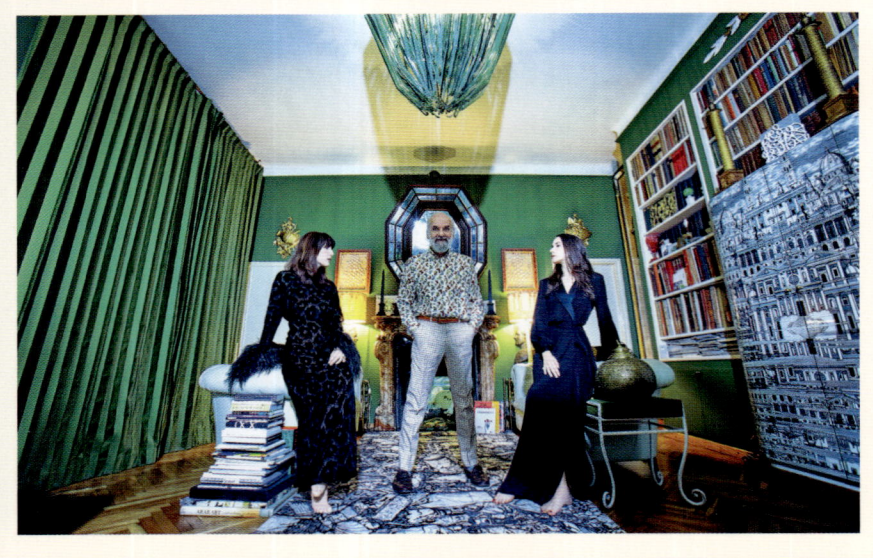

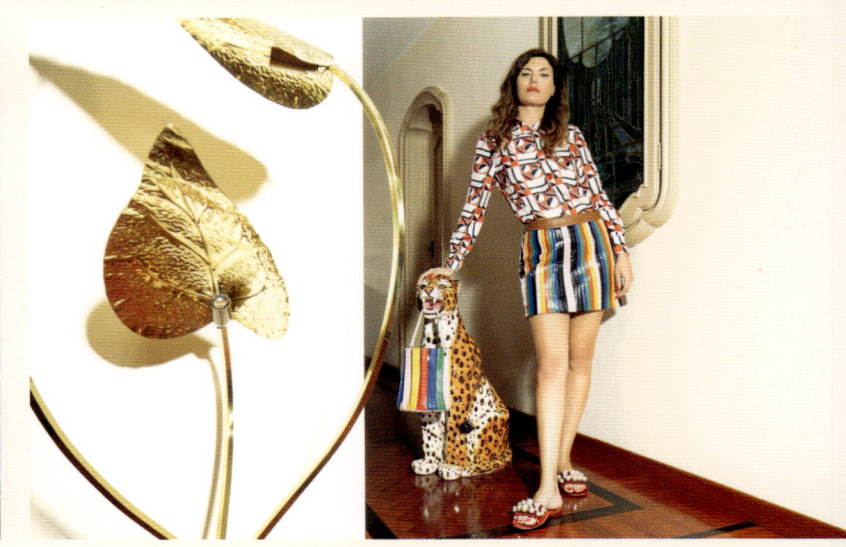

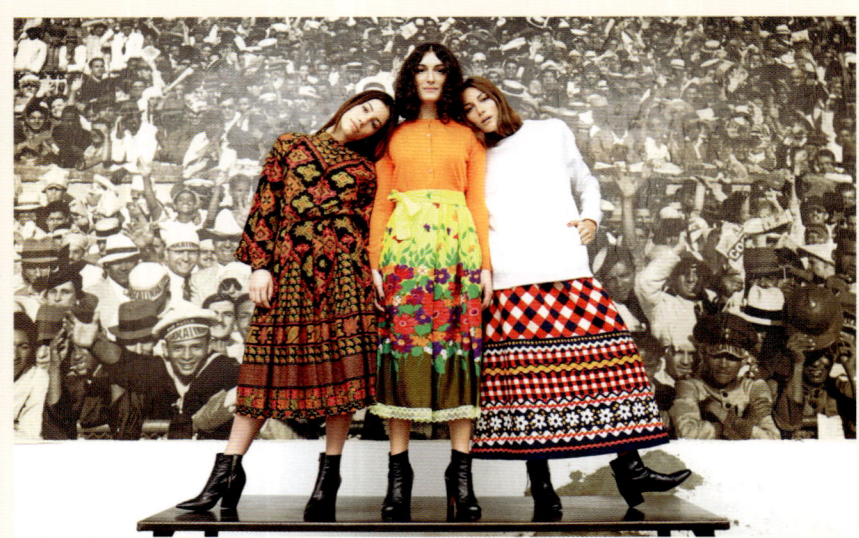

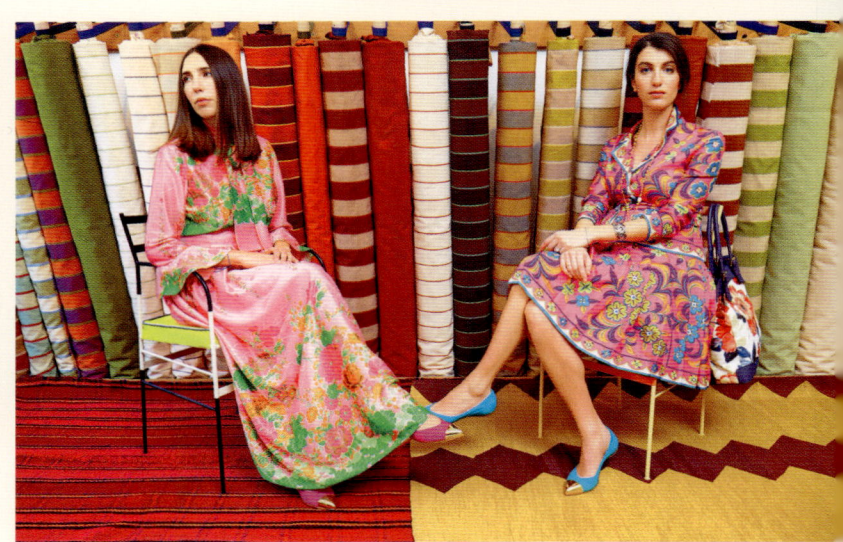

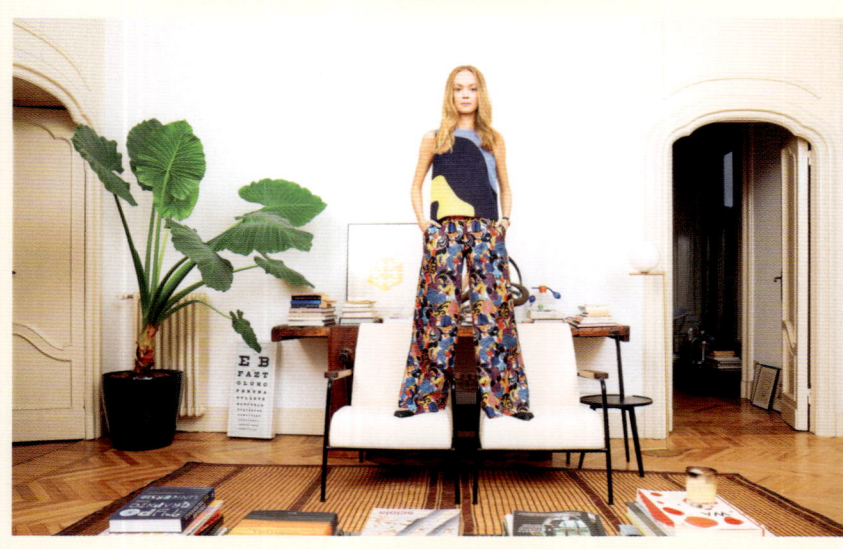

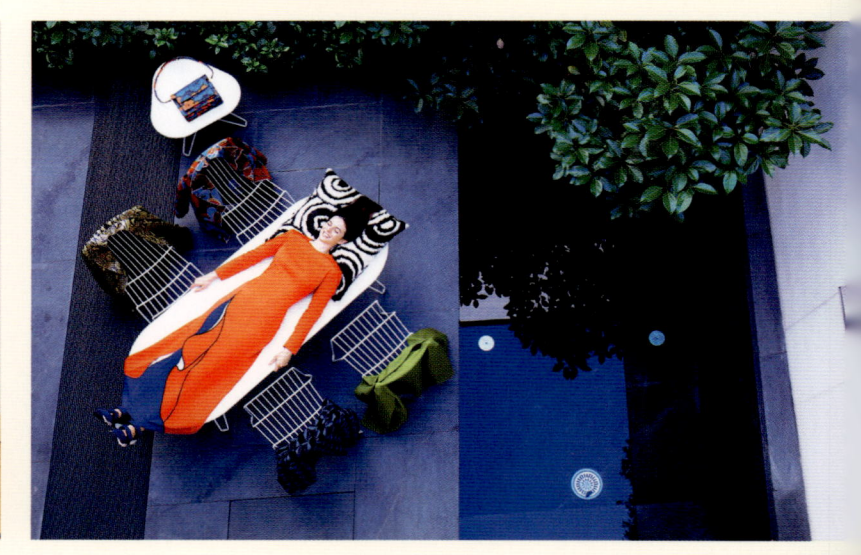

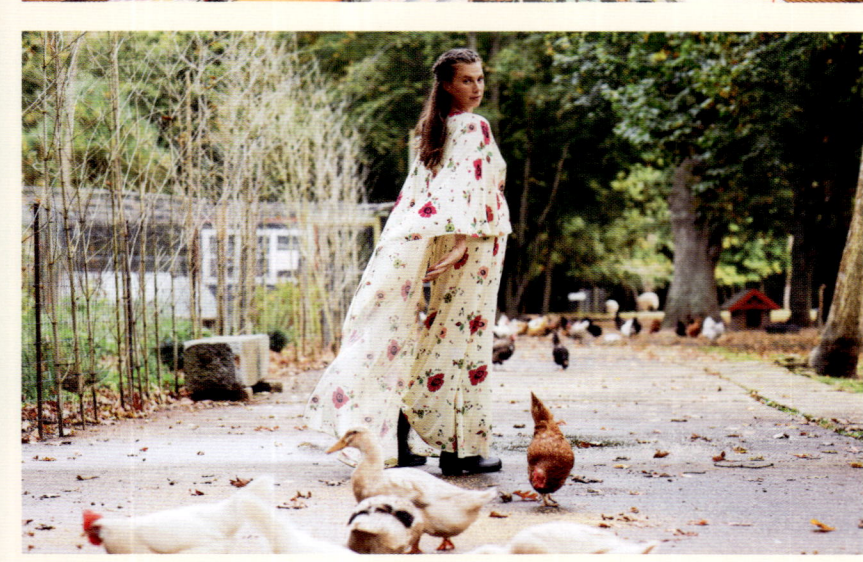

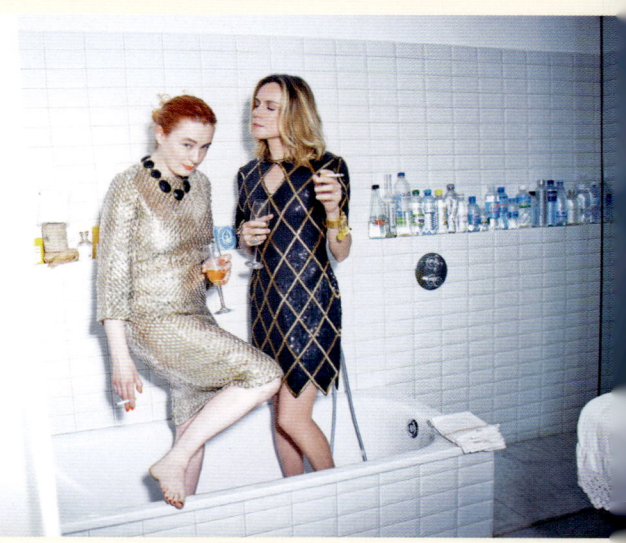

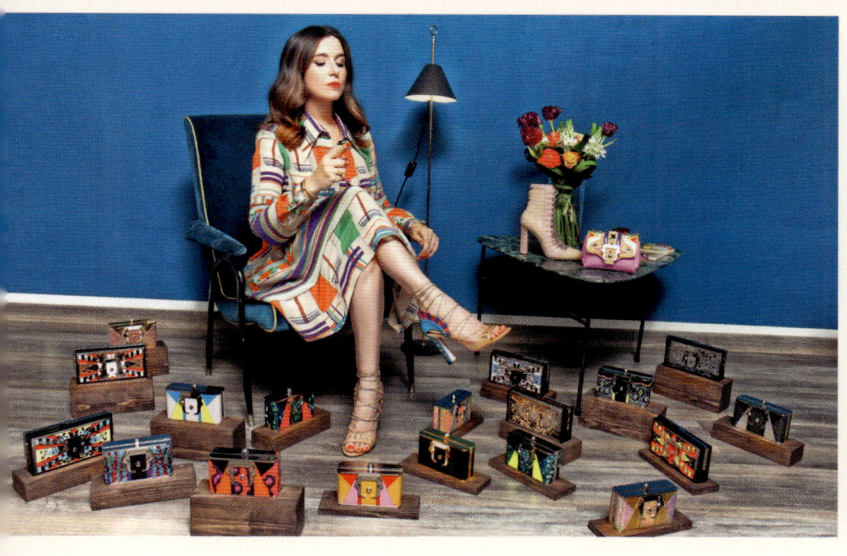

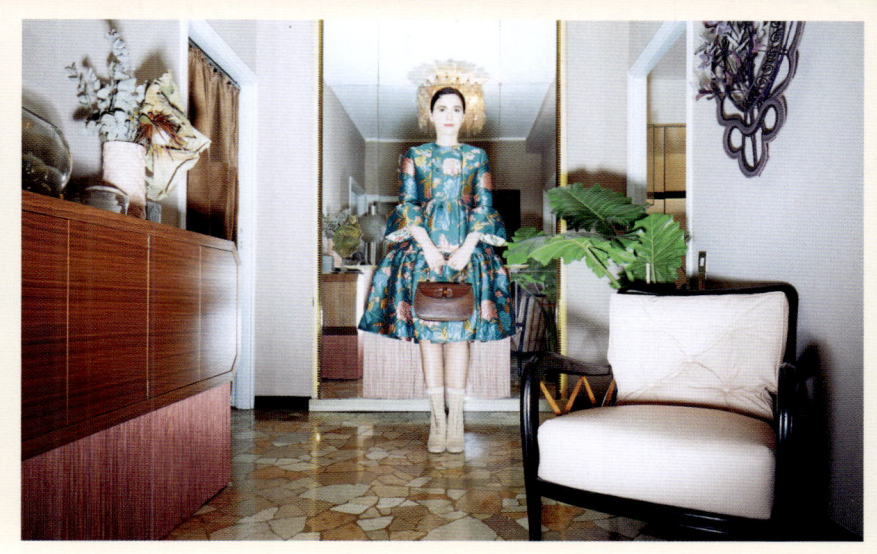

MORE GREAT GORGEOUS GIRLS *

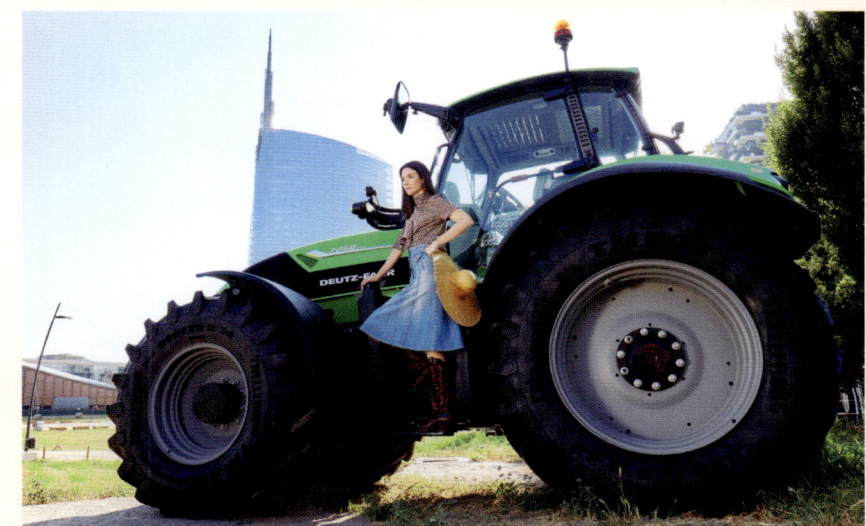

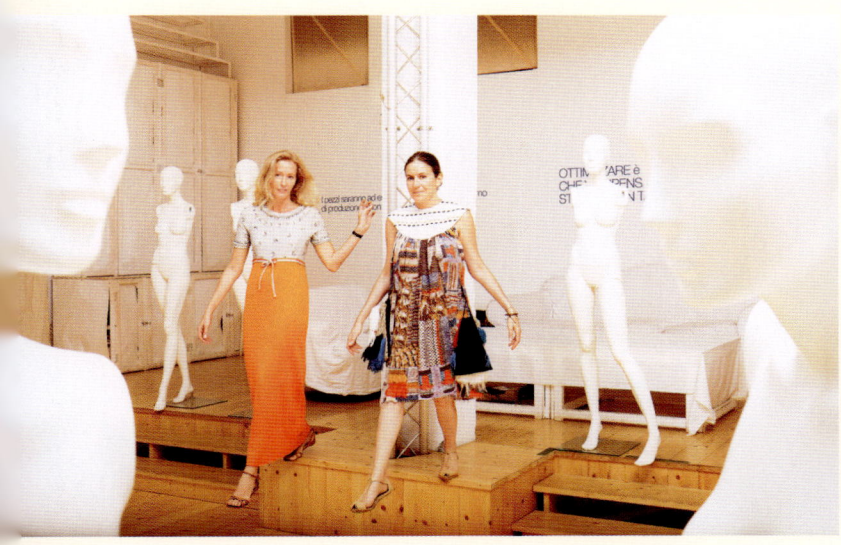

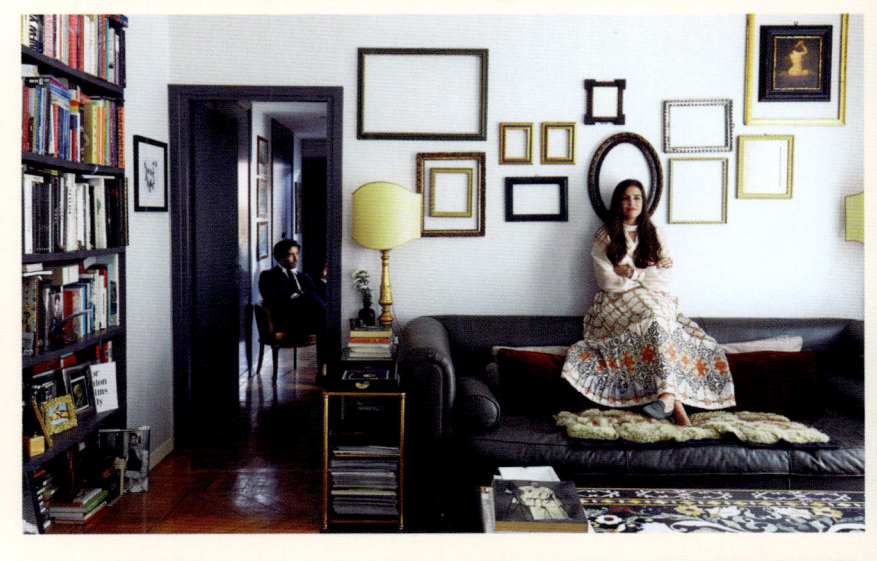

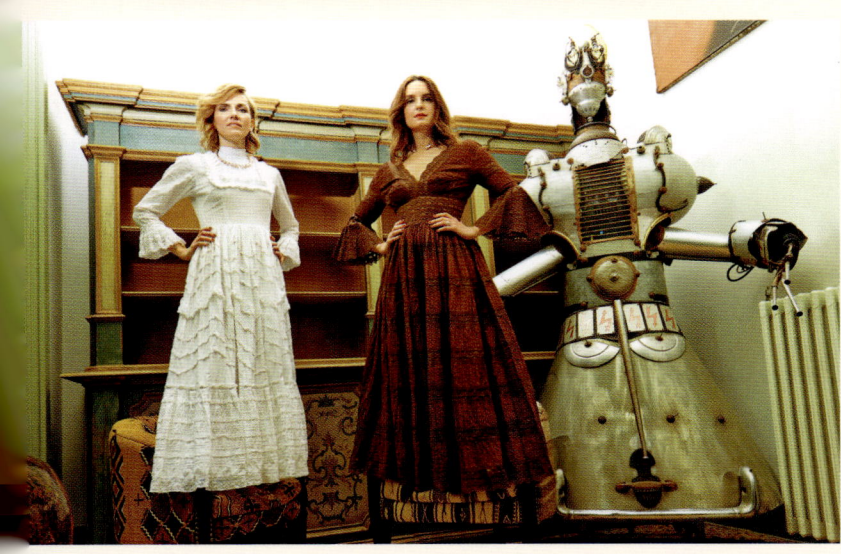

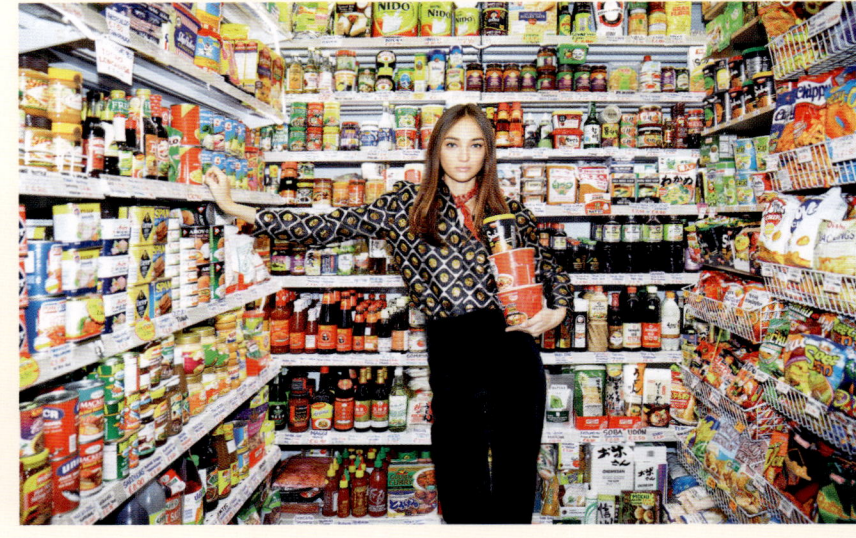

MARINA MILANO

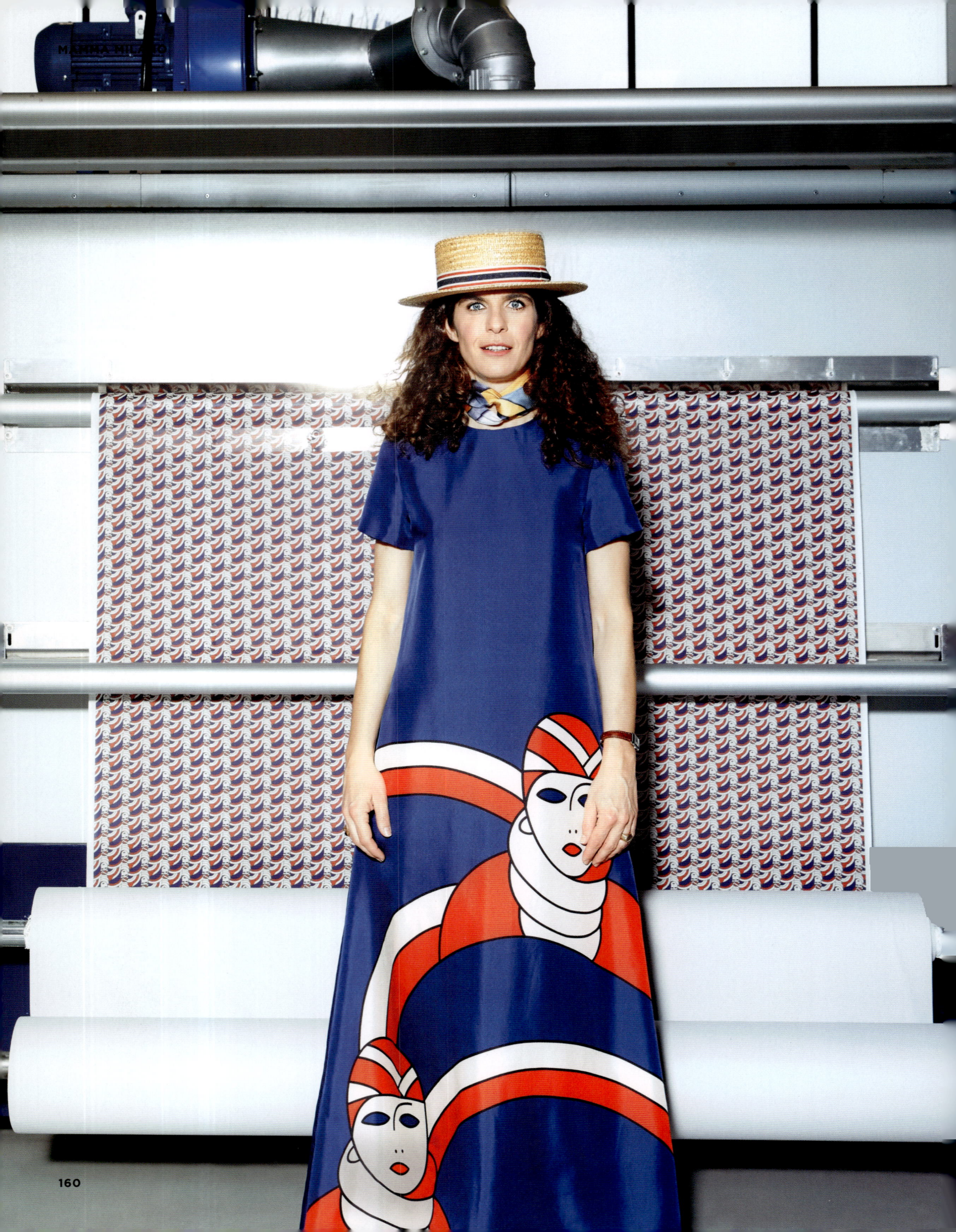

SEED #2

LET'S MAKE NEW CLOTHES!

I began by thinking that La DoubleJ could possibly become the Net-a-Porter of vintage. Guess what? No.

After one year, my lovingly collected mountain of prized antique pieces was nearly gone, and the procurement and sizing of actual vintage (twenty years or older) was just exhausting. If we landed a Holy Grail garment, we only had one to sell. Scaling was impossible. So, we had to shift and find another doorway to flow through.

Andrea would occasionally drop down to the DoubleJ playroom to get a joy kick in his otherwise heavy day. One day, as I lamented our vintage replenishment problem, he said, *"Why don't you make a new dress using vintage prints?"* Then he turned on his heel and left.

In this way, Andrea came to function as something of a trickster-farmer in my life. He would whisper something juicy into my ear, hand me the seeds, convince me to plant them, and then laugh and walk away as I was left to grow, harvest, and heave the whole darn thing on my shoulders up a hill. Everyone, I later realized, should have a trickster-farmer in their business. It's very helpful. Of course, he always showed up when things started to grow and move, which is what quickly happened. Soon enough, this seed of an idea was blowing up in my inner hothouse.

We called the Mantero family, one of Como's oldest and most prestigious silk makers, for whom Andrea had consulted years earlier. After several plates of *vitello tonnato* at their lake-view home in Como, we had a deal: I would fish out eight patterns from their archives, reprint them on new buttery silk twill, and create a brand-new dress style.

Though they'd been servicing fashion's top designers and luxury brands for 120 years, no one outside of the fashion manufacturing world had heard of Mantero. My journalist's mind whirred: why don't we put their name in our label, shine the light on these incredible craftspeople, and show the world why Italy makes the best products on earth?

CEO Franco Mantero and his sister, Lucia, loved this. In the early years, I spent days in their enormous archives, flipping through huge old books of fabric swatches and illustrations to find patterns that struck me. We started out puny with Mantero helping us on our dress production because we had no contacts or experience. Through this original seal of Italian friendship, we have since grown to become one of their biggest (and, I might add, proudest!) clients for their luxurious, Italian-made fabrics.

This partnership with Mantero became the genesis for all of La DoubleJ's future collaborations with historic Italian manufacturers, who we could also support and promote. We were loud and proud of Italy, with no plans to outsource anything to other countries. We jumped into our partner's archives, plucked the very best, and came back with it wrapped up in our DoubleJ jazz hands.

At her family's factory in Como, Lucia Mantero stands in front of actual reams of DoubleJ fabric being manufactured, wearing an early Swing Dress in our Faccine print.

MAMMA MILANO

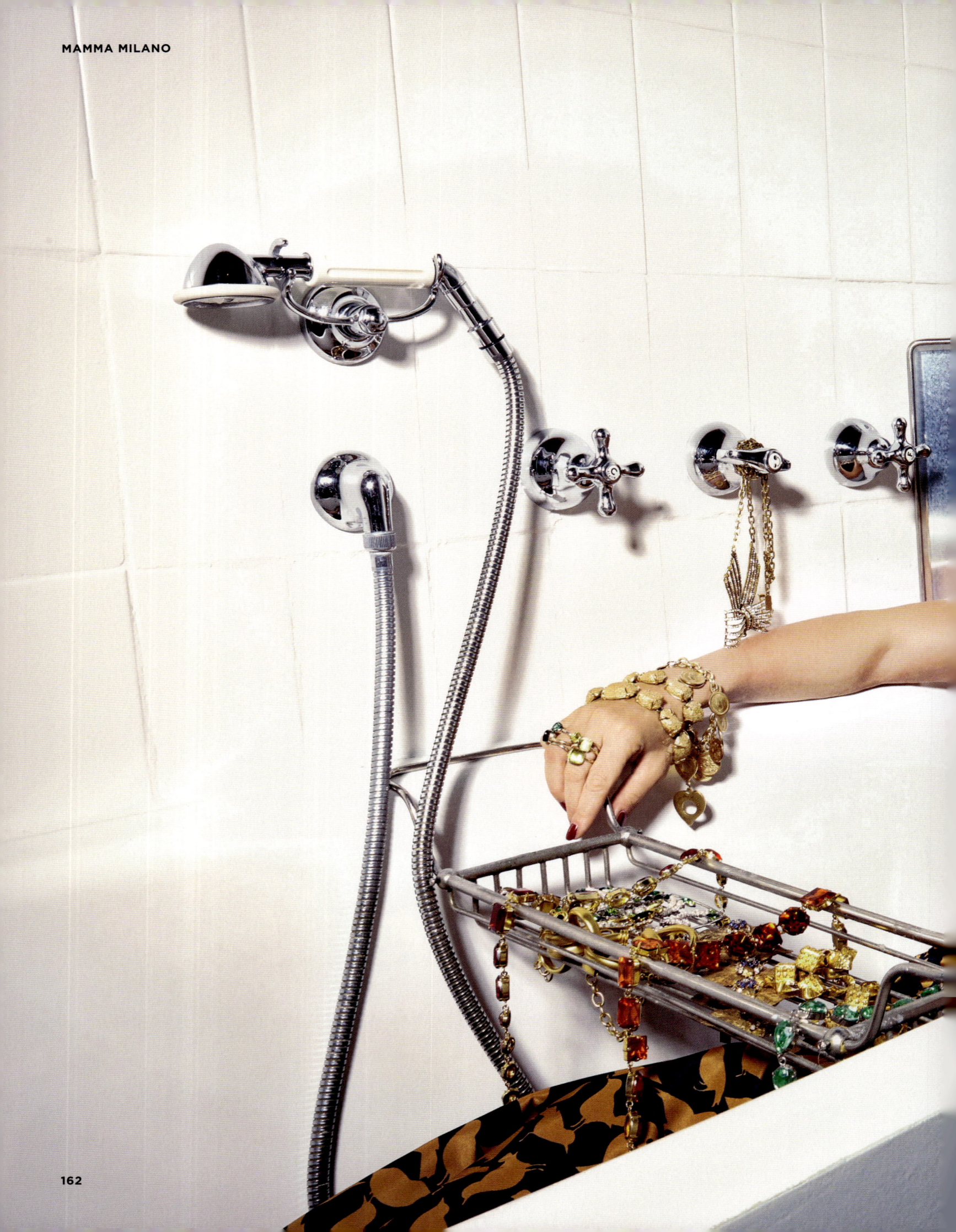

BORN TO BE WILD!

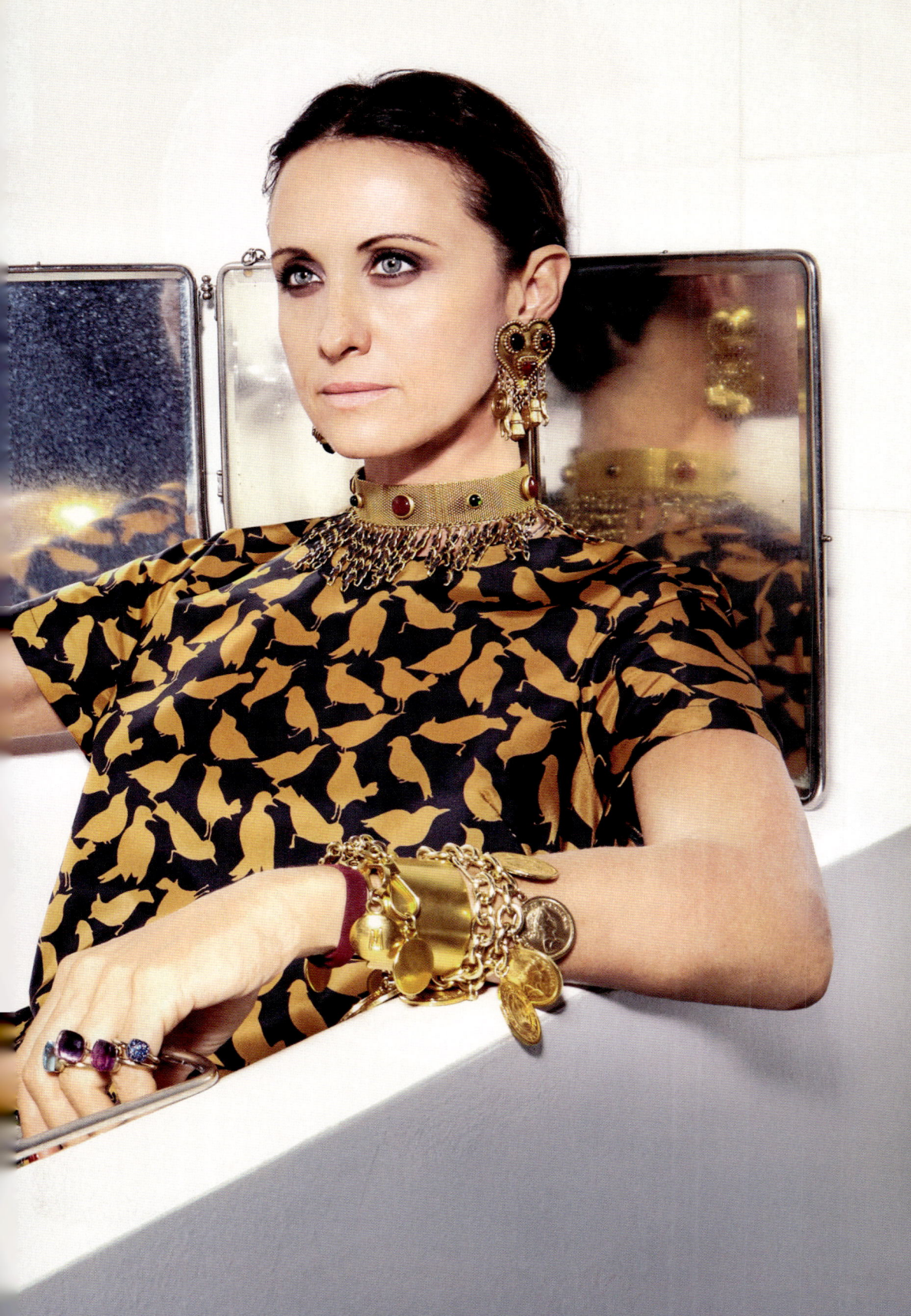

Fashion designer Alessandra Facchinetti in her bathtub in Milan, wearing one of our first new dresses with our vintage jewelry

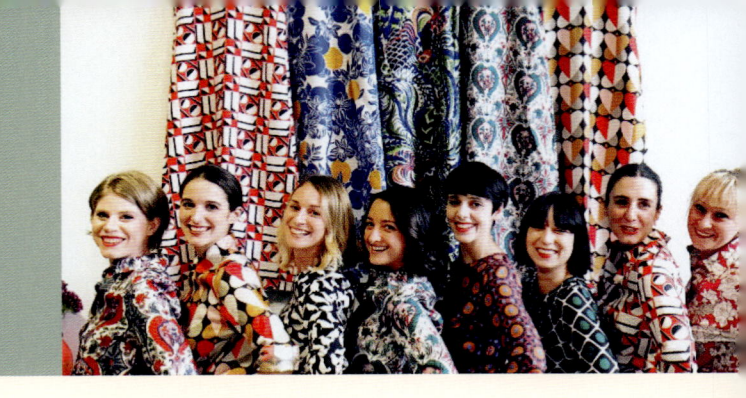

INTO THE SWING

The Swing Dress was our first dress and continues to be our bestseller. The base of it was hanging in my vintage collection. Viviana looked at it one day and announced, "This is the perfect shape!" We made a few tweaks to the shoulder cut, reduced the hip volume, added pockets, and had it printed, cut, sewn, and packed up at Mantero.

Featured in *WSJ*'s "Off Duty" and exclusive to MatchesFashion and our website, it was an instant hit because it was a multi-purpose product. You could fold it down to a handkerchief and easily pack it any bag; it fitted most body types, and could go from morning to noon to night—and from summer to winter by layering it with a thick sweater or coat. It could be worn just as easily with tennis shoes and flip-flops as with high heels and jewels; with make-up or thrown on just out of the shower.

I didn't think of it at the time, but that dress truly symbolized our entire company ethos: comfort, ease, joy, versatility, and something that makes a lot of women of different shapes look fantastic. From this point onward, this was the lens through which we made all of our products.

GODPARENT #2 SWOOPS IN

Our beloved Swing Dress made her debut during Milan Fashion Week 2016 at a small jazz club that doubled as a flower shop. A month earlier, I had called Ruth Chapman, the owner of MatchesFashion—who I'd met a few times during my journalist years—letting her know I had one humble dress in eight vintage prints that was about to birth. Was she interested?

Ruth said yes to launching the dress exclusively on her website and hosting our little party. She was yet another one of La DoubleJ's fairy godmothers. Not only did she jump unreservedly into our new product launch, but she also kept calling me and asking me what was next.

"You mean I can't just keep doing one dress?" I naively asked. "No, you cannot, I need newness every couple of months." Ruth kicked me in the production pants.

The first year, we created a total of six new silhouettes in twenty-five different prints, with no designer, no in-house product development, no factory, and no sales team. I'll never forget when I had to get on the phone and actually negotiate our markups with a retailer, not even knowing what that meant. But glittery wholesalers came to us nonetheless—Bergdorf Goodman, The Webster, Kirna Zabête, Capitol, and Le Bon Marché. All fantastic retailers who believed in small brands with big hearts.

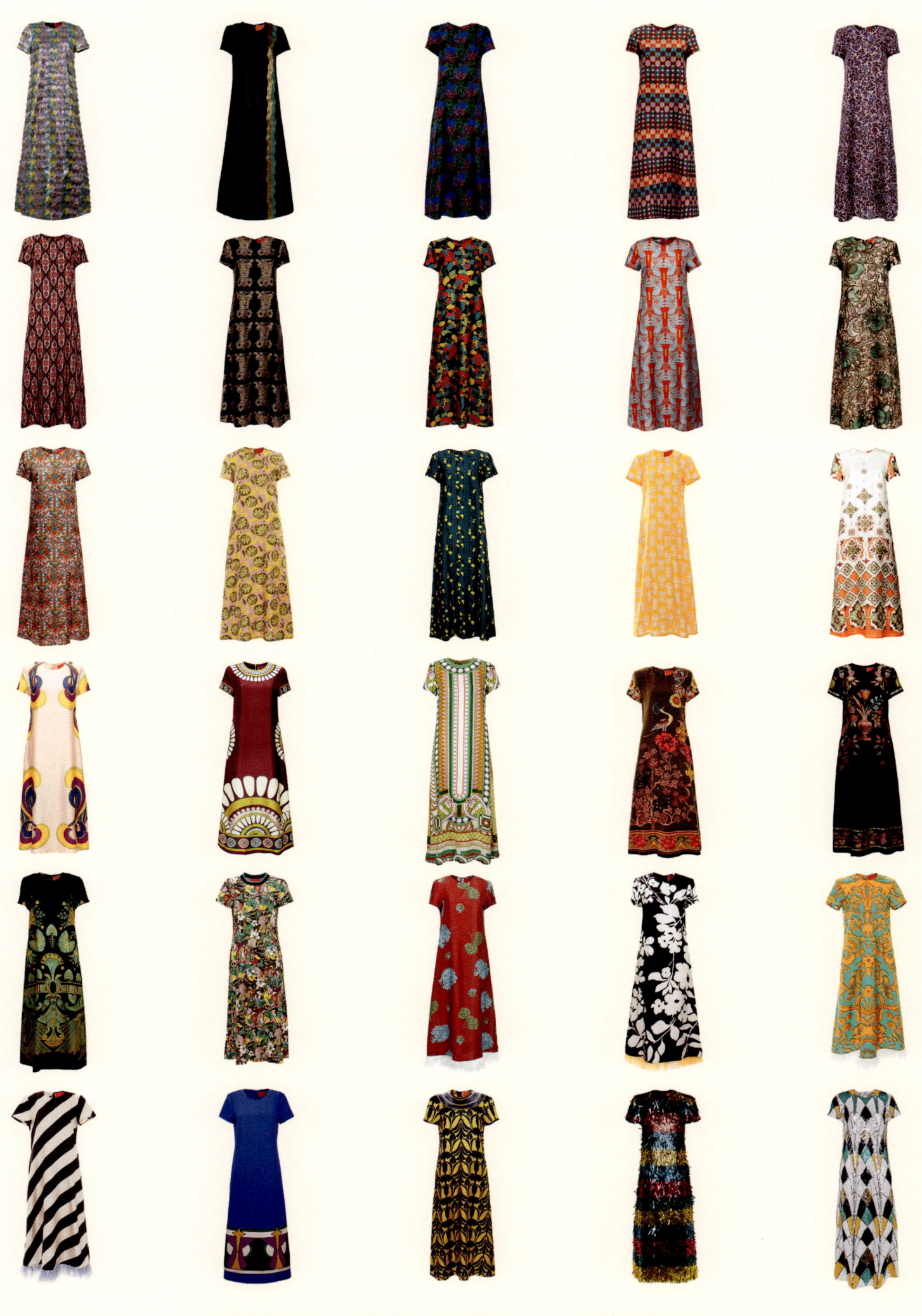

Our first and continuously bestselling model, the Swing Dress, fits absolutely everybody
Opposite, top: Beloved members of the early LDJ team

MAMMA MILANO

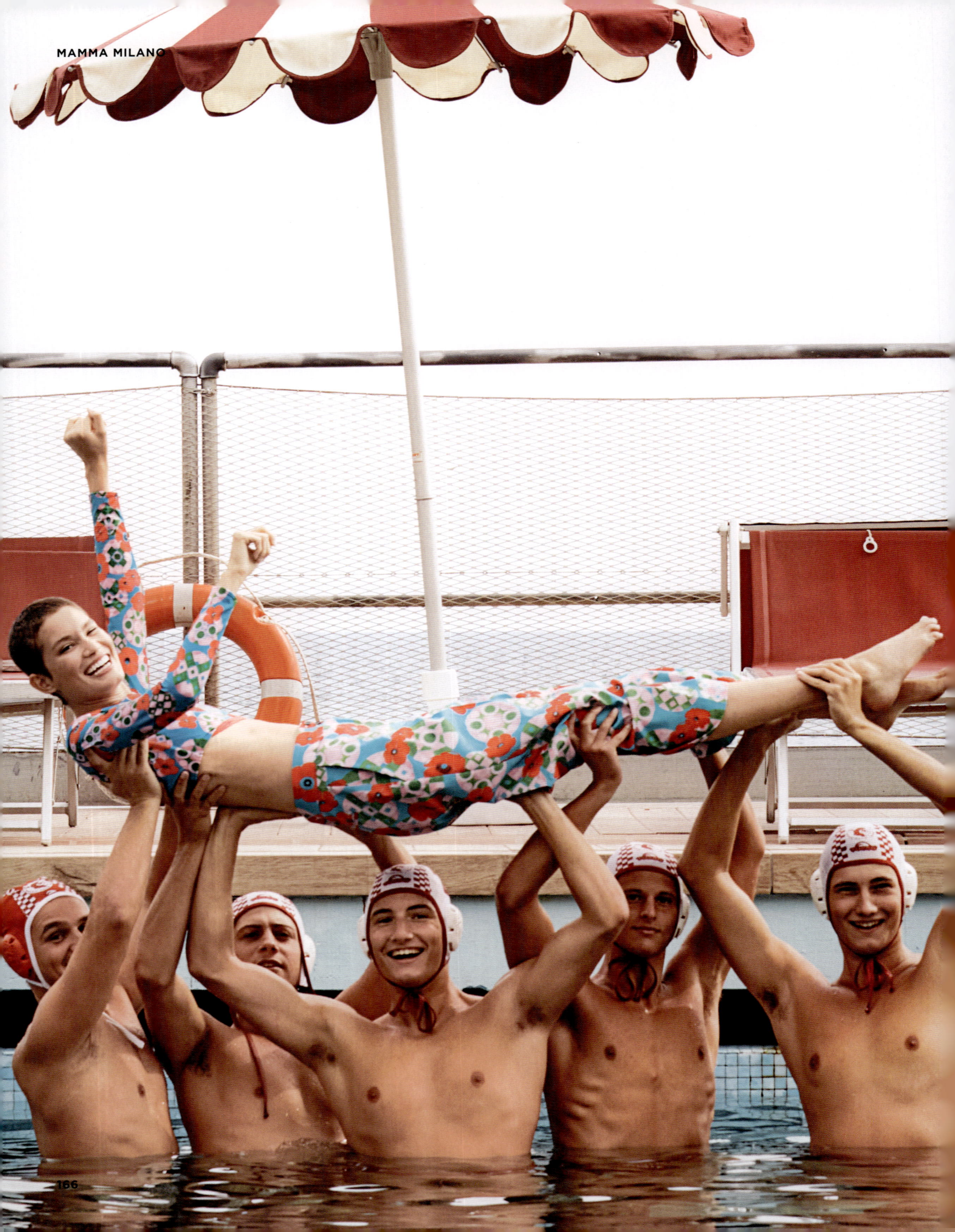

BRINGING UP BABY

La DoubleJ works because she's a living entity. I really did (and continue to) treat the company like a baby, a child conceived from two parents—Andrea and I—who were not able to have real children, but were able to merge our DNA into an entrepreneurial embryo. She came out screaming and continued to be sassy, needy, mouthy, and full of energy. I just ran after her as I would any shrieking toddler at the park. I also spoke to her and asked her frequently what she wanted. It felt very natural. And I felt incredibly protective and nurturing of this babe.

The employees all felt like sisters or midwives, and I felt their collective experience. It was always me hollering when the energy was off-balance and we were about to drown. Like any good mother, I set the tone. I decided the rules, the game plan, what we were wearing, and when everyone was going to go to bed at night. The calmer and more trusting I was, the calmer and more trusting my team was. The minute I got swallowed by my own fearful thoughts, it would amplify outwards to the whole team, burning them up in my own discomfort.

A positive mindset has been fundamental to this journey of birthing. I'm a radical seer and truth-teller. I see every problem, pitfall, blockage, and bag of density held by others. I am the first to see it, and want to fix it.

This must be done with patience and kindness—qualities at which the Italians excel, and which still give me difficulty. It also helps to have a few friends.

It was also important, once we got our wheels turning, to scratch the backs of all those who had helped glide us along in the early days. Fair energetic exchange is key in work relationships. Sometimes the exchange is monetary, but not necessarily: the most important thing—especially for Italians—is that they feel seen and recognized. I found that I could be just as generous with many of the people who had helped me out in the early days by making connections, referrals, gifts, and phone calls to the right people on their behalf. It was also extraordinarily important to let all our friends and partners know how much our success was due to their efforts, friendship, and generosity.

THEN IN FLEW A FEW GUARDIAN ANGELS

La DoubleJ was a magnetic baby. She attracted her caretakers and fairy godmothers the minute she ventured out into the world. She literally pulled people to her. Here are a few of these heavenly helpers, to whom I remain forever indebted.

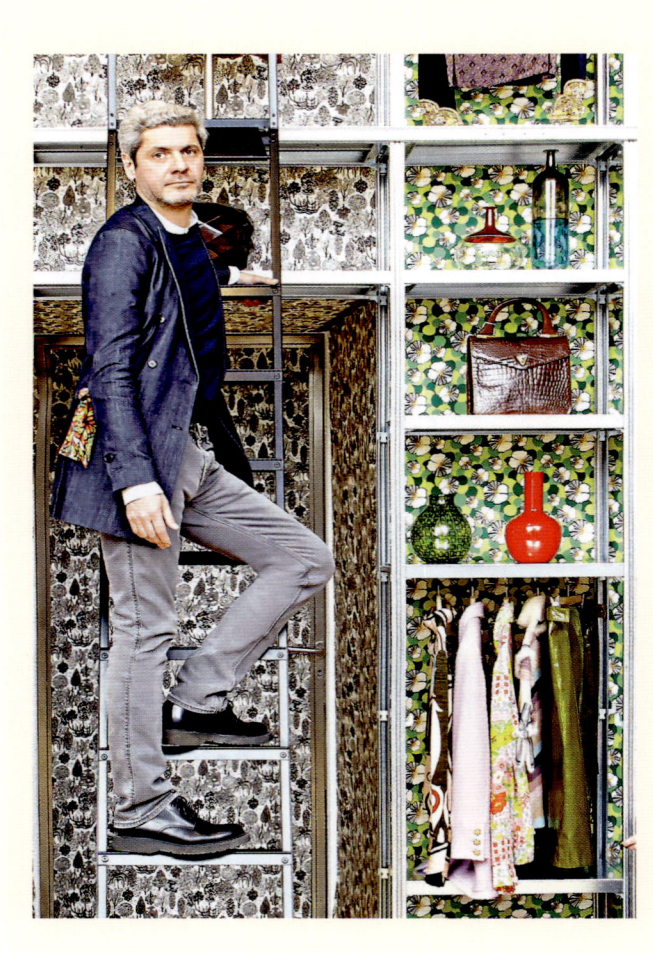

LUCA CIPELETTI

Luca Cipeletti is a talented architect and friend, whose studio was across the street from our office. He was also *completely* minimalist in his tastes. He came into our print-clashing world laughing and covering his eyes, until one day he agreed to design a magical container for our showroom that could tame the color chaos with some of his divine masculine restraint.

He called it the Wunderwall: a sensational permanent installation that ran the length of our office space featuring print-backed cubes in affordable aluminum that served as a cabinet of curiosities, as well as a space divider and dressing room. I filled it with vintage design items I had in my garage, our new and vintage clothes, as well as hand-painted pottery by Liselotte Watkins.

Later, Luca also helped me tremendously when we found our first shop in Milan, setting me up with the right contractors and helping us order and divide the space into coherent beauty.

LISELOTTE WATKINS

I met the talented Swedish artist Liselotte Watkins at—no surprise—Cucchi. She always sat with a cool Swedish crowd of creative types, and we became fast friends.

When I started the company, she was the first to pitch in. The illustrated faces that we used to cover the models' own were all hand-drawn by her, as well as the dial-a-designer illustrations of me with Giorgio Armani, Peter Dundas, etc. Liselotte was always a good-luck charm; the pottery designs she created and displayed on our Wunderwall debut were covered by the *New York Times*; she was featured as an early Great Gorgeous Girl; and she made our bed linen collection sing inside her own Milan apartment.

She has been a dear friend and fellow expat in Italy for almost two decades.

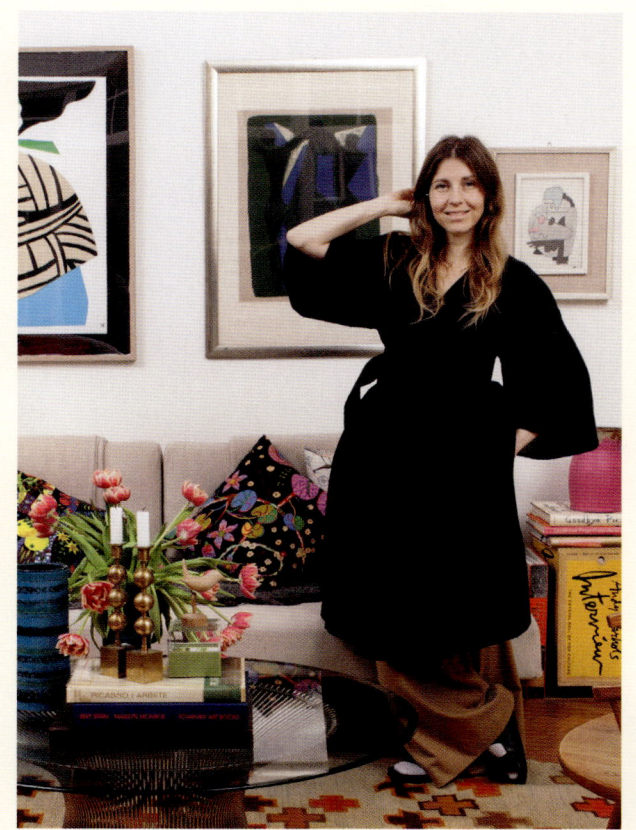

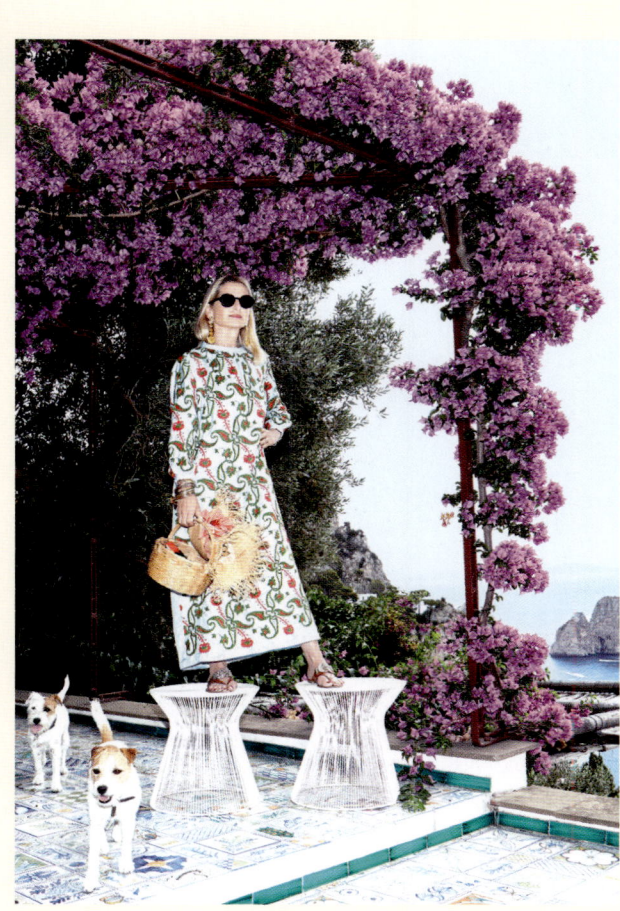

SUSANNE THUN

Susanne is an Austrian-born, Italian-based former fashion stylist and current creative muse to her architect husband, Matteo. Her personal style would give both Miuccia Prada and Manuela Pavesi a run for their money, and she could both decorate homes and entertain giant groups of people blindfolded while commanding a fleet of staff. She is a sensational creator, manager, and organizer.

This super-sophisticated woman, raised in the echelons of Milanese taste for forty years, became one of the biggest cheerleaders for me personally and for the brand. She has let us do photo shoots at her home, hosted cocktail parties for us, and invited me countless times to her magical homes in St. Moritz and Capri. She was and still is picky as hell and opinionated about everything. She would swoop into our messy, cramped offices, critique whatever collection was in progress, and then when she was done with her speech, shop like mad. She is a big sister to me and one of the company's fiercest, most protective guardian angels.

MAMMA MILANO

ANTONELLA SOLARI

Most new fashion labels struggle to get a factory on board to produce their clothes. No one wants to mess with the small-fry designers who are unreliable, disorganized, and will probably only be producing five pieces of each garment and cancelling the rest. So, it was a bit of a miracle when Antonella arrived on our doorstep in 2017, through a Mantero connection. We went for pizza dinner one night in Milan with Roberto Gigli, another guardian angel (an operations expert at many top Italian luxury brands and a friend of Andrea's, who stepped in to offer friendly consulting advice for our first years in business). When I told Antonella about my vision, she brightened, shrugged, and said, "Hey, why not? This sounds like fun. And if it doesn't work out, it's been such a nice evening together, we'll go out for another pizza." To this day, Antonella is still our primary factory—we have grown from her smallest client to her largest. And we have never gone out for another pizza.

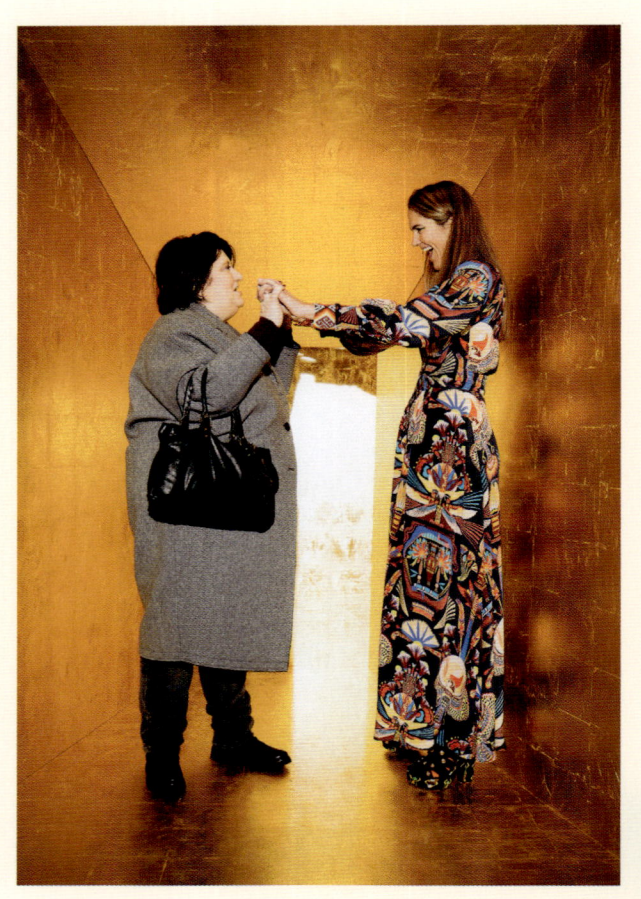

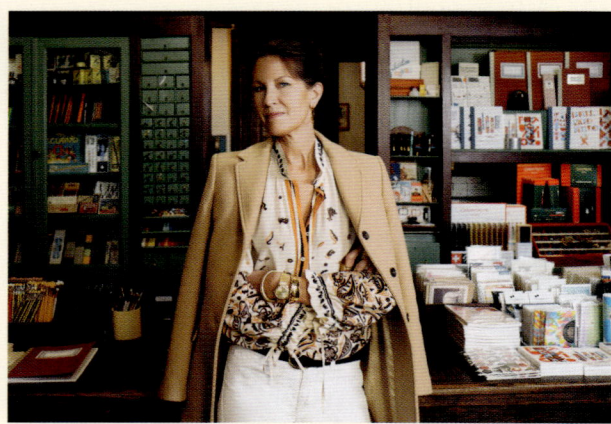

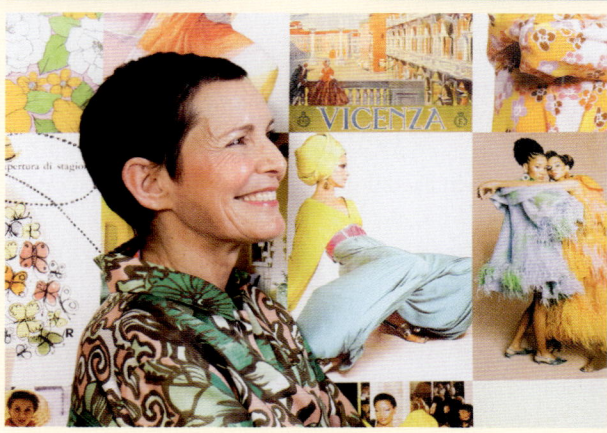

JULIA LEACH

DoubleJ would not have managed its recent wild, upward growth spurt without the wise guidance and stable grounding (in ten-inch heels no less) of magical Julia. After her arrival, Julia became the fiercely protective den woman to our growing creative team of cubs. She is the calm to my crazy, she is the voice of reason, the eye of beauty, and the heart of true kindness. Her imprint on our shops, collaborations, graphics, and takeovers has been sensational.

MAUREEN CHIQUET

When Maureen dropped out of heaven and into our store for the first time, I discovered that not only did we share a mutual love for DoubleJ's print universe, but she was also a deep spirit sister. I was elated when the former CEO of Chanel became Chairwoman of our company in 2023. Maureen's mega-experience in the hard-core world of fashion, mixed with her wise-woman approach to heart-based leadership, is rocket fuel for our brand's rapid ascent, as well as our beautiful friendship.

MARIE-LOUISE SCIÒ

A soul sister on our journey has consistently been Marie-Louise Sciò, the firecracker entrepreneur who runs an armada of glamorous Italian hotels. Marie-Louise is the perfect fusion of America and Italy—an idea exploder, a buzzing people-connector, an epic party thrower, a keen marketer, and a woman who gets things done. She has generously invited us (twice!) for pop-up shops at her beautiful Hotel Il Pellicano in Porto Ercole. She even came to Bergdorf Goodman with us to co-host our pop-up featuring her hotel bar and famous barman, Federico, who flew in for the occasion.

Marie-Louise also invited me to co-host and curate a retreat at her magical Mezzatorre Hotel on the island of Ischia with friends Rudston Steward, who led walking tours, and and Manizeh Rimer, who held yoga classes for a wonderful group of women and DoubleJ supporters, who joined us from around the world. It took place during the launch of a special collection that we designed for her hotels and her website, Issimo.

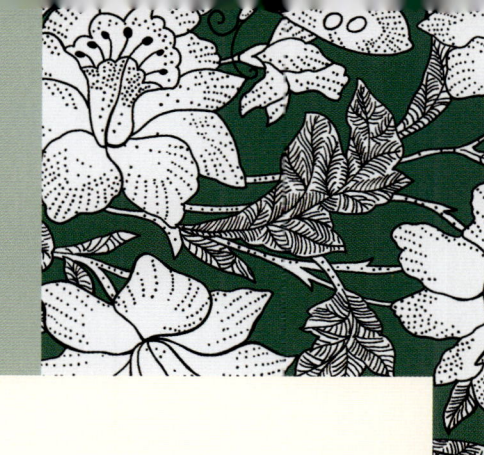

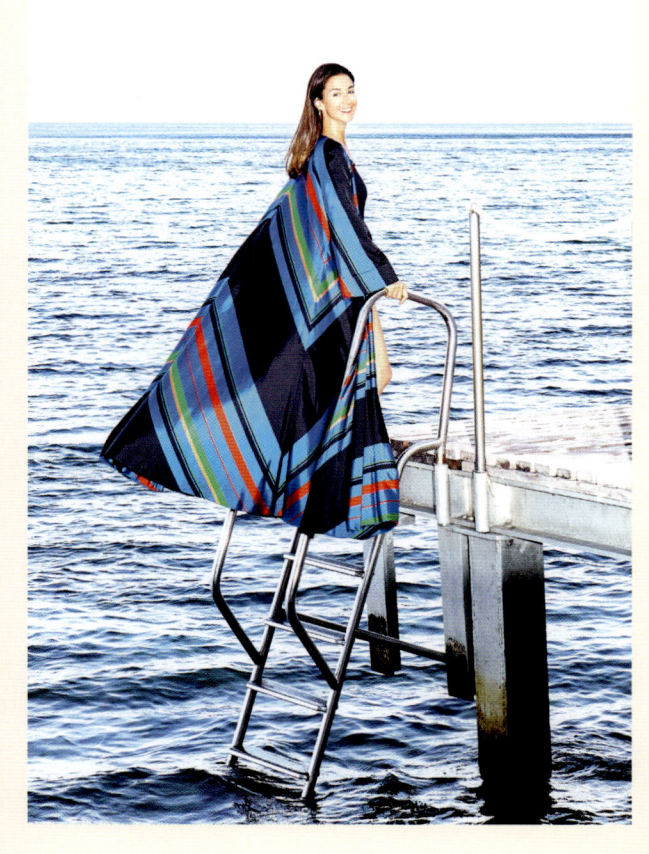

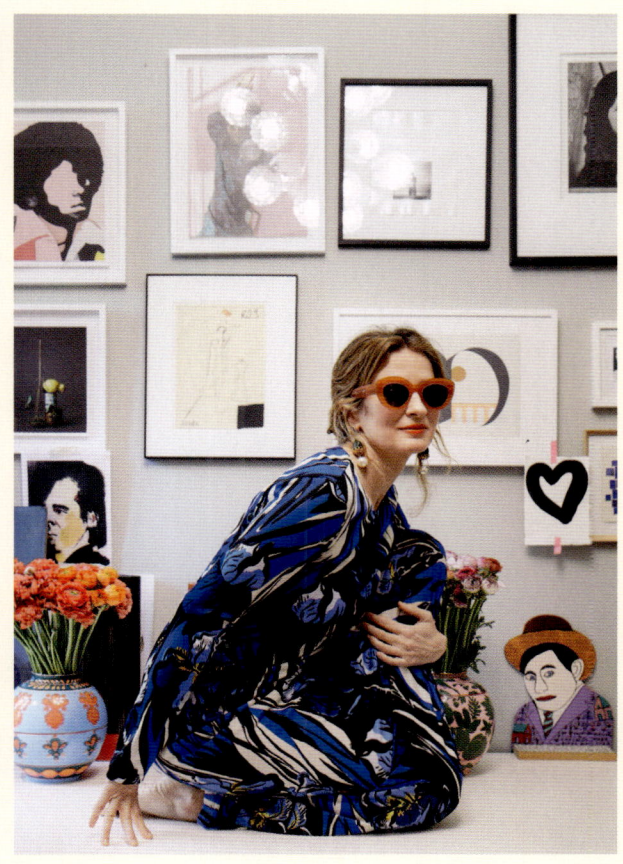

MOLLY MOLLOY

Molly Molloy, who dropped down from heaven onto my design couch directly from Marni, came for a bouncy break from the corporate slog in 2018. She was the first designer we ever had. It seemed preposterous to me that someone from such a heavy-hitting job would consider coming to work at such a puny operation as ours, but the universe has a funny way of lining up. Molly was in a place where she wanted to feel surrounded by family at work; we needed to take our designs to the next level. She came in and did it. We fell in love, became soul sisters, godmothers to each other's dogs, and dreamt about each other frequently. Three years later, when Molly came to tell me she had to leave to go full-time on her own brand Colville, my body lit up into flames. Then I literally looked up to the sky and said: *I trust this is happening for my greatest good and know this is aligned because Molly is my family. So just bring me what I need.* The universe delivered in the form of Jeanne Labib-Lamour, a sassy-pants, stylish-as-F French woman married to an Italian who loves La DoubleJ possibly even more than I do.

La DOUBLE J.

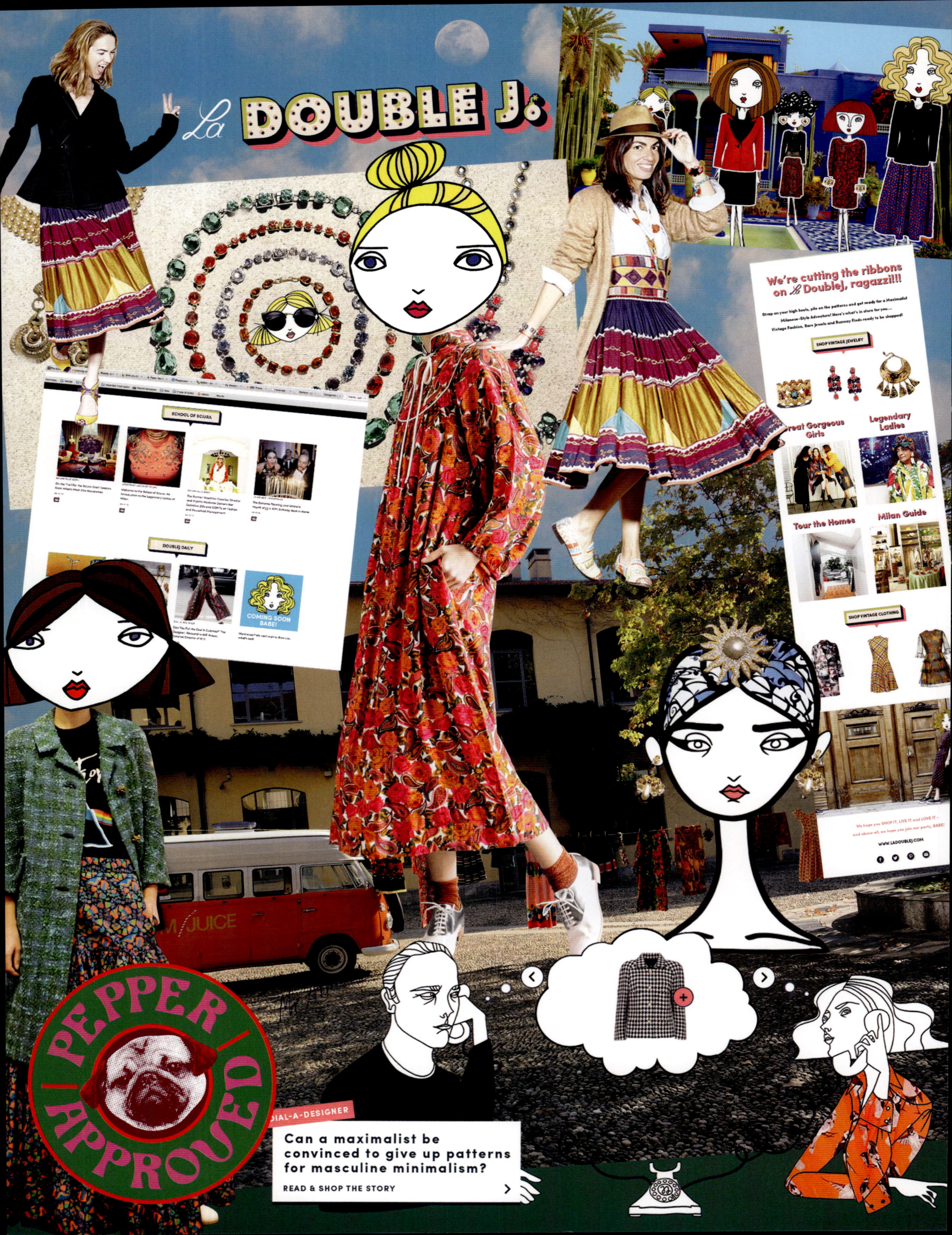

We're cutting the ribbons on La DoubleJ, ragazzi!!

PEPPER APPROVED

DIAL-A-DESIGNER

Can a maximalist be convinced to give up patterns for masculine minimalism?

READ & SHOP THE STORY

BORN TO BE WILD!

THERE'S NO ONE LIKE MY BABY

In true Italian fashion, I knew my baby was the best. There was, after all, no one like her. We had not followed the regular rules for a start-up, for a direct-to-consumer business, an online magazine, nor for a high-end luxury product.

Though we were made in the top luxury factories of Italy, we priced our product 30 to 40 percent less than other brands produced there. We had lower margins to create a fair exchange, but we also never went on sale at the end of the season. We carried over items that we loved, making sure women didn't feel that what they had just bought tanked in price or lovability. We had stringent rules for wholesalers not to promote any of their discounting online. We had no fashion shows, and we never paid any influencer to wear our clothes.

We had no investor, no placement on *Vogue* covers, and no PR person for our first three years in business, and yet we had a disorganized book stuffed with hundreds of pages of press clippings and many celebrities that somehow got their hands on the brand and wore it.

Having flown over from the depths of the true five-star fashion system, where it was my job to report on the coolest-of-the-cool designers, I actually never felt the pressure to be one. We would do things differently. I had never gone to design school, and had launched my business with vintage and content-led e-commerce. I loved a flat-level, co-creation model rather than dictating to my team from on top of the fashion ziggurat. There weren't many competitors operating at our level. I had created a new template all my own.

From the start, the La DoubleJ special sauce—vintage or new product—was bright, bold, and screaming its messages of joy. We pushed maximalism all the way: patterns were layered, mashed, mixed, and blended by the Vitamix of my own gut. The crazier the print, the wilder the color, the better. Our newsletters and homepage banners were filled with jokes, collages, and flashing GIFs. We named our products with catchy names: the Smokin' Hot Dress, Dinner at the Pellicano, and the Good Butt shorts because, you know what? They made your butt look fantastic.

Viviana was styling all the shoots, mixing vintage with new clothes on the same look, which we offered digitally for sale on our website via affiliate links. I invented verticals like Dial-a-Designer, Street-Style Milan edition, and the School of Sciura, a rolodex of information and rules for living the Italian high life in deep style.

DoubleJ was not trying to be part of the traditional fashion system, but she was fun, funny, frisky, bright, writerly, and sensationally visual. All of which were real-life elements that I derive pleasure from. This wrapped the company up in a deeply personal package. She was her own unique light signature that looked like no other.

She stepped out, and she shone.

MERGING ENERGIES: THE ART OF PARTNERSHIP

Our partnership with Mantero set the stage for an entire convoy of collaborations with some of Italy's best and, often underexposed, historic producers—such as Salviati for our Murano glass, Ancap for our porcelain, Mascioni for our linens, and Roveda for our shoes. Sometimes it was a one-time collaboration, as with Kartell, Valextra, Acqua di Parma, and Ladurée. All of these companies came to us.

Every seed that ever crossed our door I multiplied and scattered across our creative field with numerous products, events, and communication opportunities. The genesis was always simple and small: *Could you maybe just put a print on our cushion or packaging? Sure I can, and so much more!* My job was to amplify and expand and let it spin, stirring in the Divine Mother energy.

I loved working in partnership with others—a form of co-creation and sharing of talents. It's truly a feminine energetic when you hit the right balance of mutual back-scratching. I'm always really interested by who gets attracted to DoubleJ, because it's never a coincidence. When you start raising your vibration and creating at a certain frequency level, you will be calling in things that vibrate at that level and are aligned with you. There was also the mutual benefit to all. We gave fresh spins on these companies' archives or products and press opportunities, while they gave us manufacturing muscle and visibility.

Moreover, all of these partnerships manifested into product made lovingly, perfectly, beautifully, and passionately by Italians who took a month off in August and definitely sat down for a civilized lunch break every day they worked on our products. That means that every product you get at La DoubleJ has the unique energetic imprint of someone who was treated well, was paid, and who was able to relax in the process of making it.

This is not something to be underestimated. You do not want to eat or wear products that have not been made with love, as you will ingest it energetically.

SALVIATI. The oldest partner we still work with, Salviati have been blowing glass on the Venetian island of Murano since 1859. They are also our most forward-thinking partner. Their young at heart, frisky female CEO, Martina Semenzato, is flexible, creative, open-minded, and extremely excited about innovation. They came to us asking for a Salone spruce-up. We ended up creating a set of punchy, rainbow-colored Murano glasses that were such a hit, we have now developed them in multitudes of shapes, hues, and packages. There is no project too difficult for Salviati—including making exquisite, custom-made Murano glass panels for my apartment to hide a very ugly vent shaft.

ANCAP. When we found out that our first porcelain supplier in Italy was making the plate bases in Bangladesh and hadn't told us, we dumped them overnight and fell into the sturdy, reliable arms of Ancap, a sixty-year-old company based in Verona. Led by a fierce and passionate octogenarian named Claudia, Ancap was used to big numbers, and to doing white plates. They had never done a plate before that had fifteen colors on it—let alone a set of six that all featured different prints. We did a co-collaboration and put their name on the back. We pushed them beyond every boundary that they ever imagined—and they have always delivered brilliantly.

MASCIONI. Making linens the crispy, perfect Milanese way happens thanks to Mascioni, a textile expert based just outside of Milan. Our printed tablecloths, patterned napkins, and placemats are all printed, cut, and sewn by them.

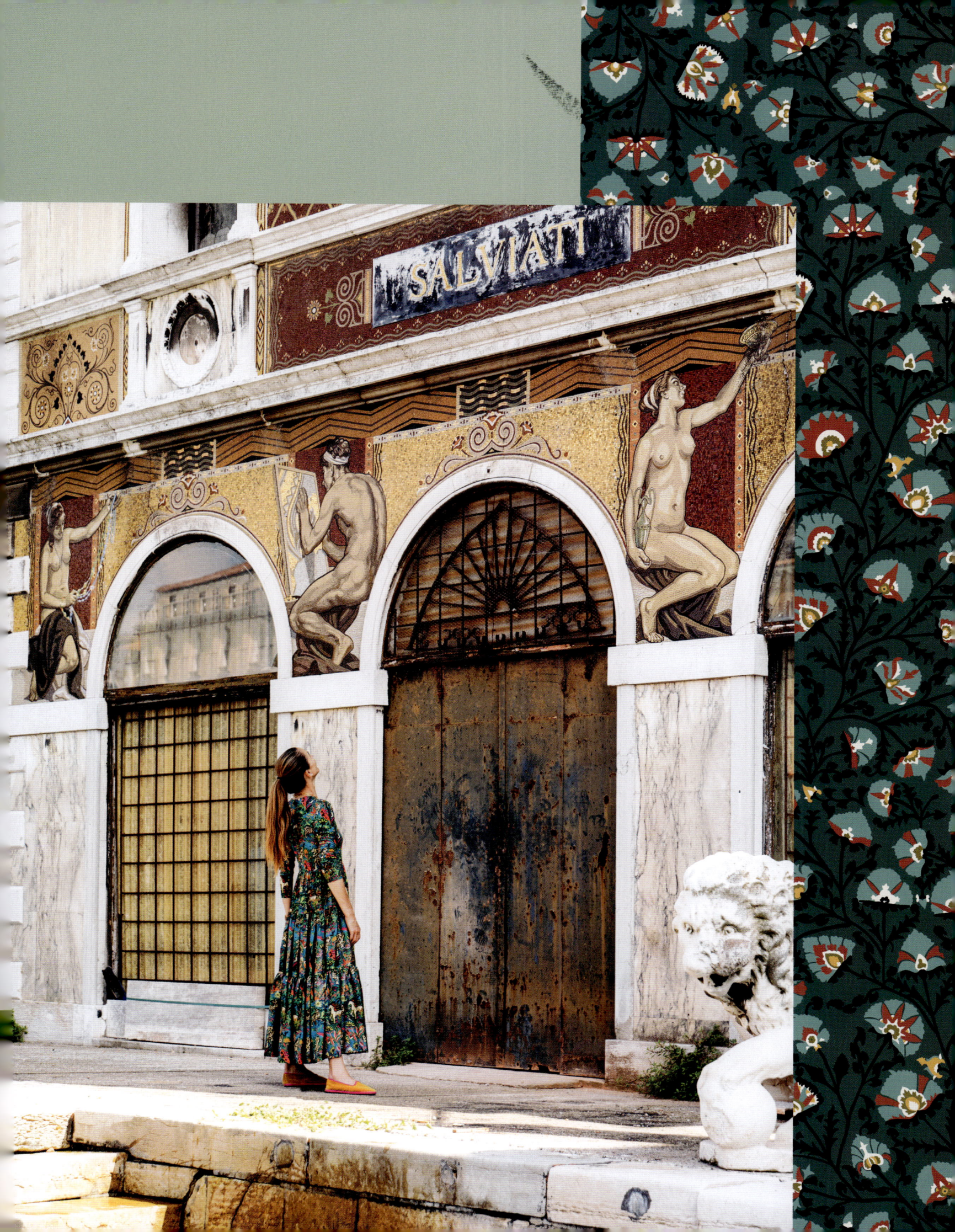

MAMMA MILANO

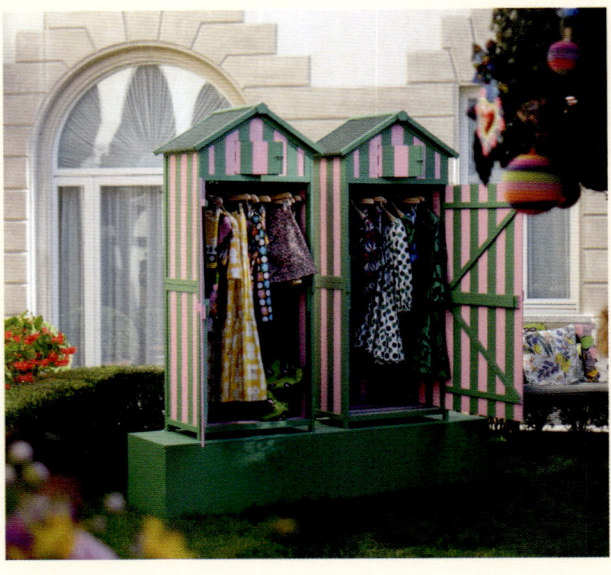

FOUR SEASONS. When they asked us to create a printed cup for their summer ice cream cart in their Milan hotel courtyard, we said yes! And then we asked if we could take over the space during fashion week—and that's how a former fifteenth-century convent came to be covered in printed pillows and couches, a striped walkway, and giant woven ornaments on every tree for two weeks.

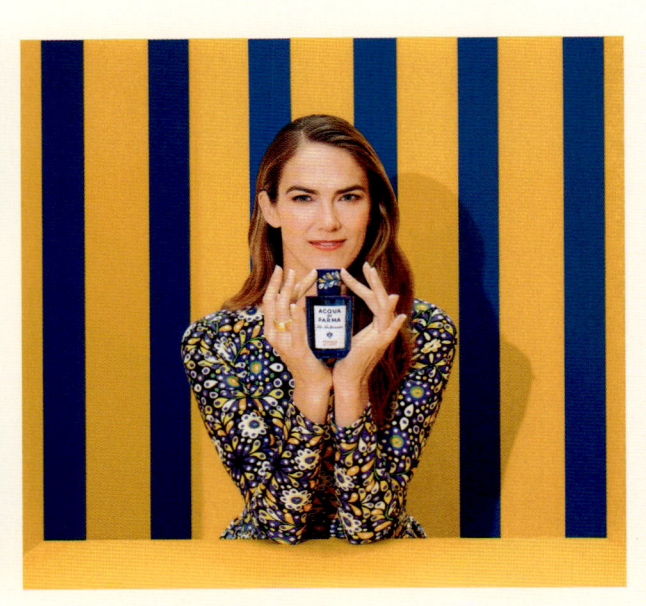

ACQUA DI PARMA. What began as an ask for a printed sleeve for their new scrub became a globally distributed "Summer Like an Italian" package, featuring beauty and fragrance products, journals, pillows, candles, swimsuits, towels, and tote bags, all lathered in one of our iconic prints. We also took over their shop during Milan Fashion Week in 2020, and used it to present our ready-to-wear collection.

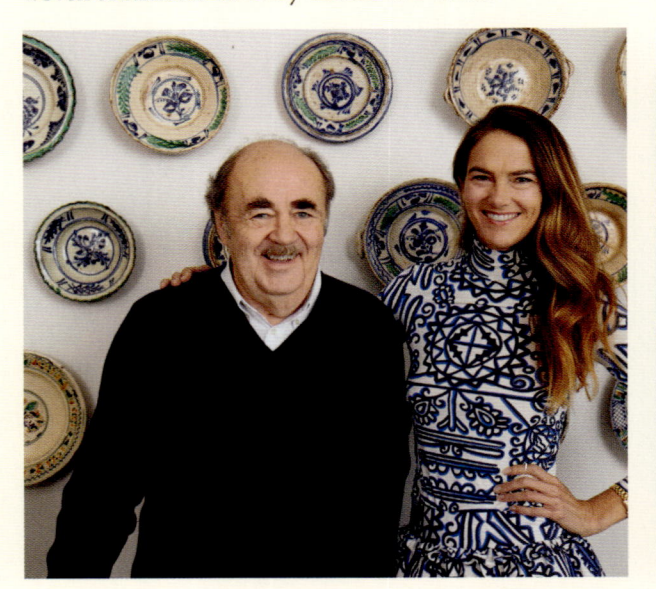

MIKI VON BARTHA & THE TRANSYLVANIA COLLECTION. When I met Miki Von Bartha, I had no idea he owned a prominent art gallery in Basel—with a back room full of antique textiles, pottery, and furniture from Transylvania. We created a fashion and homeware collection based on his sensational archives, which sold well despite launching during Covid.

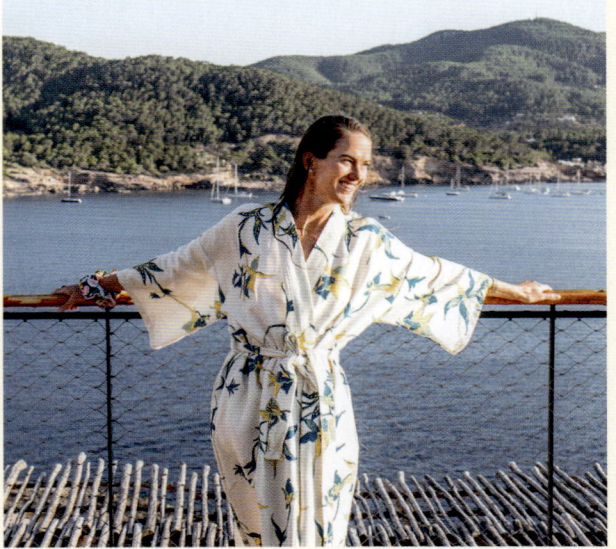

SIX SENSES. Soon after the global hospitality brand opened Six Senses Ibiza, they invited me to host a three-day wellness immersion complete with cacao ceremonies, shamanic drumming, holotropic breathing, and sound baths. For our pop-up shop, we designed our first sustainable product: a bathrobe, using organic cotton and sustainable dye, which still hangs in the rooms.

176

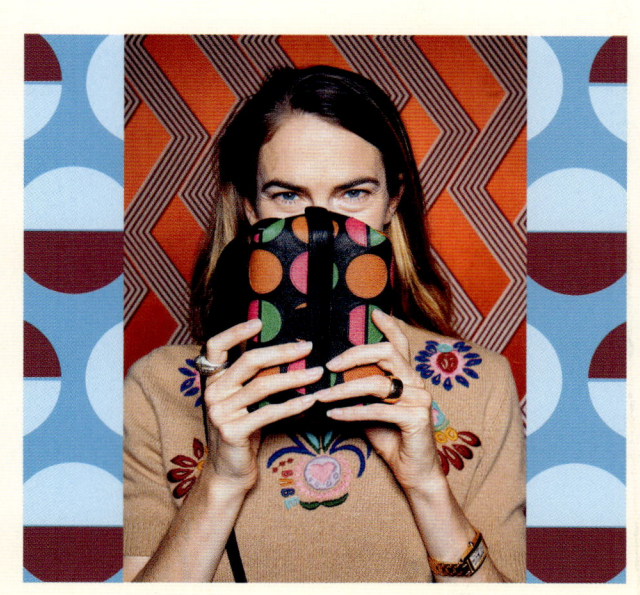

VALEXTRA. We were chosen by this venerable Milanese handbag company to bring our prints to their luxurious leathers. We created rich woven leather intarsia to mimic our patterns on several vintage styles, and we took over their Milan store with our prints and Murano glass for February 2020 fashion week, co-creating piles of fresh content that flew out across the digital ether.

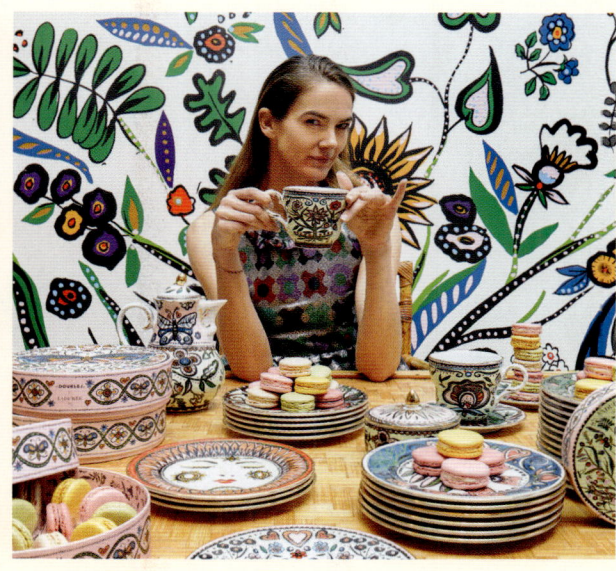

LADURÉE. Our first non-Italian partnership occurred in 2021 with this fancy Parisian patisserie. We created for them an entire coffee, tea, and dessert set, that was wrapped in Earth Mother illustrations, created by the artist Kirsten Synge Kongsli. And we designed decadent, bloom-covered printed boxes for their famous macaroons and painted a street mural for our New York takeover.

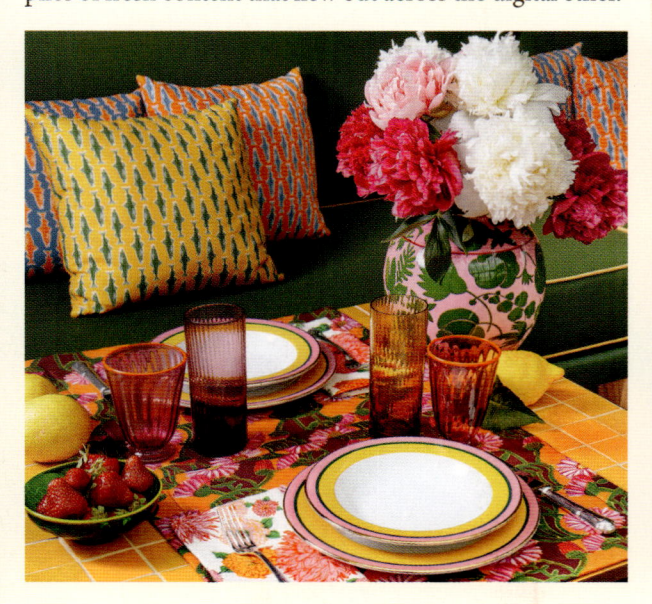

VILLA PASSALACQUA. Valentina De Santis, the joyful captain of the Grand Hotel Tremezzo in Lake Como, asked DoubleJ to design the pool and solarium areas of a new hotel opening in 2022: Villa Passalacqua. It was our first interior design project. Everything was blanketed in prints we made exclusive to the property, and complemented by tableware used by the pool and in the bar area.

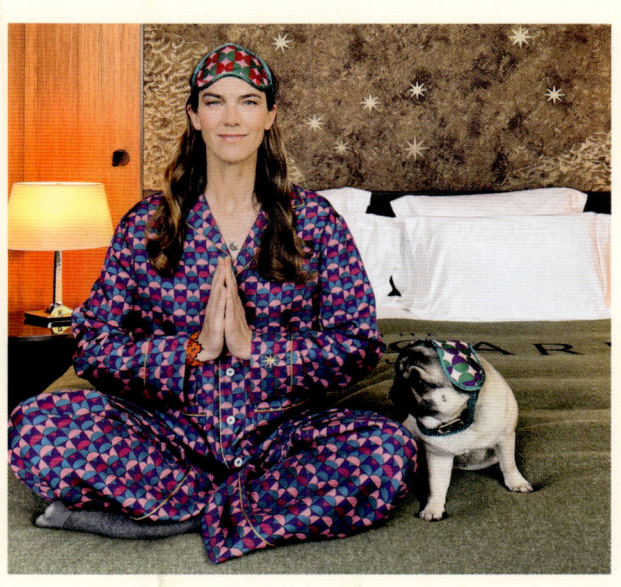

BULGARI. In 2023, we created an exclusive pajama just for Bulgari Hotels—custom-made, Italian silk-printed PJs for both men and women that they gift to every person who stays in the top luxury suites of their hotels around the world. We kicked off the program with a fun, global pajama party, that saw us jumping on beds and lounging in bathtubs simultaneously in Milan, Paris, London, and Dubai.

INTERMEZZO

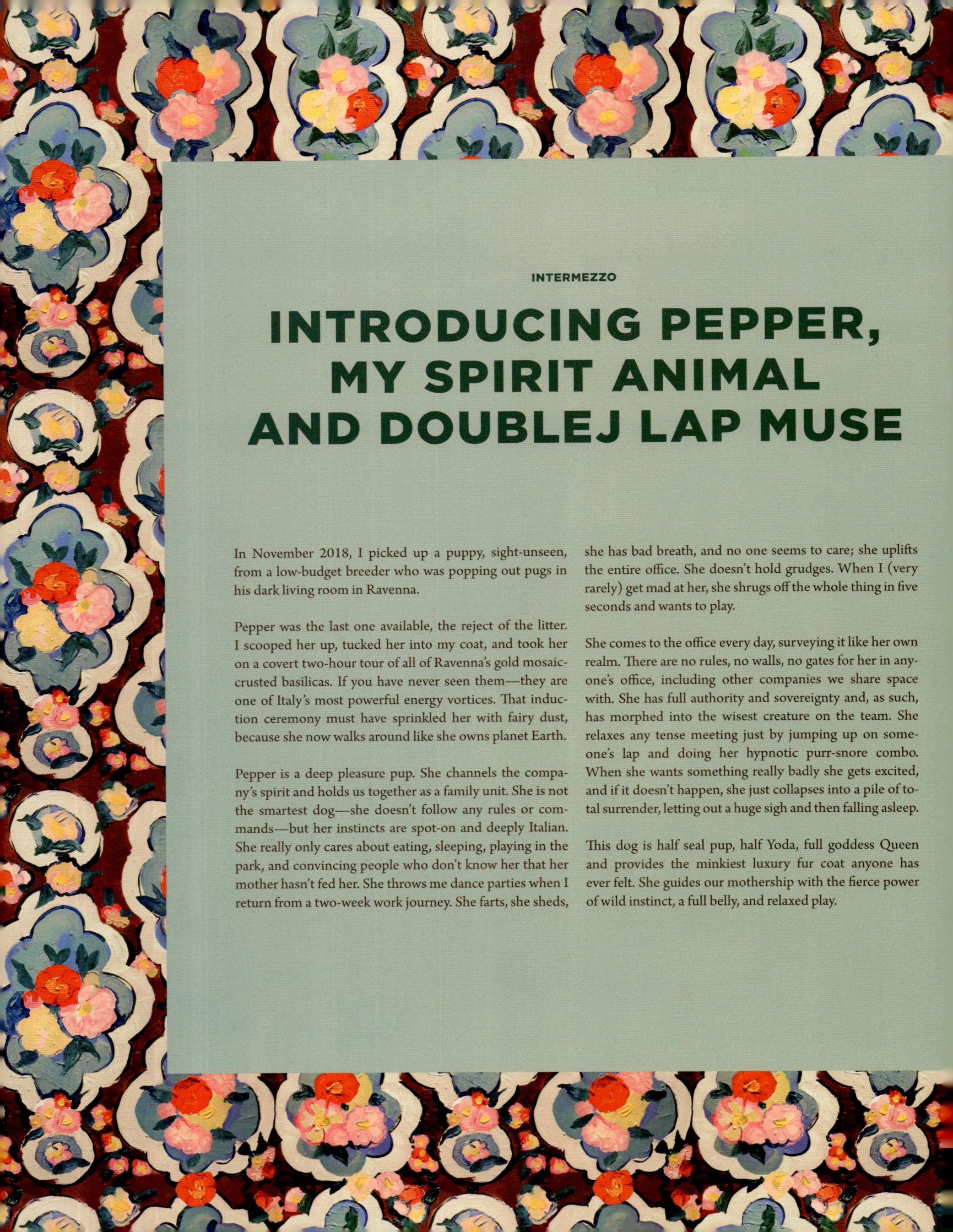

INTRODUCING PEPPER, MY SPIRIT ANIMAL AND DOUBLEJ LAP MUSE

In November 2018, I picked up a puppy, sight-unseen, from a low-budget breeder who was popping out pugs in his dark living room in Ravenna.

Pepper was the last one available, the reject of the litter. I scooped her up, tucked her into my coat, and took her on a covert two-hour tour of all of Ravenna's gold mosaic-crusted basilicas. If you have never seen them—they are one of Italy's most powerful energy vortexes. That induction ceremony must have sprinkled her with fairy dust, because she now walks around like she owns planet Earth.

Pepper is a deep pleasure pup. She channels the company's spirit and holds us together as a family unit. She is not the smartest dog—she doesn't follow any rules or commands—but her instincts are spot-on and deeply Italian. She really only cares about eating, sleeping, playing in the park, and convincing people who don't know her that her mother hasn't fed her. She throws me dance parties when I return from a two-week work journey. She farts, she sheds, she has bad breath, and no one seems to care; she uplifts the entire office. She doesn't hold grudges. When I (very rarely) get mad at her, she shrugs off the whole thing in five seconds and wants to play.

She comes to the office every day, surveying it like her own realm. There are no rules, no walls, no gates for her in anyone's office, including other companies we share space with. She has full authority and sovereignty and, as such, has morphed into the wisest creature on the team. She relaxes any tense meeting just by jumping up on someone's lap and doing her hypnotic purr-snore combo. When she wants something really badly she gets excited, and if it doesn't happen, she just collapses into a pile of total surrender, letting out a huge sigh and then falling asleep.

This dog is half seal pup, half Yoda, full goddess Queen and provides the minkiest luxury fur coat anyone has ever felt. She guides our mothership with the fierce power of wild instinct, a full belly, and relaxed play.

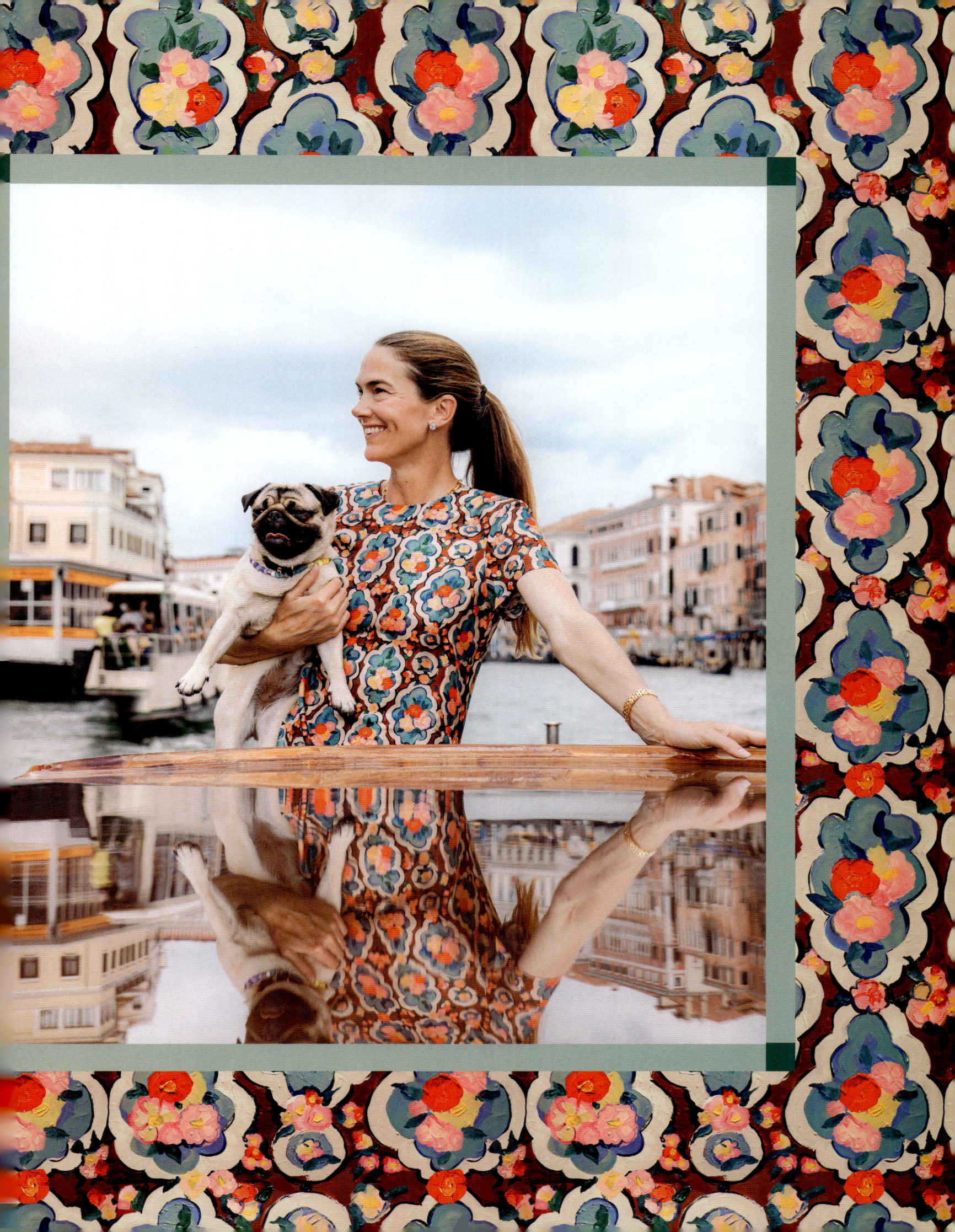

FRIENDS ✶ LOVERS
HELPERS ✶ HUGGERS

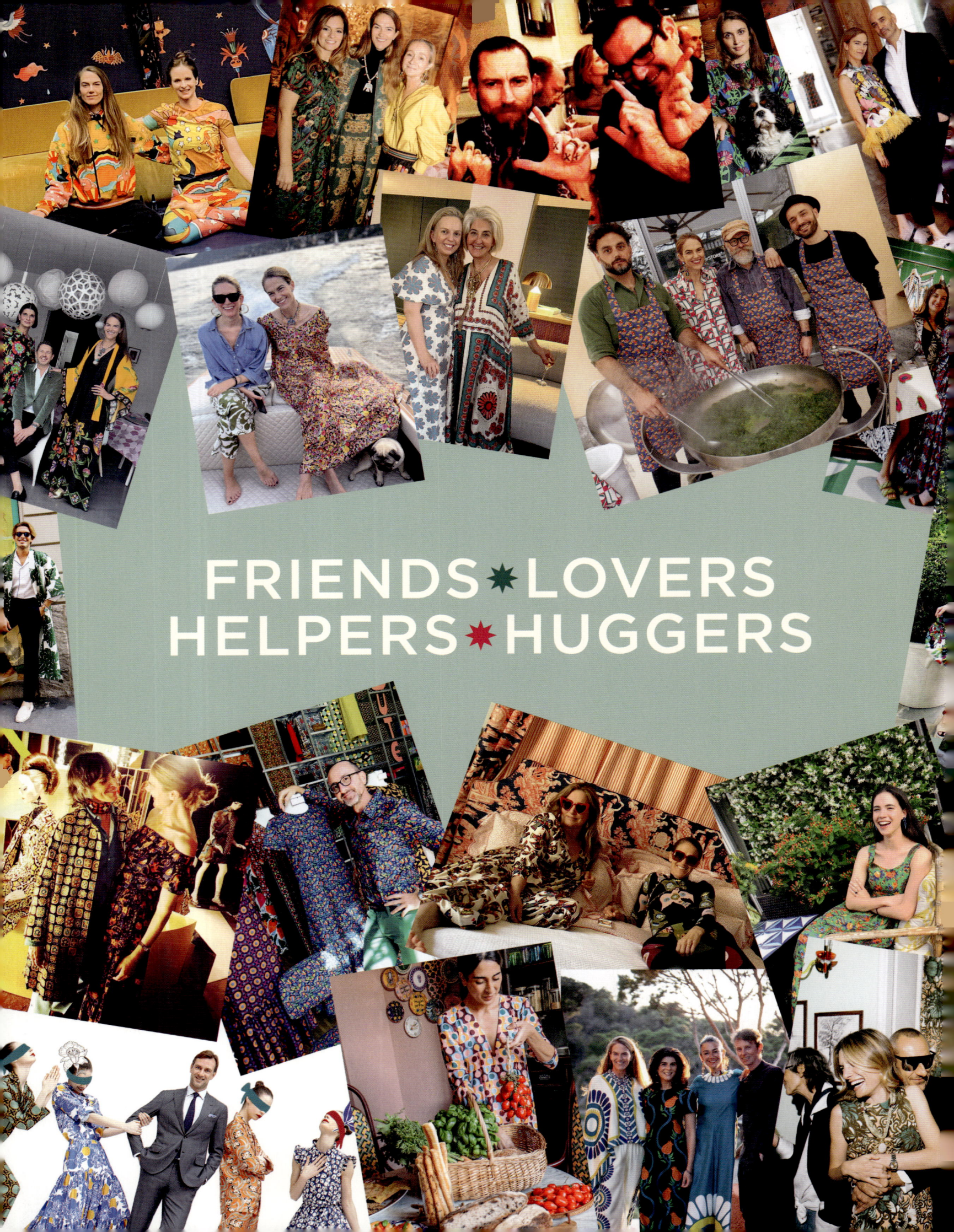

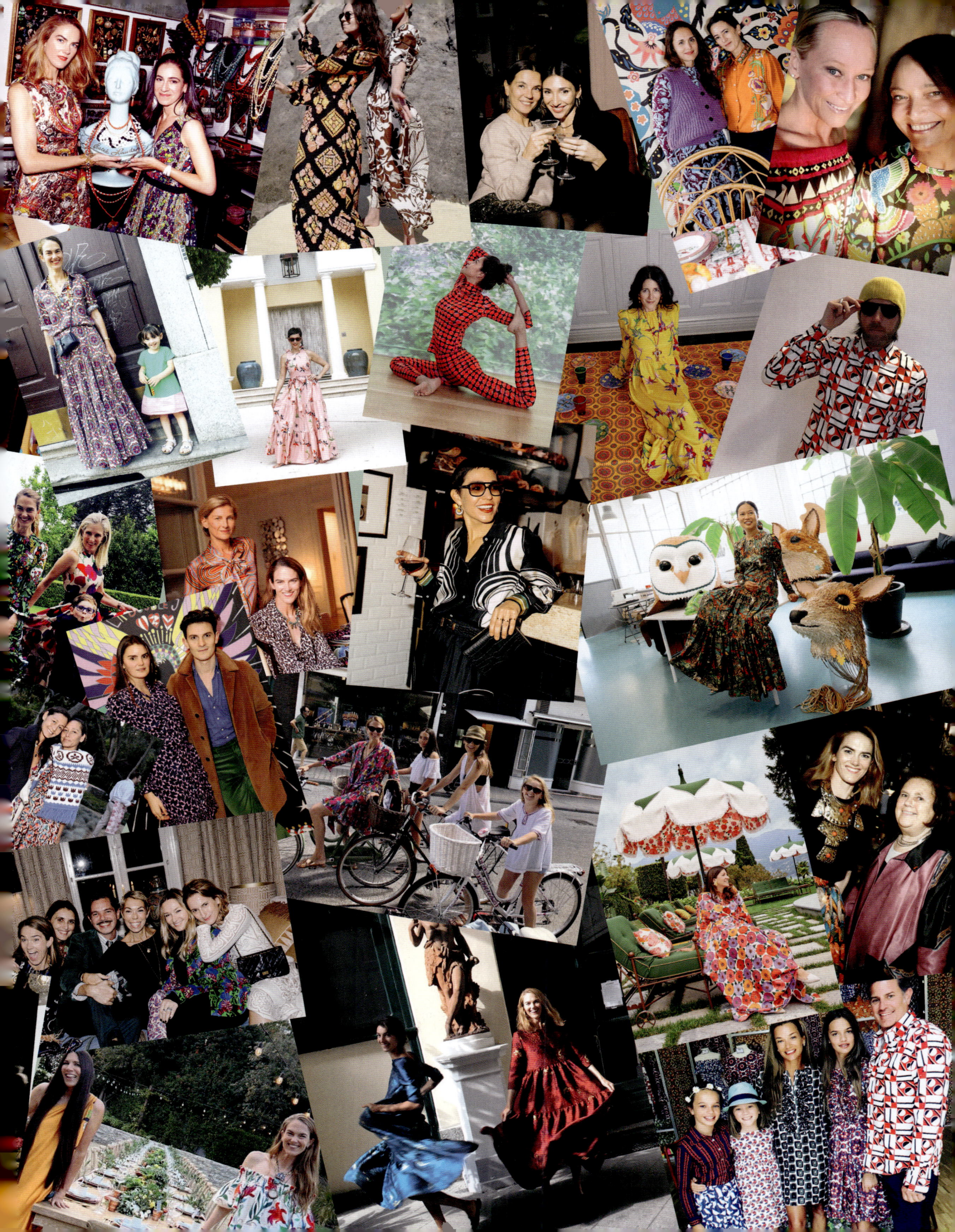

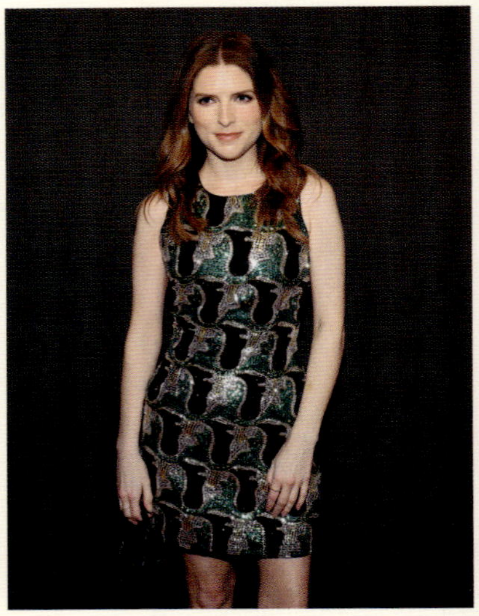

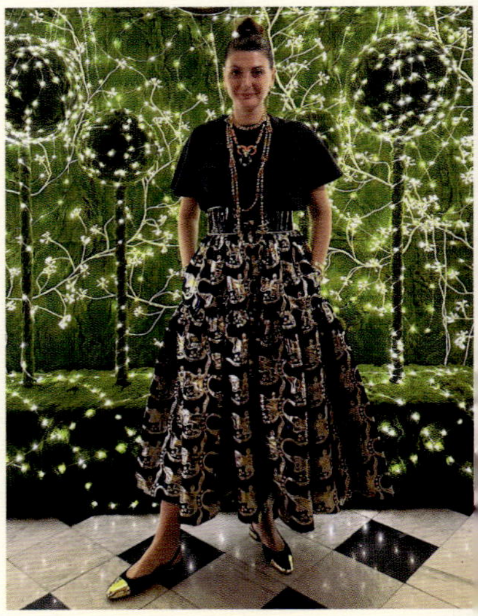

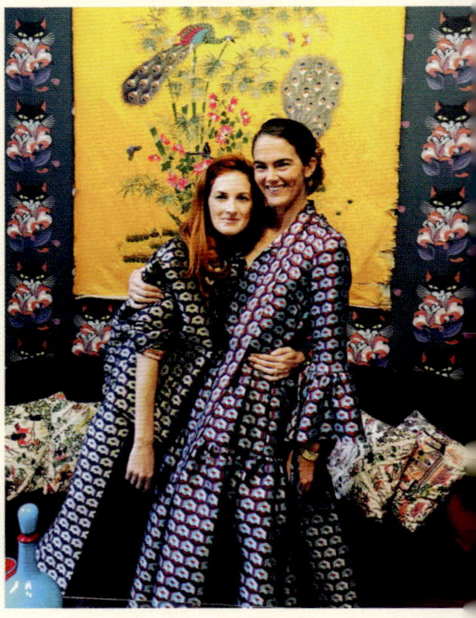

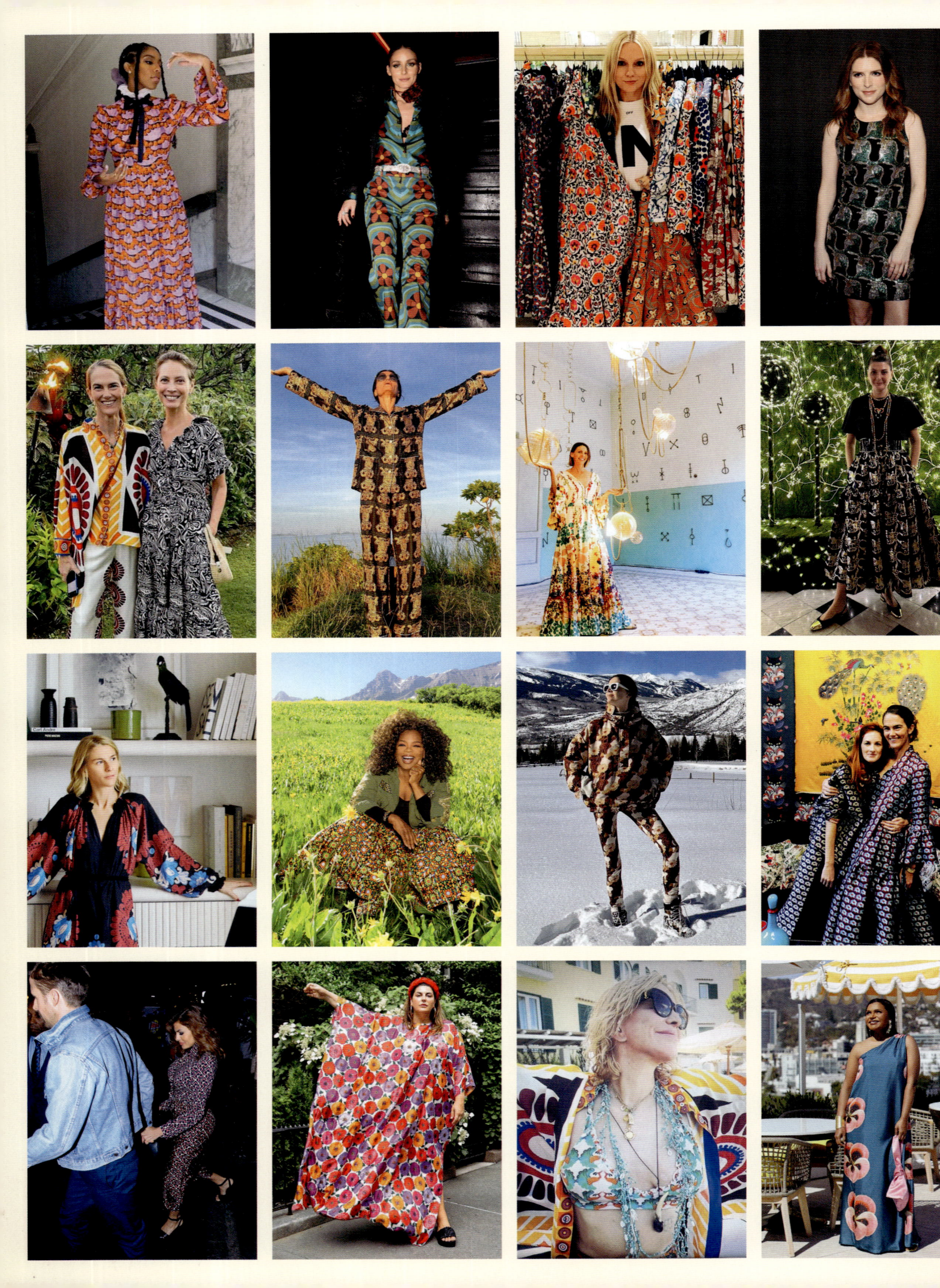

SiSTARS

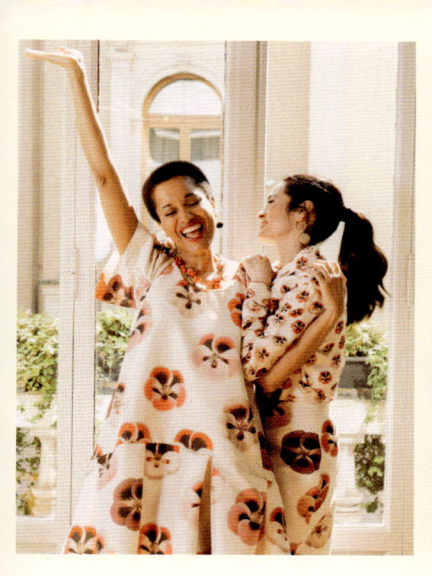

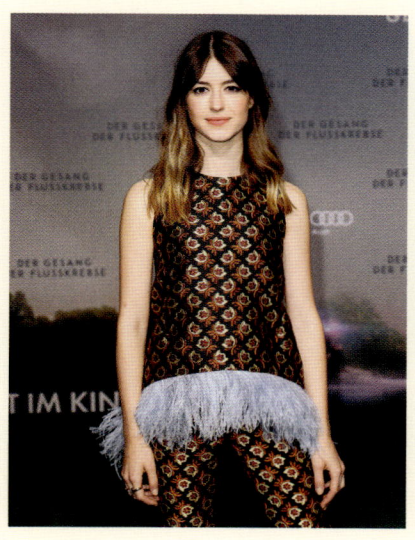

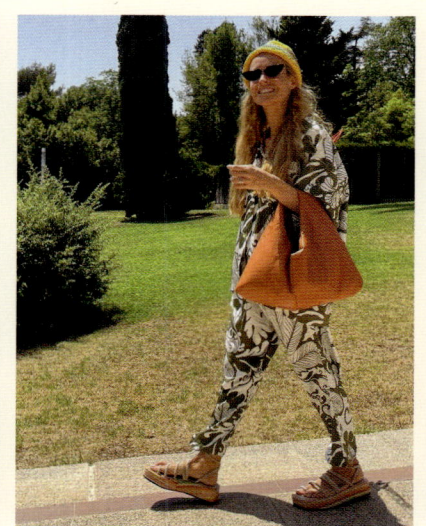

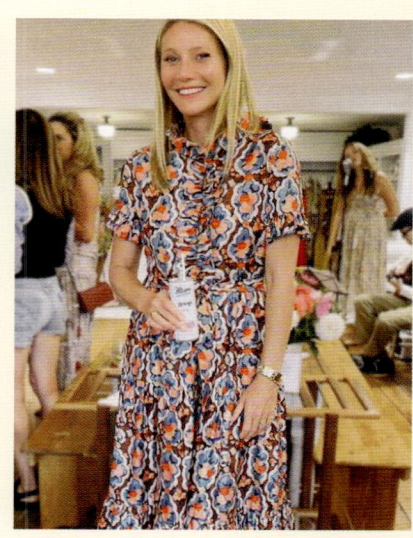

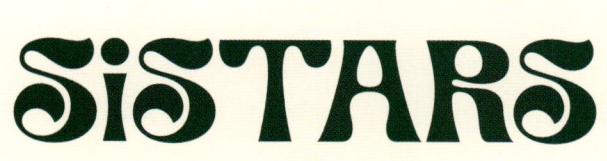

Women we love
who have supported our ascent

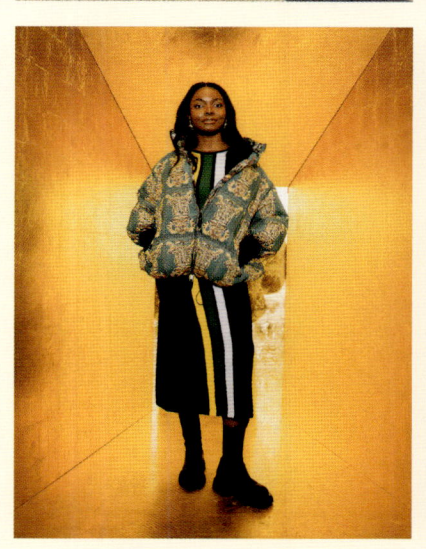

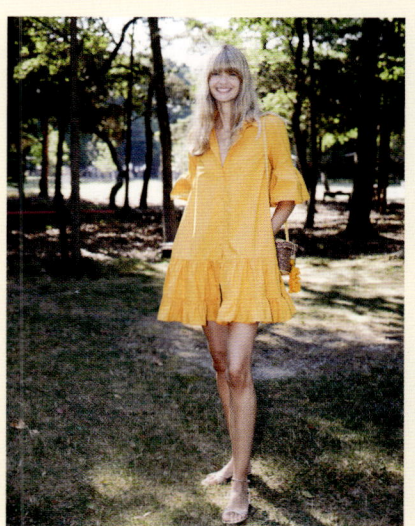

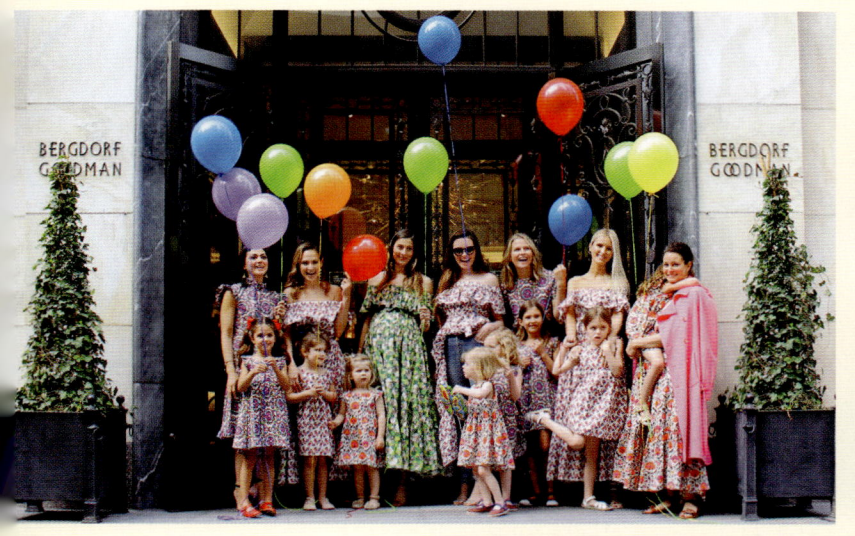

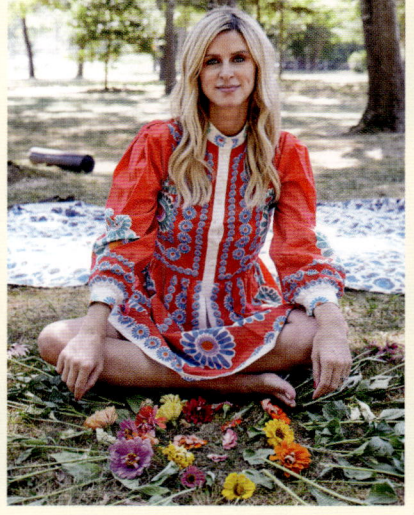

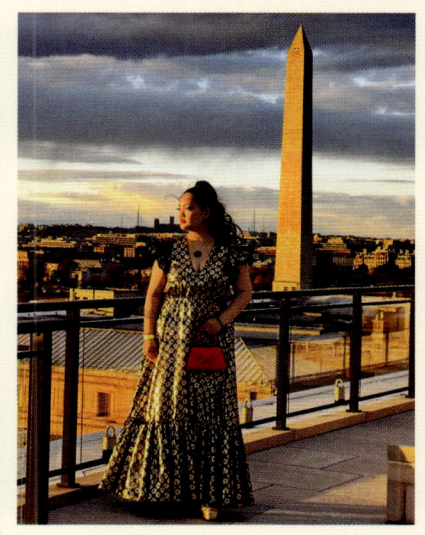

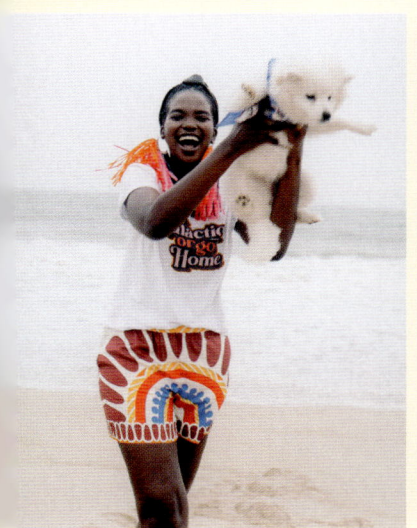

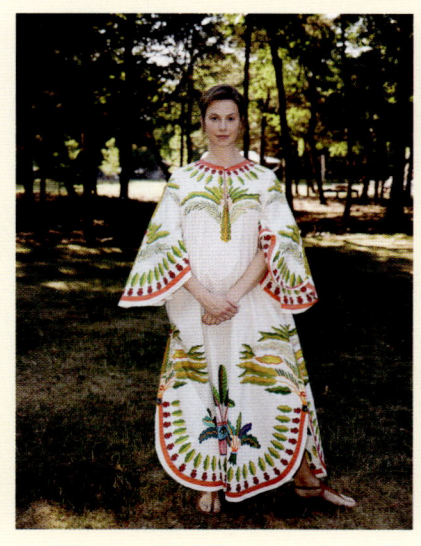

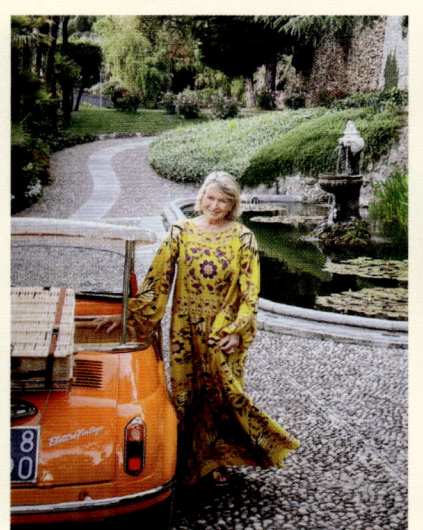

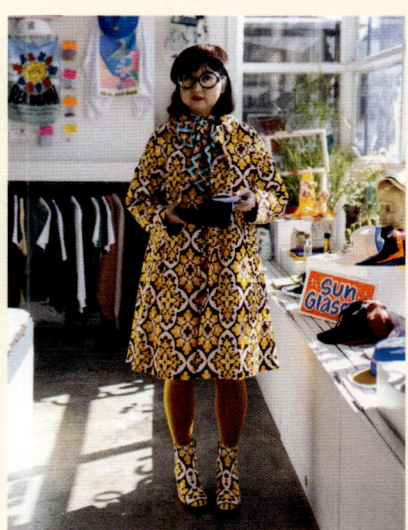

DOING BUSINESS WITH THE DIVINE MOTHER

The start of La DoubleJ was pure Divine Feminine in action, born from nothing but a dream and inner delight. I never followed any business plan. Instead, the company grew from my instincts and one strong seed—and then another. It was a stage for everything that I loved deeply in Italy. I watered this weird creation with love and joy—every shoot, every collaborator was a friend and a helper and a shepherd for this great project. It was truly a collective effort that was buoyed by a sense of playfulness and fun.

This endeavor also required a lot of masculine energy, which I freely exercised because, as I've mentioned, I was born brimming with it. First of all, I worked my ass off. Too much for the first several years—but all of that activity and action propelled things forward. I almost never took no for an answer, from *anyone*. So that was my "refusal"—a masculine trait that is often not good, but that can be helpful when you say, *No way, I don't accept a no, we can do this!*

On the other hand, I also learned that when I got a No over and over again, it was the universe sending me a message. *Back down, baby*. It is very hard for people with a lot of masculine energy to surrender. It feels like drowning in bloody defeat. And yet when we finally do, we soften, and in the softening the feminine can come back inside us and plant new seeds, new ideas, new possibilities to help us grow.

Over time, I found many ways to run the business with a big heart over a small belligerent fist, with inspiration over perspiration, with fun freak flags rather than freakouts. Every day was Bring Your Divine Mother to Work Day!

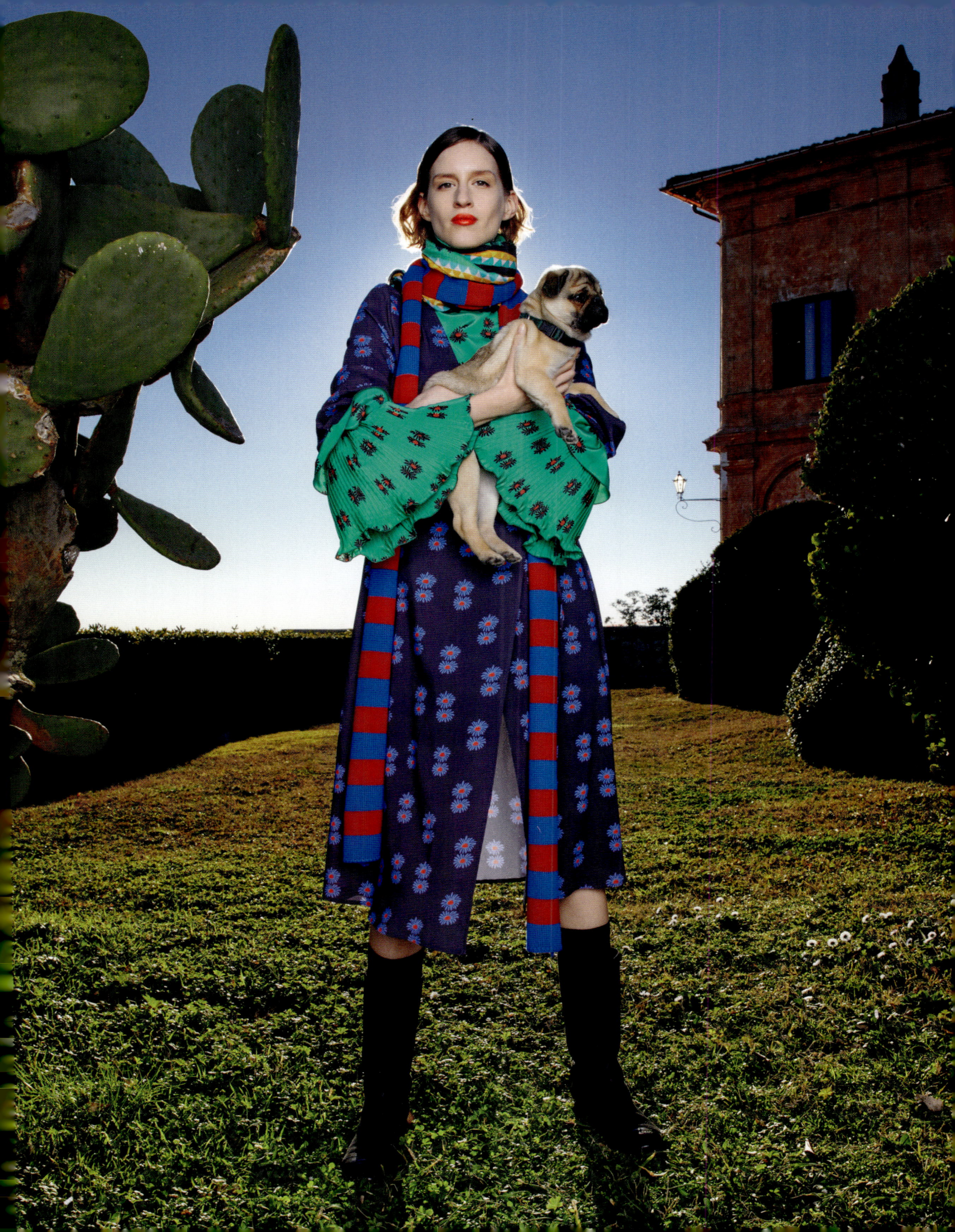

MAMMA MILANO

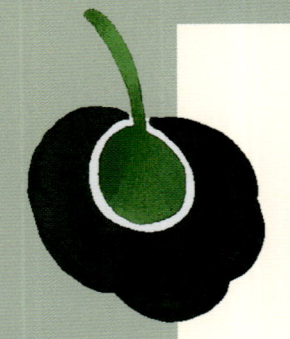

LESSON 1
IF YOU'RE BASHING YOUR HEAD ON ONE DOOR… FIND ANOTHER ONE

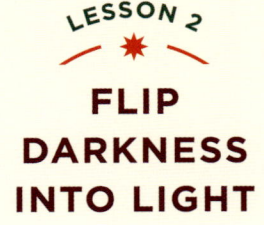

Our first business model flew and flowed… until it suddenly didn't. Rather than keep insisting that what I had in my head come to exact fruition, though, I stayed flexible and fast. I moved from a vintage sales site to building a new brand, something I never intended nor thought I could do. I didn't put up resistance but constantly refined, changed, and transformed the business, based on flow.

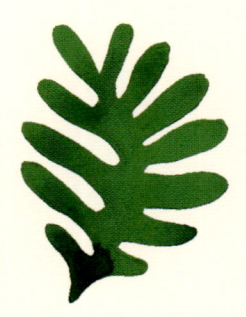

Of course, you should have objectives and work towards them. But in the process, if doors close, go to the next one and try to open it. See what happens. There's always a doorway leading to light and new opportunity. But to find it you have to stay creative. I don't mean doodling (though that can sometimes help!). I mean locating the sparkle within you that finds solutions, that is inventive, that approaches situations with curiosity and playfulness, and can imagine something new. The sparkle that is flexible and receptive enough to realize you may not even know what is for your highest good.

If you are open to it, the universe will shower you with gifts.

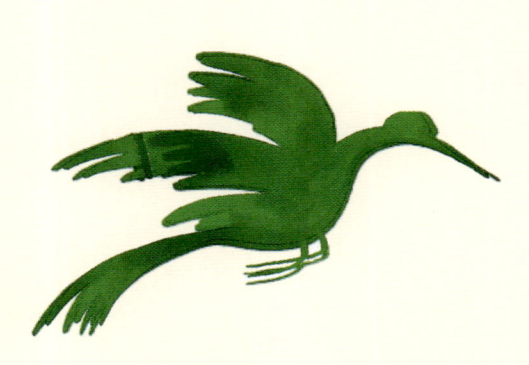

LESSON 2
FLIP DARKNESS INTO LIGHT

I'd started working with Elisabeth Manning, my energy healer, six months before La DoubleJ was born, and very quickly I began seeing the benefits of that powerful inner work. Explosive creative power pounded out of me and around me, but so did its shadow side. The company became a testing ground for every bit of progress I made on my meditation mat: employees quit before their legal three-month notice; architects, artisans, and suppliers warned, "You'll never be able to create what you want with your budget!" All of these snafus—and dozens more—were tests I had to pass to prove to myself that I can consciously create in the midst of chaos, able to transform any darkness, any density, any miscommunication into light.

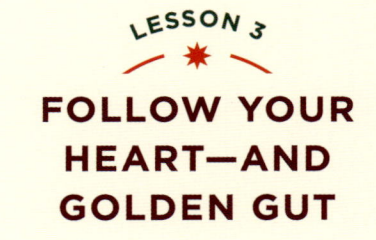

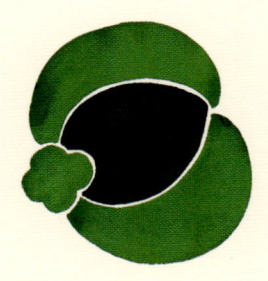

LESSON 3
FOLLOW YOUR HEART—AND GOLDEN GUT

In the end, my tortured journey to have a baby channeled my fertility into a geyser of creativity. I learned that I could be a mother to a business, to a book, to a whole gaggle of young employees who were yearning for mentorship, coddling, and growth. I learned a lot about listening to my heart and my intuition, softening my masculine cudgel rather than playing whack-a-mole with every problem.

The result is that our company is deeply guided by the sway of feminine energy—it's intuitive, mysterious, receptive. We're feelers just like Italy is; we go with the flow, just like Italians do. We bounce on the juicy waves the universe throws us. When we don't, we get slapped in the face, as happened to me many times on my road to unusual motherhood. Whenever I was behaving in a pushy, bossy, or mean way, I got smacked back into reality.

This company is a love child, and she only responds well to love and joy. To this day, not much logic drives my creative process—though of course I need our brainy businesspeople to keep me on the rails, and I listen to them and their ideas and concerns. But then I go off and start spinning in a very detached and illogical way.

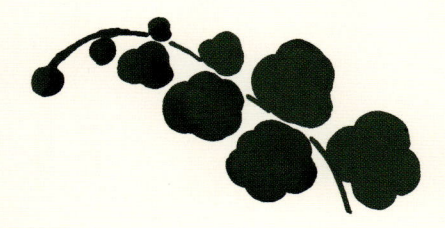

Many friends and acquaintances whose fashion companies had investors cried to me that they never had this freedom. A private equity firm is generally not set up to trust the mystery of the uncertainty of the Divine Feminine. They want results and they want them now. I always felt strangled by not having enough money, but as I look back it provided total liberty for the company and for me as its creative leader.

I truly believe the creative spark for our business comes from the heart; it comes from our golden guts. And when I see something—a new print, a new silhouette, a table setting—that is original, exciting, and alive, I feel it immediately in my body, not in my head. My cells warm up and go volcanoesque. I'll start yelling, "Winner, winner, chicken dinner!" I do it so often, it's become our company slogan (along with *Ciao, Babe! Raise your Vibration,* and *Pepper Approved*).

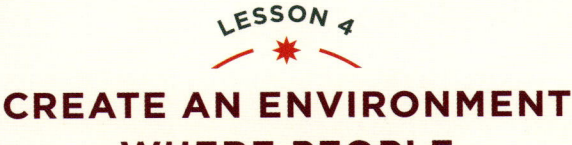

LESSON 4
CREATE AN ENVIRONMENT WHERE PEOPLE WANT TO WORK

The single biggest lesson has been keeping my head in a state of kind receivership and my body relaxed (a very feminine trait), instead of tense and tight. This means learning to hang on (and not cut out!) when the crap starts flowing in. Rather than storm off, judging things, and criticizing people, I've learned that the best thing I can do is to be a Guide and Wayshower. If I stay calm and upbeat, everyone else will move into solution mode. If I bring sunniness, joy, and humor to things that have fallen apart or become derailed, suddenly everyone else lines up behind me to follow the new lead. If I become a dictator, a bitch, start yelling, finding fault, and determined to figure out "who's responsible for the mess?" then everyone closes up and runs away.

I have veered off. I've lost my cookies. I've sunk into deep caves of misery when things fell apart. But I've also learned: I cannot hate myself for my mistakes. I must forgive myself and forgive everyone—we all fuck up. Now I know it's up to me as a leader to set the tone of amnesty and collaboration. The rule is, I sit down and talk to the person as calmly as possible with one objective: solution. How can we create something new and better in this now moment?

This is how I have been able to create ties and relationships in the workplace. It's the way I've been able to hire people for less money than they were making at other companies and been able to retain them when other big corporations come in and try to steal them. Employees feel the energy. They want this nurturing, this warmth, they want to feel valued and listened to. They don't want a hierarchical system of "who's the boss." They want to be able to talk and give their opinions. We are creating this company together by fusing the freedom and creativity of the feminine with the supportive, clear, protective, efficient power of the masculine. It is not a patriarchy. It is a collective endeavor where the Divine Masculine and the Divine Feminine energies mingle and marry, and out pops a community coming together as One.

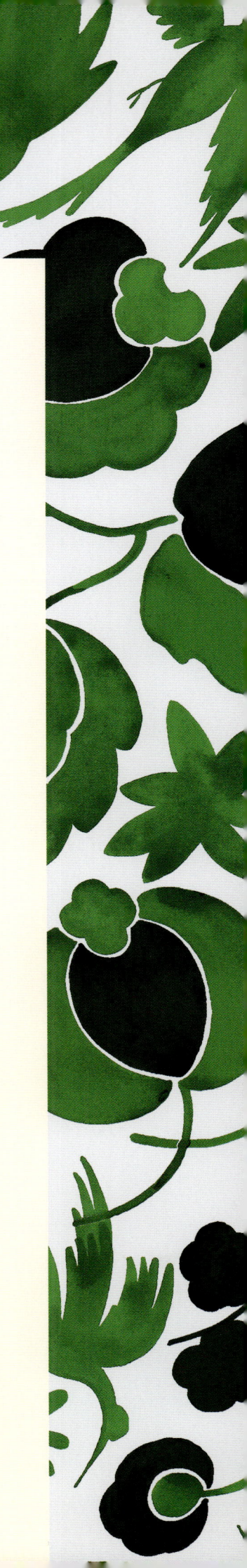

MAMMA MILANO
My High Vibration Start-Up Road Map

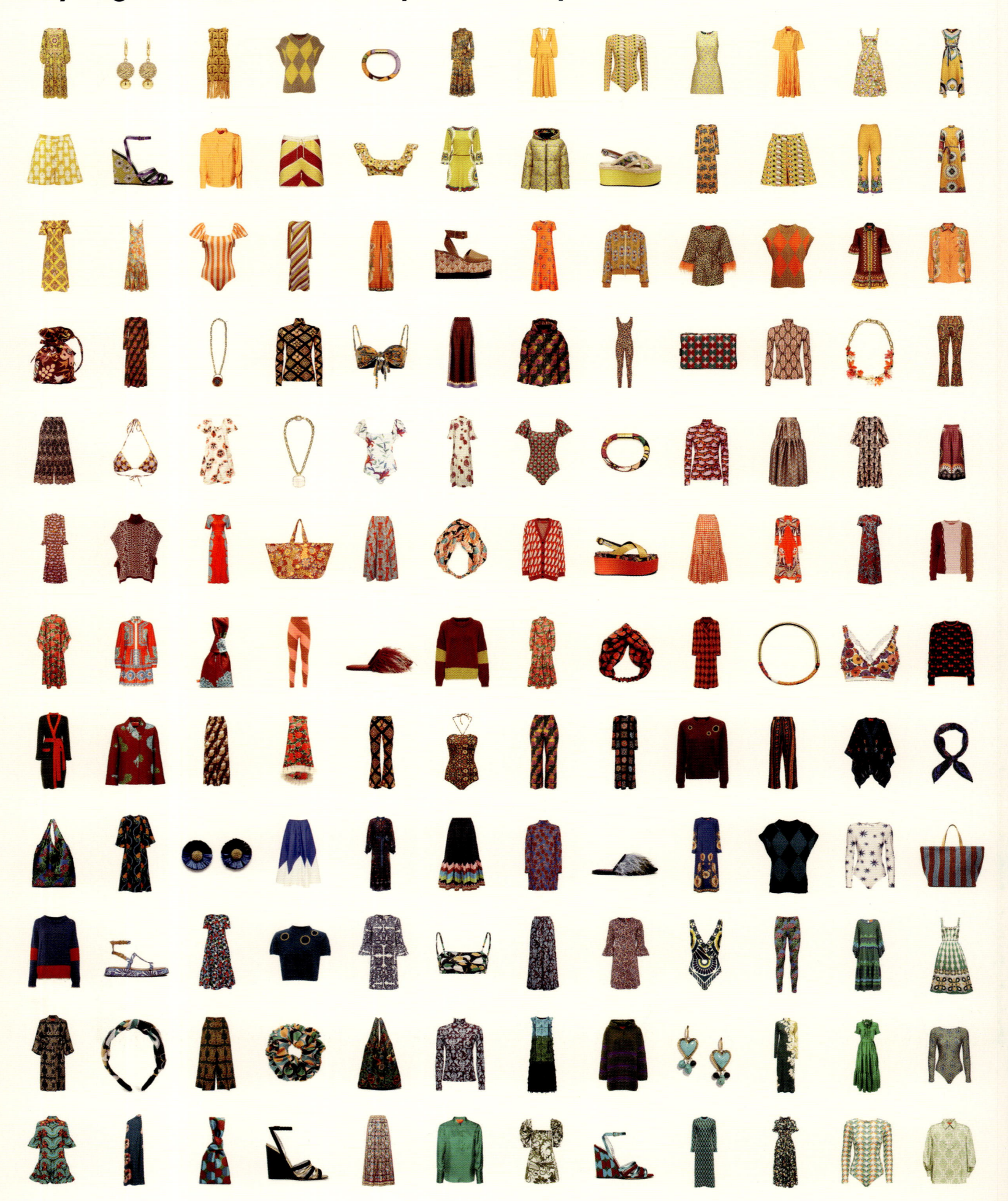

FIRST OF ALL, GO FOR IT!
Dive in and be prepared that you might not do what you think you will do. Begin at the beginning.

FOLLOW YOUR JOY CRUMBS
Don't do it for money or for fame. Do it because you love it. Go with the flow, be flexible, be humble.

BIRTH AN ORIGINAL IDEA THAT TRULY MAKES YOUR HEART PUFF
If you copy someone or something that's been done before, your project won't have the same powerful energetic signature.

EMBRACE CHAOS
The first five years will never, ever feel under control.

DON'T BANG REPEATEDLY ON DOORS THAT ARE CLOSED
Go where the energy flows. When you get shut doors, that's when you get creative. Never keep banging on a closed door. Get curious and feel around in the dark for the next one—a hole, a key, anything.

ALWAYS BE REINVENTING!
Reinventing always brings new expansion—not just of the company's coffers and reach, but also consciousness.

GET KIND AND CREATIVE WITH TRAGEDY, FAILURES, AND SHUTDOWNS
They are merely messages from the universe that a particular path wasn't meant to be, but others are, if you strap your joy rockets on again.

UNDERSTAND YOUR TALENTS AND THEN HIRE YOUR EXACT OPPOSITE
People who can do things you are incapable of (finance? project management?) are invaluable. Your potential stops at the edges of your own talent pool. Understand this and plot it strategically.

DELEGATE LATER
In the beginning, you are an eight-armed goddess. You will work every day, every night, every weekend.

YOU ARE THE MOTHER
Regardless of your gender, you are the mother of this project: you fertilized it, incubated it, and gave birth to it. Now you must nurture and nourish it before it leaves you and goes off to some amazing school. In these early years, you have to show up. You have to listen to what the baby wants. Pay attention when she screams or fights back. Do not leave her in the hands of unloving caretakers. This is a living energy being.

ONLY HIRE PEOPLE WHO CAN THRIVE IN CHAOS
Never take anyone from a big cushy job who is used to an assistant and a fleet of staff. They will hightail it out the minute they realize they too must make the coffee.

AS YOU GROW, REALIZE THAT THOSE ANGELS YOU FOUND WHO THRIVED IN CHAOS ARE NOT NECESSARILY ALSO GREAT WITH STRUCTURE
You need to bring in people who can "manage" in more traditional ways.

NEVER HIRE AN ASSHOLE
Every personality counts. Any pessimism, gossip, negativity, or criticism is going to take you and the whole team down. Be very mindful of this as you interview people. Sunny dispositions will save your life.

LEARN THE ART OF MUTUAL BACKSCRATCHING
I was the queen of barter and exchange in the early years of DoubleJ. Without much money, I constantly invented ways in which I could give creative people or other companies something they wanted. It's important to check in frequently to make sure the exchange feels fair and you both make good on it.

LISTEN, LISTEN, LISTEN
Opportunities and great ideas come from everywhere and everyone, including the intern who's never worked a day in her life. If you want to create consciously, you must be open to what other people have to say—buyers, customers, editors, your sister-in-law. You don't need to doubt what you do, but rather listen with curiosity as you consider always what you can do better.

ENCOURAGE THE YOUNG ONES TO TALK
In Italy, junior staff are not usually allowed to express their opinions in meetings. I insist on everyone sharing their opinion. They're all allowed to babble on, shrug, shake their heads, and hopefully, more often, jump up and down in joy when they like something.

IGNORE THE DOOMSAYERS
If someone is a constant naysayer and can't bring solutions, get rid of them.

DO NOT GET DRAGGED DOWN BY EMULATORS OR COMPETITORS
If you're doing great things, inevitably people will copy you. If you get enraged by this or try to smash-talk great competition, this will lower your vibration. Enjoy the giant creative field you are all sharing.

REMEMBER, YOU ARE THE MOTHER
Every time something went wrong in my business or caused me stress, worry, or frustration, I began to realize it was the result of either (i) not being clear enough in my expectations, (ii) not having the proper structure in place to support the action in question, (iii) not having the right people in the right roles. And you know what? No one was responsible for any of the above items except for me.

MAKE CRITICISM CONSTRUCTIVE
When you have your own business, you have forty-eight eyeballs that see every wrinkle and wart. You must point out the flaws, but to do it in a way that doesn't shut the other person down. Inspire them to find new ways and new solutions. It's hard. We're often taught that the only way people learn is by criticizing or punishing them. But the true gift is holding your vision in yourself, embodying what you want to see in others, and creating a bridge so people want to come towards it and you, rather than run away in fear. You want to give feedback in a way that inspires people rather than belittles or makes them feel ashamed.

REMEMBER, IT'S A VERY ITALIAN THING TO PAUSE
Wait. Listen. Pause before you react. I give myself a two-minute check-out by going into the bathroom, sitting on the toilet, and breathing. Or, I smoke a cigarette like an Italian. I remove myself from the team.

THE TEAM MUST BE SHEARED TO STAY HEALTHY
In Italy we can't just fire people when we no longer like them. It's against labor laws. This is not a bad thing. It has helped me a great deal to meet a person on a human level and figure out why they couldn't do the job. I've found myself giving life coaching advice to unproductive employees. They usually end up leaving the company on their own, once they realize they'd be happier doing something else. Carrying dead weight afflicts the whole team; you need those who love the vision, bring fresh perspectives, and are willing to work like crazy. You will survive the pruning, as well as losing people you don't want to let go of.

GIVE YOURSELF A BREAK
You're doing an awesome job. See yourself. Give yourself a pat. Everything is fine. Including if the whole operation goes down the drain.

BORN TO BE WILD!

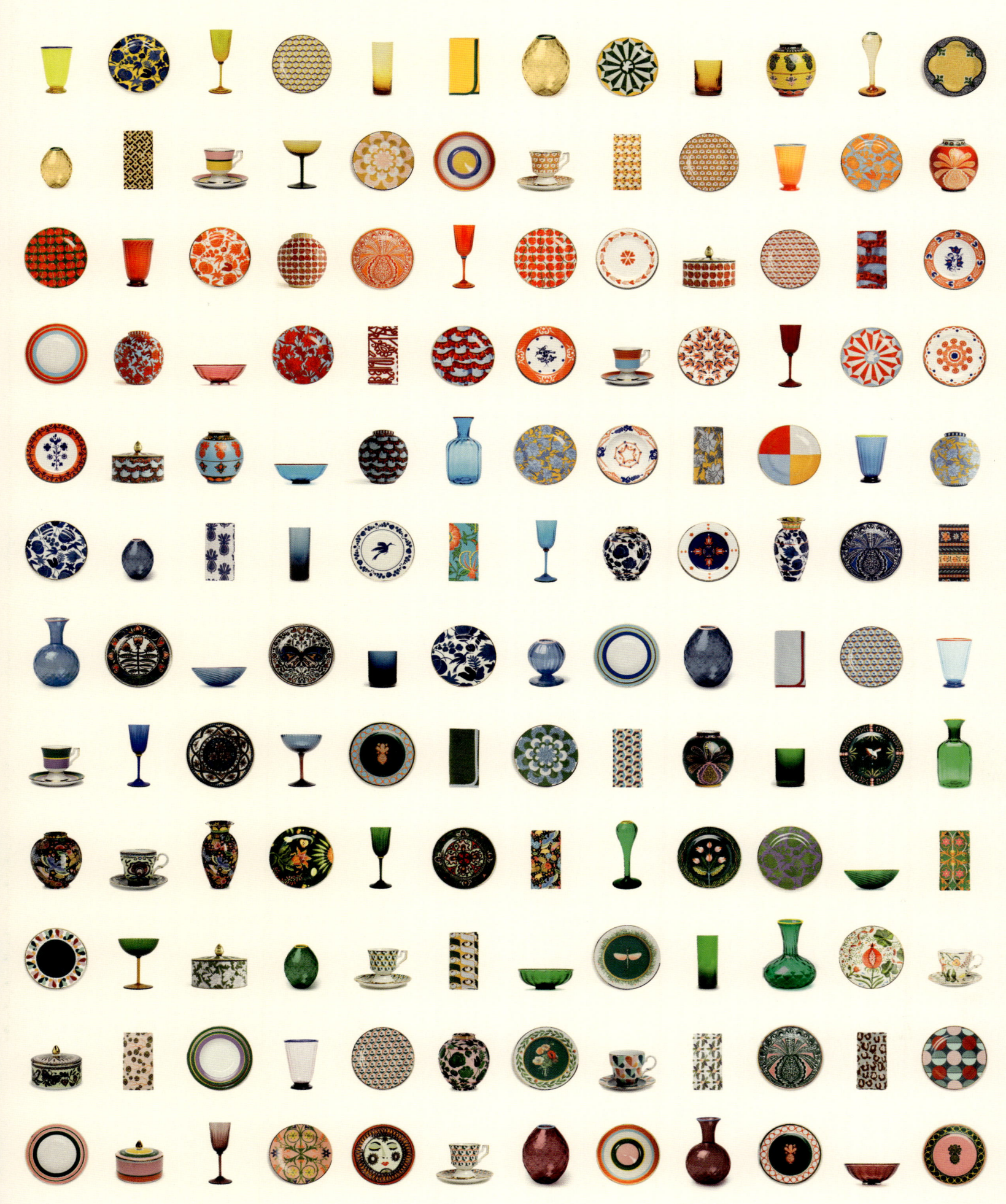

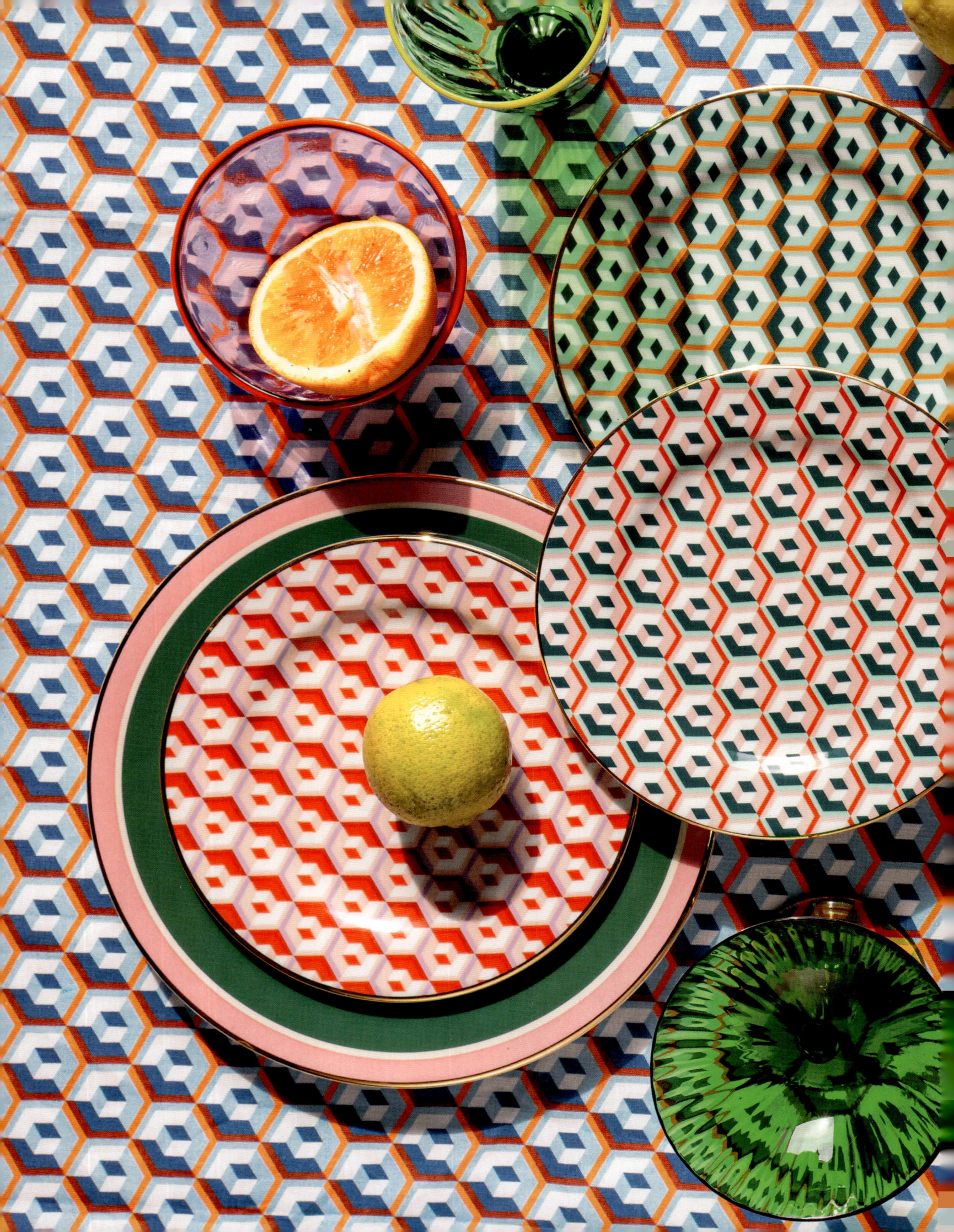

LET'S DRESS UP TABLES!

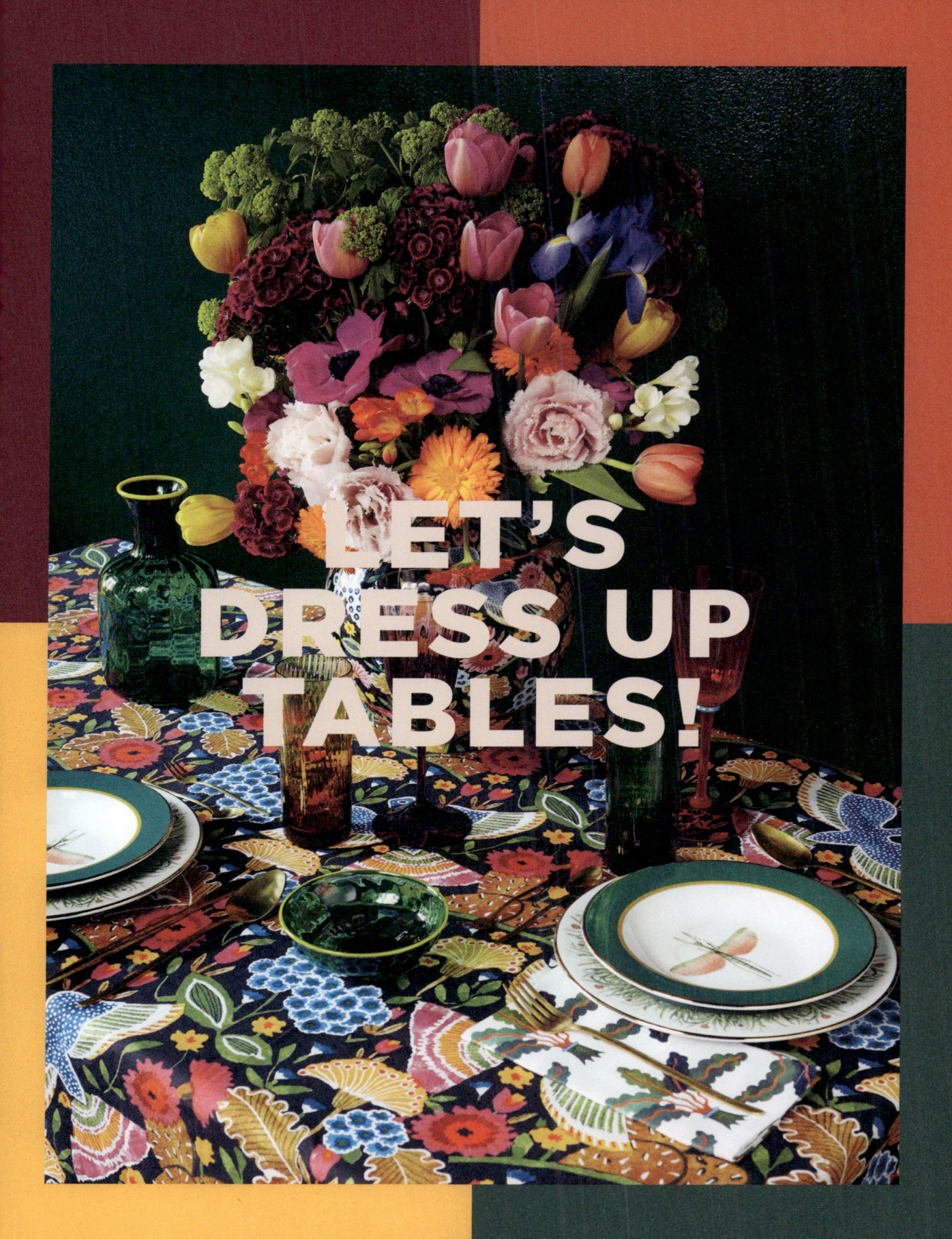

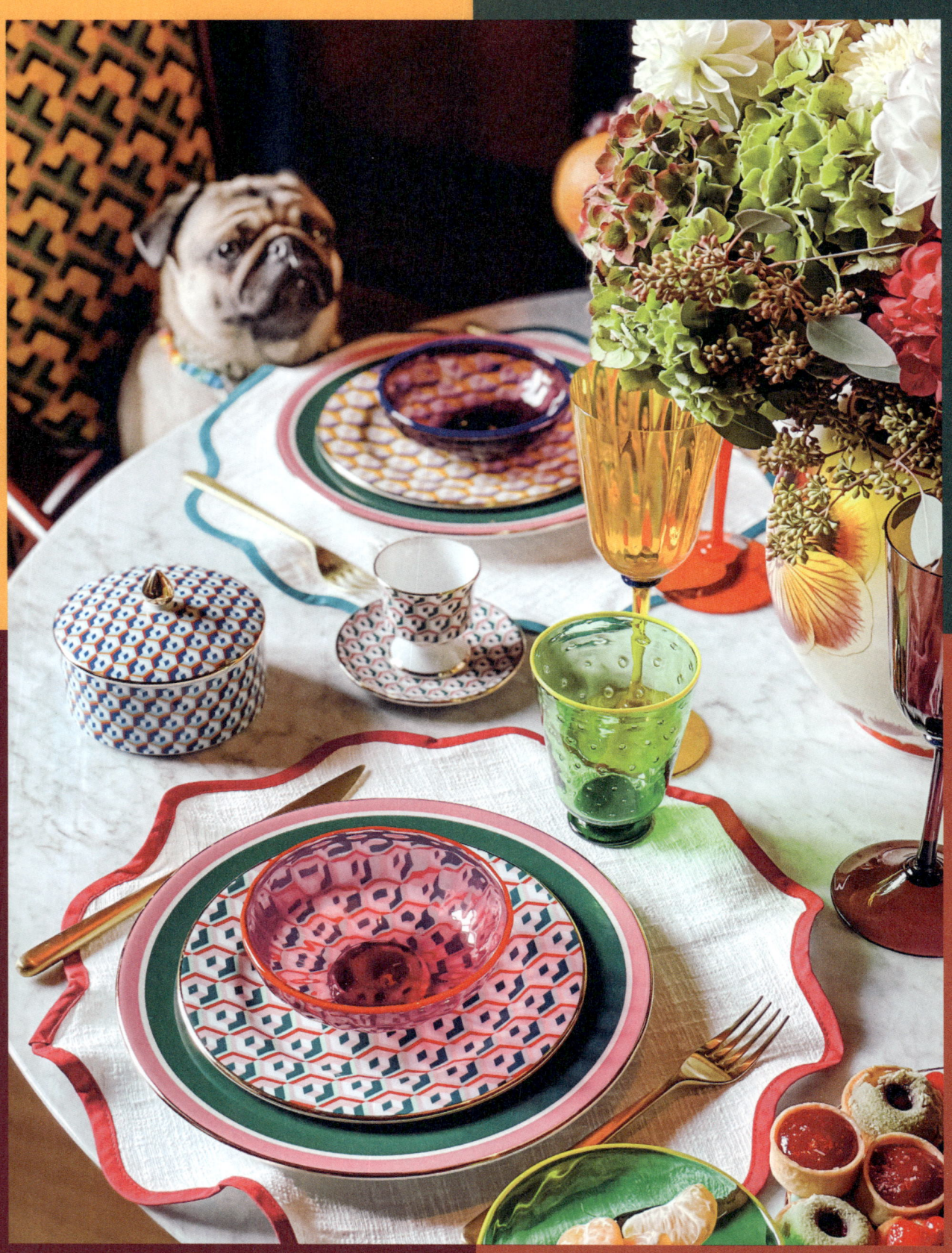

Cover: Libellula & Colombo Collections Mix & Match
Rainbow and Cubi Collections Mix & Match

The birth of our homeware was not planned, nor was it a business endeavor. Andrea told me I wasn't going to make any money on it. But I loved it and wanted to do it anyway.

It started with an event we created for Pomellato, one of many brands such as Missoni, Max Mara, and Armani who had come to me in the early years of the company to create either digital content or events for them incorporating the DoubleJ jazz hands. At this point, I didn't know where our business future would lead us, but when a paying job came in that felt right, I said yes. Pomellato asked me to curate a dinner party—from the guests, to the theme, to the happy, maximalist décor. We ended up splashing our prints everywhere that night, including across the dinner table, and everyone began to breathlessly whisper:
You should do homeware!

When we launched the collection in April 2017, we had a giant flower-filled party inside our showroom during Salone. No one was doing tablescapes like that—layer upon layer of pattern, print, table linens, porcelain plates, and wacky flowers done by our beloved Japanese florist, Sachiko. We had no PR, and our event was jam-packed. Every magazine we sent the images to covered it.

In the next five years, it seemed everyone jumped on the maximal table-top bus, but we were proud that we had put our flag on that magic mountain first.

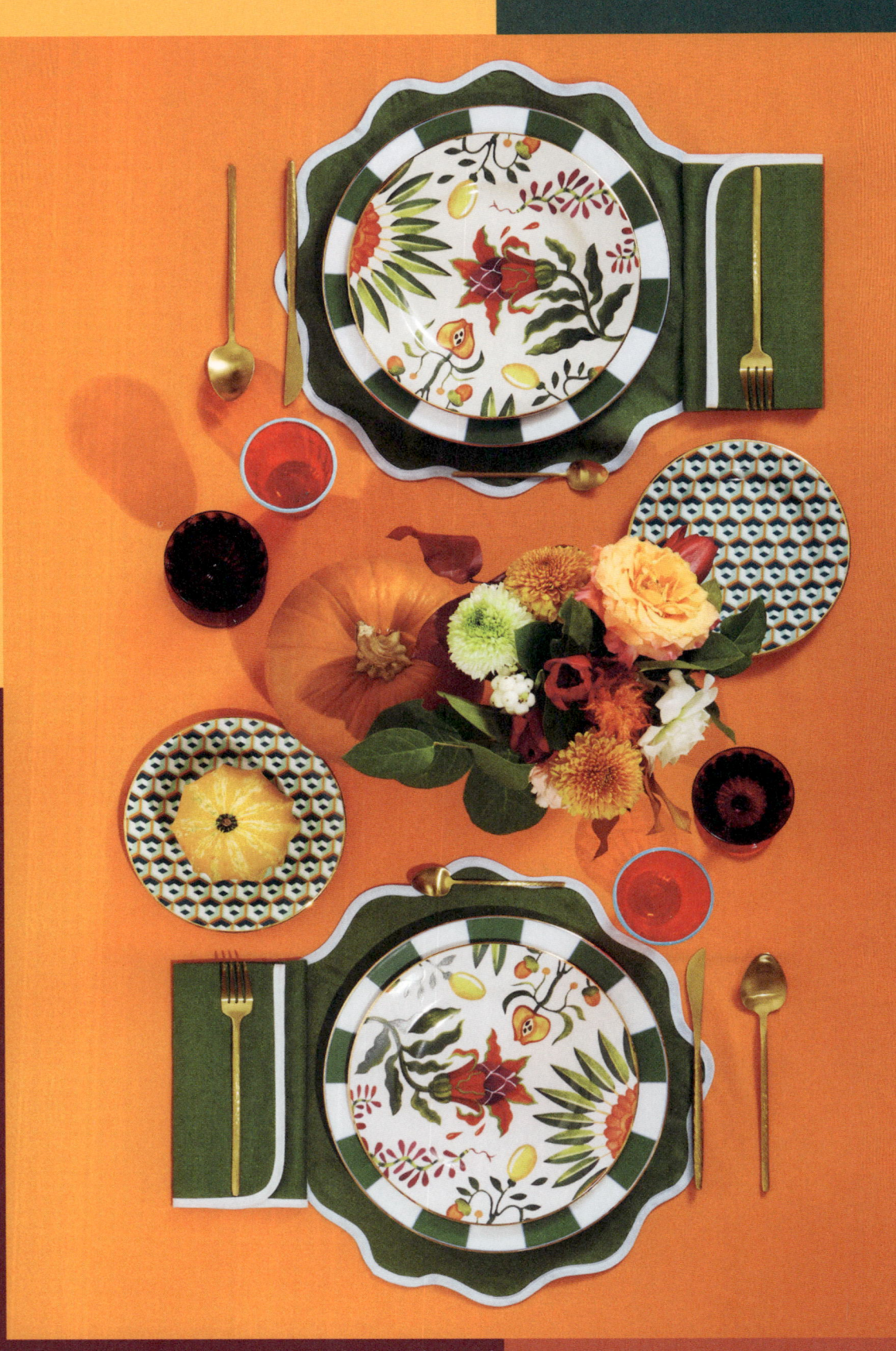

Roman Holiday, Flora and Fauna, and Cubi Collections Mix & Match

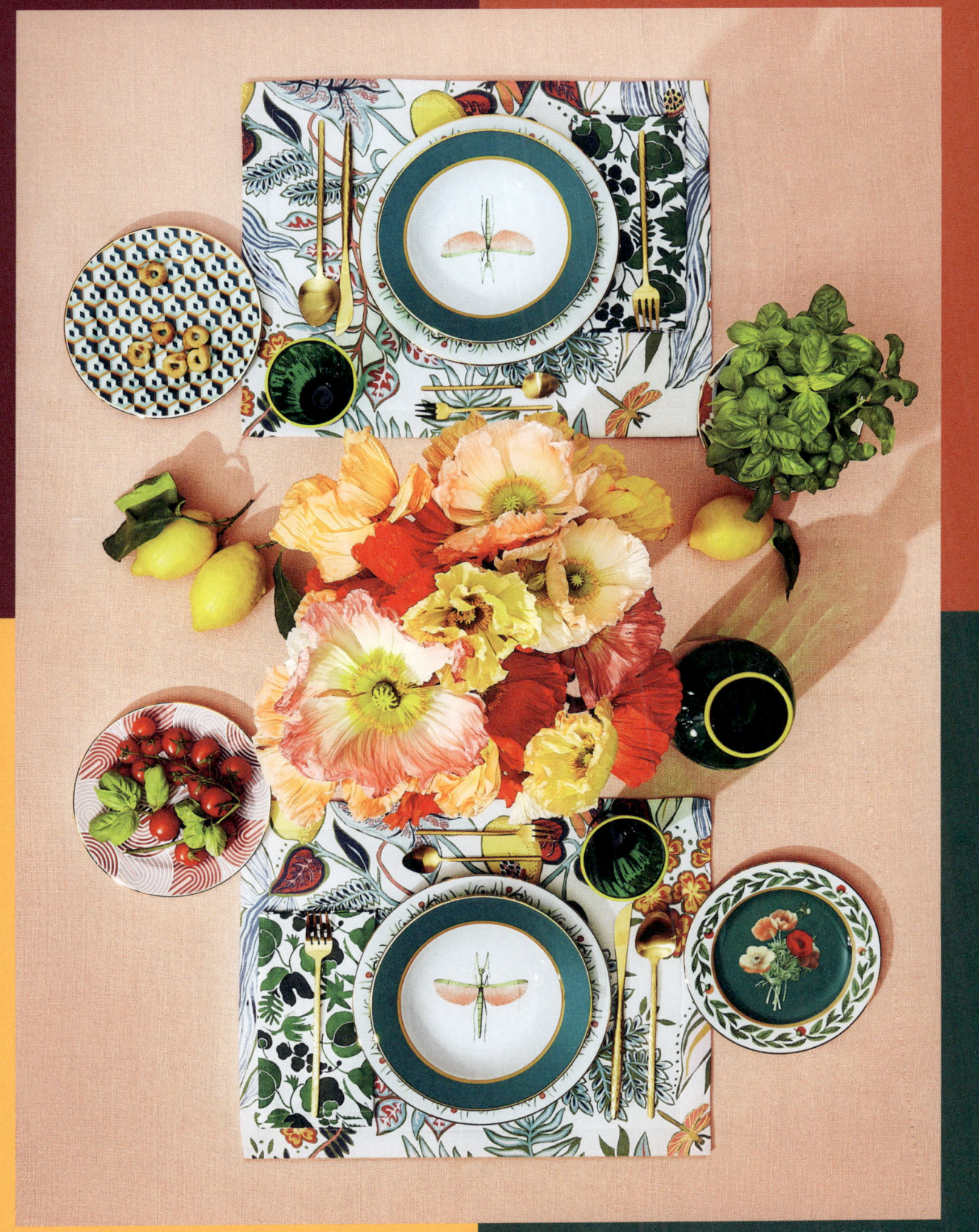

Libellula Soup and Dinner Set with Botanical Placemats

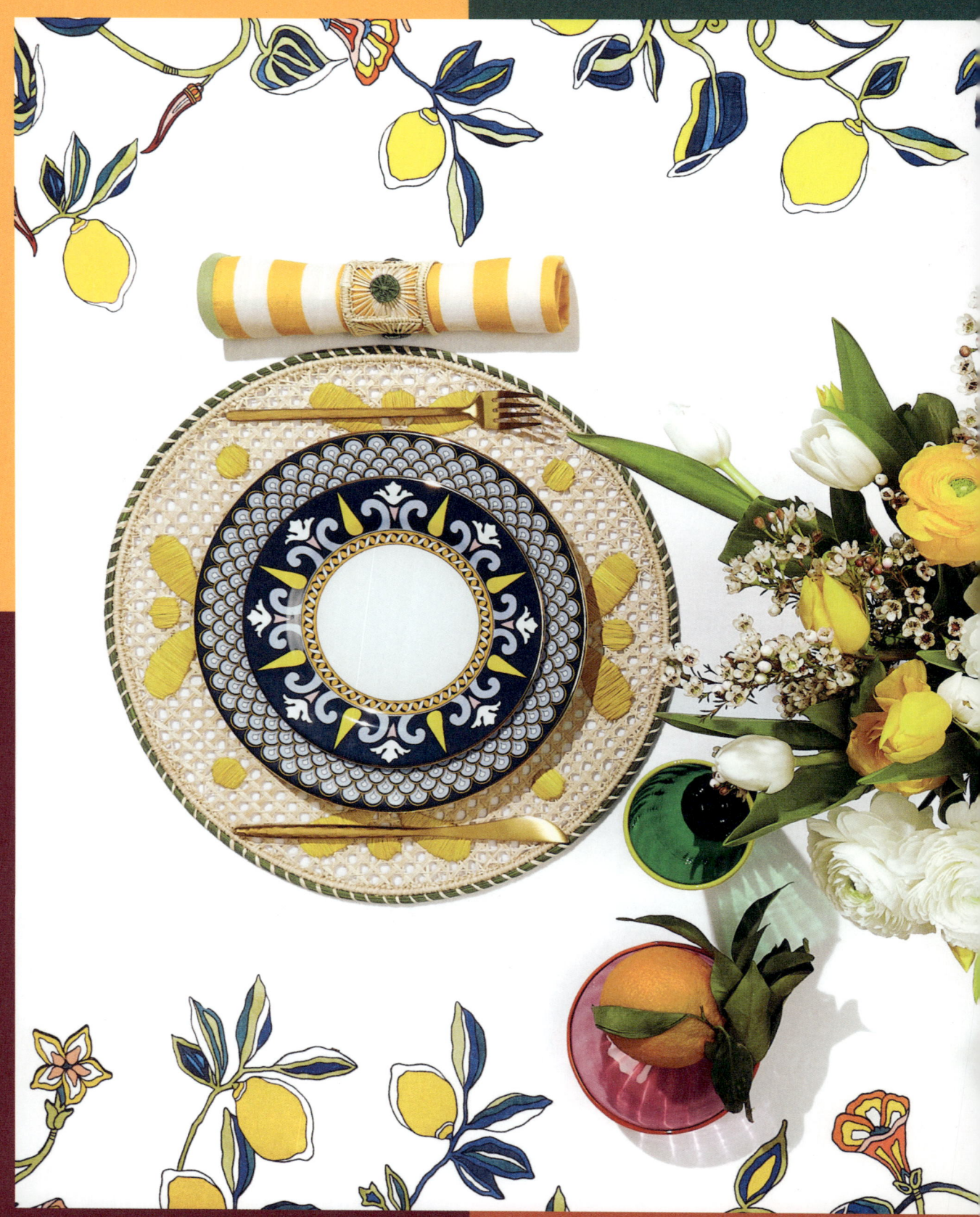

Napoli Collection

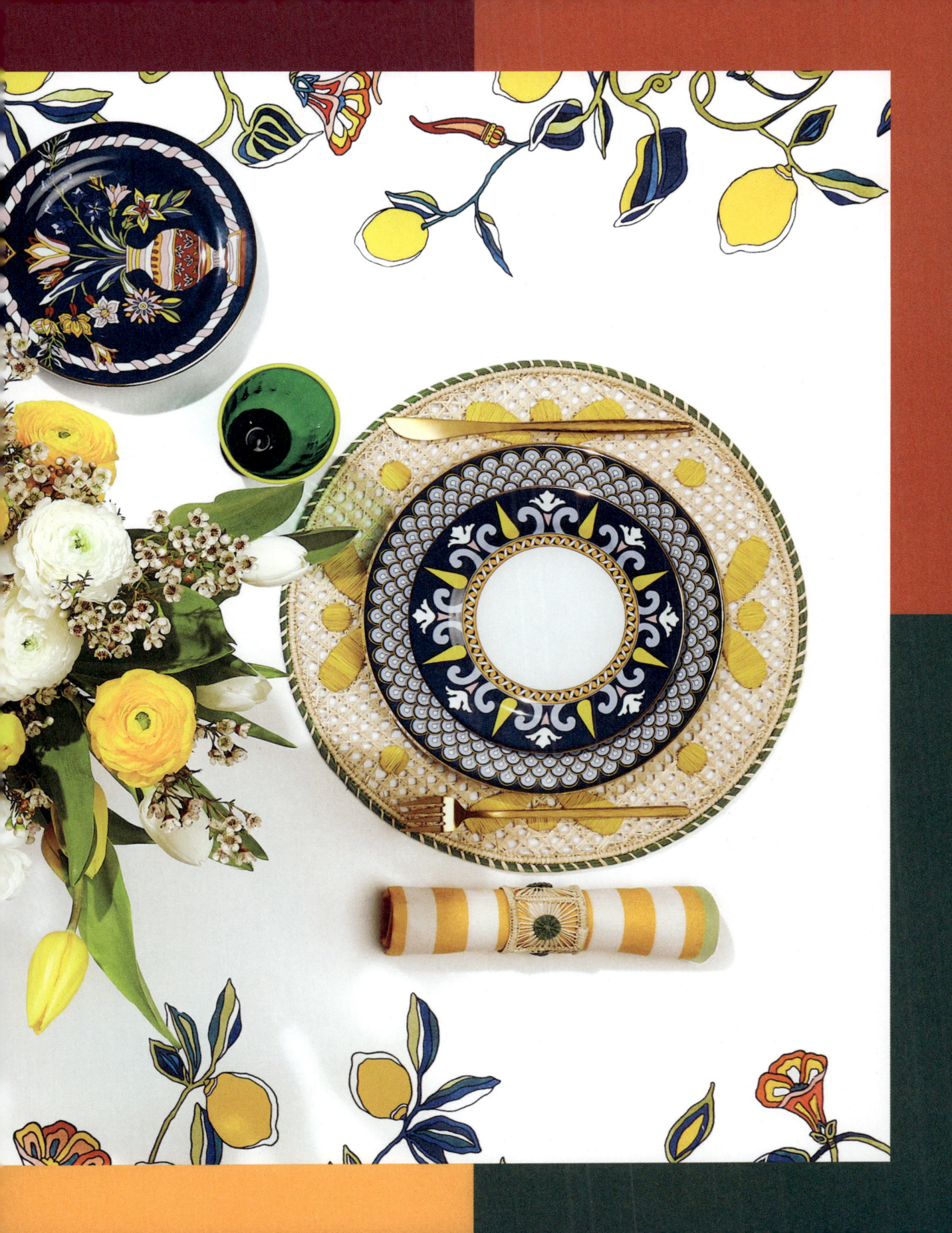

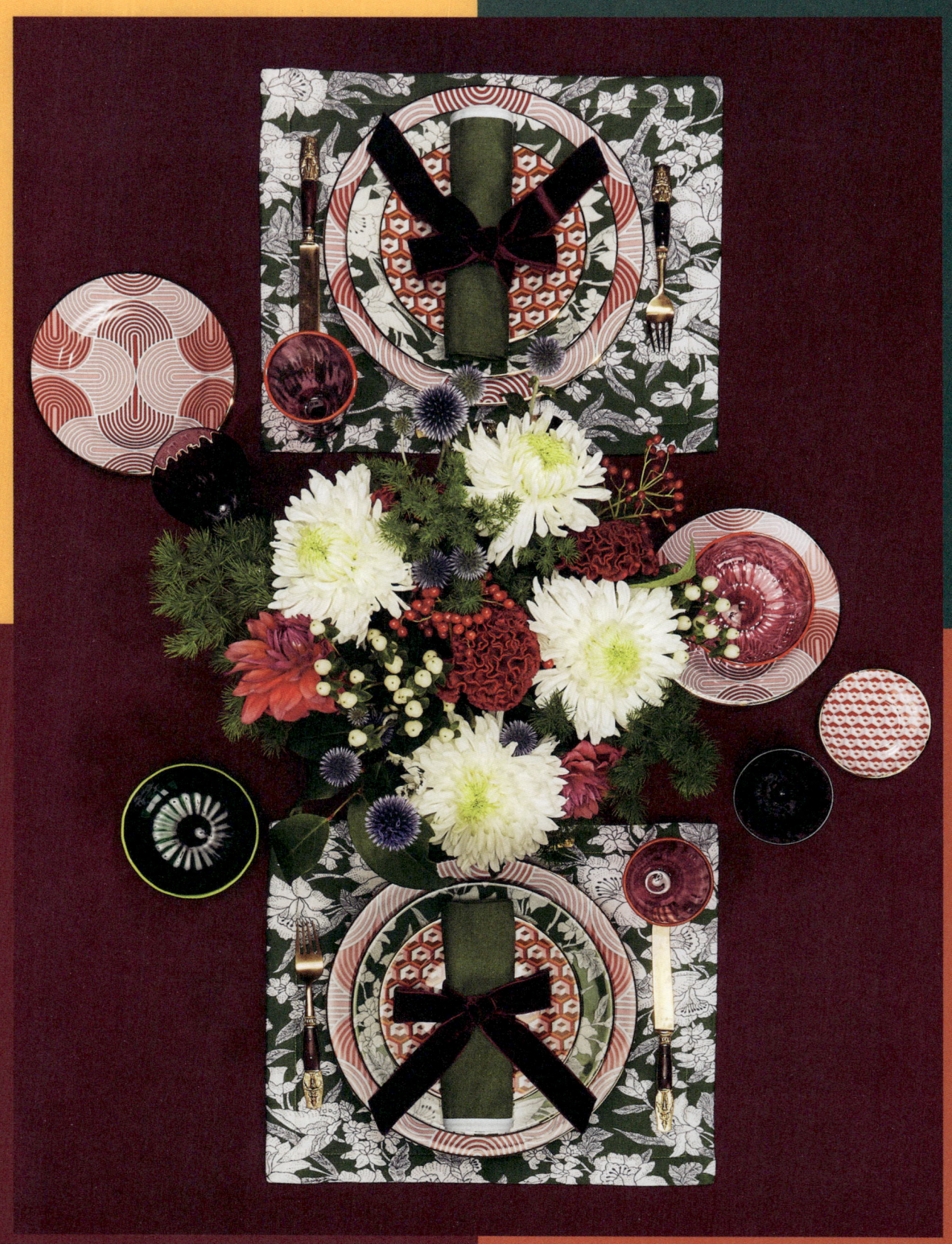

Roman Holiday, Slinky, and Cubi Collections Mix & Match

Wildbird and Cubi Collections Mix & Match

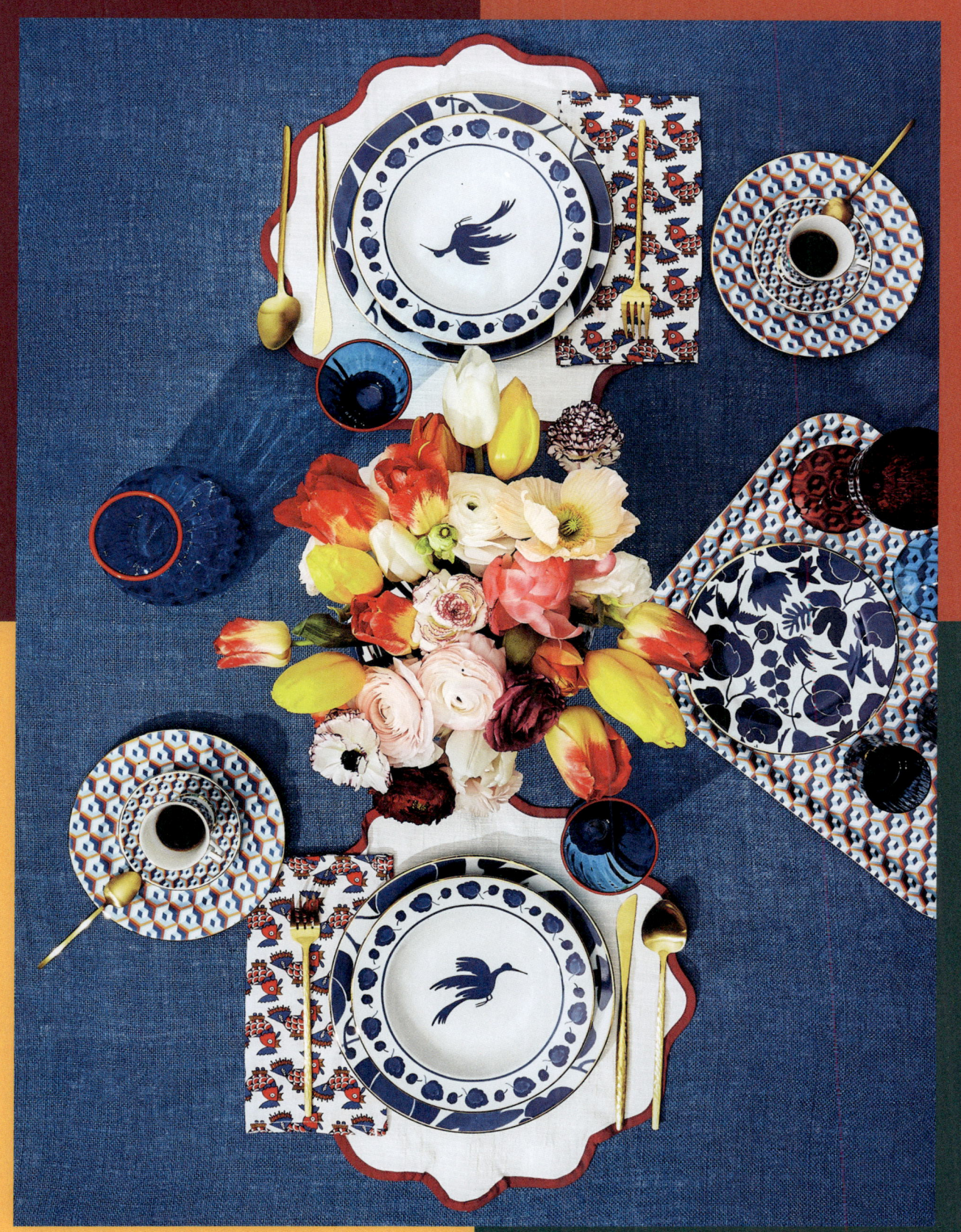

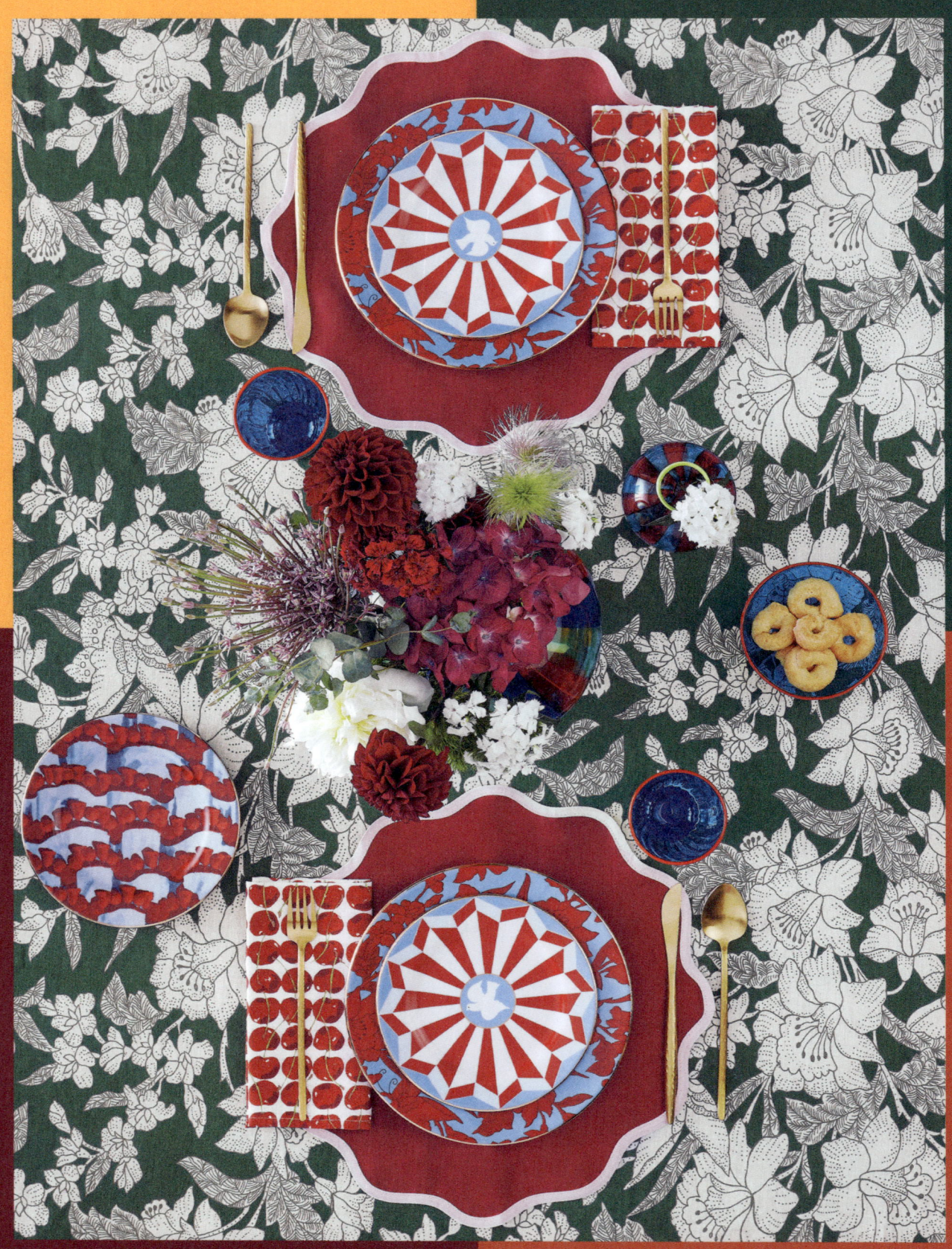

Roman Holiday Collection

Rainbow and Pineapple Collections Mix & Match

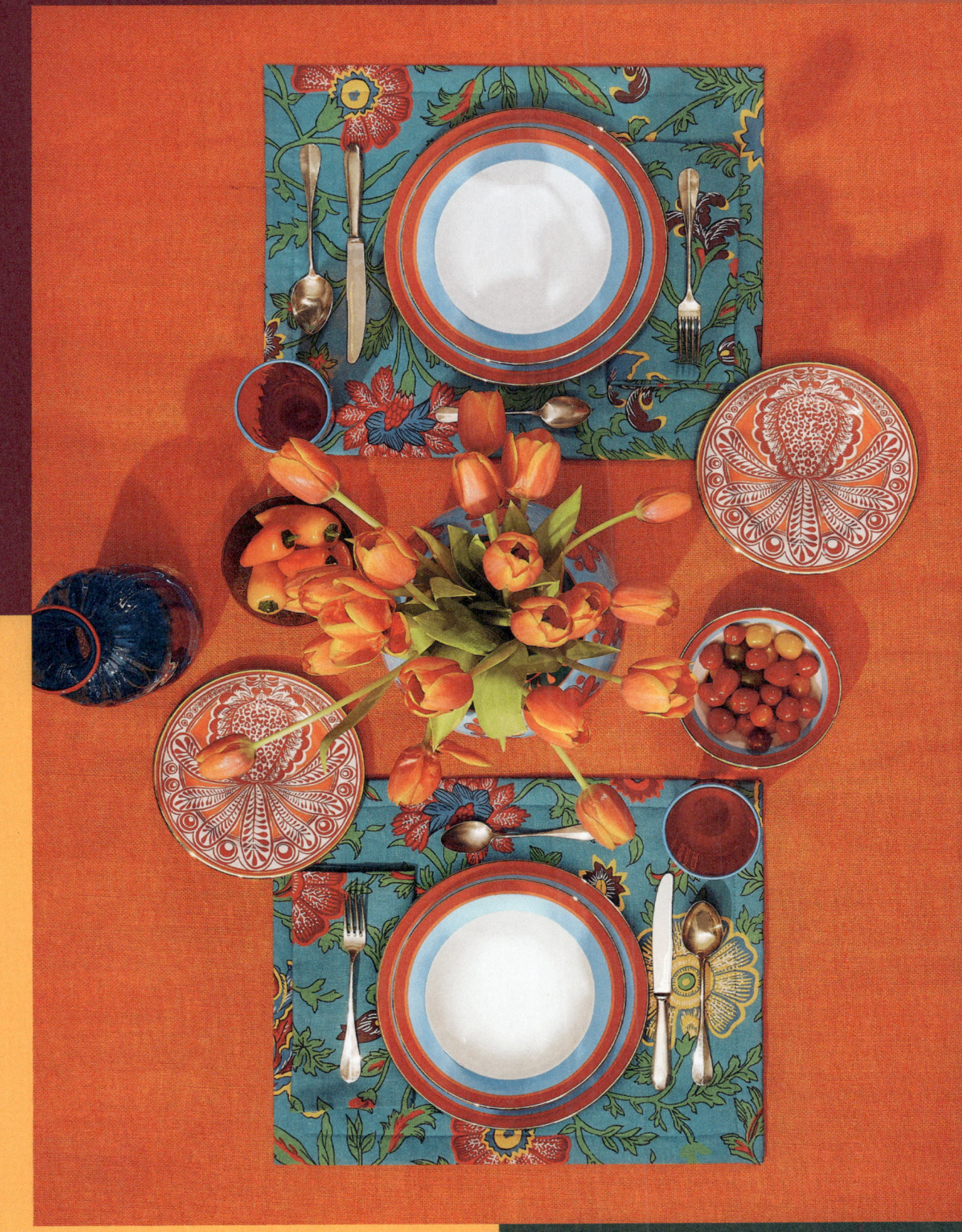

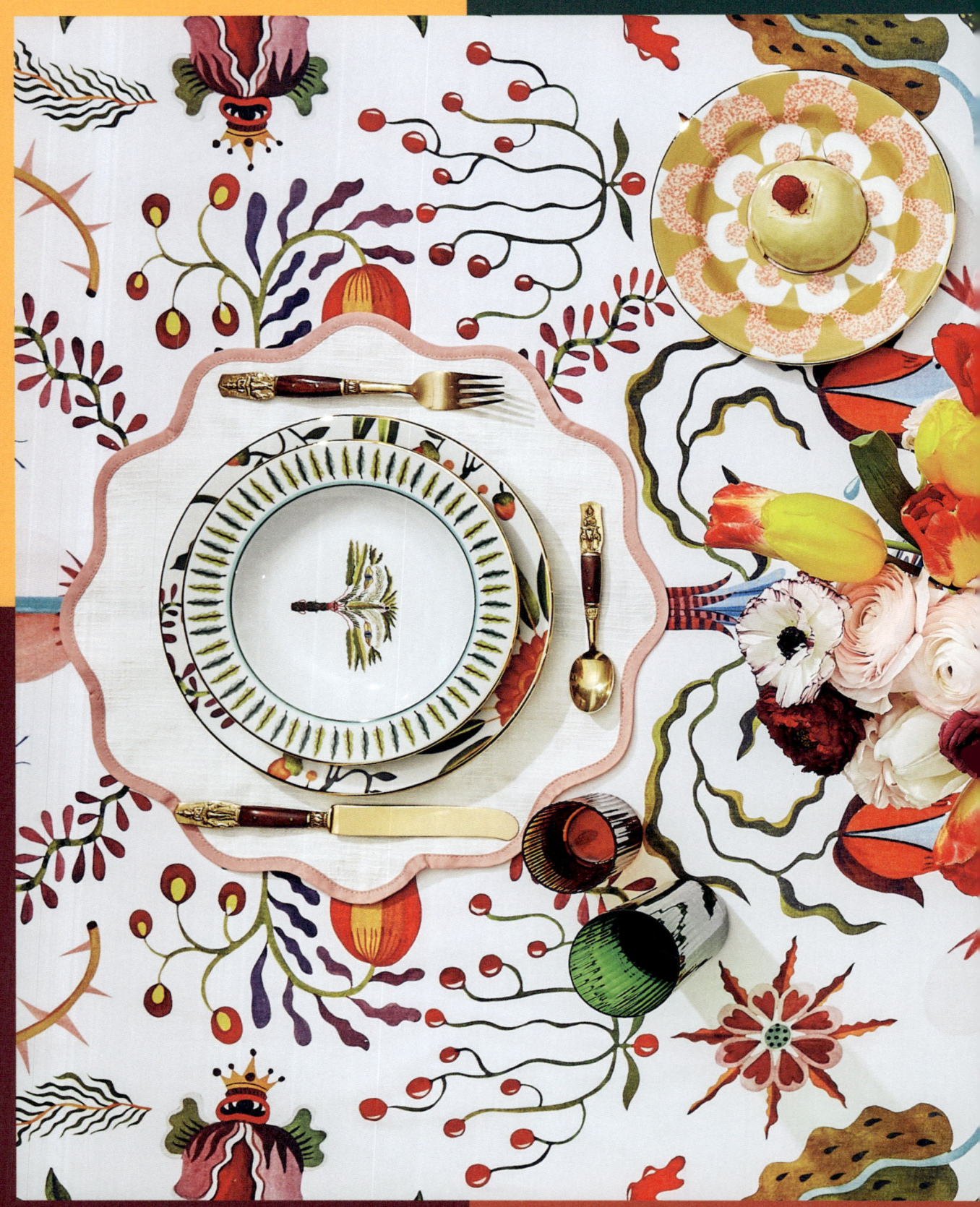

Flora & Fauna Collection

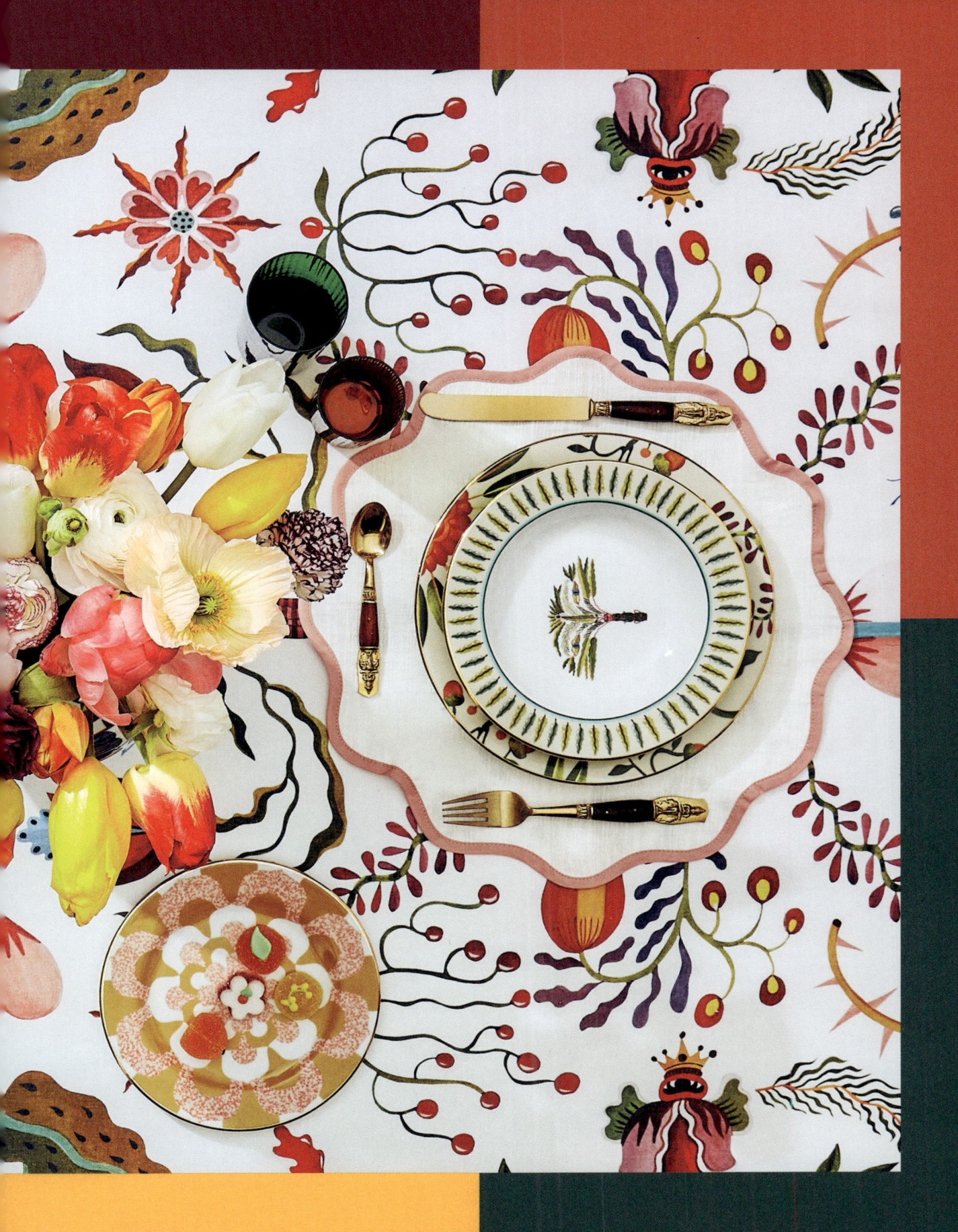

Miniscalchi and Roman Holiday Collections Mix & Match

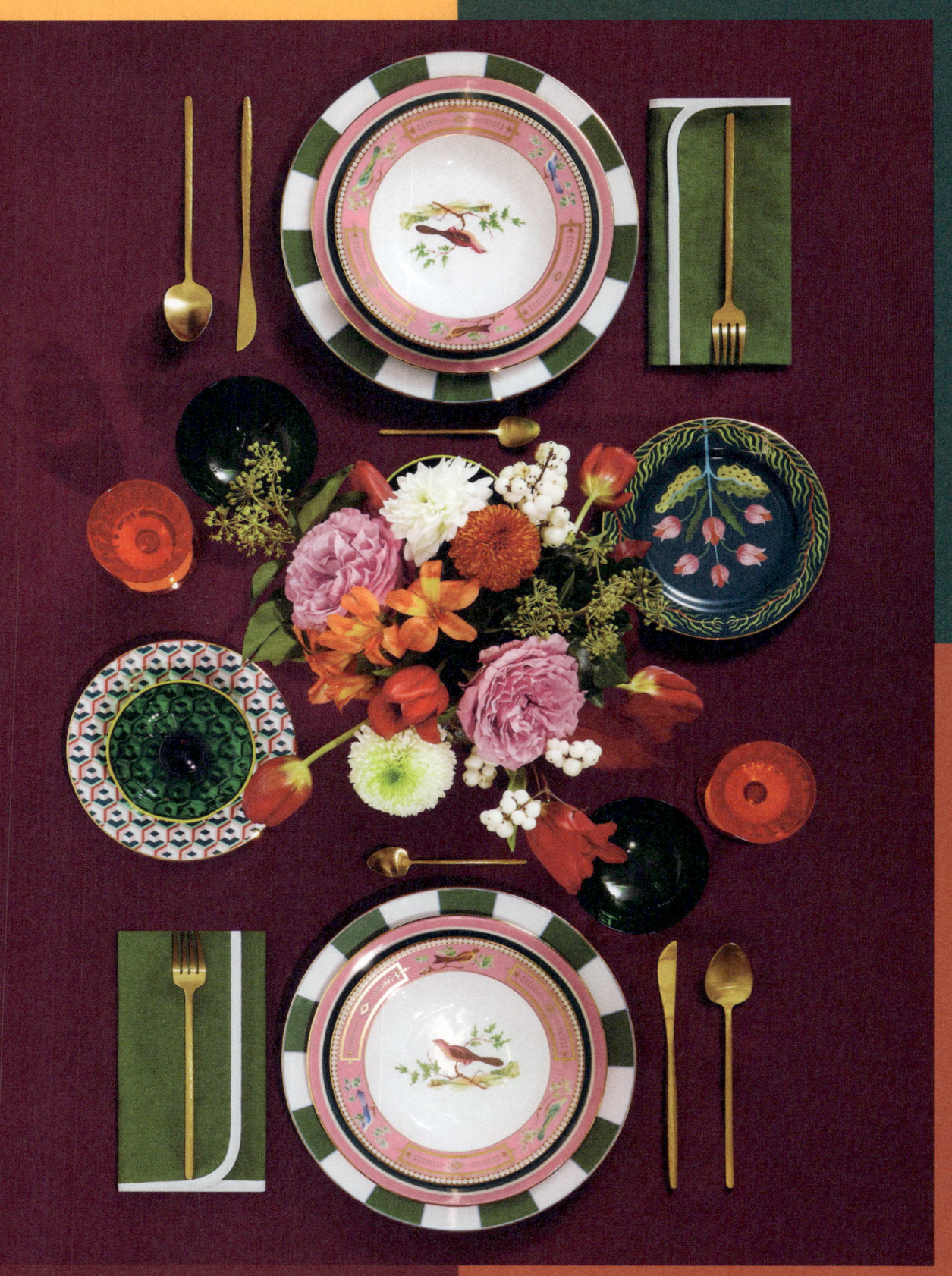

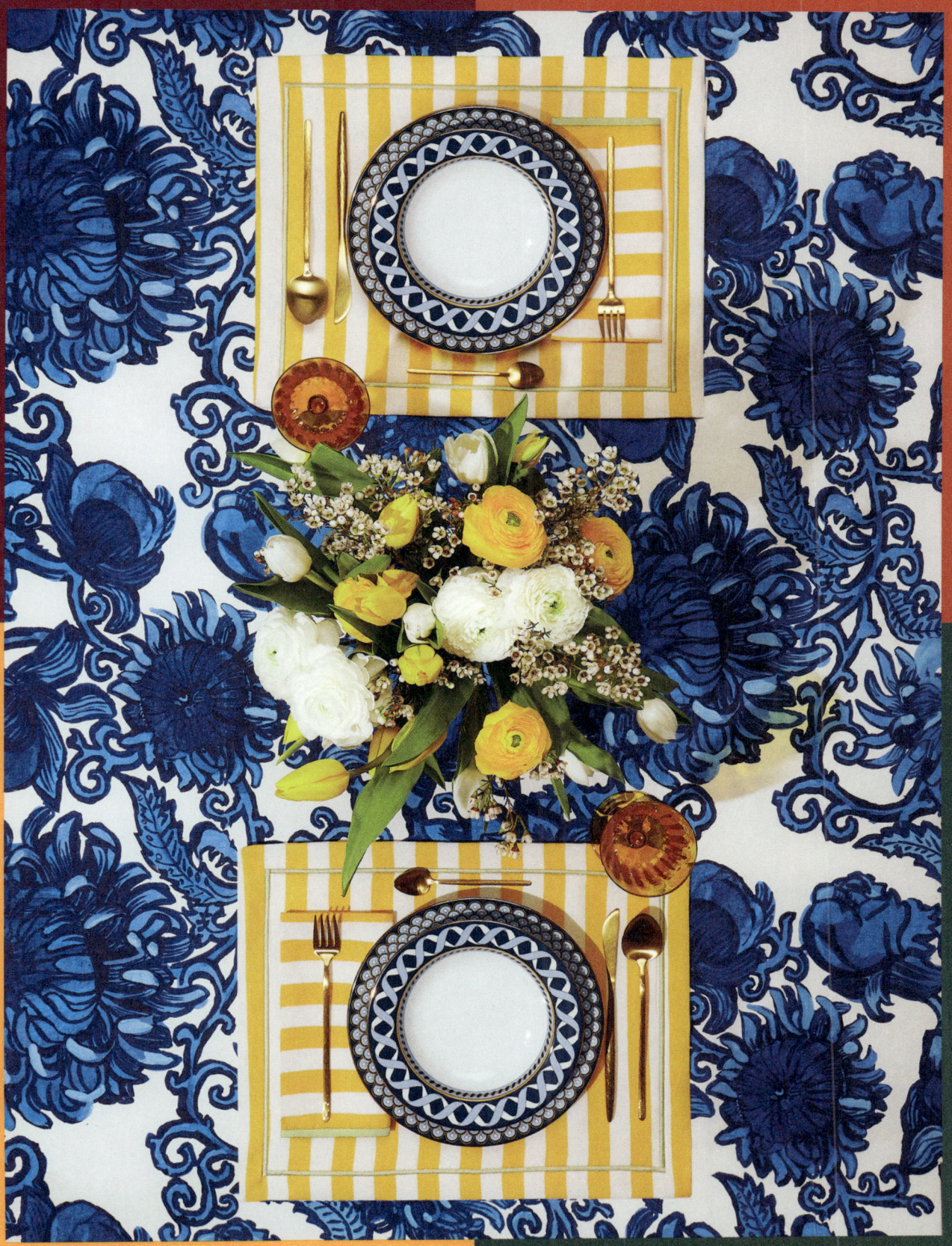

Napoli Collection
Back Cover: Wildbird Collection

READY? SET!

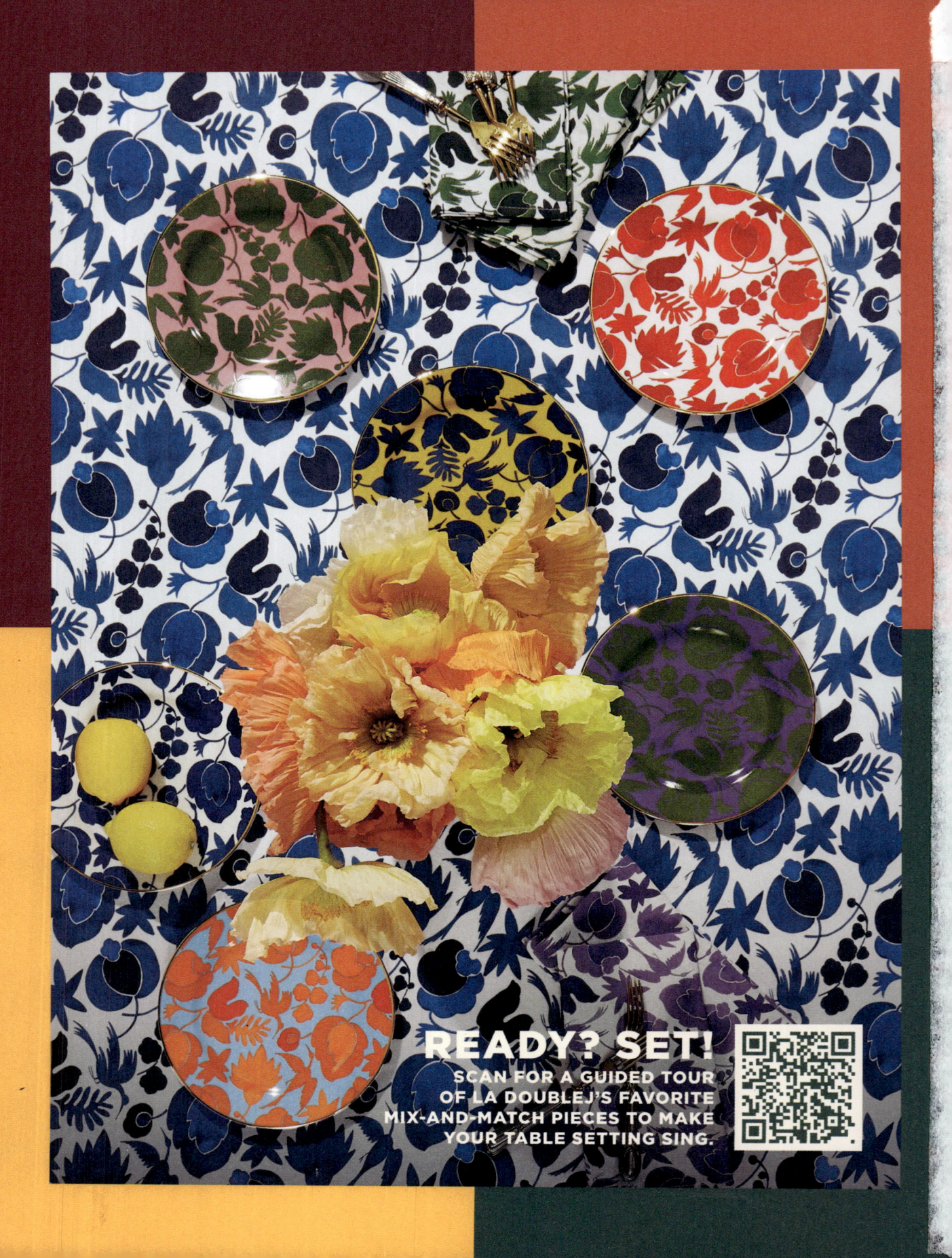

SCAN FOR A GUIDED TOUR OF LA DOUBLEJ'S FAVORITE MIX-AND-MATCH PIECES TO MAKE YOUR TABLE SETTING SING.

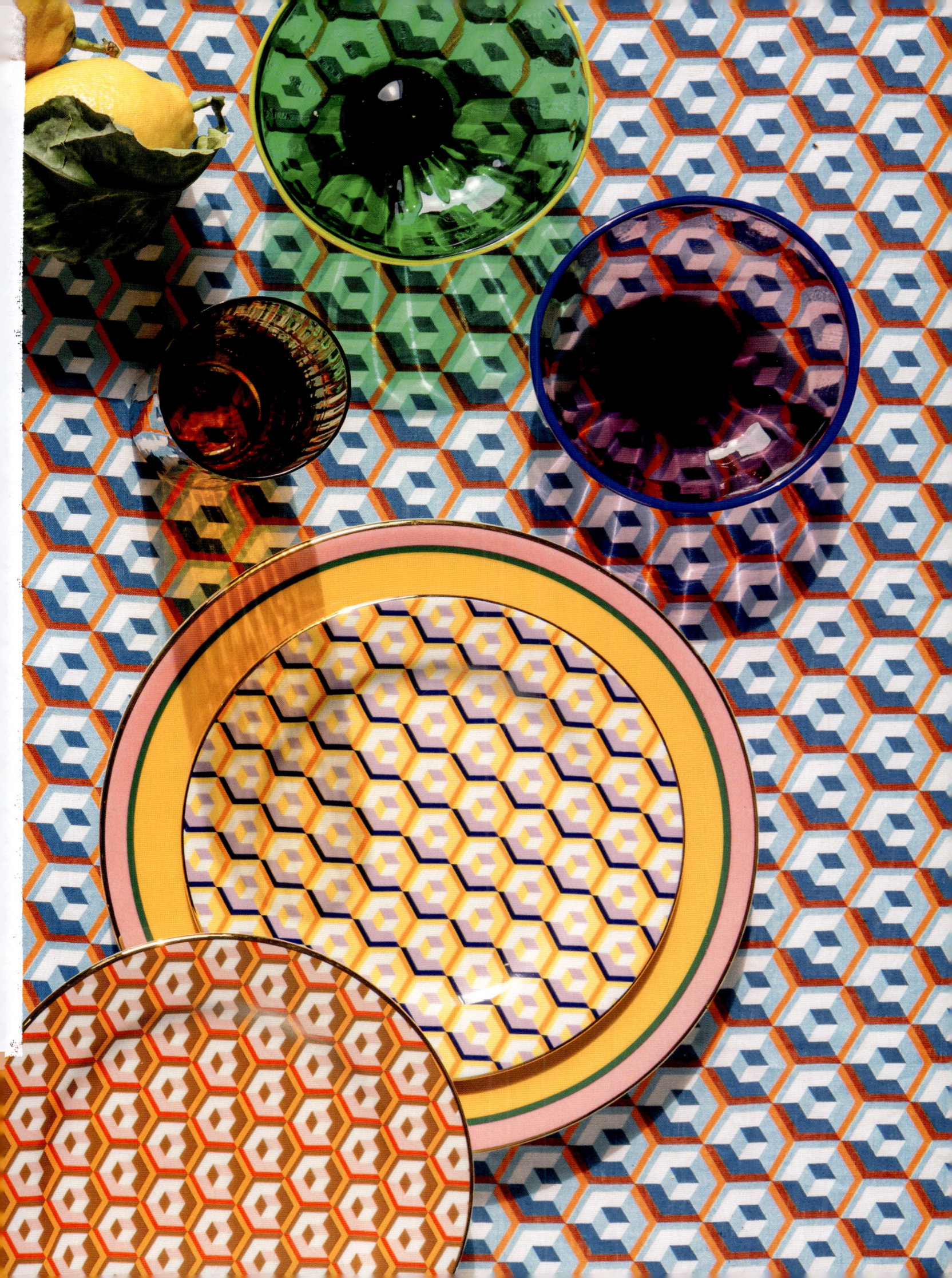

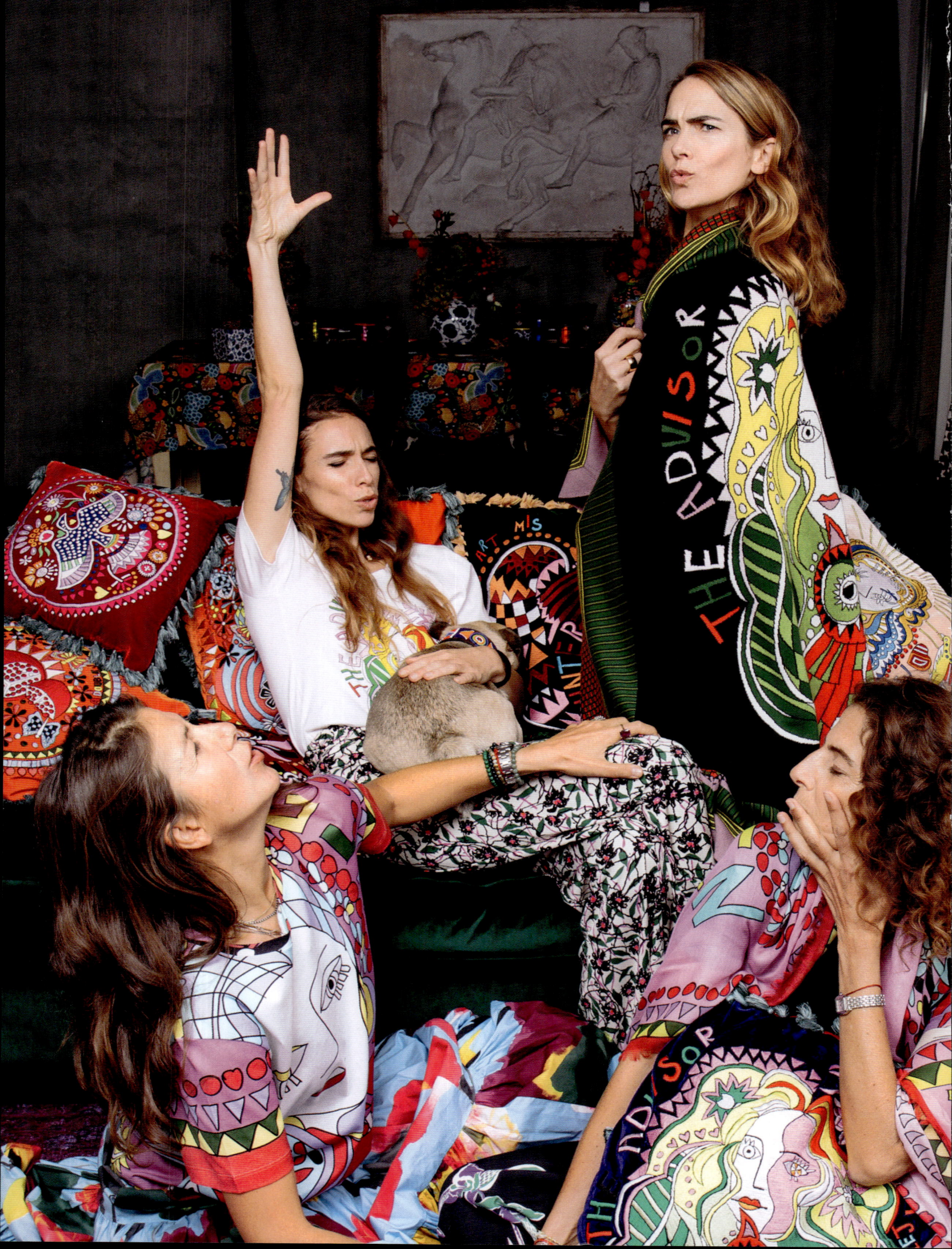

CALLING IN THE GODDESSES

In 2018, with our Greek Goddess Project, I took the first shy steps towards weaving some of the woo-woo cosmic work I was doing at home into the fabric of our company.

By this point, I had been introduced to energy healing, breathwork, sound healing, and *qi gong*, and was diving in each night to consciousness-raising books. Most intriguing to me were the sacred rites of feminine initiations that women go through as they unload their shadows and ancestral wounding and step into the light.

I had tons of tools and info on this stuff—but would anyone be interested in it? I decided to (baby) test it.

I had no idea of the psychological relevance of the Greek goddesses until my naturopath in Milan mentioned them. He described the story of the goddess Persephone, daughter of Demeter and Queen of the Underworld, who undergoes a significant psychological transformation after she is raped, kidnapped, and forced by Hades to live with him in the underworld. The wide-eyed, naive little girl who does what everyone tells her to do rises from the dark as a rich, ripe, wise woman. No one can boss her around again. The experience of darkness transforms her into a resplendent queen, an overlord of her own experience. She proves she can endure being buried in a hole by herself, using only her inner resources to discover the jewels of consciousness that are entombed in her underground psyche.

This myth is symbolic of our own inner journeys. So many of us are fearful of going below the surface of our experience. We don't want to see or feel our negative emotions, and we definitely don't want to hang out with them.

Persephone's story teaches that the opposite is true: that we find our greatest salvation and biggest growth opportunities when we are cut off from the bright sun and abundance on earth and are forced to descend into our own darkness. There, under the surface of our lives, lies all of the magic, all of the keys to who we are, what we care about, what our values are—and our true power.

The story shows the transformation that can come from embracing negative experiences, not pushing them away.

My obsession with the myth of Persephone led me to a book called *Goddesses in Everywoman* by Jean Shinoda Bolen, who explains how each goddess represents certain female archetypes that are present in every real woman on earth. The trials, the challenges, the dramas, and the victories that each goddess undergoes illuminate both their strengths and their weaknesses. These, in turn, paint a complete picture of the many aspects of the female psyche.

As I was reading and learning more about myself, I began to think that a lot of women could use these tools. So, I charged my designer Molly, who was a talented painter on the side, with designing the goddesses in a spicy way. Our goddesses looked more like abstract Picasso queens than fresh-faced Raphaels, and they provided a new, playful way of looking at these female archetypes.

MatchesFashion, always our biggest supporter and receiver of all things "weird" or new, was the first to see them. They signed up for the exclusive on homeware, plates, pillows, ponchos, swimwear, dresses, T-shirts, and handbags, and decided to throw in a launch at their fancy London townhouse, 5 Carlos Place.

I didn't want the launch to be the usual cocktail party. The goddesses deserved more. So, I invited Per van Spall, a close friend who was a *qi gong* master in Bali, to join me. As I introduced the small groups of eight to ten journalists and clients with background on the meaning of the various goddesses, Per offered them energy healing sessions, helping them to slow down, move inward, and access deeper levels of themselves so that their goddesses could come out. The event was a hit, with typically cynical, bored journalists suddenly awakened with real curiosity.

The goddesses were not a financial hit, but it was our very first spiritual voyage, and the product lived on as a sleeper favorite in our later wellness circles.

Real-life goddesses. From left: Naida Tarakcija, Giselle Bridger, and Sveva Camurati

SITTING IN THE DARK AND SWIRLING UP OUR SISTERHOOD

Covid began in March 2020 as a pure fear dump. I was literally pacing around the empty apartment in Milan that I had just moved into with a mattress on the floor and one lamp. We could not leave our homes except to go to the supermarket or pharmacy. Streets were patrolled. DoubleJ sales orders were cancelled by wholesalers left and right, not only from the new fall collection, but also from the previous collection that was already cut and sewn. Two massive global launches—Ladurée and Acqua di Parma—which were meant to explode us across multiple sales channels in Europe, the US, and Asia had to be trimmed down to bitty morsels. Many staff were panicked; some were frozen with anxiety and couldn't work at all.

At this bleak moment, I pulled out an Ayurvedic cookbook, began a massive detox, and enrolled in an online Spiritual Ascension course by Sandra Walter in Sedona, Arizona. I did morning Teams calls with the office and spent the rest of the day in absolute silence and stillness. It was the first time I'd ever spent three months by myself, and the experience rocketed me off into a completely new dimension. My editor, Scarlett, told me I should get on Instagram to discuss ways in which some of my spiritual tools could help people navigate their Covid fears. So, one morning I jumped on with an unscripted video pulled straight from my belly about what we could learn from the Coronavirus and what insights we could glean from sitting home alone. I immediately felt a new surge of energy.

I felt free and unbuckled as a river of messages came out of my mouth and onto the worldwide whatever we call it. The response was overwhelming. I received hundreds of private messages of encouragement, thanks, and requests for more advice. In that moment, I realized that what I was practicing with my teachers, healers, workshops, books, and downloads was something that our DoubleJ customer not only wanted but needed. Very soon, we began to host online virtual workshops for free for our community, introducing my roster of practitioners who have been so helpful to me along this bumpy road—and giving them a platform to share their tools. A new star constellation was born during Covid: the DoubleJ Sisterhood.

The Sisterhood is a circle-based container for our High Vibration manifesto. It is also a practical manifestation of what we mean when we talk about Divine Mother frequencies: connection, listening, feeling, sharing, and learning to expand our consciousness, together.

The activity of the Sisterhood unfolded in virtual or live circles at retreats, workshops, and across social media and podcasts. We created Spirit Tour editorials on some of our favorite Sisters; we mapped the best places to raise your vibration or expand your consciousness. This broadened further when I launched my Spirit Tickle Newsletters—jampacked with essays, Q&As, personal revelations from my own spiritual practice, and practical tips on how to start.

Once we were able to travel again, we rethought all of our events, swirling in some spirituality. Our Bergdorf Goodman pop-up shop opened with a holotropic breathwork session with a shaman; our barefoot-on-the-beach dinner with Kirna Zabête in the Hamptons featured an energy-healing circle; and we did immersive yoga with Catalina Denis in Paris. Eventually, we took the spirit show on the road with the Six Senses Ibiza retreat. I led a spiritual gathering at the Mezzatorre in Ischia with yoga teacher Manizeh Rimer, then I co-hosted a "Sacred Journey to Egypt" with my friend and high priestess, Dee Kennedy (at which most of our fellow travelers showed up in La DoubleJ).

The Sisterhood is about a shared spirit of creativity; we've expanded our circle to women creating in other fields—launching a campaign with The Selby in LA and highlighting the amazing work of designers and architects during the Salone del Mobile. The majority of our clients are women, but we feel the Sisterhood applies to anyone who wishes to sit in a circle of community, sharing, and listening.

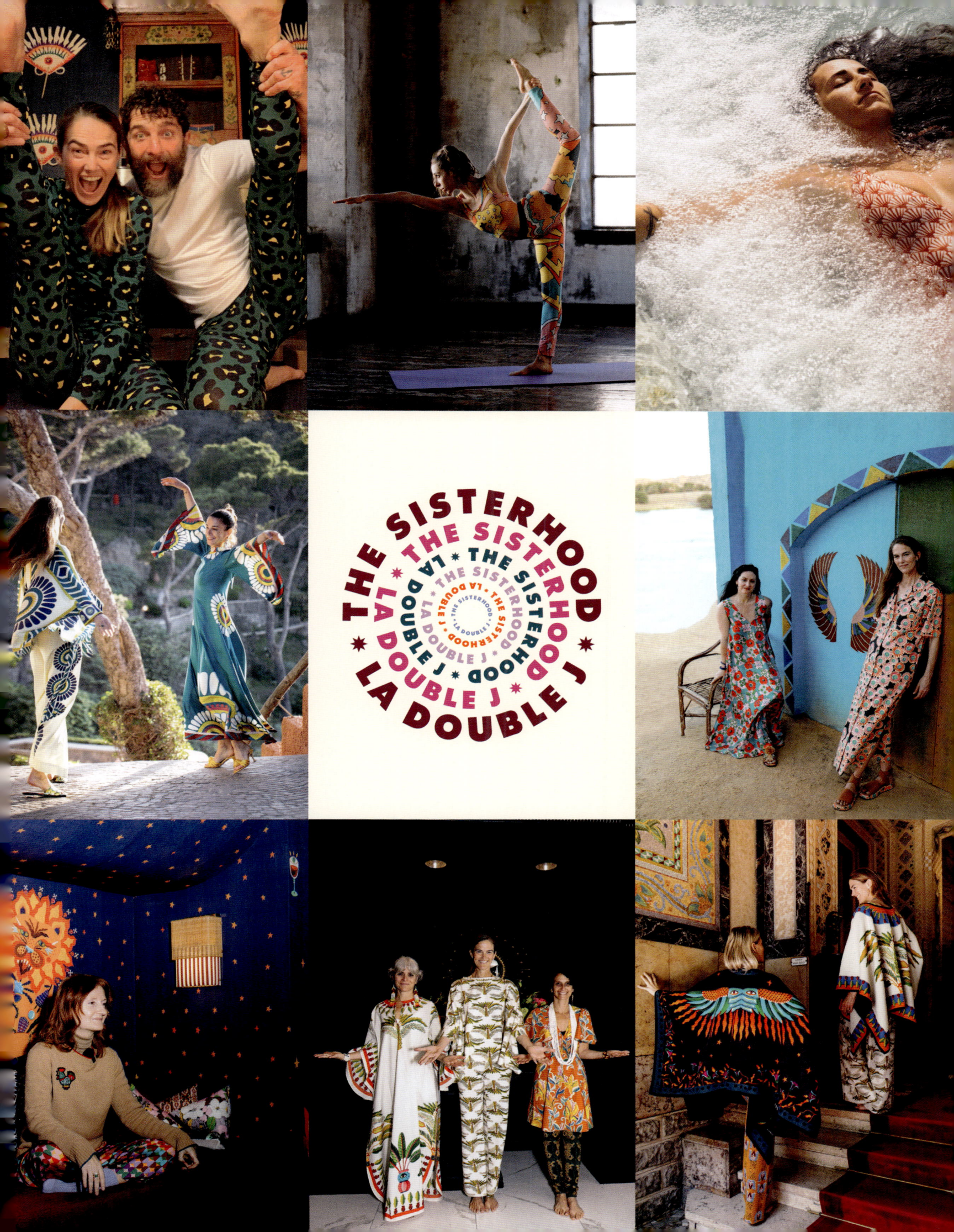

THE SISTERHOOD · THE SISTERHOOD · LA DOUBLE J · LA DOUBLE J

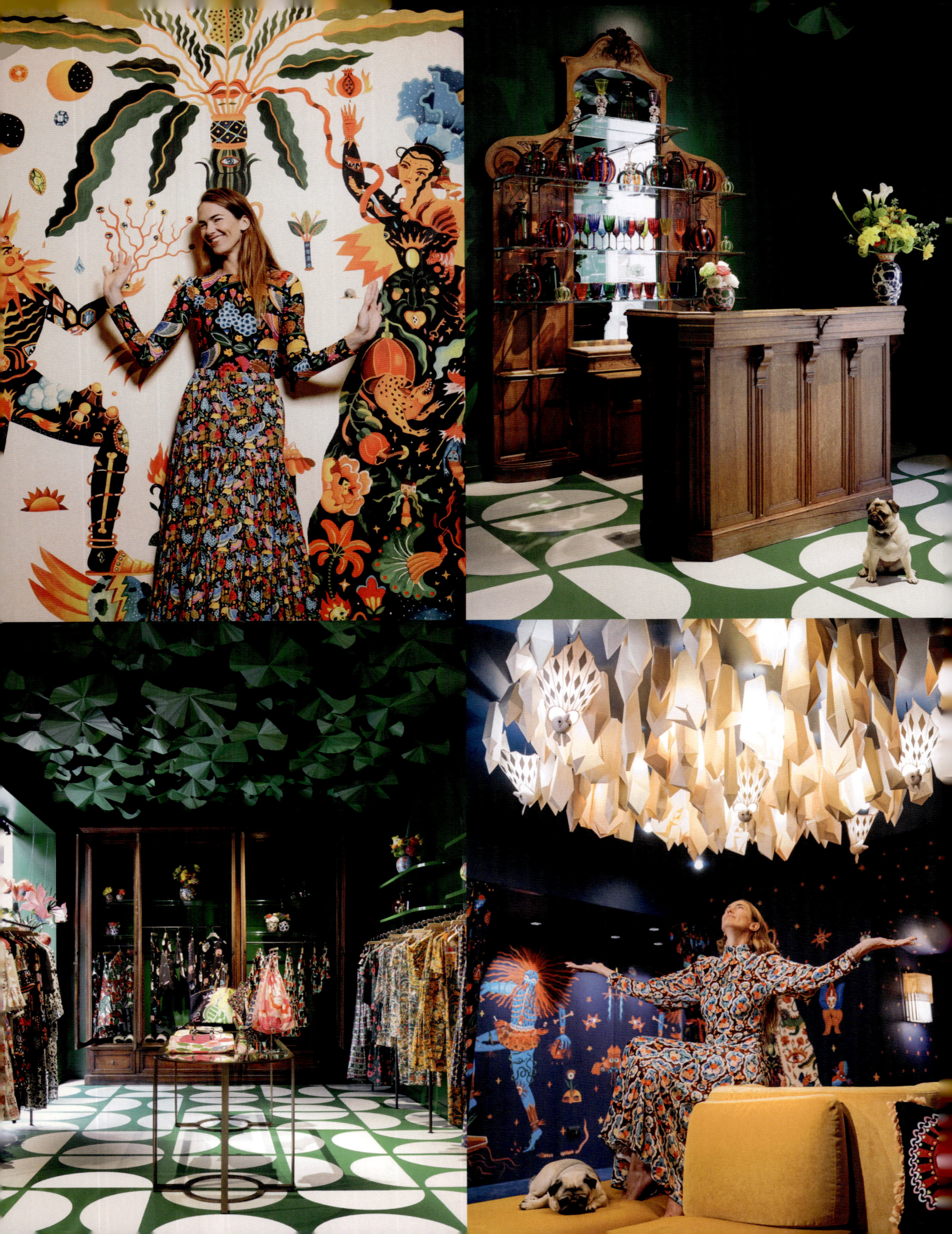

(BIG ASS) SEED #3

LET'S OPEN A STORE

A few months later, Andrea called me up and delivered his biggest, baddest seed yet. He had somehow managed during the shutdowns to secure a lease on Milan's Via Sant'Andrea, a fancypants slice of real estate next to Chanel and across the street from Bottega Veneta. *Let's open a store!* he trilled. *No effing way!* I immediately slammed back. We had somehow managed to keep sales floating on our website during Covid, thanks to my team's incredible dedication, and had not fired a single employee. But we were skin and bones, well below sales goals, and emotionally exhausted. A few weeks later, my hard "no" softened into a "maybe" and then into a begrudging *okay, let's try it*.

Once I moved into acceptance mode, I got another download. We could open a shop, but it would look and feel like no other. Andrea kept asking me to deliver "a concept" and I kept yelling back at him, *I don't have one!* Instead, I just moved where my own spiritual waters were pushing me and began unpacking a messy bag of inspiration nuggets. A few months prior, I had dug down into reading *The Kuan Yin Transmission* by spiritual guide Alana Fairchild and had grown obsessed with the five archetypes of the Divine Mother. I discovered a Romanian artist called Aitch on Instagram who I loved and cold-wrote her asking if she'd illustrate my Divine Mother archetypes—she had no idea who Kuan Yin, Isis, Green Tara, Kali were, but she'd of course heard of Mother Mary. We began a furious digital exchange of ideas over the coming months.

As always, we were on a super-tight budget; as always, I called on friends from all over. Architect Luca Cipeletti came in to chop up the place into logical spaces; Paolo Badesco and Costantino Affuso were roped in for interior design and their expert eye for vintage furniture, including a nineteenth-century bar we used as a check-out desk. The artist JoAnn Tan handmade hundreds of lotus leaves from stone paper that we used to cover the ceiling pipes to save money and to create our flower-headed goddesses in the windows. The entire downstairs floor became a Sacred Grotta dedicated to the Divine Mother, with all of Aitch's archetypes laid out by our graphics team to cover every inch of the cave-like walls, not to mention snakes, eyeballs, yonis, and other magical symbols. Our store is a wild, wacky, funny, colorful playpen of delights. Dogs and kids love it, too.

When it launched in April 2021, most people cried, *Wait, WHAT? You're opening a store right now during Covid?!* Yes, we were. Just as Milan sat empty and dark, we had yet another opportunity to cheerlead for the city and the country. When people were feeling dense and depressed, that was just the moment to turn on our own inner bright lights, shine the socks off everyone, and show the world we had faith even when everything appeared broken. We love Italy, and we were ready for this town to resurrect.

Not only did our shop not look like any other store, it also had an unintended "concept"—it was a Divine Mother vortex. I held Divine DNA workshops in the Grotta, which doubled as a VIP sales room, as well as channelings by the spiritual teacher Claudia Navone and yoga with yin master Marco Migliavacca. The space became a portal for connecting to the same feminine energy I had been cultivating all this time in Italy. We went from Mamma Milano as our muse to off-planet mystical priestesses who were channeling the very same energy.

Although our shop is designed to sell merchandise, it became a bigger opportunity to anchor and engage with the Sisterhood. More and more it's clear that I do not just want to sell a woman a dress. I am happier if I can get her to start meditating, introduce her to a new *pranayama* breath technique, hook her up with an energy healer, get her to open her heart space, and put her in touch with her intuition—all topics of our Zoom webinars and in-store workshops.

Opposite: Some of the most high-vibration corners of our store

CIAO CIAO!! ENDINGS AND BEAUTIFUL BEGINNINGS

I certainly could never have expected where this journey, which began one desiccated, infernal Milanese summer, would carry me. And Mamma Milano is still bouncing me along on her loopy rainbow path. Did I mention I now love Milan? I truly do.

Being bathed in that gratitude is certainly what has made my experience as a founder that much brighter and more abundant. The baby known as La DoubleJ is now a full-fledged teenager, and she is prancing around like the best of them, wearing a miniskirt and glittery eye shadow, taking selfies, and sass-talking her parents all day long. We love her, though, and have been quick to adjust ourselves to her more mature tastes.

Our company events—with retailers, editors, and clients—have morphed from traditional parties with cocktails and people standing around chatting into deeper realms of inspiration. I always think, *how can we plug this group of people into a higher-realm energy circuit?* We bring in sound and energy healers, breathwork specialists, or a side dish of meditation and yoga, to almost every gathering we do. Even our company off-site started with a sharing and meditation circle before we jumped into reviewing numbers and celebrating ourselves.

And we haven't stopped collaborating: from our furniture collection with The Socialite Family in Paris, to our takeovers of Sotheby's London HQ, as well as cafés in New York and restaurants in Milan, which we dressed in head-to-toe print for fashion week. We've hung a bat installation in our downstairs *grotta* (where we now have a resident yogi), and we use our shop windows in Milan to highlight the angels, aliens, and spirit animals that are a guiding force in our creative wave.

We are now sold in nearly 200 stores globally; our e-commerce business ships to countries on every continent in the world (except Antarctica!); we make four collections of ready-to-wear per year, two homeware collections, and countless capsules and exclusive products for friends and retailers. We are a swirling pod of non-stop creative energy.

Another swerve I didn't foresee: Andrea and I didn't make it as a couple. After eighteen years together, we split up. Everyone told me I was a fool to keep working with my ex-husband, but I shooed off the naysayers. I knew that both he and I were deeply committed to co-parenting our baby and made a vow to take her all the way—to Princeton if she so desired. Since 2018, Andrea has taken on a much more active role within the company. He was responsible for creating our highly modern business model that blends twenty-first-century e-commerce know-how with his financial smarts and deep industry understanding, all of which has kept us dancing with ourselves, ahead of the competition. For many years, he served as a strategist and part-time CEO. Trickster-farmer that he is, he keeps handing me seeds to plant. He has become one of the key reasons for our continued success. I could not do this without him. Thank you dear, darling Ciccoli.

Ciccoli, Pepper, and me

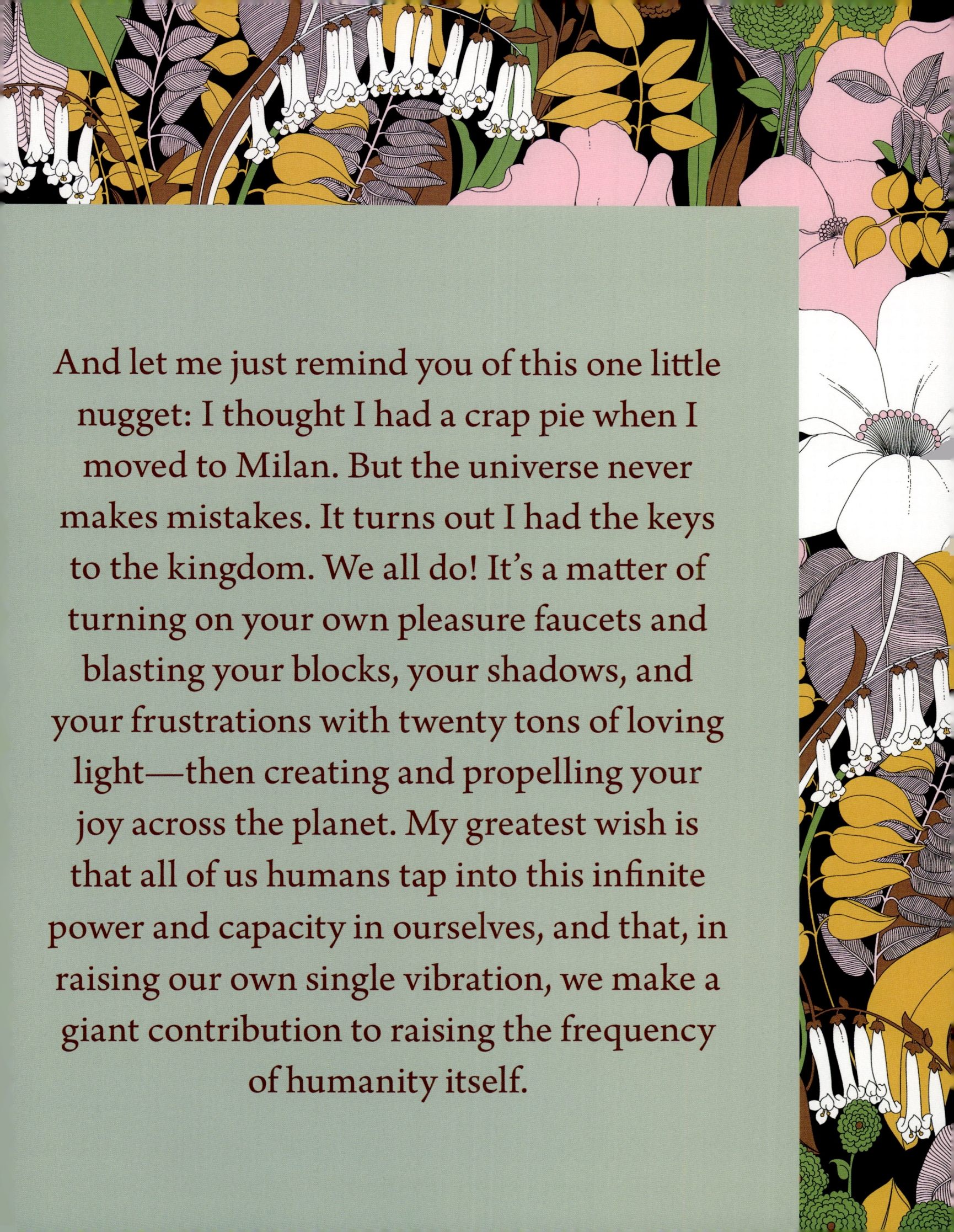

And let me just remind you of this one little nugget: I thought I had a crap pie when I moved to Milan. But the universe never makes mistakes. It turns out I had the keys to the kingdom. We all do! It's a matter of turning on your own pleasure faucets and blasting your blocks, your shadows, and your frustrations with twenty tons of loving light—then creating and propelling your joy across the planet. My greatest wish is that all of us humans tap into this infinite power and capacity in ourselves, and that, in raising our own single vibration, we make a giant contribution to raising the frequency of humanity itself.

RAISE
VIBRA

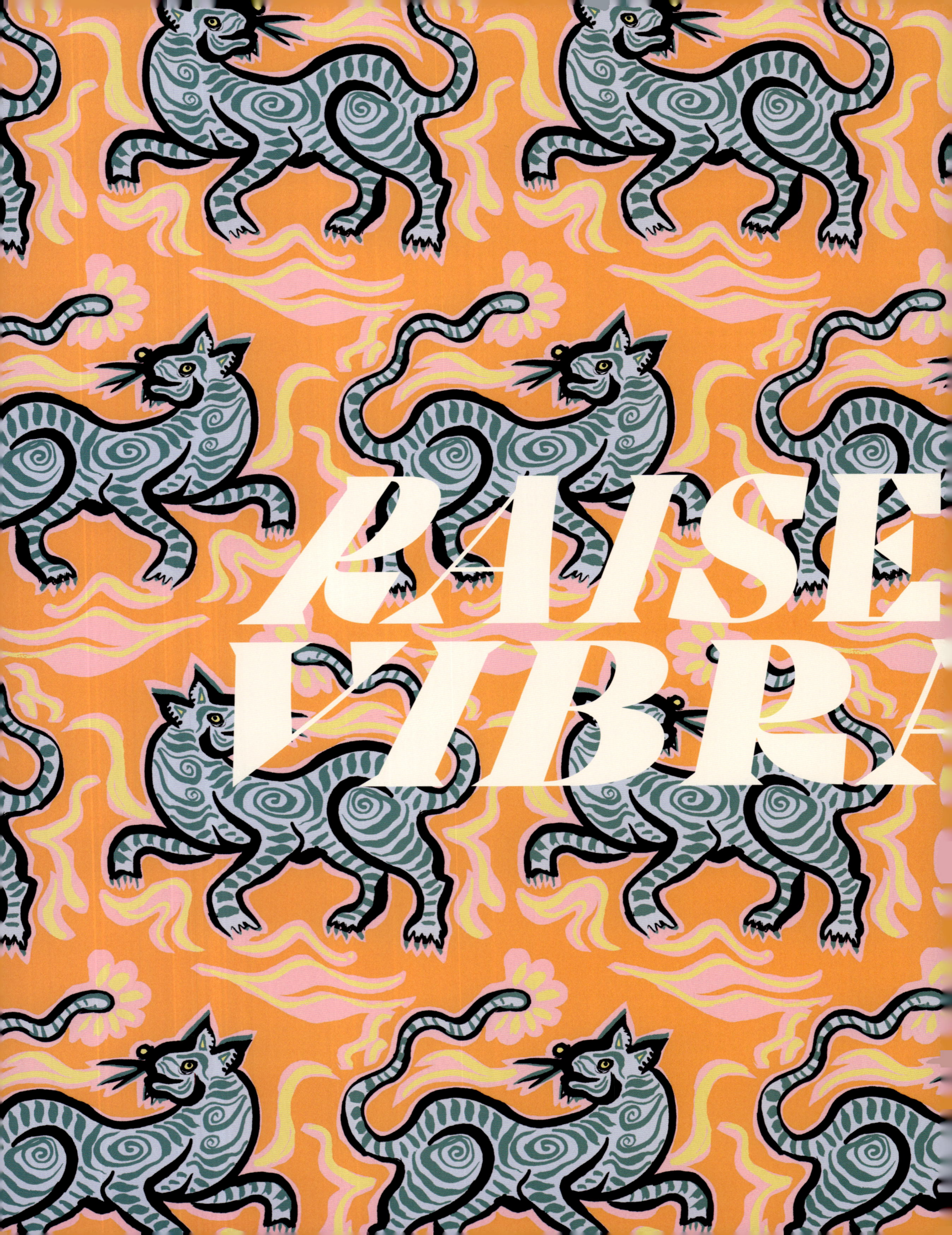

YOUR
ITION

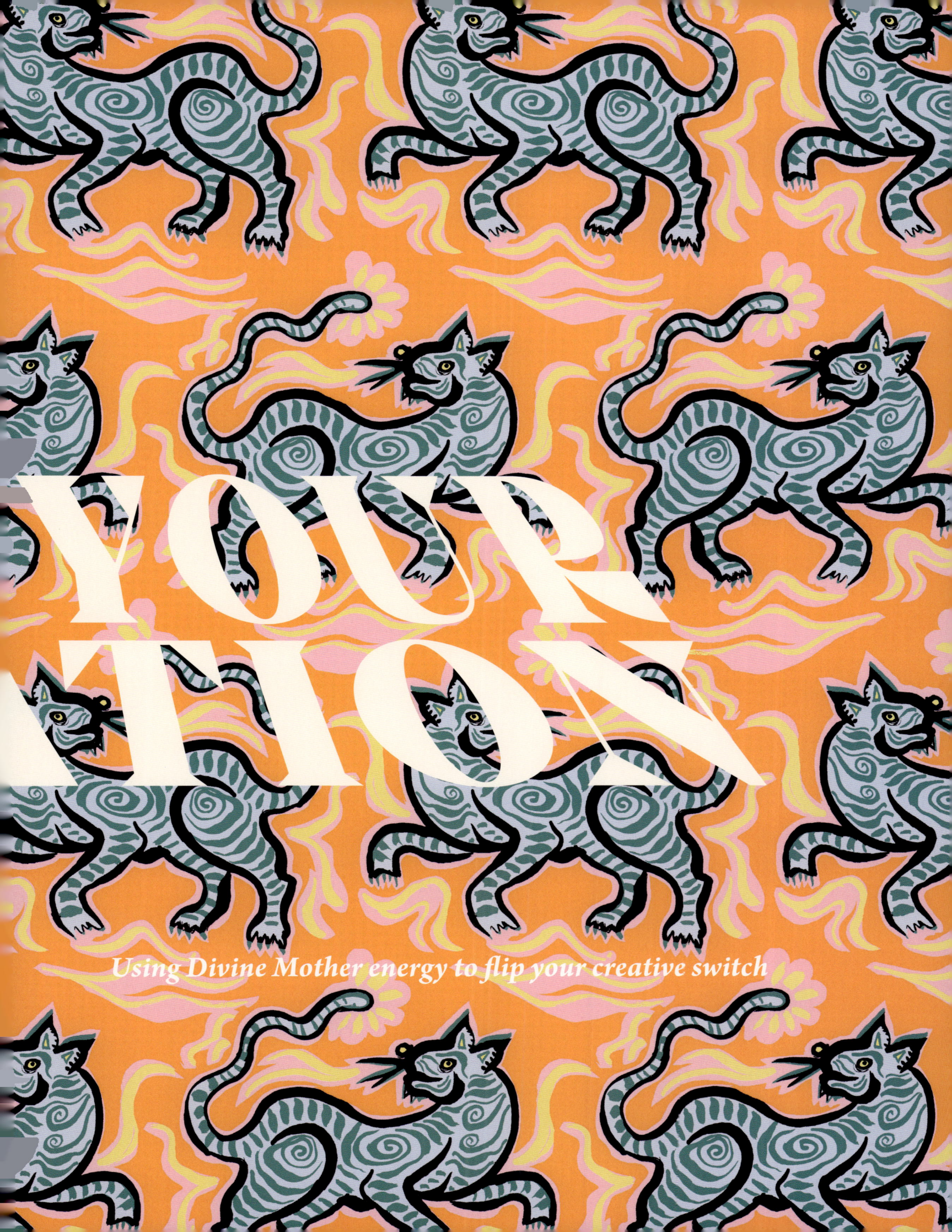

Using Divine Mother energy to flip your creative switch

WONDER POWERS —ACTIVATE!

We are all here on planet Earth to expand ourselves creatively, to follow our own unique spirits into the world, and to watch them manifest. If I—an American without a single contact, no cooking skills, zero friends, and no career—could create all of this in a foreign land, in Italy, what can other women do? All of it, and more.

Our goal at La DoubleJ is to refract our kaleidoscopic energy to help women feel juicy and amazing, to feel confident to shine, and be seen, rather than hide their light behind drab invisibility cloaks. We want our global community to seek joy inside and out, to crack open their hearts with wonder, and to be the goddesses they truly are.

We also want to be a kick-starter to help women trust and tap their own swirling creative impulses, whether it's starting a company, writing a novel, or laying a beautiful table—to give birth to their own beautiful moments and ideas, and to keep an open nature and a passion for discovery.

How does all of this really work, and how can it be applied to you? The first thing to understand is that this magic of the Divine Mother, or Mamma Milano—or whatever you want to call her—is a force. She is everywhere you look. You just need to apply the basics of energy work. Fortunately, you don't have to move across the planet to make it happen.

This work starts with how you treat, handle, and care for yourself, and then how you broker, nurture, and repair relationships with family, friends, lovers, co-workers. You can start this wherever you are—in the supermarket in London, in a skyscraper in New York, in your Parisian *pied-à-terre* with the plumber. What we're doing, wherever we are, is raising our vibrations while calling in the Divine Mother frequency that prepares our inner ground for new growth.

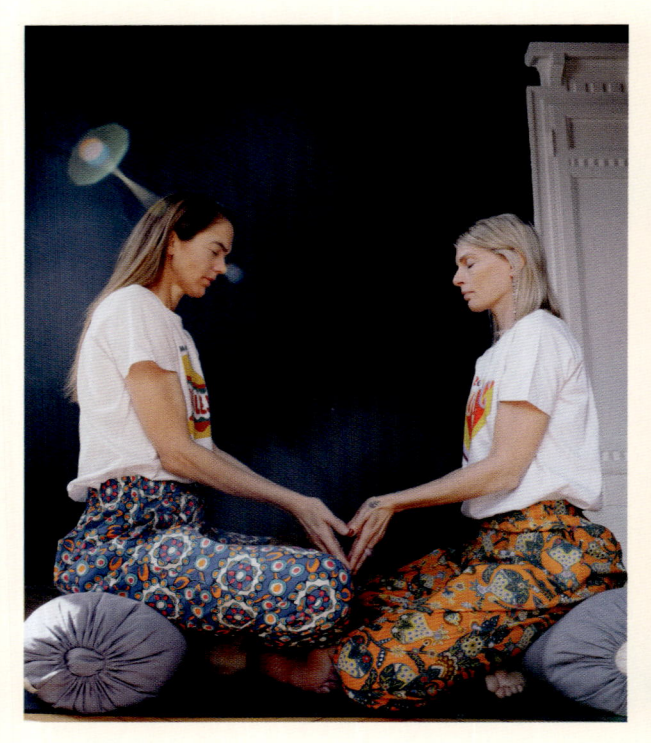

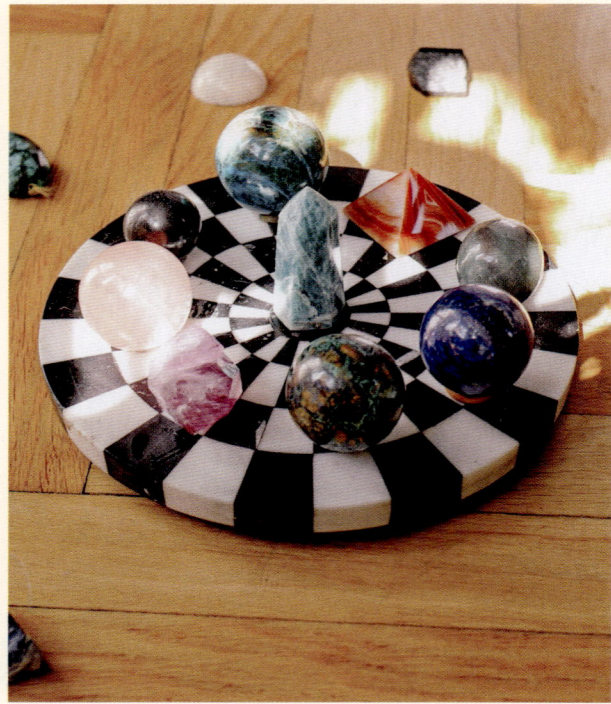

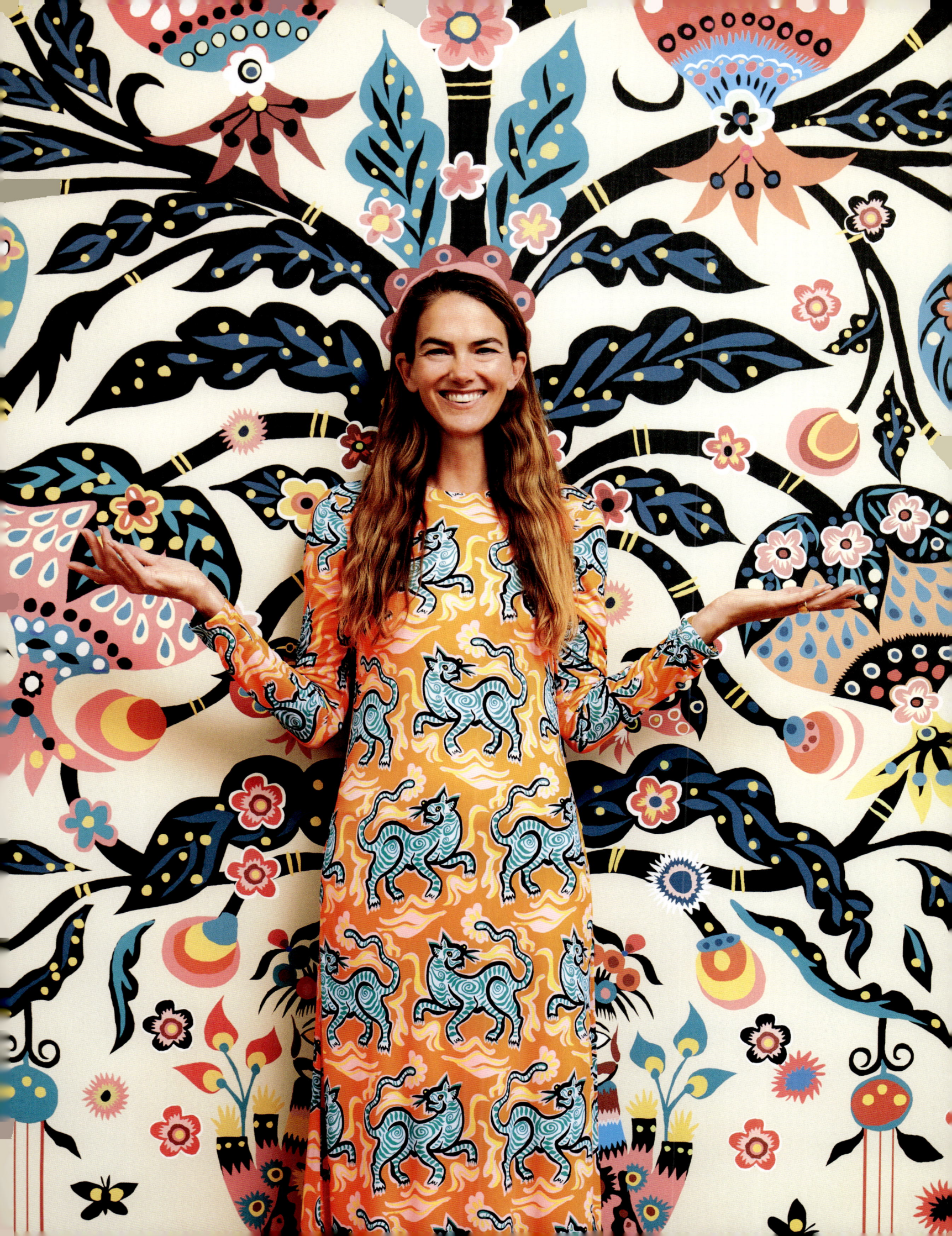

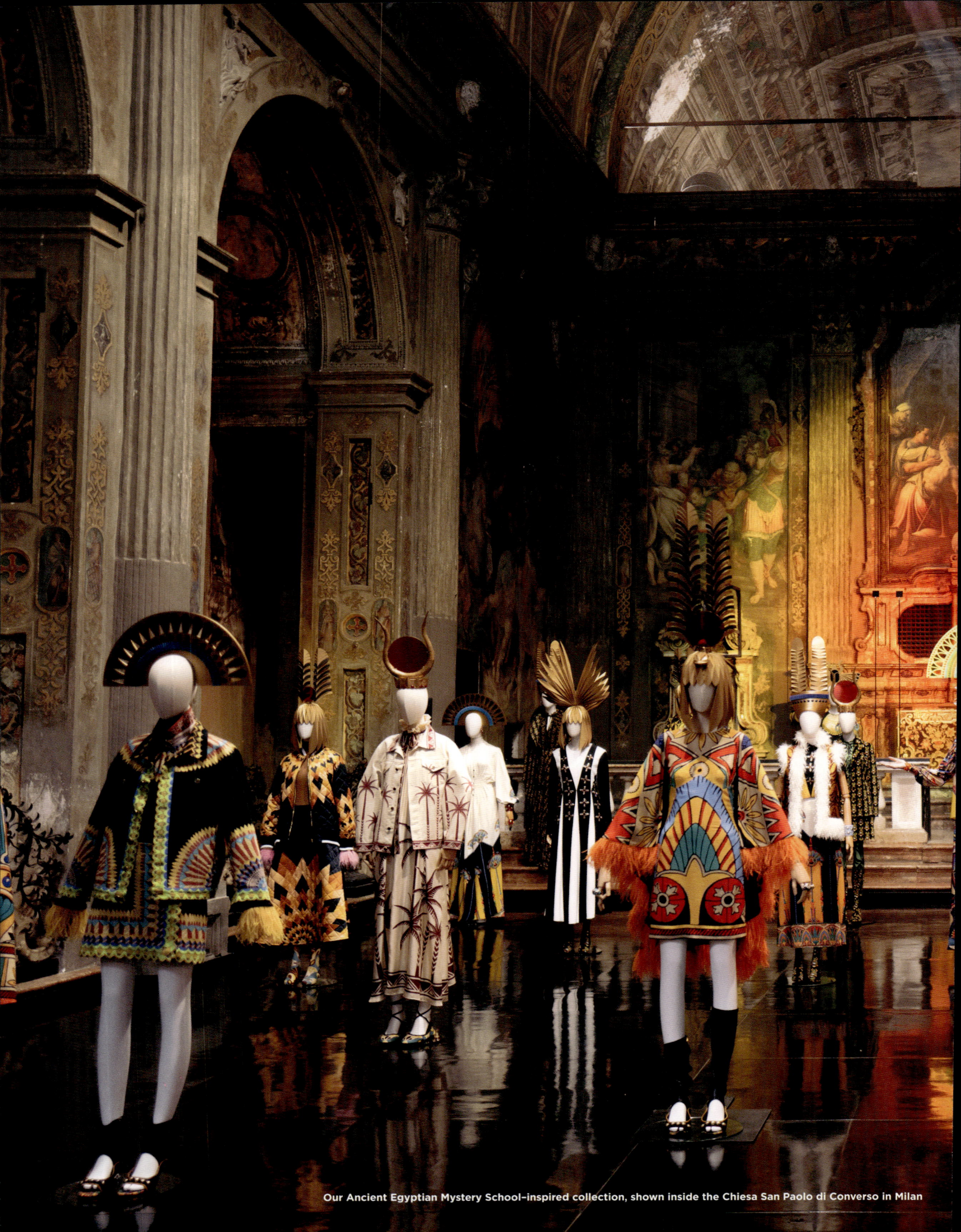

Our Ancient Egyptian Mystery School–inspired collection, shown inside the Chiesa San Paolo di Converso in Milan

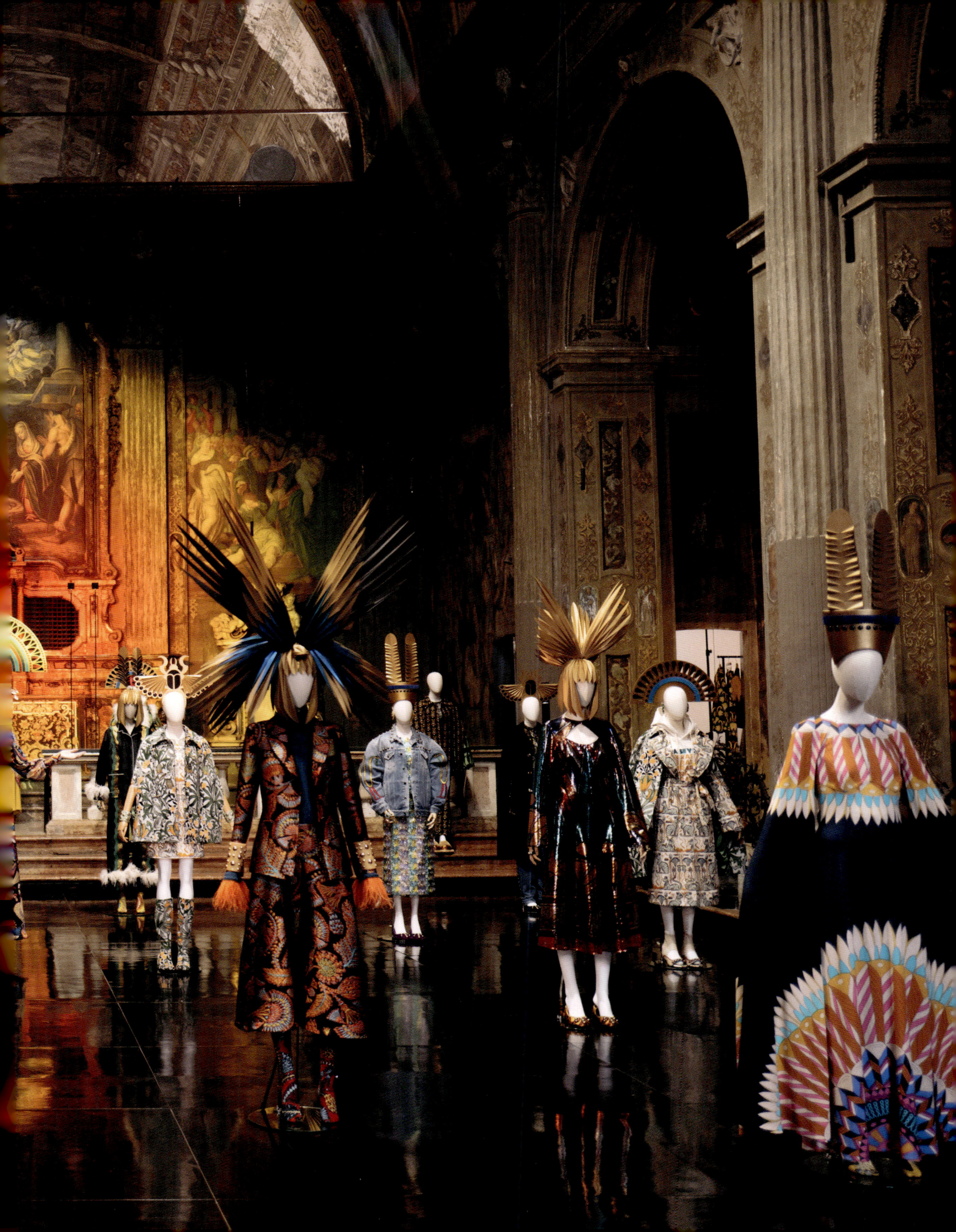

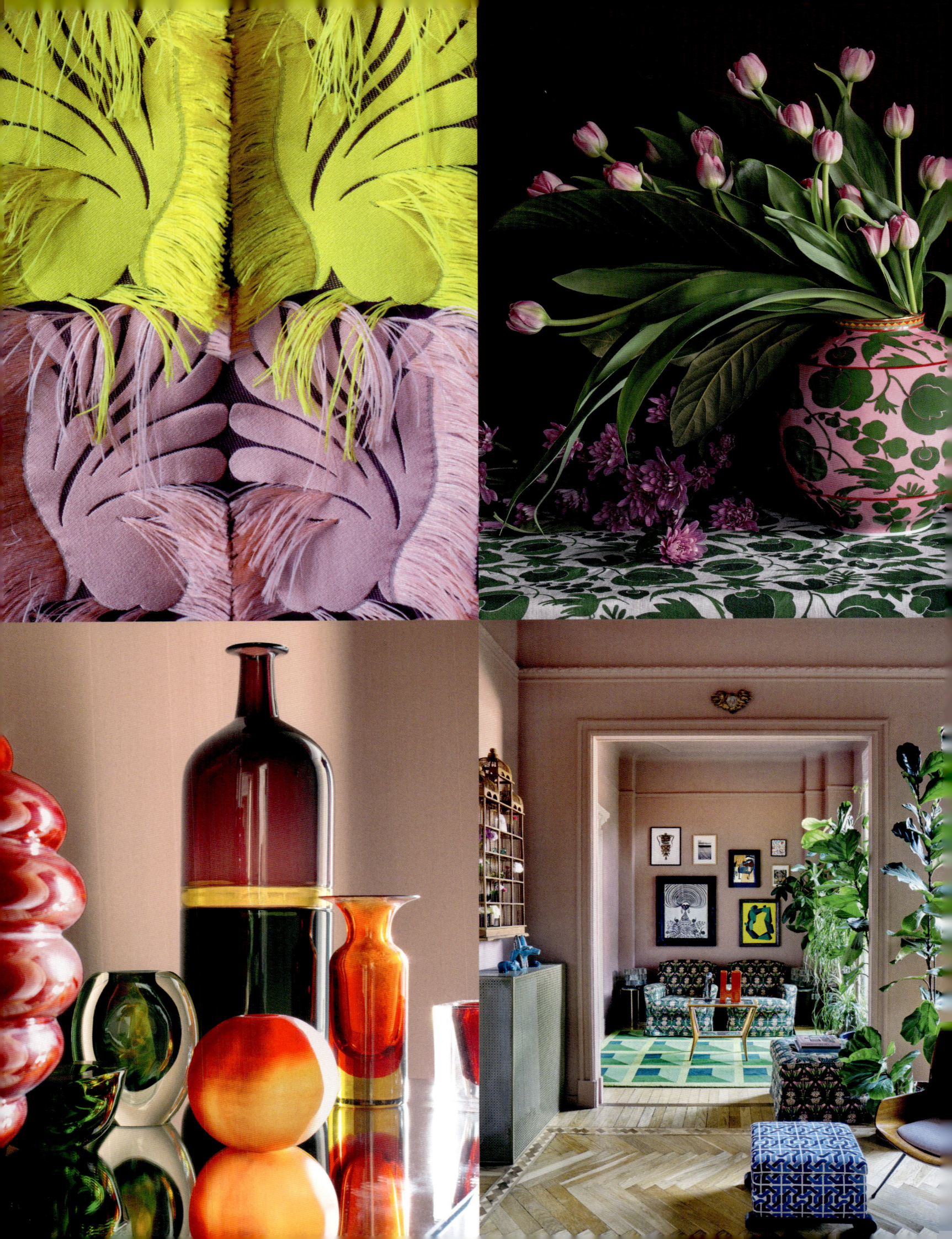

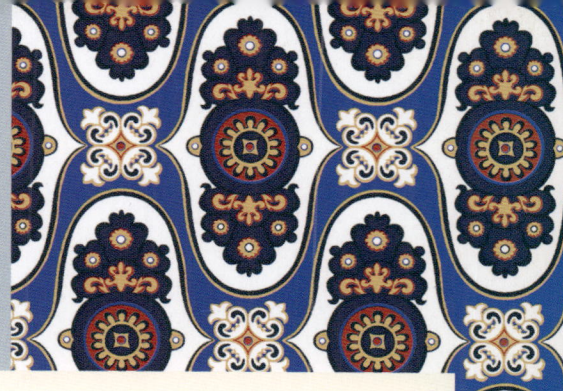

GET CREATIVE WITH COLOR

This notion of high-frequency energy feeds the motherlode idea behind La DoubleJ's toe-tapping prints and feel-good fashion: color has vibrational energy, too, and the power to transform moods and minds.

I have long used color and print as a way to flex my creativity and shoot out wild and wacky expression. I find dressing in color to be liberating; it is an unbuckling of my most expansive self that gets me out of my cage. This isn't an exact science and you really don't need to know a thing about color theory. You just need to know that, *Jeez, I feel like a vixen in my pink pants!* Or, *I feel powerfully grounded in my red dress.* It's very much about your own experience with color. How does it speak to you?

Here's a trick: When you are feeling your most frisky, sassy, and light—like you've just won a little lottery in some life pursuit—stop, close your eyes, and ask, *What does that look like? Does that look like black?* Probably not. See the color that's there, and put it on as a visual marker and a manifestation of your inward state of joy.

Obviously, not everyone wants to wear bold colors head to toe or to mix five prints like I do. There are degrees of maximalism that you can safely dip into. Maybe it's just a printed shirt you'll throw under your black suit armor, or a set of patterned napkins on an all-white table with simple flowers. Go with what feels good in your body. Fashion is just one outward creative manifestation of yourself.

LET'S GET VIBRATIONAL

"Raise Your Vibration" is not just a cute company motto. It is our galactic mission, an expansion of my own personal spiritual practice.

What does it mean? Let's start with the basics. Everything in the universe possesses an energy quotient, from the tiniest atoms to the most massive stars. Humans—with our sacks of skin, feelings, thoughts, hearts, chakras, spirits, and souls—are not exempt. All of it pulsates with vibrating energy. Energy exists on a frequency spectrum, from low levels that are dark and dense to high levels that are light and bright.

The vibrational frequency of all energy can be manipulated and morphed—this energetic is actually decided by us. We control it with our own free will. Shit may happen, emotions course through our bodies, but how we react to the crap storm is us taking our energetic field into our own very capable hands. It is done first by becoming aware that energy is swirling around you always, then deciding you want to raise your vibration, then moving into that frequency.

So, "raising your vibration" means moving your energetic scale from the heavy, sluggish, bottom rung of the ladder—which is where we often reside in our day-to-day, stressful lives—to the luminous top of the ladder, governed by the energy of love, one of Mamma Milano's biggest tanks. When you do that, you are more connected to your most expansive creative self, and your true higher self that is linked to the great power socket of the universe: source itself.

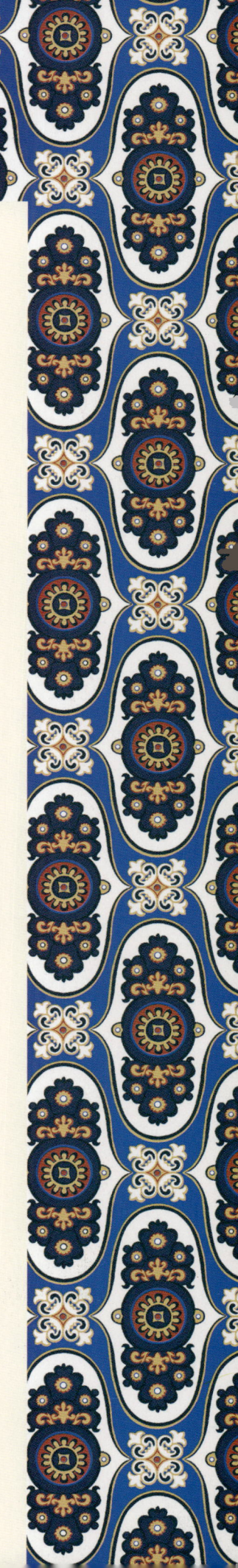

ACTIVATE YOUR CHAKRAS

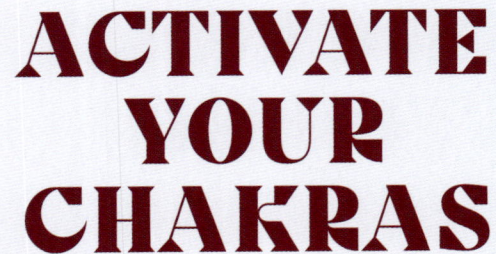

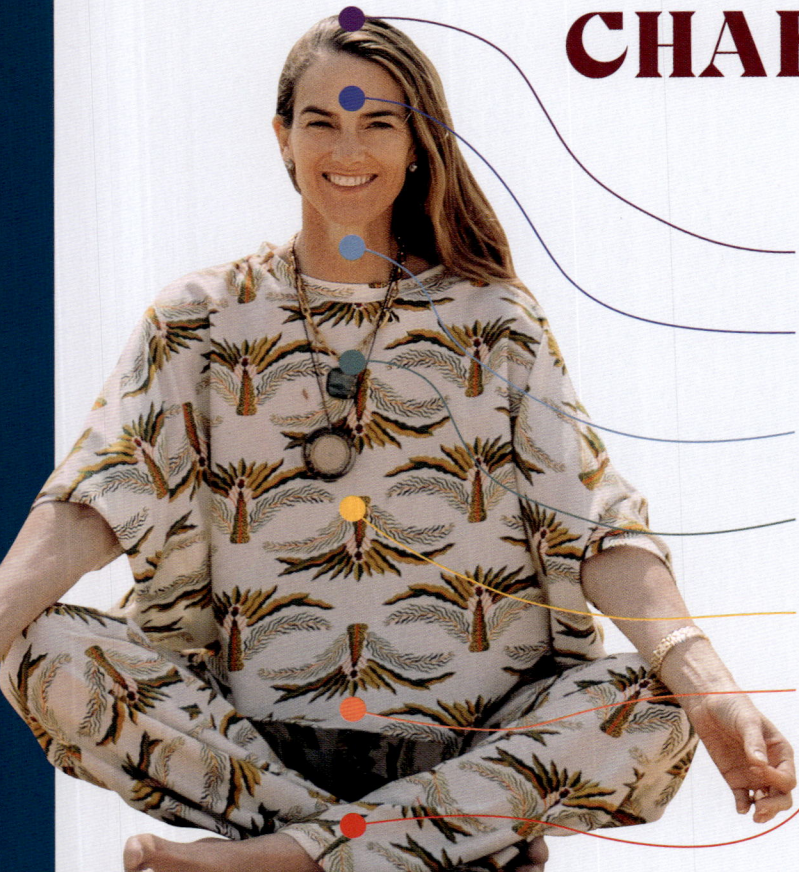

CROWN CHAKRA: DIAMOND VIOLET
Claircognizance, higher realms of consciousness

THIRD EYE CHAKRA: INDIGO BLUE
Intuition, inner sight, clairvoyance

THROAT CHAKRA: LIGHT BLUE
Speaking your truth

HEART CHAKRA: GREEN OR PINK
Love, forgiveness, passion, connection

SOLAR PLEXUS CHAKRA: YELLOW
Inner motor, fire, will center

SACRAL CHAKRA: ORANGE
Creativity, fertility, self-worth

BASE CHAKRA: RED
Safety, belonging, grounding

When you go into your feeling senses and leave your mental faculties behind, you're slipping back into the Divine Mother's fruitful juices. You're allowing your intuition to turn on, and you're accessing different realms of consciousness. While you're here, you might also be aware of your energy body. You have an invisible, highly sensitive bubble of light that surrounds your physical shell and anchors inside it through your meridians (which your acupuncturist taps into) and your chakras.

Anyone who's taken a yoga class is familiar with these swirling vortexes of energy that move vertically from the root of the spine to the crown of the head. It's no coincidence that each chakra is associated with a different color—each color, and each energy center, vibrates at a different frequency. Each chakra corresponds to a life-force element that is vital to mental, emotional, and spiritual health. Some chakras are underused, some are overused, others are clogged or slammed shut. You can open, cleanse, unclog, and expand these energy centers using your breath, intention, meditation, and energy work—alone, or with a healer. You can also activate them by wearing colors or crystals that correspond to them.

At the end of the day, there's a very good reason why you feel so good in your vixen pink pants.

DUMP YOUR HEAD WHEN YOU'RE GETTING DRESSED

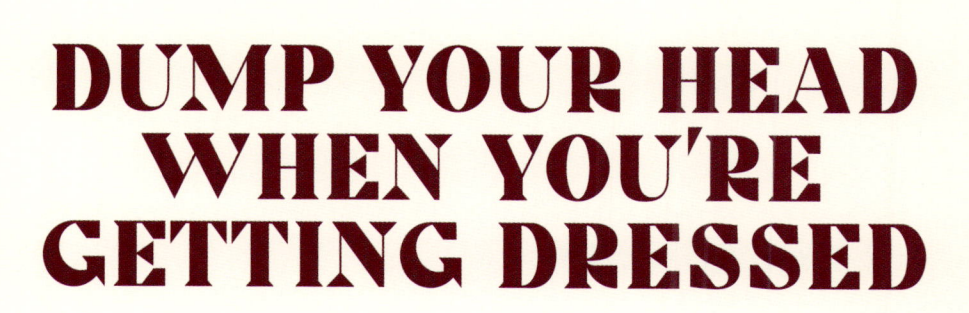

How do you put together colorful outfits or prints without looking like a car crash? I've noticed that the mind isn't very helpful in this process. I smash together prints like a food processor, throwing everything in to create an artful mix. But I realized that my body is also deeply involved, activated like a finely honed kinesiology test. When I put something on—or looking at new print patterns or dress designs in the office—and my body freezes or my stomach tenses up, it's not right. If I get a blood-rush of bouncing pleasure or feel like jumping or tapping my feet, it's a hard yes. My body's somatic intelligence is a superpower antenna that's plugged into the Divine Mother mainframe.

You can use this approach for bigger decisions in your life. Your body is a wise machine, constantly messaging you with information. Its software program is way smarter than the little digital computer in your head—which is helpful, of course, but shouldn't be the master of creative decisions. Try using your somatic feelers as you're getting dressed. Does it sit well in the stomach? Has it gotten your heart hot and open? Then go for it! My invitation is to bring meaning to how you dress yourself. Clothing made in a sweatshop or by slave labor is not going to emit a high frequency of energy. Honor yourself and this ritual of dressing. But do not become consumed by it, either. Your spiritual/energetic expansion is about finding your highest potential, which is a soul force, not a closet full of designer clothes.

There are actually a few ways we *can* use our logical heads in this endeavor. I tend to put two prints of different scales together, with the larger-sized print on the bottom half of my body. Geometrics are often a great compliment to floral prints. When you wear vintage clothes, add hyper contemporary accessories to avoid looking like a *nonna*.

Lastly, don't be afraid of originality in your own genius. Fashion culture tells you what you need to emulate, but what you really need to do is tap into your own joy faucets. It might look very different from what you see on others—and this is a good thing.

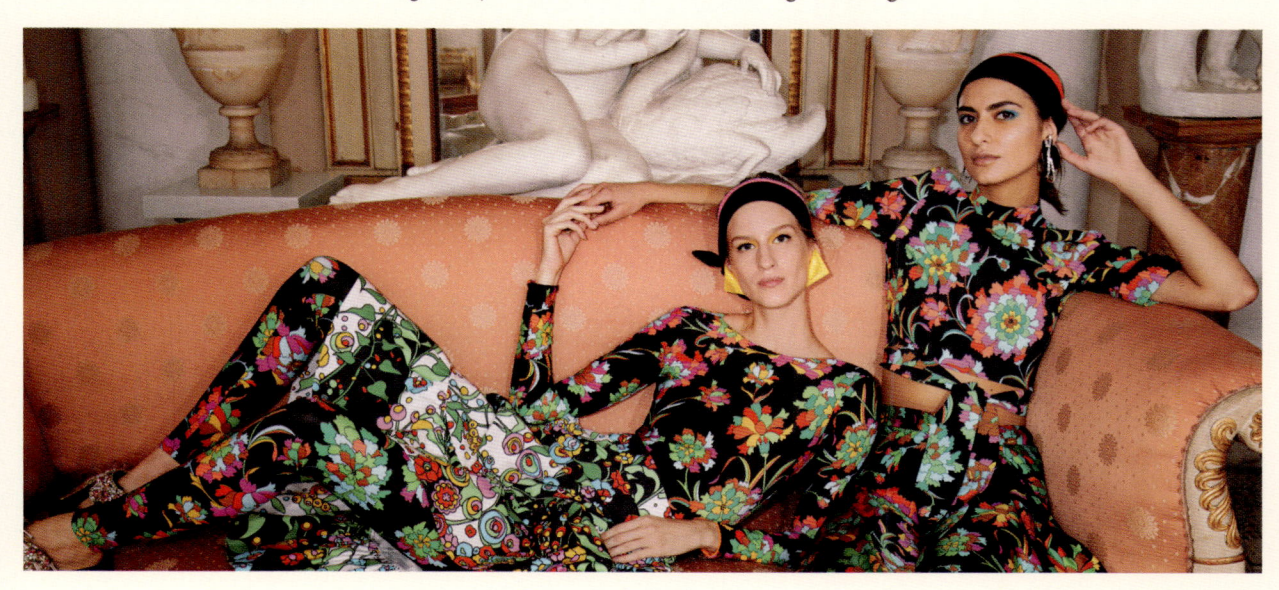

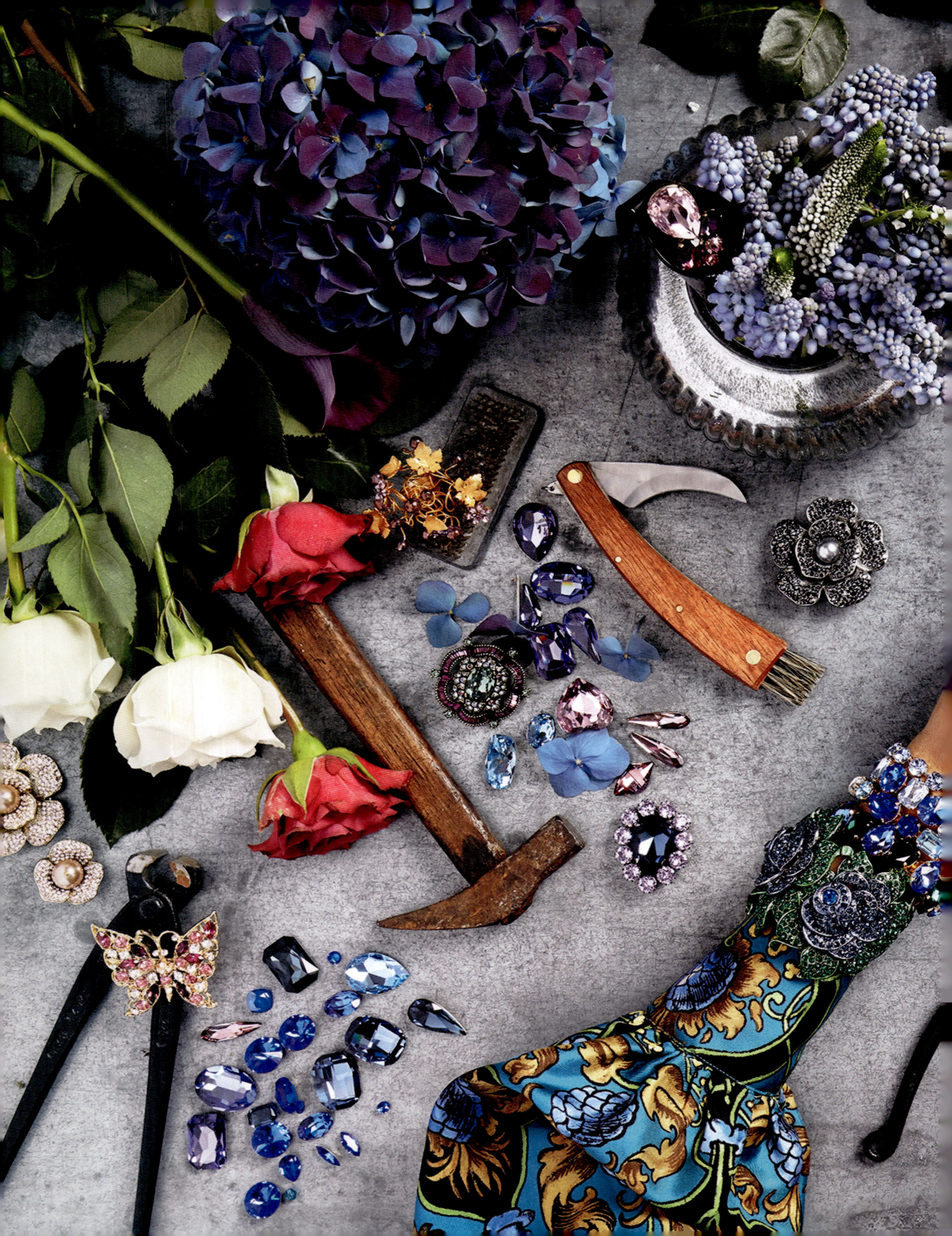

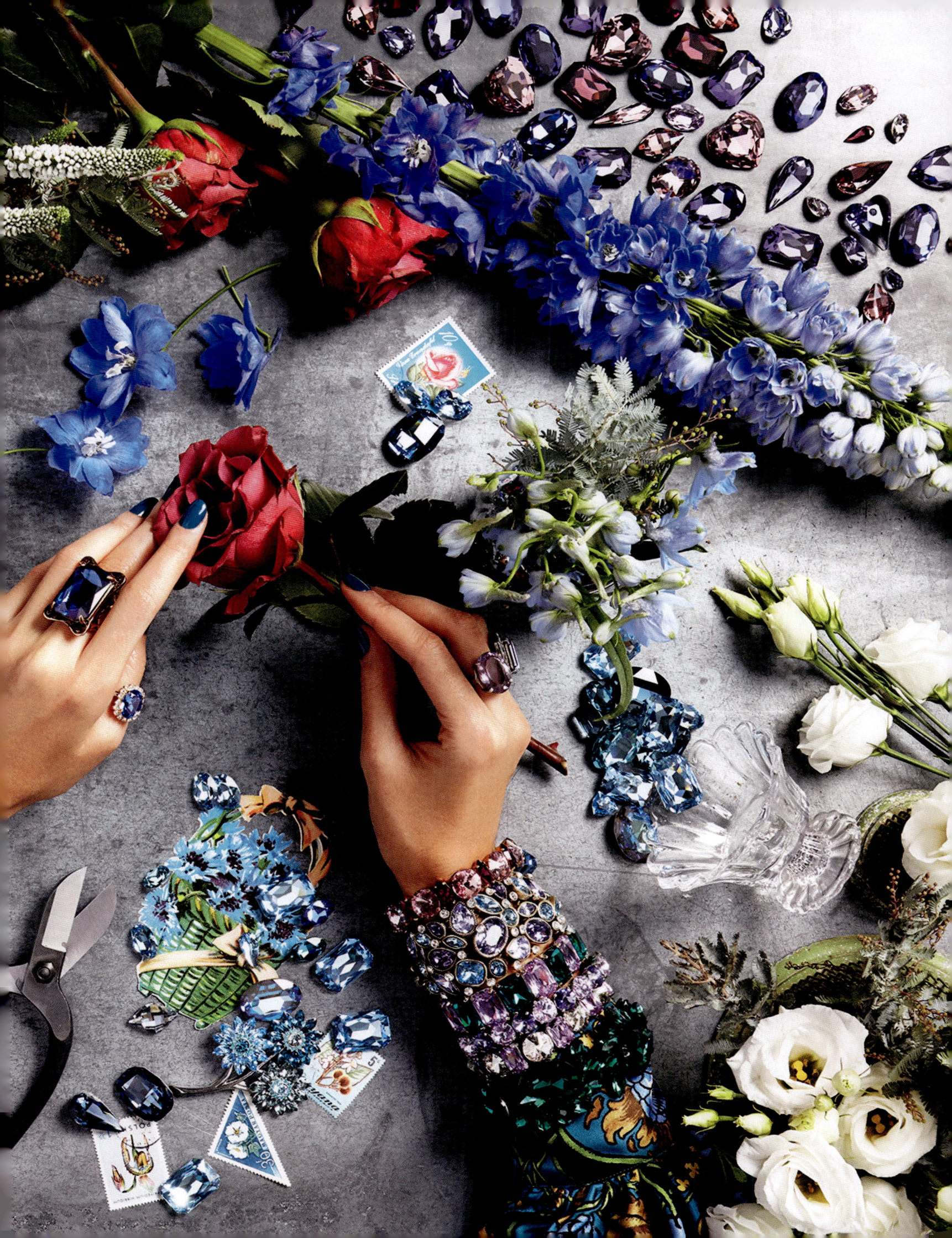

FLIP YOUR OWN CREATIVE SWITCH

There are many other ways besides getting dressed to Raise Your Vibration, and part of your job as a conscious creator of your own life is to develop an arsenal of skills for this. (For a few more tips from my own practice, scan the square across the page.) Once you've scrubbed up your energy, it will be much easier to create consciously. Creativity is a golden doorway to your highest self. But conscious creativity is a step further; it involves aligning with your innate gifts, mining your inner joy, and bringing into the world something that hasn't been seen before. I did this unwittingly at La DoubleJ by following the two things that drove me crazy with pleasure: vintage, and the Italians. When I swirled it all up and served it in my multicolored, maximalist package, it firecrackered into unique life.

One thing that came naturally to me—and is important if you want to create anything, be it a business or a brunch buffet—is uniqueness. Every crumb of an idea, product, message, and package needs to be authentic to you. This is your own singular voice, your own special sauce. Discovering this is not done through the brain. You need to use your heart and your stomach when you're putting the ingredients together and building your recipe. It must be your own unique egg that you're going to crack open. And that germ cell must come uniquely from you, the Mother.

So true creativity, just like true style, is not imitating anyone. I've found myself arching my neck over into someone else's creative backyard and wondering if I should be more like them. No, no, I should not. And neither should you. It becomes imitation. When you imitate, you become mediocre, and you lose the frisson of fresŸess. So how do you create something genuinely new and true to you? It happens with a mixture of balls, naivete, and playfulness. It bubbles forth from the heart center.

Conscious creation also requires that you never create from a place of fear. The minute you start thinking, *will people like this?, will I sell this?, will anyone follow me on IG?*, then you start compromising your vision, and you will not create something that is aligned with your highest good and with the highest outcome. You must stay focused on your core love, your heart's belief, or you will chop off your baby's legs. The genius is holding your miracle baby up above the swirl of chaos and fear, and using your own mamma legs to run in the right direction.

But creativity cannot be put on a leash and pulled to a place it doesn't wish to go. It must be let loose and run wild. Let it leap across the field of your mind, let it whirl and dance and shake itself. It is dying to come up and out of you. This can manifest as a magnificent fashion show filled with fantasy and wonder, or a wild, messy, improvised invention in the kitchen, or a drawing that goes out of control, a paintbrush that strokes off the page, a dance you do in your underwear with your hair whipping around in luscious circles. This is letting your hips move the way they are dying to, your heart expanding outside of your body, and your energy pouring forth from your hands like hot water jets.

Let yourself vibrate with this raw buzzing energy source. This is how you connect with the Force of Source.

Also, stop comparing! Stop with the jealousy that someone has it better, easier, bigger, and more beautiful and bountiful than you do. If you experience scrolling envy, use it to your advantage—ask yourself what it truly represents. If the answer is that she just looks effortless, glamorous, or she's got it all together, then go inside your own system and ask how *you* can recreate that feeling of effortless glamour. It won't be by carbon copying her, because you'll just dilute it and lose the sizzle. You'll start your own fire when you spark the synapses within your own unique creation station. Imagine what that energy of "ease, glamour," etc. feels like refracted through your prism and put into practice.

To penetrate true creativity, close your eyes and let your heart explore. There is fantasy, there is whimsy, there is dreaming. This is what we need more of. Otherwise we are just making plain, unbuttered toast.

You also need patience and trust. This is about having faith that if your creation is really aligned for your highest good, it will come through. If it's not, you'll find it next round. You must believe this, or it won't work. You will also need time, space, and stillness. During Covid, it was scary to live in the void. As a maximalist, I'm scared of emptiness and total stillness. It's not my natural state, but it is the state of the Divine Mother. This is where her creations are birthed: in absolute black, uncertain silence.

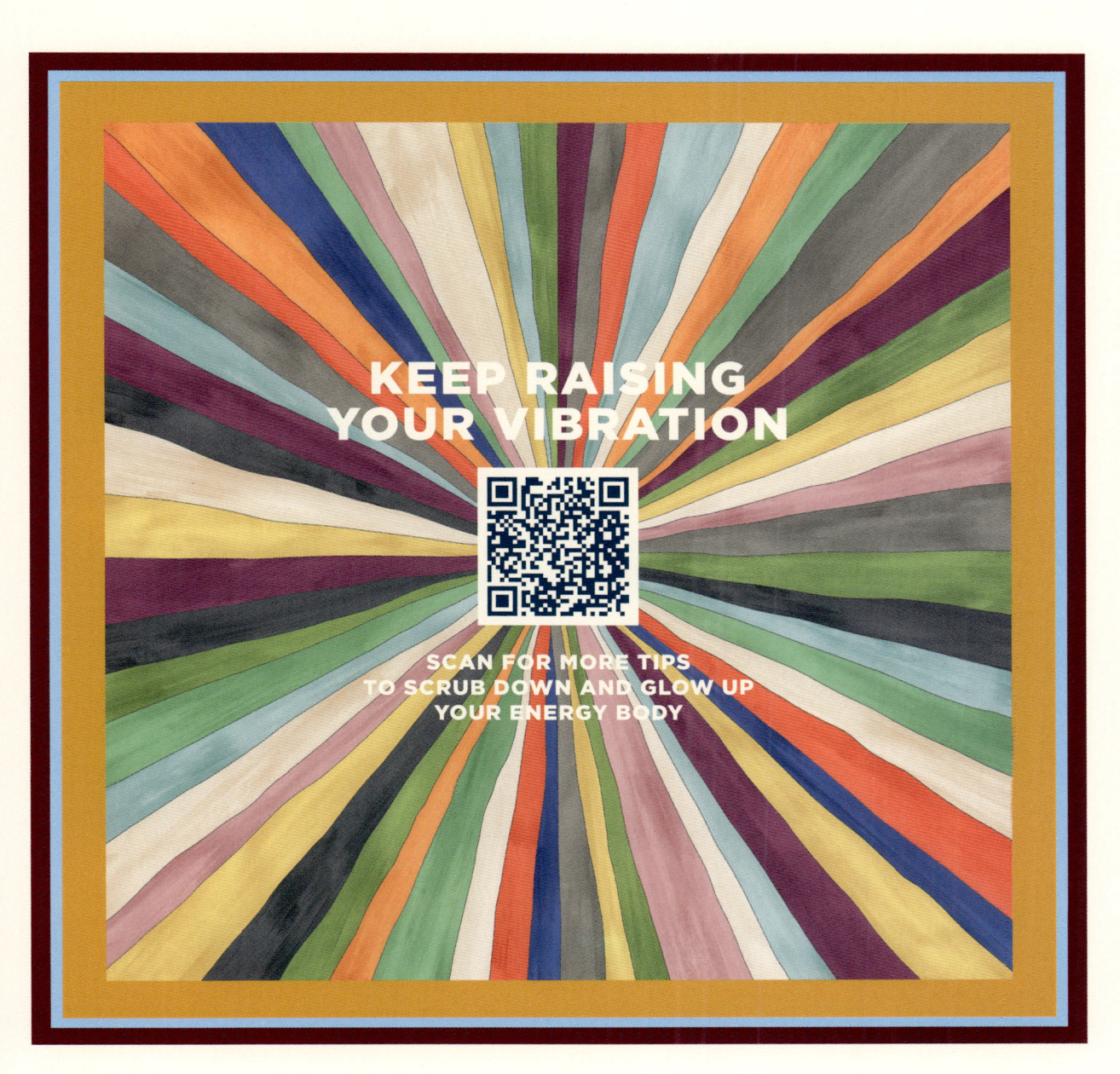

KEEP RAISING YOUR VIBRATION

SCAN FOR MORE TIPS
TO SCRUB DOWN AND GLOW UP
YOUR ENERGY BODY

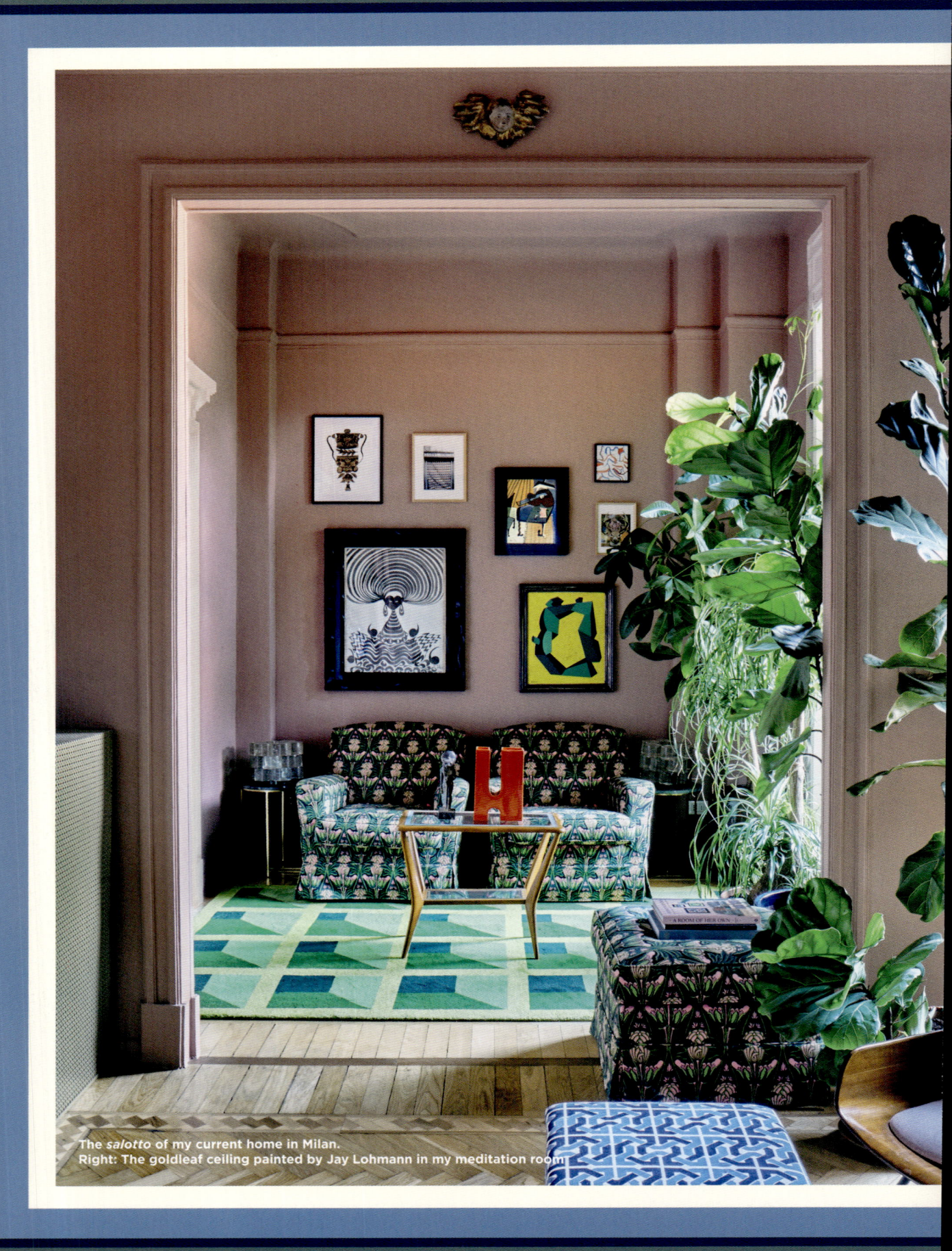

The *salotto* of my current home in Milan.
Right: The goldleaf ceiling painted by Jay Lohmann in my meditation room.

RAISE YOUR VIBRATION

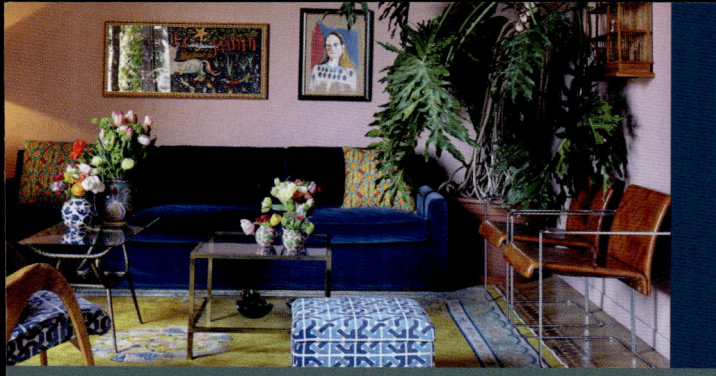

BIRTHING A NEW HOME FROM THE DEEP VOID

No one really likes to step into the void. I know I don't, even though I understand its powerful, universal law of creation. But sometimes I'm forced to do it, and I can tell you without a doubt that if you play with the darkness and don't fight it, something magical will sprout up.

This is what happened during Covid, when I moved into a new apartment one week before Milan's draconian lockdown. I was newly divorced, all alone with one couch, a mattress on the floor of the bedroom, two lights, and a couple of coffee tables. I could not go out to vintage fairs or charity shops to do my shopping and decorating of my home. I was forced to sit and pause with the emptiness and muteness of my apartment for three months.

After a few weeks of pouting and stomping my feet on the *terrazzo* floors, I finally just surrendered to the simplicity and vacancy in and around me. I did my daily work calls on Zoom and spent the rest of the time in deep meditation and spiritual courses I took online. I sat for hours with my pile of crystals in one of the guest rooms I'd consecrated as a meditation room. I was inside a dark, empty womb where I unknowingly planted and fertilized a new way of life. The conditions were perfect; I just had to trust and wait.

Every once in a while, I'd drop a seed for a future bloom: ordering furniture from online auction sites, calling an upholsterer for a job he'd complete in four months' time, laying out all of my vintage jewelry on the floor, only to discover it would all look so great hung on the bathroom wall (once the handyman could leave his house!), inviting the artist Jay Lohmann to sneak out of his Milan home to come paint gold stars on my meditation room ceiling, and commissioning the Norway-based artist Kirsten Synge Kongsli to illustrate some collages I'd found in Bali for wallpaper in the dining room.

I couldn't see anything—except those gold Byzantine stars, which I identified as my guardian angels in this process.

I could not run to the finish line in victorious relief, but the forces of creation were flickering nonetheless.

The darkness turned out to be a marvelous teacher and incubator; this black space I had feared turned out not to be barren at all.

Lucious life was simply waiting to come through in its vibrant, energy-tinged color and patterns.

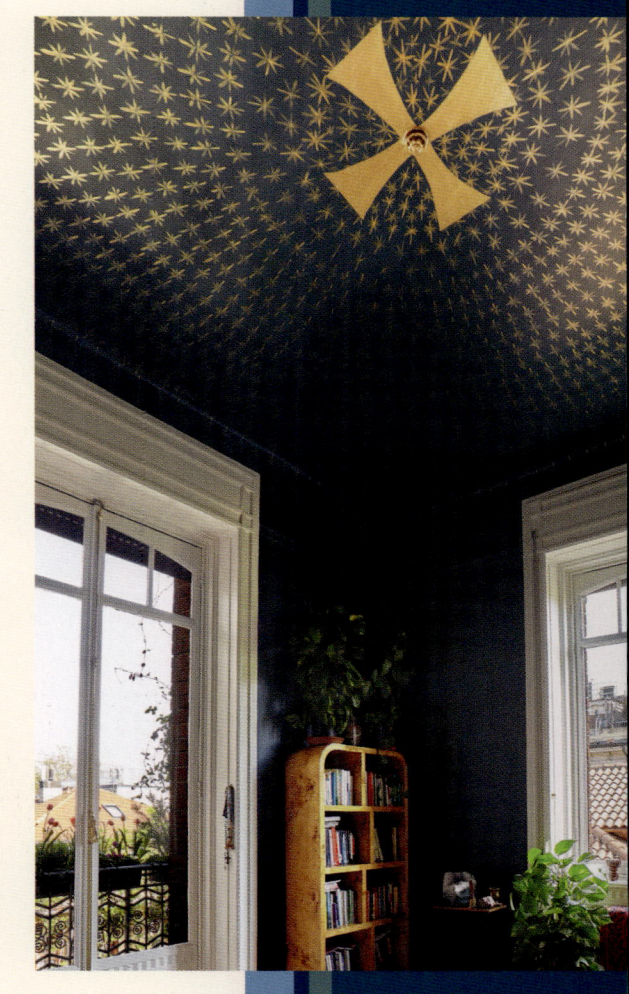

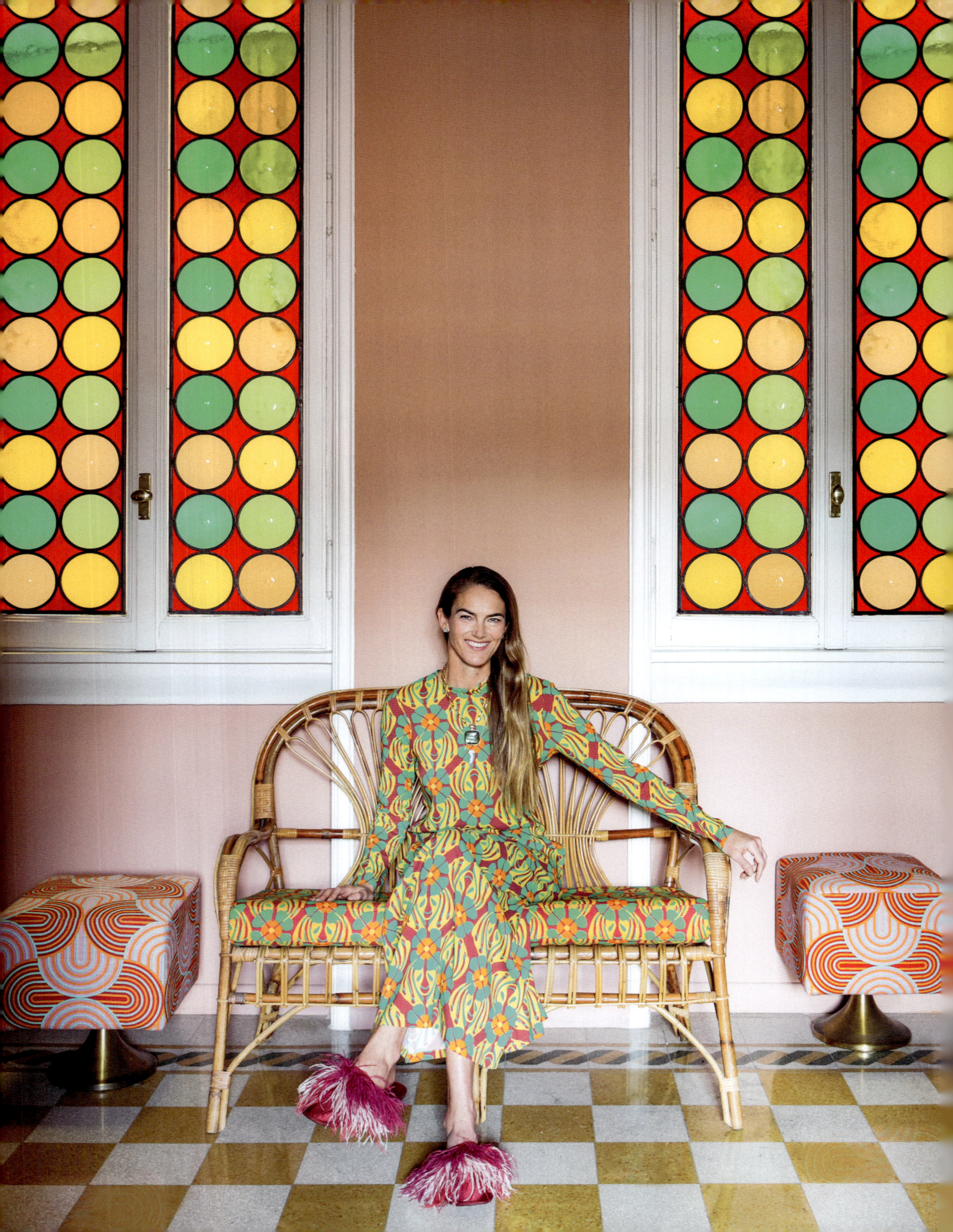

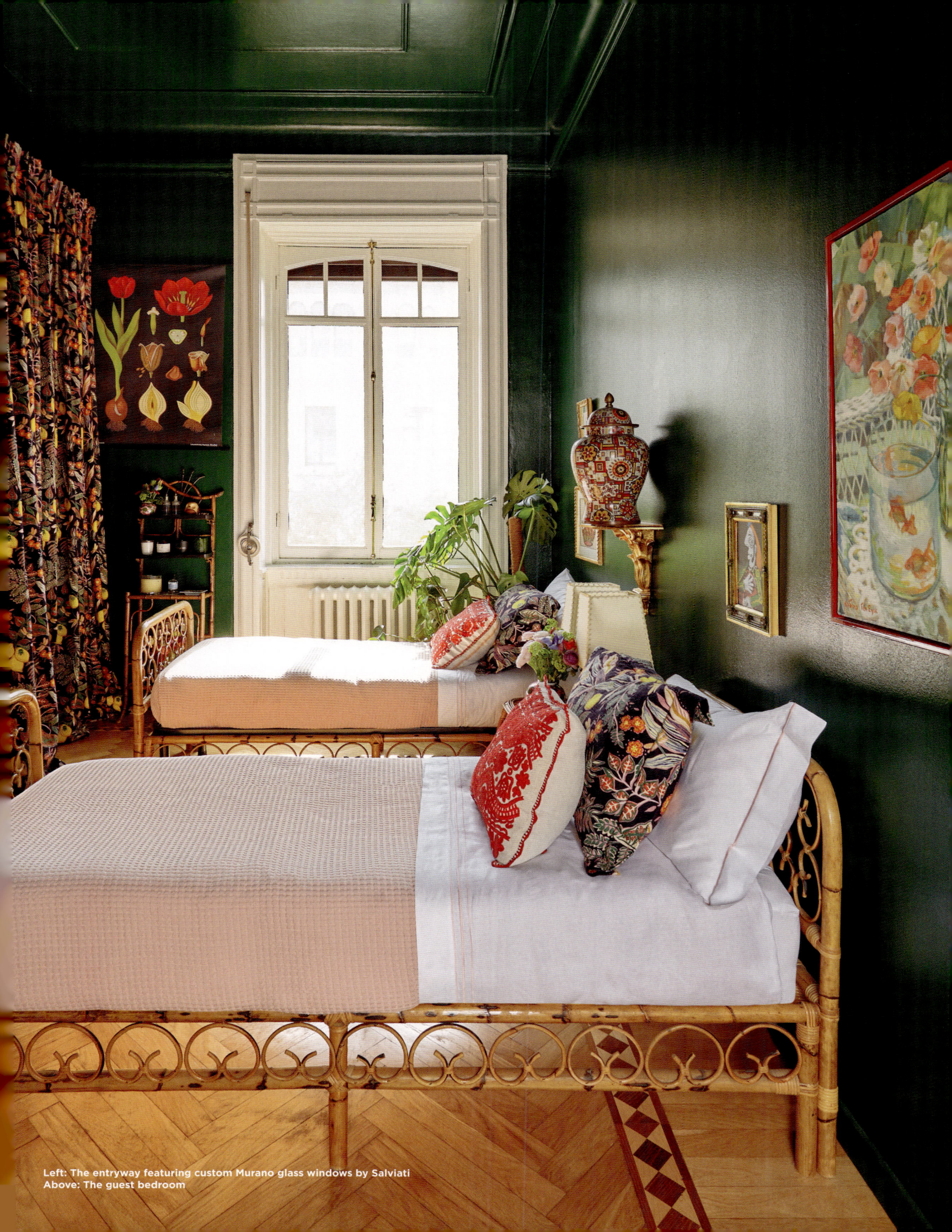

Left: The entryway featuring custom Murano glass windows by Salviati
Above: The guest bedroom

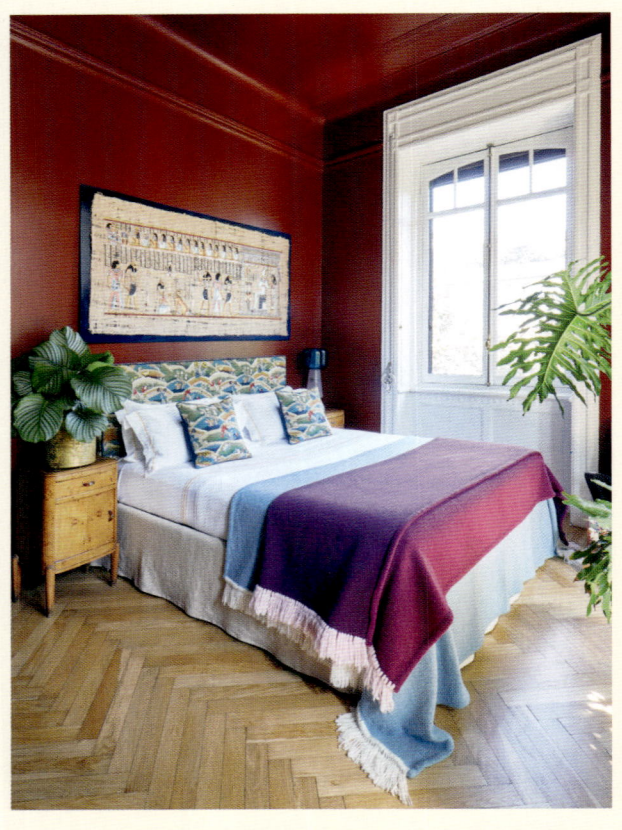

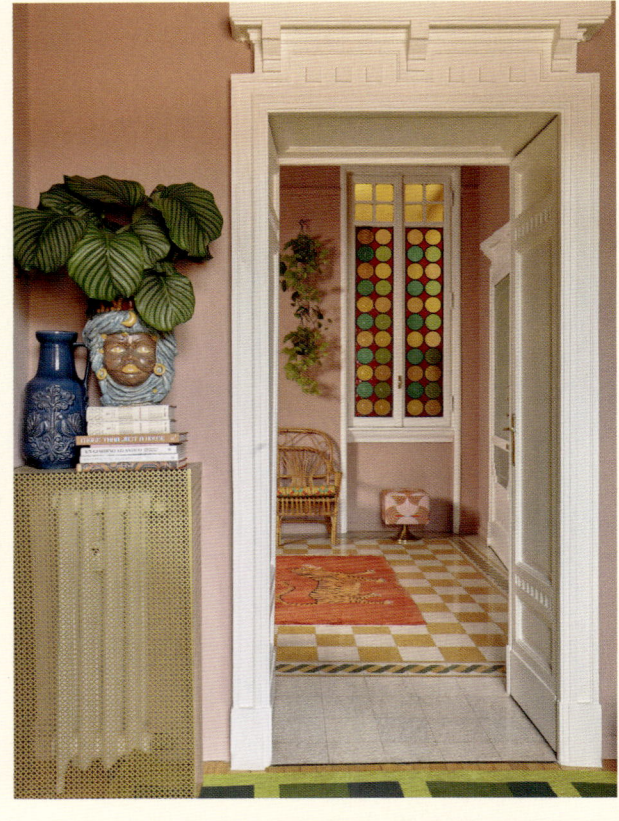

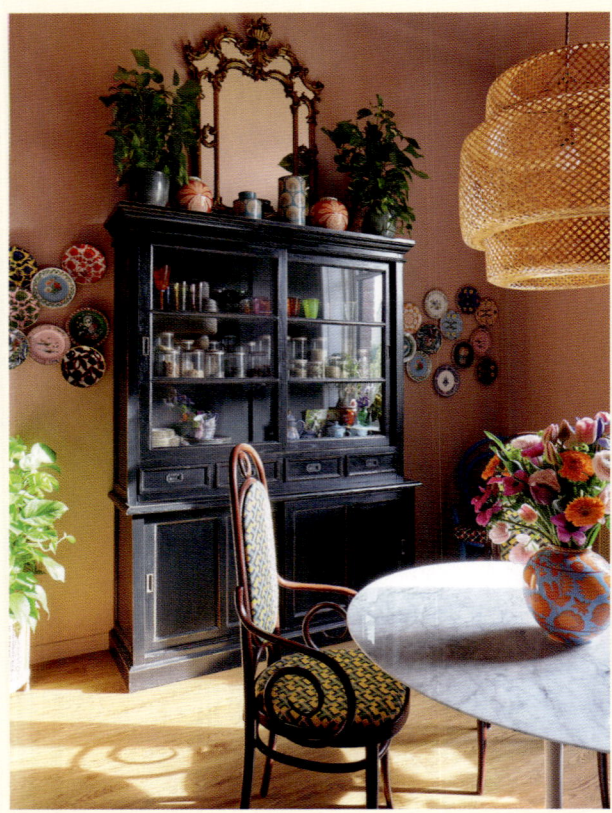

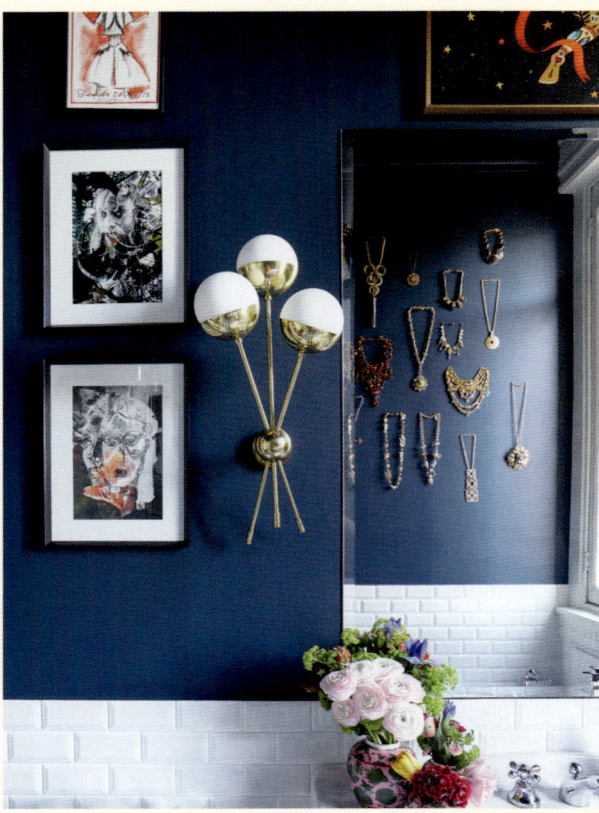

MAMMA MILANO

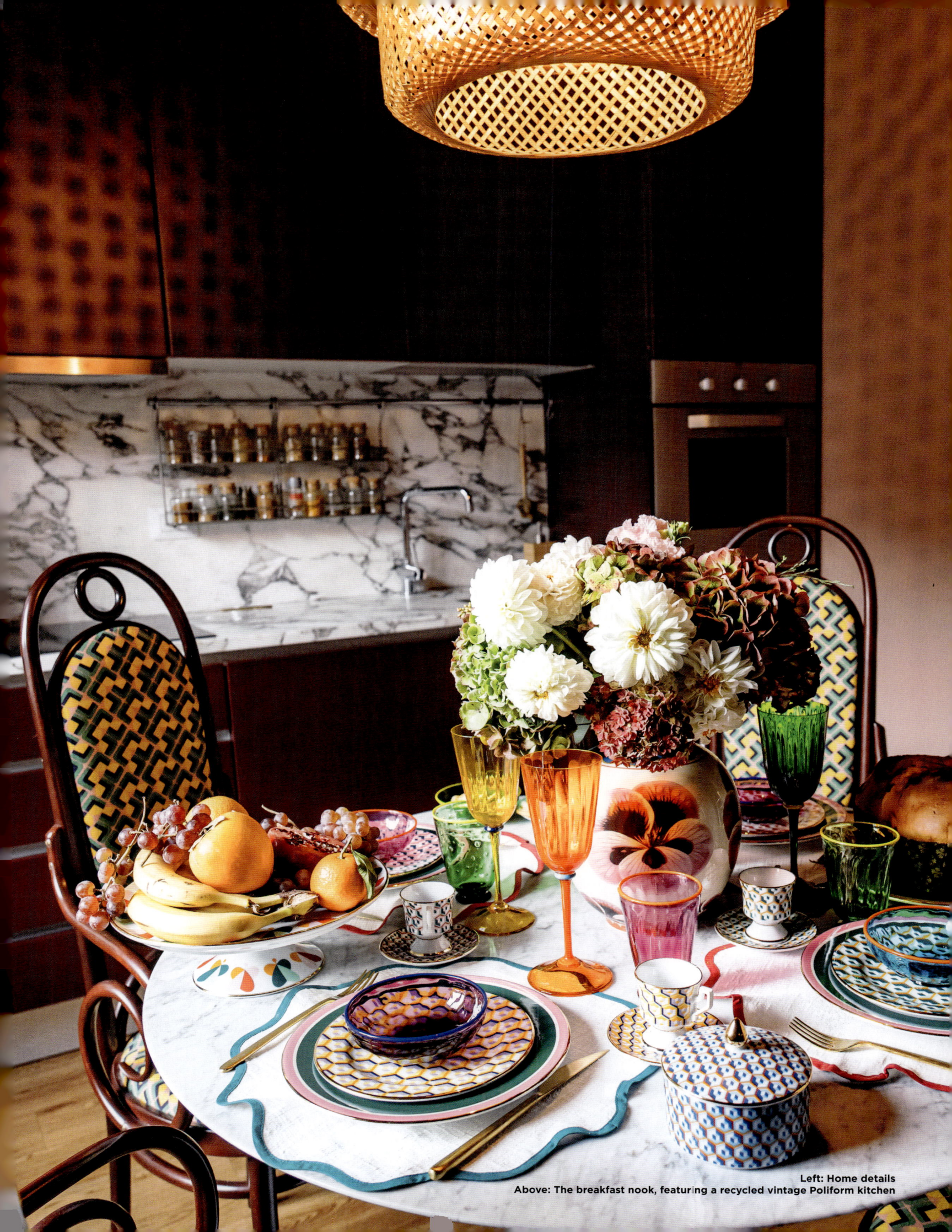

Left: Home details
Above: The breakfast nook, featuring a recycled vintage Poliform kitchen

My altar at home.

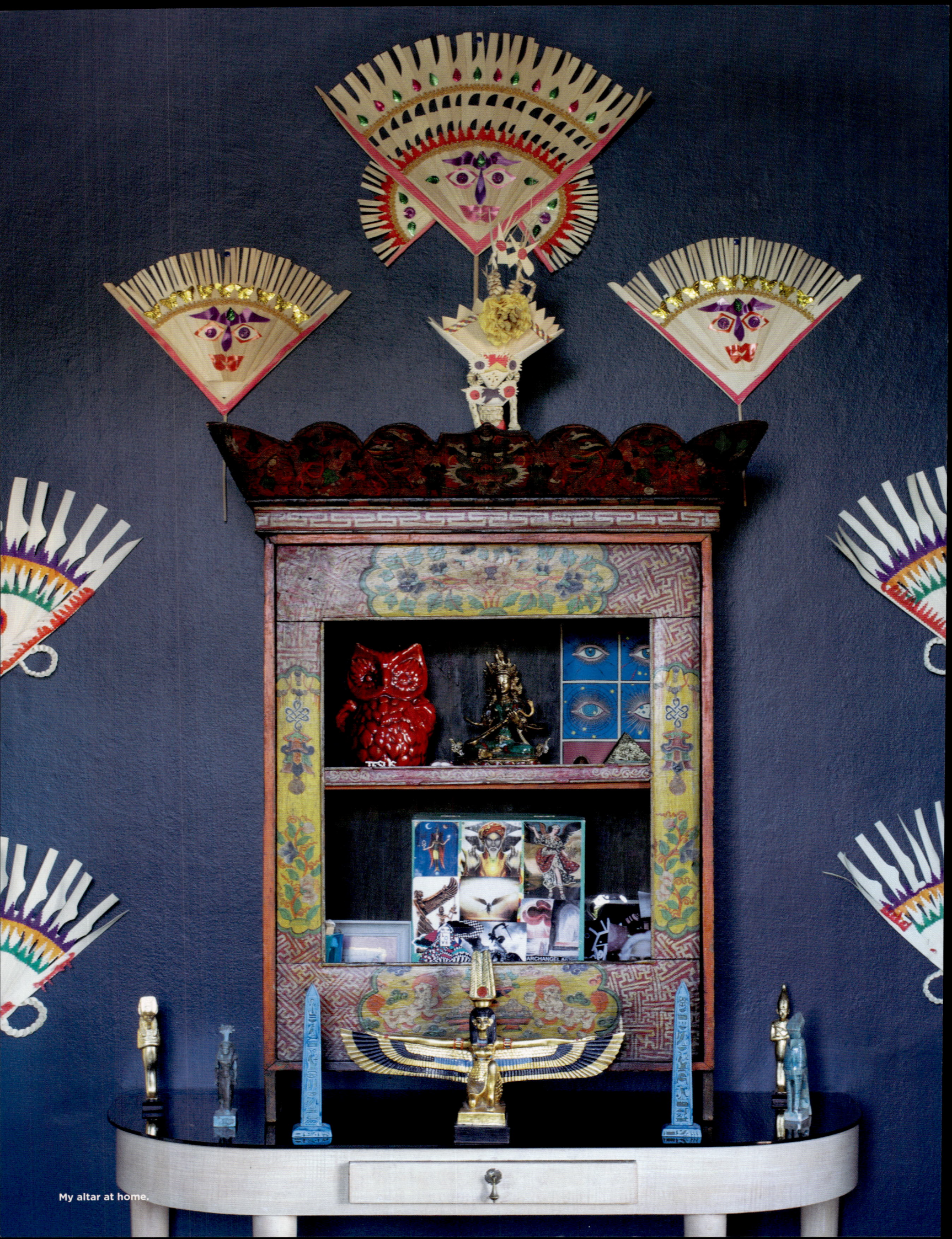

A FEW LAST WORDS FROM MAMMA MILANO

As you embark on this journey of stepping into the unknown mystery of your own fabulous creations, remember to listen to the wise whisper of the Divine Mother. Her gentle, quiet voice is infused with deep wisdom and can be heard best in stillness, in nature, next to trees, and floating in the liquid magic of water. She is your guide, and she wishes to lead you.

Soften your belly, your jaw, and your heart, and melt into the uncomfortable pool of uncertainty that she exudes. You will not be able to control her, and you will not be able to be her boss. Instead, stand with humility in front of her and bow to the great, dark unknown, however that may present to you. Allow yourself to see the truth and good in yourself, in others, and in all things. Allow yourself to speak your truth and do it with kindness.

As you surrender, befriend your fear and your anxiety, even as they burn in your blood. Welcome them as beloved, wanted guests in your inner home who you actually want to sit and speak with. This is the true nature of the Divine Feminine, this is the sacred place you create within yourself to allow all of your magnificence to come through and around you.

And when all else fails… *DAI!* Hug a pug and eat a plate of homemade Italian pasta.

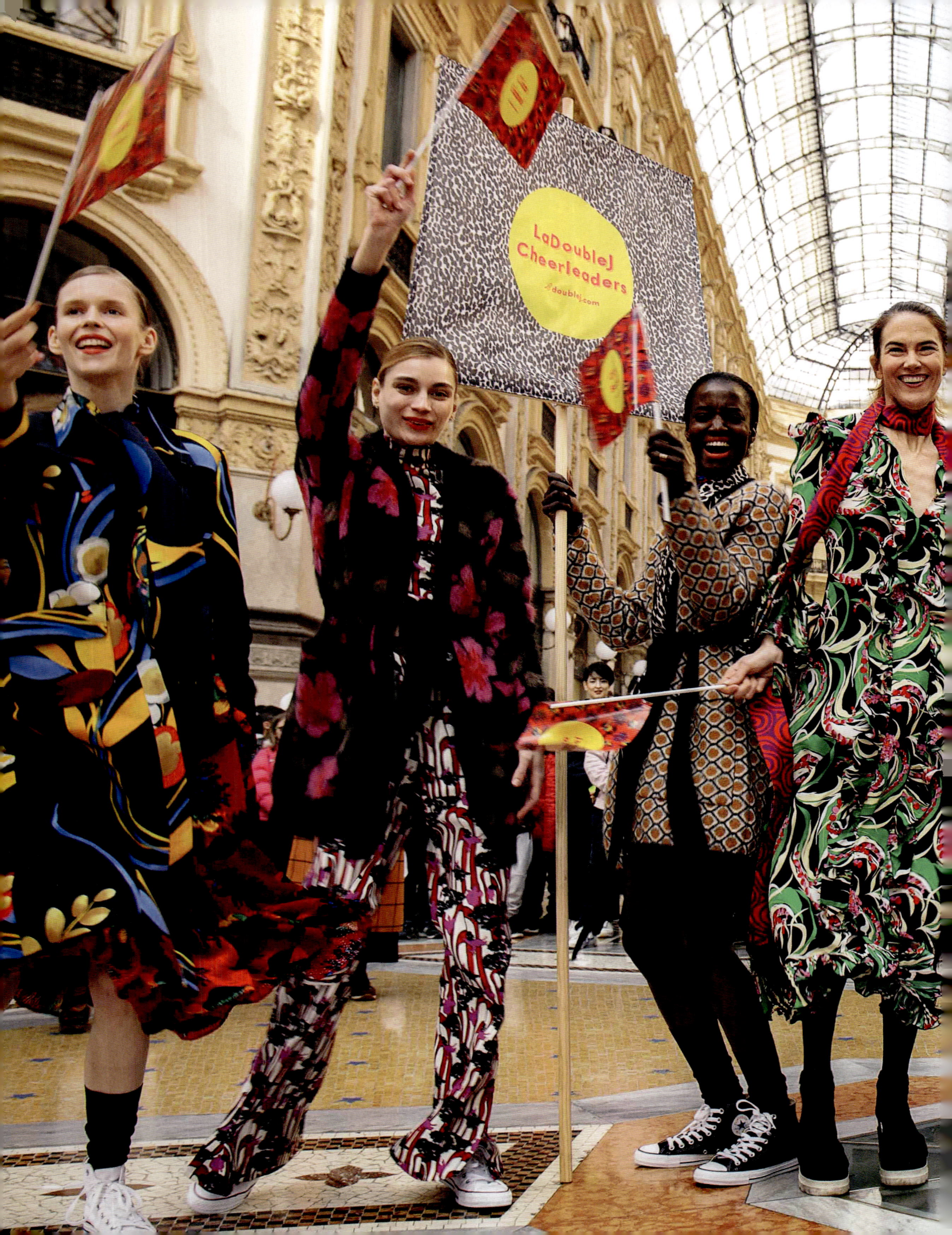
LaDoubleJ
Cheerleaders
doublej.com

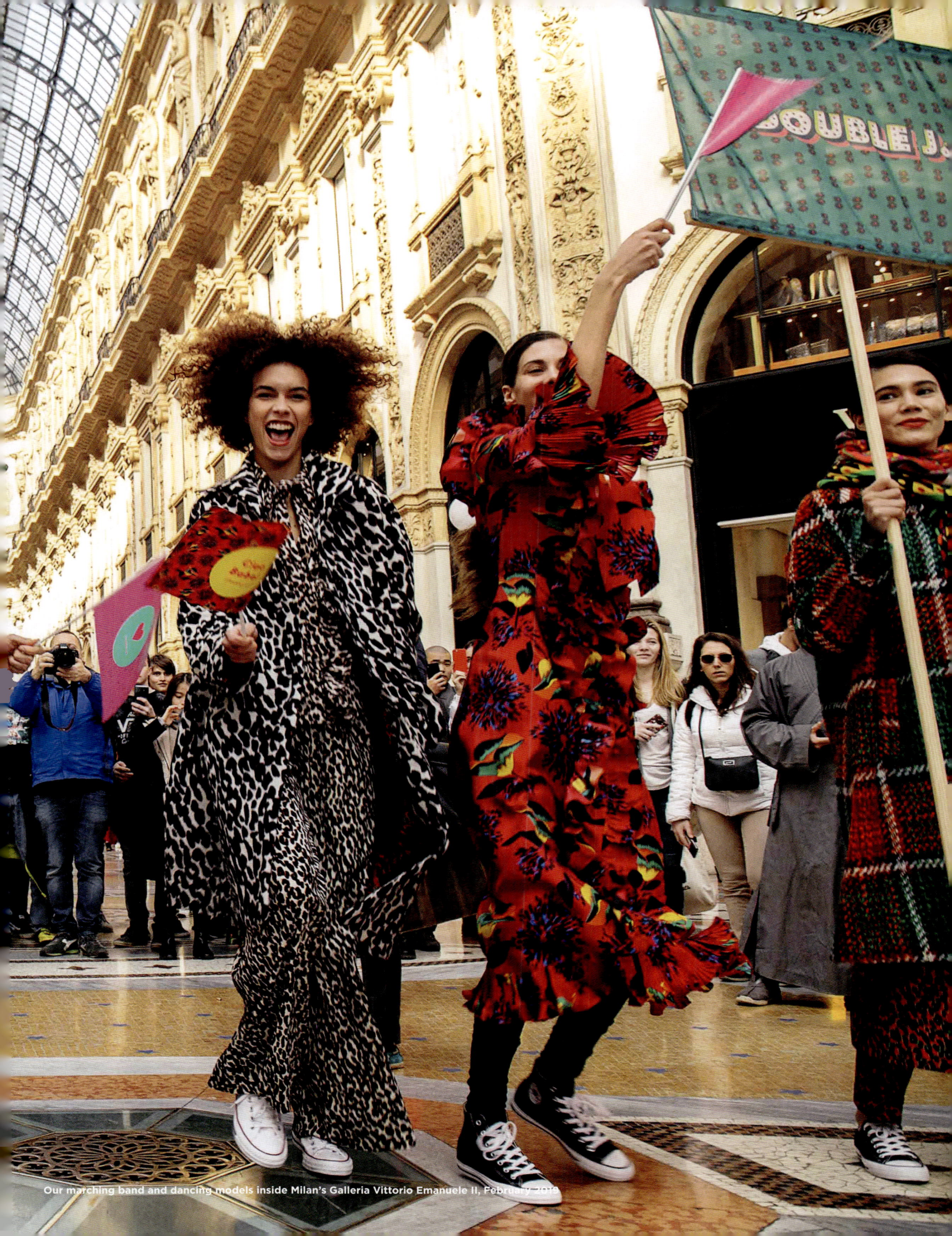

Our marching band and dancing models inside Milan's Galleria Vittorio Emanuele II, February 2019

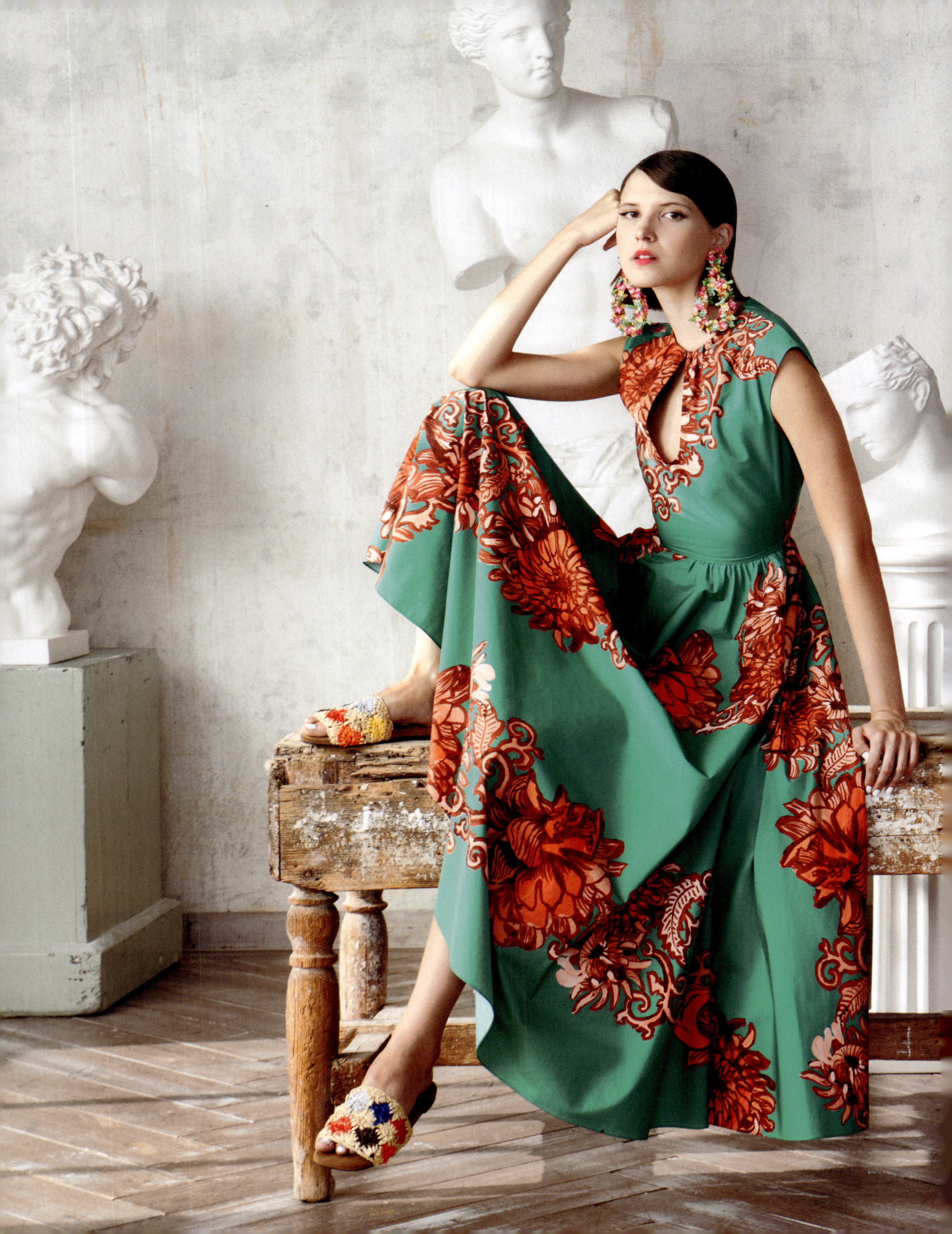

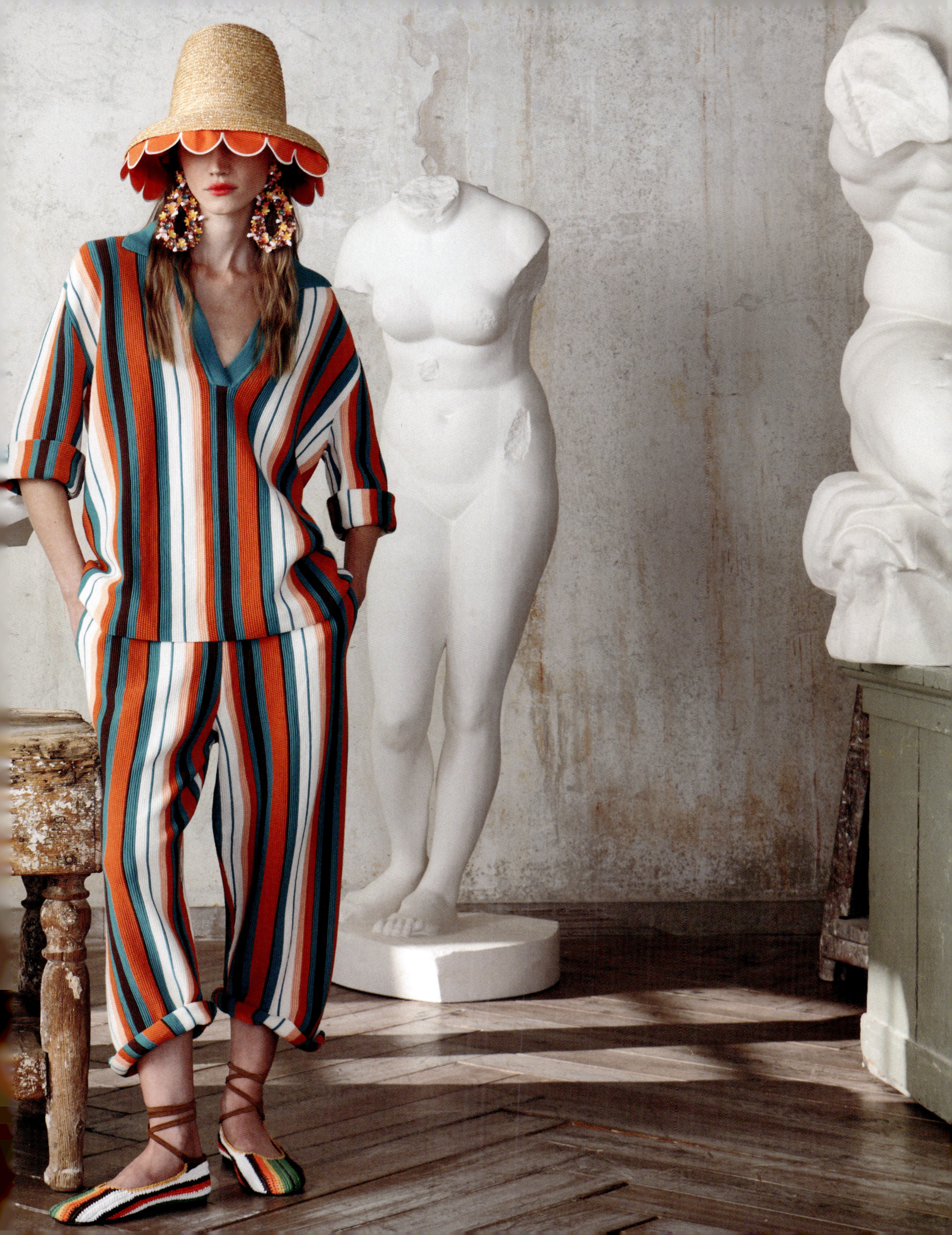

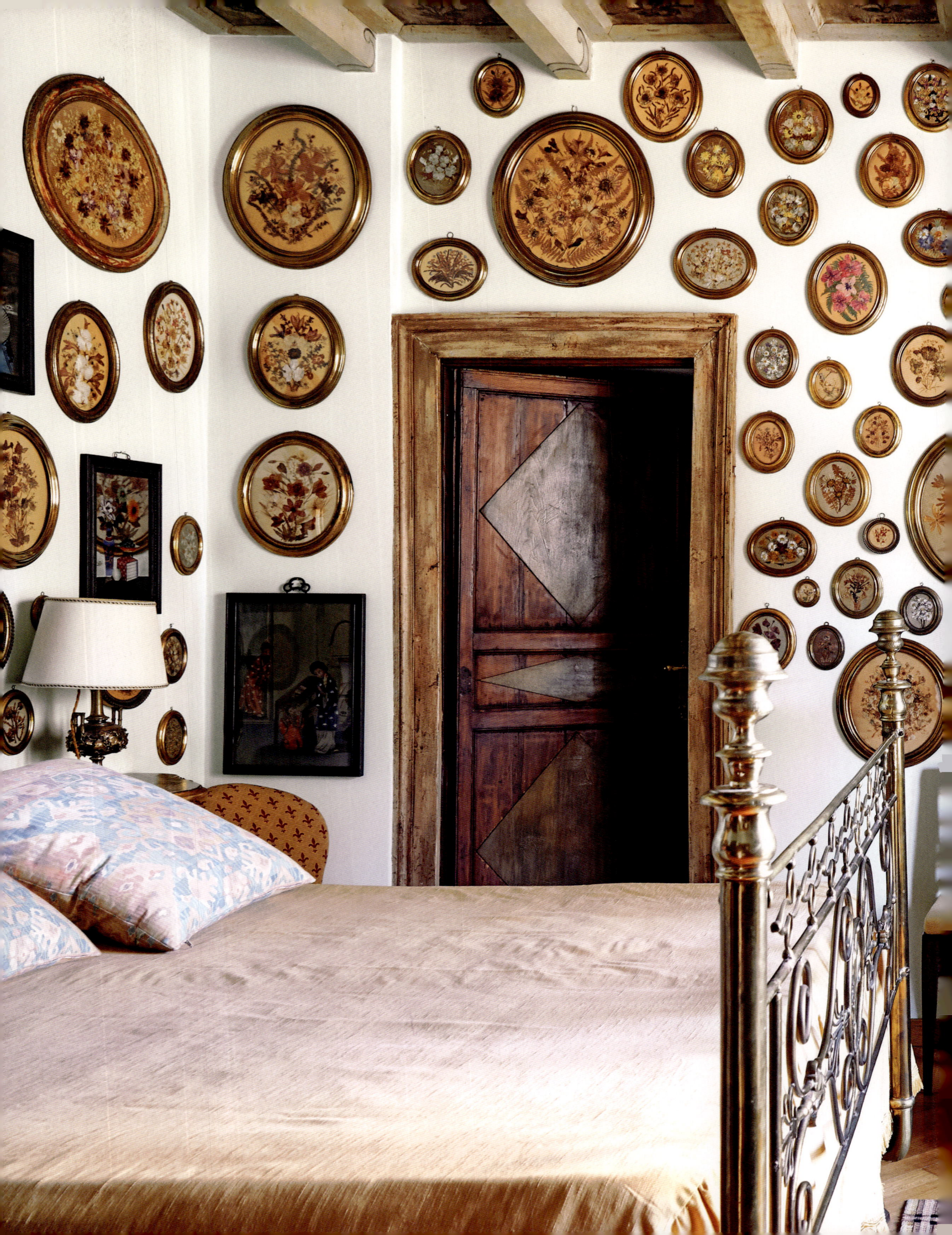

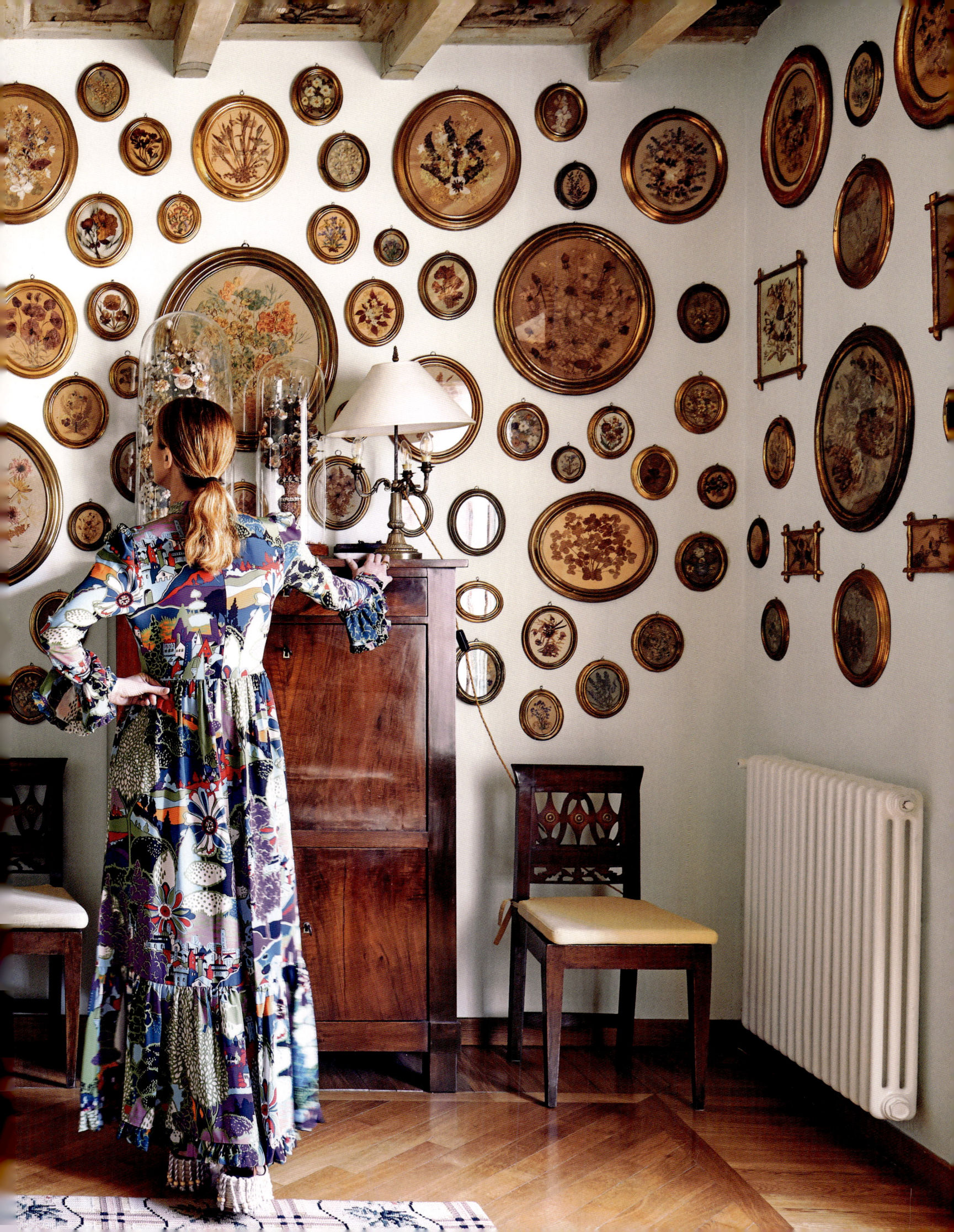

GRAZIE!!!!!!!!

Gratitude is one of the great heart tenderizers and a potent power source. In my spiritual practice, I've learned how to (try to) be grateful for all of the itchy, scratchy moments in life as a kick-start to higher consciousness. But then there's the easier form of gratitude, which comes from acknowledging all of the people and experiences that have brought ease, joy, support, and love into our lives. Mamma Milano is one such project!

This book has had so many beautiful midwives who've helped me deliver her kicking into the world: I would like to start by thanking *Alex Postman*, my wonderful editor who consistently channeled the Divine Masculine on this project, from cutting and containing to anchoring in logic, analysis, and structure—grounding my otherwise spinning vortex of ideas and words. As Alex lovingly remarked towards the end, "We were elephant mammas, gestating our baby for twenty-two months!" Right along for this long, wondrous delivery was the brilliant *Julia Leach*, our guiding light in her vision for what this Big Baby could look like and, as always, bringing calm to my chaos, and clear yin to my always explosive yang ways. *Laura Capsoni* was the most magical book designer we could ever have conjured, and she became part of the DoubleJ family as she sat for months with us inside of our home in Milan, next to *Dorothé Lenaerts*, our eagle-eyed art director of great taste, who worked tirelessly on this project. I cannot thank you four enough. I love you, dear sisters!!!!

I also wish to thank every single DoubleJ employee—past, present, and future, through all of the lifetimes, timelines, dimensions, and realities of this mystical creation. From *Claire* and *Meredith*, my very first two official employees, to *Alberto Zanetti* for his incredible photos (many in this book), sisters *Viviana Volpicella*, *Riley Viall*, and *Jeanne Labib-Lamour*, and the wonderful managing directors (*Sabine Brunner*, *Roberto Falchi*, and *Luca Voarino*) who have shepherded our project as she's grown from peanut to full-scale operation. I extend this circle of gratitude to every single light being—designer, marvelous merchandiser, super salesperson, e-comm specialist, PR maven, content wiz, finance phenom, freelance photographer, stylist—who ever set foot inside our doors. I am so indebted to you all and I'm sorry for all the moments I might have lost my Higher Self. I truly love you all.

Inside the DoubleJ family, I would like to thank *Andrea Ciccoli* and *Christian Musardo*, partners in the Level Group who gestated DoubleJ from the very beginning and gave her a crib to live in and a lifeline with their e-commerce juice. Ciccoli, thank you for always being by my side to protect our *bambina piccola*, and for loving and supporting creativity as much as I do. We've both driven each other crazy and, guess what? We forgave, we survived, we soared, we loved along the way. *Alberto Biagetti*, you have been not only a DoubleJ cheerleader and generous friend to me, but also someone who has guided our ship and done incredible design work for us.

We have talked about *Mantero* inside the book, but I'd also like to point out that the prints we have chosen for our covers were taken from this historic Italian company's archives, not to mention one that I fell in love with that was an etching on their great-grandfather's eighteenth-century villa in Lake Como and was lovingly redrawn, first for our clothing and now here on these pages. *Moritz*, *Lucia*, and *Franco, siete stupendi. Grazie, grazie.*

A big shout out to my cheerleader in book-building, the firecracker *Andy McNicol*, who knows exactly what people want to read. From Vendome, I wish to thank *Beatrice Vincenzini*, who came to me with quite a specific idea on the book she'd like from me, but then graciously accepted a very different one. We all also loved working with the sharp-eyed *Miranda Harrison*, who never skipped or missed a single beat. Your collective feedback and guidance to me as well as your dedication and enthusiasm were precious gifts.

Lastly, I bow to the greatness that is Italy and the feisty, fabulous Italians themselves. I am sorry for all of the times I lost faith. I am sorry for all the times I screamed at you, criticized you, and might have even cursed you.

Please forgive me.
Thank you.
I love you.
For real.

Love,
J.J.

ACKNOWLEDGEMENTS AND PERMISSIONS

PHOTO CREDITS

Felipe Cordeiro: 2–3, 85, 170 top left | Alberto Zanetti: 4–5, 37, 41, 42, 55, 94, 104–105, 106, 123, 124–125, 131, 134, 136–137, 138–139, 140, 141, 142–143, 144–145, 146, 147, 148, 149, 150 top, 151, 156, 157, 158, 159, 160, 162–163, 168, 169, 171 top left, 176 top right, 177 top right, 205 | Mariela Burgos: 6–7, 62–63, 64–65, 68 right, 71, 110, 111, 116–117, 127, 175, 177 bottom left, 179, 192–193, 197 bottom right, 198 bottom right, 221, 228–229 | Filippo Bamberghi: 10, 74–75, 78, 81,198 top right, 198 bottom left, 218 | J.J. Martin: 12, 59 top, 182 | Amina Marazzi Gandolfi: 20–21, 25, 26–27, 47, 48–49, 82–83, 166, 226–227 | Lucas Possiede: 28, 29, 30 left, 30 right, 170 bottom right, 176 top left, 197 top center, 198 top left, 200, 204, 206–207, 224–225 | Barbara Franzò: 31, 60, 217, 220 bottom left and right | Camilla Alibrandi: 38–39 | Nick Mele: 57 | La DoubleJ: 58, 70–71 top, 90, 97 top left, 97 top center, 97 left center, 97 right center, 97 bottom center, 97 bottom right, 150 bottom left, 153, 164, 176 bottom right, 177 bottom right, 180–181,182, 197 top left, 197 bottom left, 197 bottom center, 212–213, 219 | Asia Typek: 62–63, 89 | Phoebe Cowley: 66–67 | Torvioll Jashari: 68 left, 176 bottom left | David Cicconi: 69 | Courtesy of Capasa: 70 | Alice Dotto: 86 | *New York Times*: 97 top right | Style Du Monde: 97 bottom left | Cynthia Matthews: 101 | Serena Eller Vainicher: 102 top, 102 bottom left, 102 bottom right, 103 | Massimo Listri: 114 | Alessandro Grassani/ *New York Times*: 112–113 | Josh Shinner: 118, 120, 122 right | The Coverture: 119 | Mattia Lotti: 121 | *ELLE Decor*: 122 left | Jeanne Perotte/TSF: 133 | Phil Oh: 138 left | Claudia Quadri: 154–155 | Genevieve Garruppo: 158 bottom left | Henrik Blomqvist: 171 bottom right, 177 top left, 185, 194, 211 | Courtesy of Jobi Manson: 197 top right | Susan Mariani: 197 center left | Mostafa Ahmed: 197 center right | Robyn Lea: 208, 216, 220 top left, 222

Page 34 in order of images:
Lucas Possiede | Lucas Possiede | La DoubleJ | Lucas Possiede | La DoubleJ | La DoubleJ | La DoubleJ | La DoubleJ

Page 35 in order of images:
Lucas Possiede | La DoubleJ | Lucas Possiede | La DoubleJ | Lucas Possiede | La DoubleJ | La DoubleJ | La DoubleJ | La DoubleJ | La DoubleJ | La DoubleJ | Filippo Bamberghi | La DoubleJ | La DoubleJ | La DoubleJ | La DoubleJ

Page 182 in order of images:
Courtesy of Jessica Williams | Deonté Lee | Courtesy of Laura Brown | Courtesy of Getty Images | La DoubleJ | Courtesy of Maryam Malakpour | Mariela Burgos | Courtesy of Giovanna Battaglia | Mariela Burgos | Courtesy of Renata Zandonadi Quaglia | Ruven Afanador | La DoubleJ | Courtesy of Getty Images | Courtesy of Katie Sturino | Courtesy of Courtney Love | Courtesy of Mindy Kaling

Page 183 in order of images:
Lucas Possiede | Courtesy of Getty Images | Courtesy of Blanca Miró | Courtesy of Gwyneth Paltrow | Zev Starr-Tambor | Felipe Cordeiro | Courtesy of Alex Sweterlitsch | Zev Starr-Tambor | Courtesy of Amanda Nguyen | Courtesy of Getty Images | Zev Starr-Tambor | Courtesy of Martha Stewart | Todd Selby

Inserts:
Insert 1
Mariela Burgos: 1, 4–5, 16 | Asya Tipek: 6–7 | Alberto Zanetti: 8–9, 10–11 | La DoubleJ: 15

Insert 2
Mariela Burgos: 1 | La DoubleJ: 2–3, 4–5, 8–9, 12, 15, 16 | Claudia Zalla: 6, 11 | The Coverture: 7

Insert 3
Mattia Lotti: 4, 15 | Chiara Quadri: 5, 6, 7, 9, 13 | Alberto Zanetti: 8, 10 | Andrea Wyner: 11, 12, 14

Insert 4
Mariela Burgos: 1, 2, 4, 5, 14 | Barbara Franzò: 6–7, 8, 9, 10, 11, 12–13, 15, 16

Page 119: Text adapted from "House Tour: Inside a Fashion Writer's Breathtaking Milan Apartment," *ELLE Decor*, Hearst Magazine Media, Inc., January 2015

Each of the La DoubleJ archival prints featured on our three unique covers has been sourced from and lovingly provided by our friends at Mantero Seta in Como.

Mamma Milano: Lessons from the Motherland
First published in 2023 by The Vendome Press
Vendome is a registered trademark of The Vendome Press LLC

www.vendomepress.com

VENDOME PRESS US
PO Box 566
Palm Beach, FL 33480

VENDOME PRESS UK
Worlds End Studio
132–134 Lots Road
London, SW10 0RJ

Copyright © 2023 The Vendome Press LLC
Text copyright © 2023 J.J. Martin

All rights reserved.
No part of the contents of this book may be reproduced in whole or in part
without prior written permission from the publisher.

Distributed in North America by Abrams Books
Distributed in the UK, and the rest of the world, by Thames & Hudson

Every effort has been made to identify and contact all copyright holders
and to obtain their permission for the use of any copyright material.
The publisher apologizes for any errors or omissions and would be grateful
if notified of any corrections that should be incorporated
in future reprints or editions of this book.

ISBN 978-0-86565-434-2

Publishers
Beatrice Vincenzini, Mark Magowan, and Francesco Venturi

Editors
Alex Postman and Miranda Harrison

Production Director
Jim Spivey

Designer
Laura Capsoni

Library of Congress Cataloging-in-Publication Data
available upon request.

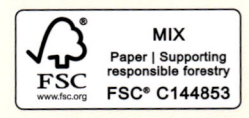

Printed and bound in China by RR Donnelley
(Guangdong) Printing Solutions Company Ltd.
First Printing